Nurse's Manual of

LABORATORY TESTS
and
DIAGNOSTIC PROCEDURES

Nurse's Manual of

LABORATORY TESTS
and
DIAGNOSTIC PROCEDURES

Louise M. Malarkey, Ed.D., R.N.
Professor and Chairperson, Department of Nursing
College of Staten Island, Staten Island, New York

Mary Ellen McMorrow, Ed.D., R.N., C.C.R.N.
Professor, Department of Nursing
College of Staten Island, Staten Island, New York

W.B. SAUNDERS COMPANY
A Division of Harcourt Brace & Company

Philadelphia London Toronto
Montreal Sydney Tokyo

W.B. SAUNDERS COMPANY
A Division of Harcourt Brace & Company

The Curtis Center
Independence Square West
Philadelphia, Pennsylvania 19106

Library of Congress Cataloging-in-Publication Data

Malarkey, Louise M.
    Nurse's manual of laboratory tests and diagnostic procedures /
Louise M. Malarkey, Mary Ellen McMorrow. — 1st ed.

        p.   cm.

    ISBN   0–7216–3774–4

    1. Diagnosis, Laboratory—Handbooks, manuals, etc.
2. Diagnosis—Handbooks, manuals, etc.   3. Nursing—
Handbooks, manuals, etc.
    I. McMorrow, Mary Ellen.   II. Title.
        [DNLM: 1. Diagnosis, Laboratory—nurses' instruc-
tion. QY 4 1996]

    RB38.2.M34   1996   616.07′54—dc20

    DNLM/DLC   95-17715

Cover Art: Artist's representation of blood cells being analyzed by Coulter's proprietary VCS technology, which uses volume, conductivity, and laser light scatter to identify and differentiate blood cells. (Courtesy of Coulter Corporation, Miami, FL.)

Nurse's Manual of Laboratory Tests and Diagnostic Procedures   ISBN   0–7216–3774–4

Printed in the United States of America.

Last digit is the print number: 9   8   7   6   5   4   3   2

This book is dedicated to our families, with love
To Frank, Valerie, Christopher, and Travis
and
To Charles and Alison

LMM

❧

To the two Marys in my life,
My mother and my daughter

MEM

REVIEWERS

Tina K. Allen, R.N., M.S.N. Troy State University, Montgomery, Alabama

Stella B. Bellarts, Ed.D., R.N., M.N. University of Portland, Portland, Oregon

Cheryl J. Cassis, R.N., M.S.N. Belmont Technical College, St. Clairsville, Ohio

Leslie A. Dickson, R.N., M.S.N. Lincoln Land Community College, Springfield, Illinois

Ellen Stoetzner Duke, M.S.N., R.N., C.C.R.N. Angelina College, Lufkin, Texas

Patricia A. Gallagher, R.N., M.S. Waynesburg College, Waynesburg, Pennsylvania

Margaret M. Gingrich, R.N., M.S.N. Harrisburg Area Community College, Harrisburg, Pennsylvania

Ann Putnam Johnson, Ed.D., R.N., C.S. Western Carolina University, Cullowhee, North Carolina

Rhonda Johnston, R.N., M.S., A.N.P. University of Southern Colorado, Pueblo, Colorado

Nancy Kupper, R.N., M.S.N. Tarrant County Junior College, Fort Worth, Texas

Charlene J. Morris, R.N., M.S.N. Austin Community College, Austin, Texas

Jacquelin S. Neatherlin, R.N., Ph.D., C.N.R.N. Baylor University School of Nursing, Dallas, Texas

Carol J. Nelson, R.N., M.S.N. Spokane Community College, Spokane, Washington

Kathleen LeClear O'Connell, R.N., M.S.N., A.N.P. Indiana University-Purdue University Fort Wayne, Fort Wayne, Indiana

Susan L. Smith-Prather, R.N., M.S. Tidewater Community College, Portsmouth, Virginia

Karen L. Then, R.N., B.N., M.N. University of Calgary, Calgary, Alberta, Canada

Norma J. Uremovic, R.N., M.S.N. St. Joseph Medical Center, Joliet Junior College, Joliet, Illinois

Timothy L. Wren, R.N., M.S. Clarkson College, Omaha, Nebraska

P R E F A C E

This book was written by nurses and for nurses. During the planning, organization, and writing of this text, the questions uppermost in the authors' minds were: What does the nurse *need* to know about a test? And what would a nurse *want* to know about a test? There is an exhaustive (and exhausting) base of knowledge concerning many of the tests in this book. The authors have attempted to analyze and synthesize this knowledge and to convey clearly the information that is most relevant to the practice of nursing.

Since the book is designed for nurses, the organizational framework is based on body systems. This organization provides for the concentration of knowledge about laboratory and diagnostic tests for a particular body system, and the material can be integrated readily into the clinical situation, with the nurse taking into account the needs of the patient who must undergo one or more of these tests or procedures.

The systems approach makes this book compatible with the major texts that are used for the education of the nursing student. This book complements and supplements the knowledge provided by nursing faculty in the classroom and clinical settings. It can be used throughout the nursing curriculum because of the integration of nursing considerations across the life span. Normal test values, when established, are provided for all age groups.

Part I provides a general discussion of the nurse's role and responsibilities in laboratory and diagnostic testing, with a particular emphasis on the patient-nurse interactions that are involved in the testing process. This section also includes the procedures and measures that are used to collect specimens. Parts II and III address the multisystem laboratory tests and procedures that are used to assess the anatomy and physiologic function of many organs and body systems. Part IV concentrates on laboratory and diagnostic testing of specific body systems.

Throughout the book, each test and procedure is presented with a consistent format. The background information helps the learner understand what the test is, how it is performed, and how it relates to the clinical state of the patient. In addition, there is a clear and concise explanation of why the test is usually performed. The conditions that produce abnormal results are listed, as are the factors that interfere with the accuracy of the test or procedure.

Another major strength of the book lies in the delineation of the nurse's role in the specific test or procedure. Emphasis is placed on the patient's education and preparation for the test. Nurses who are employed in hospitals, home health agencies, and outpatient settings will find this content relevant to their practice. The tables of potential complications and the appropriate nursing assessments are a vital feature for the nurse at the bedside and for the nurse who prepares the patient for discharge after outpatient testing.

Congruent with current nursing practice, a unique feature of this book is the identification of quality-improvement measures. The careful preparation of the patient, accurate collection of the specimen, and arrangements for delivery of the specimen to the laboratory all are measures that promote high-quality performance. When the steps of the process are performed correctly, the results are more cost-effective and minimize distress to the patient. Quality-improvement measures prevent needless repetition of tests or delay in making an accurate diagnosis. Accurate and timely performance may also shorten the length of the patient's hospitalization.

We hope that by consolidating and organizing complex data into a usable resource for the practicing nurse we have also made an appealing and helpful text for the nursing student.

LOUISE M. MALARKEY
MARY ELLEN McMORROW
DEPARTMENT OF NURSING
COLLEGE OF STATEN ISLAND
STATEN ISLAND, NEW YORK

ACKNOWLEDGMENTS

The authors are indebted to many professional and personal friends, whose support and encouragement have made this book possible. But first, we wish to express appreciation to all our students, the younger and older enthusiastic future nurses. Their questioning and quest for knowledge was limitless and served as an ongoing source of stimulation for us.

To our co-faculty members, past and present, we are deeply grateful for your support. It is a pleasure to work with nursing educators who remain committed to excellent teaching and the communication of nursing knowledge.

Both of the authors gratefully acknowledge the dedication, creativity, knowledge, and skill of Thomas Eoyang, Vice President and Editor-in-Chief, Nursing Books, at W.B. Saunders Company. As our editor, his ability to stimulate the desire to publish and then nurture its growth was inestimable and humbly appreciated. This book would not exist without his continuous encouragement and belief in the authors. The authors also wish to thank Terri Wood, Associate Developmental Editor. Her warmth, intelligence, and willingness to help made the publication process a pleasure.

Last, but of prime importance, the authors wish to thank their families, who sacrificed many a night and weekend to watch us read mountains of articles and reference materials and struggle with newly acquired computer skills. We cherished each phone call and inquiry about our efforts, always accompanied by encouragement to continue.

CONTENTS

PART I

NURSING RESPONSIBILITIES IN LABORATORY AND DIAGNOSTIC PROCEDURES

CHAPTER 1

The Nursing Role

There are two broad areas of nursing performance involved in laboratory tests and diagnostic procedures. The first area pertains to the procedure itself and the nursing measures that ensure completion of the testing in a timely and accurate manner. The second area concerns the nursing interactions with the patient who must undergo the diagnostic test or procedure. The nursing process is used to organize patient care and meet the patient's needs.

The nursing role in patient care for individuals undergoing diagnostic tests and procedures may be direct or indirect. Often, it involves an interdisciplinary approach to the planning and implementation of care.

Direct care is provided by the nurse when the patient is hospitalized or enters an outpatient setting for performance of the laboratory or diagnostic test. The nurse may perform some aspects of the care or supervise paraprofessional workers in the delivery of care, particularly during the pretest and posttest periods. For some of the more complex or invasive tests, a nurse is present during the procedure to provide care to the patient and assist the physician who performs the test.

Indirect care often occurs when the patient is at home for the pretest and posttest phases of the diagnostic testing. The nurse may have responsibility for guiding or instructing the patient in preparing for the test or in recovery after the test. The patient performs self-care, or a family member assists the patient according to the instructions that are given.

In many instances, diagnostic work is an interdisciplinary function that involves coordination and communication among the nurse, several physicians, and technicians of the laboratory, radiology department, or diagnostic specialty units. The nurse's role is often pivotal in the transmission of information to and from the testing center. The nurse must explain specific laboratory or diagnostic pretest requirements to the patient or must perform specific pretest procedures on the patient. Additionally, the specific needs or problems of the patient are

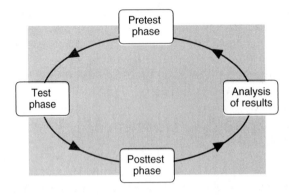

FIGURE 1–1. The cycle of laboratory or diagnostic testing. Both the nurse and the patient are involved in each phase of the cycle. After the results are analyzed, the cycle may be restarted for additional tests or procedures that have been ordered.

explained to the testing center personnel. The goal is to accomplish the diagnostic work accurately, safely, and in a timely manner.

The process of laboratory or diagnostic testing can be conceptualized as a cycle that has four phases of operation: (1) the pretest phase, (2) the test phase, (3) the posttest phase, and (4) interpretation of the results (Fig. 1–1). During each phase, there are appropriate nursing roles and responsibilities for the test or procedure as well as appropriate aspects of nursing care for the patient.

PROCEDURAL ROLE AND NURSING RESPONSIBILITIES IN LABORATORY AND DIAGNOSTIC PROCEDURES

Pretest Phase

SCHEDULING OF A DIAGNOSTIC TEST. This involves communication among the individual who prescribes the test, the patient, and the individual who performs the test. The nurse or unit coordinator is often responsible for accurate transcription of the orders, completion of the requisition form, and scheduling of the test.

When multiple tests are prescribed, there is sometimes a need to prioritize the test schedule because the method of conducting one test can interfere with the results of another test. For example, x-ray studies that use iodinated contrast medium are performed before x-ray studies that use barium contrast material. This timing is necessary because residual barium remains in the intestine for several days and its opacity obscures the view of the other tissues, such as the biliary tract and abdominal vasculature. Likewise, blood tests that use a radioimmunoassay method of analysis must be performed before or 7 days after a nuclear scan because the radioisotopes of the scan would interfere with the radioimmunoassay method of analysis of the blood and alter the test results.

When these interfering factors involve tests performed by a single department, such as the laboratory, the priorities are routinely sorted out by the laboratory personnel. When the interfering factors involve two departments, such as the laboratory and radiology departments, the nurse consults with the departments to clarify the priorities and to plan appropriately.

Critical Thinking: The patient has evidence of abdominal trauma and shock after a car accident. Which laboratory and diagnostic tests take priority in the assessment for fluid volume deficit related to abdominal hemorrhage?

Some priorities in scheduling are determined by the acuity of the patient. Particular test results are needed rapidly for the assessment of the patient's status, for correct medical diagnosis and treatment, or for evaluation of the patient's response to treatment. Particular blood tests may be performed serially, for example, every hour for 4 hours; at frequent intervals such as daily; or immediately (STAT). The request may specify the urgency and the desired times for the tests.

The nurse monitors each situation, ensuring that the tests are performed on time and that the test results are reported to the physician or posted in the patient's chart, or both, as quickly as they become available. When a test is ordered with an immediate or urgent priority, the laboratory or diagnostic unit is notified by phone, the scheduling arrangements are confirmed, and the tests are completed as requested. With modern laboratory technology, some test results, such as serum electrolyte levels or a blood chemistry panel, can be analyzed in minutes, and the results are available almost immediately. Analyzing other tests can be time-consuming, and some final results may not be available for several days or more.

Nonroutine or special tests must be scheduled in advance. For example, positron emission tomography, a nuclear scan, is performed in special medical centers on a particular day of the week because the radioisotopes are made in a special laboratory, with the use of a cyclotron to split the atoms. Once the radioisotopes are made, they are rushed to the nuclear medicine department of the nearby test center because the nuclear material has a half-life of only a few hours. Before there is radioisotope decay, the preparation is administered to the patient and the radiographic films are taken rapidly.

Whenever there are questions about scheduling, priorities, the availability of the test, or even the type of specimen container to be used, the nurse can consult the printed hospital reference manual or communicate with the appropriate laboratory or diagnostic unit for assistance.

REQUISITION FORMS. These forms must be completed accurately because they are often the only form of communication used to request a test and they are part of the identification process that ensures that the correct test is performed on the correct patient. The requisition form is used to request the specific test, including the time and date that the test should be performed. It contains the patient information, including the patient's name, identification number, and hospital room, and the name of the physician. Some agencies require additional information, such as the patient's birth date, to help ensure correct identification.

The requisition slip includes additional information that is appropriate to the test as determined by the physician or the individual who prescribes the test. Examples include the patient's age and gender, date of the last menstrual period, gestation of the pregnancy in a pregnant woman, pertinent medical history, or the suspected diagnosis. The information is used in the analysis of the specimen and in the interpretation of the results.

Test Phase

The procedural responsibilities of the nurse vary considerably with different tests, and they vary somewhat among different institutions or units within an institution. When the specimen collection is performed by the physician or technician, the nurse may have only indirect responsibility for ensuring that the test is performed, that the specimen is labeled properly, and that it is sent to the laboratory.

If the hospitalized patient must go to the radiology department or a special diagnostic unit, the nurse ensures that the patient care is completed and that the patient is prepared for transport to the unit. Equipment, such as intravenous lines and drainage systems, is determined to be functional and secured properly. The patient's chart goes with the patient.

In some cases, the nurse is directly involved in the collection of specimens. This may include the collection of blood, urine, stool, and culture specimens, as well as assistance with the collection of a sample of tissue or other body fluids. In these processes, the nurse shares in the responsibility for maintenance of quality controls, the proper performance of the equipment, and accurate identification of the patient.

Critical Thinking: What are the potential risks when the laboratory specimen is obtained from the wrong patient or the specimen container is labeled incorrectly?

IDENTIFICATION PROCEDURES. It is essential to perform a correct identification before collecting the specimen, before starting a diagnostic procedure, and by labeling the specimen container before it is transported to the laboratory. To identify the patient, the person who performs the test compares the data on the patient's identification band (name, room number, bed number, and other data) with the data on the requisition slip. Also, the patient is asked to state his or her full name. If the patient cannot respond, the staff nurse or a relative is asked to verify the identity (Jacobs et al., 1990).

Once the specimen is obtained, the label is compared with the requisition slip and the patient's identification band. All three must be identical. Before leaving the patient's bedside or the examining room, the nurse applies the label to the specimen container. For specimens of tissues or body fluids, the labels and requisition slips must identify the source of the specimen.

QUALITY CONTROL. This often refers to the calibration or testing of instruments and the analysis of control specimens that ensure accurate measurement. Today, the concept has expanded in scope, and quality control is part of a more inclusive quality assurance program (Handorf, 1994). Quality control and quality assurance activities are used to assess for human and mechanical problems in diagnostic testing. The goal is to prevent or eliminate problems that interfere with the accuracy and reliability of test results (Bjerkan and McKelvy, 1991).

In clinical laboratory testing, quality control measures are maintained in the preanalytic, analytic, and postanalytic phases of the testing process (Johnson, 1992). This means that the laboratory works to detect and eliminate error in the actual analysis of the specimen and in the steps that precede and follow the analytic phase.

Nursing is usually involved in quality control efforts that are part of the preanalytic phase. Activities include preparation of the patient before the test, testing or calibration of the diagnostic equipment, and ensuring that specimen collection requirements and special requirements for the storage or transport of the specimens are met. In the procedural aspects of quality control, the nurse minimizes or eliminates many of the interfering factors that would affect the accuracy and validity of the test and its results.

Throughout this text, quality controls that pertain to nursing are identified. They include special requirements in the collection, storage, and transport of specimens. They also include restrictions and requirements the patient must follow before the test, optimal times for particular specimen collections, and special conditions, such as sterility, the use of preservatives, and temperature controls that protect the specimen from contamination or deterioration.

ALTERNATIVE-SITE TESTING. This is a new and rapidly evolving aspect of laboratory testing. In the past, a central laboratory and its subsections were housed in a single location, often in a hospital or single community location. Today, there is a growing move toward decentralization, with an increase in the sites of laboratory services inside the hospital and outside the institution as well. The reasons for decentralization are politically and economically driven in part, but technologic developments also constitute a strong factor. The development of miniature, computerized, portable, hand-held analyzers has brought laboratory testing and analysis nearer to the patient. This change in the past 3 to 4 years has resulted in a proliferation of testing sites and has created changes in the role of the nurse, laboratory technician, other health care professionals, paraprofessionals, and even the patient. The technology of the future is going to increase these trends and practices.

The rapidity of change has resulted in confusion in terminology and responsibilities as well as some conflict or resistance among professional workers. Handorf (1994) describes the testing that is performed outside the central laboratory in terms of two basic and overlapping concepts (Fig. 1–2). Alternative-site laboratory testing refers to choices about where laboratory testing is performed. Point-of-care testing includes alternative testing sites outside the central laboratory, but it specifically refers to methods of testing and analysis that bring the laboratory services nearer to the patient. Point-of-care testing and its subconcepts are pertinent to nursing because they involve changes in the nursing role, nursing procedures, and nursing practices.

POINT-OF-CARE TESTING. This type of testing, also known as near-patient testing, brings laboratory testing and analysis to the patient or to the bedside. In many cases, satellite laboratories are established near or next to operating rooms, intensive care units, and emergency rooms. Sometimes there is a desktop analyzer that is used in a clinic, an ambulatory care setting, a physician's office, or even the patient's home. With this new technology, automated analyzers are used to perform certain laboratory tests rapidly and with increased efficiency (Rabbitts, 1993; Schembri, 1992; Rock, 1991).

In critical care units and other hospital settings in which patients are acutely ill, the common tests that are performed and analyzed at the bedside include determination of blood gases, potassium, sodium, ionized calcium, creatinine

Critical Thinking: You are informed of the hospital's plan to decentralize the laboratory services and that your staff nurses will perform some of the laboratory tests on the nursing unit. What strategies can be used to help the staff work toward successful implementation of the plan?

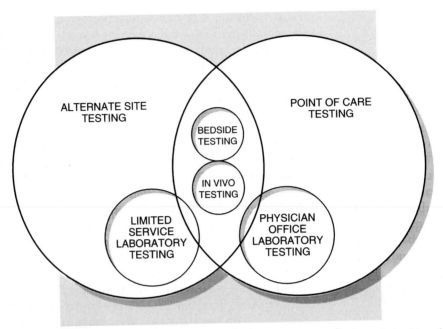

FIGURE 1–2. Alternative site laboratory testing. The diagram represents the interrelationships of terminology in the description of laboratory testing outside the traditional central location of the laboratory. (With permission from Handorf, C.A. [1994]. Background—Setting the stage for alternate-site laboratory testing. *Clinics in Laboratory Medicine, 14,* 455.)

kinase, osmolarity, and glucose levels; prothrombin time and other coagulation studies; and determination of the hematocrit value and other hematologic studies (Woo and Henry, 1994). These automated analyzers use whole blood rather than serum, and the test results are available in a few minutes. When the patient is critically ill, many tests are performed at frequent intervals. In addition to other laboratory test responsibilities, the nurse must ensure that all the results are charted in the correct order and time sequence.

Point-of-care testing eliminates the delays caused by the transport and processing of specimens and the transmission of test results back to the clinical unit. When the patient is critically ill, these test results reflect the patient's current or real-time blood values. In contrast, the centrally located laboratory produces test results 1 hour to 1 day later. When pathophysiologic changes occur rapidly, the test results may not be current or useful by the time they are transmitted to the patient's unit.

BEDSIDE TESTING. This is one category of point-of-care testing and refers to the testing that is performed with small hand-held instruments that analyze the patient's blood in a few minutes. The phrase "bedside testing" is inadequate because the specimen is obtained and the blood analyzed wherever the patient is located, including the home or workplace. The patient may be the one who performs the test as part of self-care responsibilities.

Glucose testing is the first well-established procedure for bedside testing. Other instruments have now been developed for bedside testing, including those that measure electrolytes, blood gases, and coagulation ability. There is also an instrument that screens the urine for the drugs of abuse (Jones, 1994).

With the glucose test as an example of bedside testing, the procedure is as follows. The blood glucose is measured by the hand-held analyzer, with the fingerstick method being used to obtain blood from a diabetic patient. This reading of the blood glucose level provides current data that are used to determine the next dose of insulin or to monitor the patient's response to diabetic medications. This point-of-care testing may be performed at the patient's bedside or may be used by the patient in the home for long-term monitoring of blood levels.

EXPANDED NURSING ROLE. Point-of-care testing involves an expanded role for nurses that overlaps with that of the laboratory technician. The nurse may collect the blood sample, perform the analysis, and produce the test results. When the diabetic patient uses the glucometer, the nurse may have to teach the patient these same functions or evaluate the patient's performance and accuracy in using the equipment. In addition, nurses are involved in the selection and maintenance of the equipment located in the patient care units (Bickford, 1994).

With point-of-care testing, there can be significant "operator error," producing invalid test results. The most common reason for error is insufficient training of nonlaboratory personnel in the use and proper function of the equipment, lack of calibration of the analyzer at regular intervals, and lack of emphasis on quality control assessment (Roby et al., 1993).

To maintain accuracy, laboratory instruments are calibrated daily. In addition, the function of the equipment is evaluated, and a quality control check is performed to measure the accuracy of test results every day. This may be carried out by the laboratory personnel or by the nurse. The biomedical department of the hospital usually is responsible for periodic maintenance of the equipment so that ongoing function is ensured (Baer and Belsey, 1991).

When the agency or patient care unit uses point-of-care testing, quality control measures are taken to ensure accurate performance by the personnel (Handorf, 1994). A written protocol for equipment use is developed. Personnel are trained and evaluated on a routine basis. These requirements are now incorporated into the regulations of the Joint Commission on the Accreditation of Healthcare Organizations (JCAHO) and other professional accrediting organizations (Travers et al., 1994).

In some institutions, laboratory technicians are responsible for point-of-care testing; in other places the nurse, as the provider of direct patient care, uses the automated analyzers. As part of the cross-training approach that is being used in hospitals, the nurse who uses this equipment must have formal training, certification that the training has been completed satisfactorily, and periodic reevaluation of performance. Because of the turnover or rotation of nursing staff, the nurse manager of the unit must monitor the ongoing staff needs for continuing education (Roby et al., 1993).

For the integration of point-of-care testing equipment into nursing units, the best outcome occurs when laboratory personnel coordinate with nurses and physicians to develop and maintain a quality assurance program. Without the training of nonlaboratory personnel, there is a high incidence of inconsistency of performance and inaccurate test results.

INFECTION CONTROL–BARRIER PRECAUTIONS. These precautions must be used when obtaining or handling a specimen of blood or body fluids. Gloves must be worn during the collection. If splashing or contact with a mucous membrane is anticipated, the nurse wears a mask, protective eye wear, and a gown or protective clothing in addition to the gloves.

All specimens of blood or body fluids are placed in the correct containers with tightly fitted lids to prevent leakage during transport of the specimen to the laboratory. After the completion of the procedure, the gloves and disposable clothing are removed and discarded. Hands are washed with soap and water.

Precautions are taken to prevent the puncture or cutting of one's own skin with a contaminated needle, scalpel blade, or sharp instrument. To prevent needlestick injury, the needle and syringe unit is disposed of in the puncture-resistant container. The needle is not recapped, broken, bent, or removed from the syringe because of the risk of accidentally puncturing the hand.

Special reusable needles, such as those for a spinal tap or aspiration of a joint, are placed in puncture-resistant containers for transport to an area where they are cleansed and sterilized. After use, reusable instruments and diagnostic equipment are also cleansed and sterilized or disinfected according to standardized procedures.

The use of universal blood and body fluid precautions is based on the premise that all patients are potentially infectious and there is a risk of transmission of infection after exposure to blood or other body fluids. The precautions are used to protect all health care workers against blood-borne pathogens, including human immunodeficiency virus (HIV).

Posttest Phase

TRANSPORT OF THE SPECIMEN. The specimen is generally transported to the laboratory as soon as possible; however, some laboratory or pathology specimens become unstable within a short interval after they are collected. Specific factors, such as exposure to sunlight, warming, refrigeration, and exposure to air, can cause alteration or deterioration of particular specimens (Brunzel, 1994). As soon as the specimen is collected, quality control measures are used to protect it. The specific requirements and quality control measures are presented in the individualized tests located in Part IV of this volume.

For many blood tests, the untreated specimen begins to deteriorate within a few hours. To prevent this problem, the blood must be centrifuged and the serum extracted. With proper temperature control, serum has a longer period of stability than that of blood and can be stored for a specified period. The nurse

---

TABLE 1–1

CRITERIA FOR REJECTION OF AN UNSATISFACTORY LABORATORY SPECIMEN

Improper labeling of the specimen
Lack of a label on the specimen
Improper collection of the specimen
Lack of a preservative
Delay in delivery of the specimen to the laboratory
Improper preservation of the specimen
Improperly completed requisition form
Insufficient volume or quantity of the specimen
Inadequate pretesting preparation of the patient

---

ensures that all specimens are delivered promptly to the laboratory for prompt processing, storage, and analysis.

When a fresh tissue sample must be analyzed for cytologic features, the specimen cannot be placed in fixative or preservative. Because the specimen will dry out after some exposure to the air, it may be delivered directly into the hands of the pathologist or technician as soon as it is obtained. This coordination of activity provides immediate transport and tissue preparation so that the quality of the specimen is maintained.

Some specimens are obtained in the home and then transported to the laboratory. Other specimens must be mailed or transported to a reference laboratory in another city or another part of the country. In these situations, there is an automatic delay before the specimen can be analyzed. General measures to protect the specimen from damage or deterioration include careful packaging, keeping blood cool and away from sunlight, extracting the serum from the cells by centrifuge, and adding a preservative tablet to urine samples. Specific directions are also provided by the laboratory, or they are included in the test kit and its mailing envelope.

REJECTION CRITERIA. When an unsatisfactory specimen is delivered to the laboratory, rejection criteria are applied. The causes of rejection are presented in Table 1–1. The nurse can help ensure acceptance of the specimen by collecting a sufficient quantity, by compliance with the written protocol of the test, and by careful labeling of the specimen container.

Critical Thinking: On your nursing unit, you note that several recent laboratory specimens were rejected as "unsatisfactory" and the tests had to be repeated. Is there a pattern to the errors? What steps can be taken to prevent future problems?

Analysis of the Results

REFERENCE VALUES. Normal values, or reference values, are often presented in a range from the lower to the upper limits of normal. The reference values are used to interpret the results of the test, assist in making an accurate diagnosis, and evaluate the patient's response to treatment.

The reference values for a test vary with the different methods of analysis and different quantitative measurements that are used. For example, the test that measures the 5′-nucleotidase enzyme may be reported with different numeric reference values. The results can have different measurements, and the values are reported as units per liter (U/L), units per milliliter (U/mL), units (U), or Bodansky units. The nurse can use the reference values in this text as a general guide, but the reference values provided by the laboratory that performed the test are the most appropriate values for interpreting the findings in the clinical setting.

For some tests, there is no normal value because the particular substance should not be present at all. When it is not present, the result is described as negative. When it is found, the result is abnormal. The finding may be described as "present" or "positive," or it may be measured with a numeric value that quantifies the amount.

The phrase "possible panic value" refers to a test result that is extremely abnormal and indicates that the patient's life or health is in imminent danger. Identification of these extreme abnormalities helps the nurse and physician differentiate between abnormal results and the critical extremes that indicate a crisis.

VARIABLES. The normal reference values are determined by research studies that use human subjects with varying characteristics. These include the variables of demographics, age, sex, and race. Some of the tests, however, have additional reference values for particular groups of individuals because their normal values are influenced by differences in physiology.

Age differences create distinct sets of reference values for some tests. At one end of the life cycle, some reference values are different for the fetus, newborn, and child. In children, there are some tests with different reference values at distinct ages within the years of childhood development. At the other end of the spectrum, age differences result in some variation of reference values in the older adult or geriatric population (Melillo, 1993 *a* and *b*). For example, hormonal values in the postmenopausal woman are measurably different from those in the younger adult woman. Unfortunately, although it is obvious that there are physiologic changes in the older adult, there are relatively few published research studies that identify the normal ranges of test results for the geriatric age group (Jacobs et al., 1990).

Gender is another variable that produces some difference in the reference values for men and women. When differences occur, the variations are probably due to increased muscle mass in men and differences in hormones and hormone secretion between men and women (Henry, 1991).

Additional variation in the reference values for some tests are due to differences in body weight, posture (whether the patient is lying down or seated at the time of specimen collection), and pregnancy.

SI UNITS. The International System of Units (Système International, or SI, units) is a system that reports laboratory data in terms of standardized international measurements. This system of measurement is currently used in a number of countries, with the goal of worldwide use in the near future. Throughout this text, whenever possible the reference values are presented in conventional units and also in SI equivalents.

PATIENT-NURSE INTERACTIONS IN DIAGNOSTIC TESTING

Dimensions of Nursing Care

The range of interactions between the patient and the nurse varies considerably with the complexity of the test or procedure. Blood tests that use specimens of blood, urine, or feces require some nursing intervention to ensure adequate patient preparation and quality control standards in the collection, storage, or transport of the specimens. Diagnostic procedures, however, require increased interaction with the patient, particularly when the procedure is invasive. Nursing responsibilities involve physical and psychosocial dimensions of patient care, with particular concern for the patient's safety.

Patient-nurse interactions involve direct or indirect care in the pretest, test, and posttest phases of the diagnostic procedure. The nursing process is applicable as a guide to the identification of the patient's needs and the development of the appropriate nursing interventions that lead to a positive outcome (Fig. 1–3).

CHANGES IN HEALTH CARE DELIVERY. These changes have resulted in shorter hospital stays for patients. Shorter periods of hospitalization limit the time for direct care during the acute phase of illness. For the acutely ill hospitalized patient, numerous diagnostic tests or procedures are often scheduled during a concentrated period. In addition to the routine pretest and posttest assessments of the patient, the nurse assesses the actual or potential complications that are related to the invasive diagnostic procedures.

The changes in health care delivery have also resulted in many diagnostic tests being performed on an outpatient basis while the patient continues to live at home (Macpherson, 1993). The patient has been given greater self-care responsibility for pretest preparation and posttest recovery. The direct nursing interactions with the patient are often of short duration and may be limited to a brief pretest phase, the test phase, and the immediate posttest phase.

When a diagnostic procedure is performed in the outpatient setting, the patient receives pretest planning information and instructions regarding any special requirements that are necessary before or after the procedure. The clearly

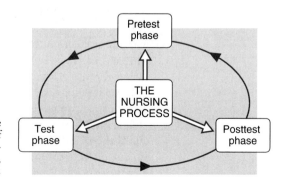

FIGURE 1–3. Application of the nursing process. In each phase of diagnostic testing, the nursing process is applied to provide safe, accurate, complete, and effective nursing care.

stated instructions are given to the patient or the family member who assists with the patient's care. If the instructions are complex, they should be given in writing so that the patient can refer to them as needed. Additionally, the patient needs the address and location of the laboratory or diagnostic unit as well as the time and date for which the test is scheduled.

In procedures requiring sedation or light anesthesia, the patient is instructed in advance that a responsible individual will be required for transportation home at the end of the test. When there is a possibility of a delayed complication in the posttest period, the patient receives instruction so that he or she will recognize abnormal symptoms and will notify the physician if they occur. All these measures are designed to provide continuity of care, even when the patient is some distance from the health care provider.

PEDIATRIC PATIENTS. Modifications in communication and safety measures are required for pediatric patients. These measures should be compatible with the age and behavior of the child. When explanations can be understood, time is taken to prepare the young child for the test or procedure. Honest, friendly explanations help the child cope with and endure the test. The child may fear pain, injections, or the large equipment of the radiology department or may fear the strangers who perform the test. Explanations are given simply and briefly. In some cases the parents help prepare the child and provide the calming reassurance (Torres, 1993).

Infants or active small children usually require restraints to protect them from harm and to maintain immobility during the test or procedure. The choice of restraint is based on the particular need; these restraints are used for tests that are of short duration. The choices include a sheet restraint, a mummy-style restraint, or a special commercial restraint that holds the patient in a particular position.

When the procedure requires a prolonged period of immobility, sedation is often used for infants and small children. Because of the young age, the child cannot be expected to remain still for a long time. The procedures that use sedation in children include nuclear medicine scans, computed tomography, magnetic resonance imaging, electroencephalography, echocardiography, and some ultrasonography procedures. Chloral hydrate, given orally or rectally, is the most frequent method of sedation (Nelson, 1993; Cook et al., 1992). When other diagnostic procedures are painful or distressing, sedation or anesthesia is used.

GERIATRIC PATIENTS. These individuals may have specific needs that are age-related or caused by a specific disease process. For the confused or depressed patient, instructions may need to be given slowly or repeated several times. The patient may have a hearing deficit or difficulty in understanding speech or language. Alternative communication measures may include written pretest and posttest instructions, inclusion of a family member in the communications, or providing an interpreter to help the patient.

The elderly patient may take a considerable number of different medications, and some of them can interfere with particular laboratory tests. The physician is consulted regarding any alteration in the medication schedule, such as withholding the medication for a specified period.

Frail, elderly patients are at risk for injury from a fall. The common underlying problems include visual impairment, stiffness, weakness, mental confusion, dizziness, and the effects of medication. Care is taken to prevent accidental injury or a fall by assisting the patient out of the wheelchair and onto or off a gurney, examining table, radiography table, or toilet.

The elderly individual is often uncomfortable when lying on an x-ray table for a long time. The table is hard and the patient's joints are often stiff with arthritis. The room is usually cool, and some older patients complain about the cold temperature. It may not be possible to change the patient's position during x-ray studies or other diagnostic procedures because of the requirements of the test; however, warm blankets are usually provided so that at least the discomfort of chilling is removed.

Pretest Phase

NURSING ASSESSMENT. This assessment consists of the appraisal of the patient's physical and psychosocial status in relation to the requirements of the test. Pertinent findings in the psychosocial and physical history include any problems with the patient's vision, hearing, mobility, and comprehension of instructions. Current medications are listed. When iodinated contrast medium will be used in the radiologic study, the nurse looks for any history of allergy to shellfish, iodine, or a previous reaction during a radiology test. Allergies to foods and medications are also documented. If a female of childbearing age needs an x-ray study, she is questioned to determine whether there is any possibility of pregnancy.

Vital signs are taken to establish baseline values, particularly for invasive procedures, or when contrast medium, sedation, or anesthesia is used. The infant's or child's weight is recorded when the dose of medication or contrast medium must be calculated according to body weight.

For the purposes of consent, the patient is assessed for knowledge about the procedure, the pretest preparation, and other information that has been explained by the physician.

Critical Thinking: In the pretest assessment, what types of patient behaviors are indicators of altered thought processes? How can the nurse intervene to promote the successful completion of the patient's pretest preparation?

The nurse assesses the patient for signs of anxiety or fear. The cause can be apprehension about the test or procedure, or it may be fear of abnormal test results that indicate serious illness. If there are signs of distress, the nurse asks about the cause or source of the anxiety.

The nurse also reviews the laboratory and other diagnostic test results, and these results are placed in the patient's chart. Some tests, such as prothrombin time, complete blood count, chest radiograph, and electrocardiogram, must verify a health clearance before some of the more invasive diagnostic tests are undertaken.

NURSING DIAGNOSES. Once the nursing assessment is completed, the nurse formulates nursing diagnoses that are appropriate to the patient who will undergo a procedure. The pretest-phase nursing diagnoses are presented in Table 1–2.

TABLE 1–2
PRETEST-PHASE NURSING DIAGNOSES

Nursing Diagnosis	Defining Characteristics	Related Factors
High risk of injury	Presence of risk factors such as developmental age, psychologic factors, or physical factors such as sensory or motor deficit	
High risk of infection– allergic reaction	Presence of risk factors such as altered immune function, history of chronic illness, impaired oxygenation of tissues, external factors such as allergens, infectious agents	
Altered protection	Presence of risk factors such as altered clotting factors, immunosuppression, myelosuppression, or altered cardiovascular status	
Impaired verbal communication	Speaks a foreign language, speaks with difficulty, disorientation, inadequate understanding	Cultural, developmental, or age-related factors
Anxiety	Presence of increased tension, uncertainty, fear of unspecific consequences, cardiovascular excitation, facial tension, quivering voice, insomnia	

EXPECTED OUTCOMES. During the pretest period, the expected outcomes include the following:

1. When sedation or anesthesia is anticipated, the patient arranges with a family member or friend to provide transportation home from the ambulatory test center.

2. The patient is free from all signs and symptoms of infection.

3. The patient communicates any history or allergic reaction to iodine, other allergens, and medications.

4. The patient's vital signs, coagulation studies, and other blood profiles remain within normal limits.

5. The patient requests information or clarification regarding the test and any special measures required in preparation for the test.

6. The patient, a family member, or a significant other demonstrates comprehension of the test and its preparation requirements.

NURSING IMPLEMENTATION

Notify the physician of abnormal pretest results that indicate infection, clotting abnormality, fever, or irregularity in the vital signs. The diagnostic procedure may be postponed until the abnormality is corrected.

If the patient has allergies to food, medication, or contrast medium, post the allergy warning sticker on the outside of the patient's chart.

Provide the pretest instructions in a way that is understood by the patient. Pretest instructions often include the discontinuation of food and fluids for a specific period. They may also involve modification of activity or the temporary discontinuation of one or more medications for a specified period. Some abdominal or intestinal tests require a cleansing of the bowel by enema or cathartic, or both.

When indicated, obtain the patient's signature of consent for the test or procedure. The patient should have received the physician's explanation of the procedure, the method of performing the test, and the potential risks involved. If the patient cannot give consent because of age or physical or mental impairment, obtain the signature of the person who is legally responsible for the patient's health care decisions. Once the consent form is signed and witnessed, enter it into the patient's chart.

Provide reassurance or information, as needed, to help reduce the patient's anxiety. Communicate with and assist the patient in an attentive and caring manner.

NURSING EVALUATION. The pretest phase is completed successfully when the patient

- has followed all the pretest instructions accurately
- has blood values, vital signs, and temperature measurement within normal limits
- appears calm and accepting about the test

Test Phase

NURSING ASSESSMENT. The nursing assessment during the test phase begins with the correct identification of the patient and verification of the procedure and the particular area that is to be tested (such as right or left leg, arm, breast, lung).

Monitoring of the physiologic status of the patient is carried out by a variety of measurements, depending on the complexity of the procedure and the use of

TABLE 1–3
TEST-PHASE NURSING DIAGNOSES

Nursing Diagnosis	Defining Characteristics
High risk of impaired skin integrity	Disruption of the skin surface Presence of internal or external risk factors, including skin compression, trauma, immobility, or compromised peripheral circulation
Decreased cardiac output	Variations in blood pressure readings, arrhythmias, color changes of the skin and mucous membranes, decreased peripheral pulses, dyspnea
Gas exchange impairment	Anxiety, cyanosis, restlessness, dyspnea Risk factors: administration of sedative analgesic medications, contrast medium, and potential allergic reaction
High risk of infection	Presence of risk factors such as inadequate primary defenses and performance of invasive procedures
Pain	Verbal communication, moaning, crying Nonverbal communication, such as guarding behavior or grimacing
Anxiety	Verbalization of the feelings about the test or its potential findings

sedation or light anesthesia. Ongoing assessment of the patient may be performed through observation, repeated monitoring of vital signs, pulse oximetry, cardiac monitoring, or, in pregnant patients, fetal monitoring.

The nurse assesses the skin for signs of infection or trauma, particularly at the site of intended venipuncture (Borris, 1992; Fleishman, 1992). The chart is also reviewed for the most recent laboratory findings and the pretest vital signs.

The nurse observes the patient for signs of discomfort, including shivering, trembling, pain, and tension. The patient is asked how he or she feels to encourage communication of any problems or concerns.

NURSING DIAGNOSES. Once the nursing assessment is completed, the nurse formulates nursing diagnoses that are appropriate to the patient who undergoes the procedure. The test-phase nursing diagnoses are presented in Table 1–3.

EXPECTED OUTCOMES. During the test period, the outcomes include the following:

1. The patient maintains adequate skin circulation and tissue perfusion.

2. Cardiopulmonary stability is maintained, with vital signs and results of monitoring devices in a normal range.

3. The puncture wound or incision remains clean and free from infection.

4. The patient expresses any pain or discomfort, including the location and characteristics of the sensation.

Critical Thinking: When an invasive procedure is planned, what are examples of external and internal risk factors that could result in impaired skin and tissue integrity?

5. The patient describes any feelings of anxiety and helps identify the cause of those feelings.

NURSING IMPLEMENTATION

Position the patient correctly for the procedure. Use padding, supportive devices, or restraints to promote safety and protect the patient's tissues against injury.

Continuously monitor the patient's cardiopulmonary status, including assessment of skin color and integrity, vital signs, breathing status, and level of consciousness. Keep the emergency cart in a nearby location.

Ensure that all invasive equipment is sterile or has been properly cleaned and disinfected. Before the skin is punctured or opened, ensure that the skin is appropriately cleansed. Draping the area with sterile towels may also be indicated.

Offer reassurance through verbalization or physical support, particularly when the patient appears distressed by the procedure. Administer prescribed pain medication as indicated.

NURSING EVALUATION. The test phase is completed when the patient

- demonstrates normal cardiopulmonary function as measured by normal vital signs and normal readings on all monitoring devices
- maintains normal skin color and tone, with palpable peripheral pulses
- experiences a lessening of pain, anxiety, or discomfort
- has a clean, dry dressing with no signs of renewed bleeding, hematoma, swelling, or redness

Posttest Phase

NURSING ASSESSMENT. The assessment is focused on the patient's physiologic, emotional, and mental status after the test is completed. Physiologic assessment is essential after an invasive procedure, sedation, or anesthesia. The nurse assesses the expected alterations that occur because of the procedure or medications and also the potential complications.

When cardiac monitoring, fetal monitoring, and pulse oximetry are used during procedures, they are usually continued into the posttest period until the results remain stable in a normal range. Vital signs are taken to ensure that the hemodynamic status remains stable.

When an invasive neurologic, cerebrovascular, or peripheral arterial study is performed, there is a risk of complications from an allergic response to the contrast medium as well as a risk of an embolus to a more distal location. Neurovascular assessments are performed to assess the integrity of the distal arterial blood flow and the responses of the neurologic tissues that are supplied by that blood flow. Vital signs also are monitored frequently to identify any untoward changes in cardiorespiratory status.

The nurse also uses observation to perform many assessments. When the diagnostic procedure is invasive, the nurse examines the site of the incision, penetration of the needle, or insertion of the instrument. The tissue is examined for signs of swelling, discharge, bleeding, or discoloration. Some pain or soreness may be present because of the incision or the manipulation of internal tissues. The nurse asks the patient to describe and locate the pain or tenderness. Sometimes the patient does not have immediate pain because of the lingering effects of the anesthetic or narcotic-analgesic medications. The nurse also examines the dressings. They are normally clean, dry, and intact.

The nurse can usually perform an emotional assessment by asking general questions about how the patient feels and observing the patient's responses. Most patients are relieved to have completed the test and are ready to return to their hospital rooms or to their residences. If there has been a period of fasting, they often express the desire to eat.

The assessment of mental status is appropriate when the patient has received sedation or anesthesia or after a cerebrovascular invasive test. The nurse assesses consciousness and alertness as well as clarity of speech. During the initial recovery from sedation or anesthesia, the patient may be somewhat confused or drowsy, with diminished affect. As the medications are metabolized and excreted, there is increasing responsiveness and clarity of thinking.

Prior to discharge, the patient who has had an invasive procedure is assessed for knowledge about continued requirements for care at home until healing is complete. The patient may be able to perform self-care, or there may be a need for family assistance for the remainder of the day. Assessment for infection or inflammation continues for several days because the symptoms take time to develop. The patient or family member is taught to continue this assessment at home.

NURSING DIAGNOSES. Once the nursing assessment has been completed, the nurse formulates nursing diagnoses that are appropriate to the patient during the posttest phase of care. The posttest-phase nursing diagnoses are presented in Table 1–4.

EXPECTED OUTCOMES. During the posttest period, the outcomes include the following:

1. The patient sustains oxygenation and tissue perfusion, including circulation to the extremities.

2. The patient maintains adequate cardiac output.

3. The skin remains warm, with normal color and no evidence of swelling or bleeding.

4. The patient does not fall or experience trauma.

5. After medication is administered, the patient expresses relief from pain.

6. The patient remains infection-free at the site of puncture or incision.

7. The patient, family member, or significant other verbalizes understanding of posttest instructions regarding patient care.

NURSING IMPLEMENTATION

After the completion of a diagnostic procedure in which sedation or a light anesthesia was used, position the patient on his or her side to maintain a

---

TABLE 1-4
POSTTEST-PHASE NURSING DIAGNOSES

Nursing Diagnosis	Defining Characteristics
Alterations in tissue perfusion: cerebral, cardiopulmonary, peripheral	Changes in skin temperature or color, blood pressure changes, decreased peripheral pulses, changes in mental status
Pain	Communication about pain or discomfort Alteration in muscle tone, movement, or facial expression Distracting behavior, such as moaning, grimacing, and crying
High risk of injury	Presence of risk factors such as immobility, developmental age, sensory-motor deficit
High risk of infection	Presence of risk factors such as microorganisms, immunosuppression, broken skin
Knowledge deficit regarding care after procedure	Verbalization of the problem

---

patent airway. Oxygen may be administered, and the intravenous fluid replacement continues until the patient is able to drink fluids orally.

Administer the prescribed pain medication as needed. To help relieve discomfort, encourage the patient to change positions. Provide support with pillows.

Maintain sterile technique in the assessment of the wound or in changing the dressing.

To prevent a fall or an injury, assist the patient off the x-ray or examining table; also help the patient to the bathroom or with dressing in street clothes, as necessary. The patient may be stiff, in pain, or drowsy or may have diminished mental acuity as the result of the medication or procedure.

Prior to discharge, instruct the patient about any additional restrictions that are recommended. There may be instructions regarding activity, bathing, resumption of medication, the intake of fluids, or the care of the incision.

Inform patients that the physician will discuss the diagnostic results with them as soon as this information is available. The patient with sutures is instructed to make an appointment with the physician for the evaluation of the incision and removal of the sutures.

Critical Thinking: After the diagnostic procedure is completed, your patient will go home. Identify the strengths and limiting factors in the patient's life that could affect the course of recovery. What modifications of the discharge plan can help promote a successful outcome?

NURSING EVALUATION. The posttest phase is completed when the patient

- demonstrates normal vital signs, responsiveness to questions, and normal skin color and temperature
- experiences a lessening of pain, anxiety, or discomfort

- has a clean, dry dressing with no signs of renewed bleeding, hematoma, swelling, or redness
- verbalizes his or her understanding of the postdischarge instructions

REFERENCES

Baer, D.M., & Belsey, R.E. (1991). Bedside testing: New requirements from the JCAHO. *RN, 54*, 19–22.

Berkowitz, J.F., et al. (1992). Diagnostic imaging: Special needs of older patients. *Geriatrics, 47*, 55–62, 65, 68.

Bickford, G.R. (1994). Decentralized testing in the 1990's: A survey of United States hospitals. *Clinics in Laboratory Medicine, 14*, 623–650.

Bjerkan, D.L., & McKelvy, B.W. (1991). Covering the bases with a new QA program. *Medical Laboratory Observer, 23*, 43–47.

Borris, L.C. (1992). Complications of heelpad punctures for blood sampling in the newborn. *Neonatal Intensive Care, 5*, 63–64.

Brunzel, N.A. (1994). *Fundamentals of urine and body fluid analysis*. Philadelphia: W.B. Saunders.

Cook, B.A., et al. (1992). Sedation of children for technical procedures: Current standards of practice. *Clinical Pediatrics, 31*, 137–142.

Fleishman, A.R. (1992). Clinical considerations for infant heel sampling. *Neonatal Intensive Care, 5*, 62–63.

Handorf, C.R. (1994). Background—Setting the stage for alternate site laboratory testing. *Clinics in Laboratory Medicine, 14*, 539–558.

Henry, J.B. (1991). *Clinical diagnosis and management by laboratory methods* (18th ed.). Philadelphia: W.B. Saunders.

Jacobs, DS, et al. (Eds.). (1990). *Laboratory test handbook*, (2nd ed.). Baltimore: Williams & Wilkins.

Johnson, R.L. (1992). Flow cytometry from research to clinical applications. *Clinics in Laboratory Medicine, 13*, 831–852.

Jones, B.A. (1994). Testing at the patient's bedside. *Clinics in Laboratory Medicine, 14*, 473–492.

Macpherson, D.S. (1993). Preoperative laboratory testing: Should tests be routine before surgery? *Medical Clinics of North America, 77*, 289–308.

Melillo, K.D. (1993a). Interpretation of abnormal laboratory values in older adults: Part 1. *Journal of Gerontological Nursing, 19*, 39–45.

Melillo, K.D. (1993b). Interpretation of abnormal laboratory values in older adults: Part 2. *Journal of Gerontological Nursing, 19*, 35–40.

Nelson, M.D. (1993). Guidelines for monitoring and care of children during and after sedation for imaging studies. *American Journal of Roentgenology, 160*, 581–582.

Rabbitts, D.G. (1993). Point of care testing: Needs and cost benefit analysis. *Clinical Laboratory Science, 6*, 228–230.

Roby, P.V., et al. (1993). The laboratory outside the laboratory: Our role in point-of-care testing. *Clinical Laboratory Science, 6*, 222–224.

Rock, R.C. (1991). Why testing is being moved to the site of patient care [Special issue]. *Medical Laboratory Observer, 23*, 2–5.

Schembri, C.T., et al. (1992). Portable simultaneous multiple analyte whole-blood analyzer for point-of-care testing. *Clinical Chemistry, 38*, 1665–1670.

Torres, L.S. (1993). *Basic techniques and patient care for radiologic technologists* (4th ed.). Philadelphia: J.B. Lippincott.

Travers, E.M., et al. (1994). Consolidating ancillary testing in multisystems. *Clinics in Laboratory Medicine, 14*, 493–524.

Woo, J., & Henry, J.B. (1994). The advance of technology as a prelude to the laboratory of the twenty-first century. *Clinics in Laboratory Medicine, 14*, 459–472.

CHAPTER 2

Specimen Collection Procedures

Three of the major sources of specimen samples are blood, stool, and urine, with the greatest number of tests performed on blood. The laboratory performs biochemical and microscopic analysis of these body substances to provide objective data about the patient's health and to identify disease processes.

In collection procedures, accurate technique is essential to obtaining a valid specimen and to preventing injury to the patient. In addition, quality control measures are used to maintain accuracy in the identification of the patient and the specimen, in the method of obtaining the specimen, and in the transportation of the specimen to the laboratory.

LABORATORY TEST PROCEDURES

BLOOD COLLECTION: ARTERIAL PUNCTURE

(BLOOD)

Synonyms:

Background Information

Arterial blood specimens are obtained for blood gas studies, including the measurement of oxygen, carbon dioxide, and pH. The assessment of arterial blood is usually performed on the patient who has an actual or a potential problem with oxygenation. The nursing diagnoses may include ineffective airway clearance, ineffective breathing patterns, and impaired gas exchange.

The procedure of arterial puncture is technically more difficult than that of venipuncture, but arterial blood is far more accurate for the measurement of oxygenation throughout the body. The usual site of the arterial puncture is either the radial or the brachial artery; the radial artery is preferred. Although the femoral artery can be used, there is a greater risk of hemorrhage at that site.

Before an arterial puncture of the radial artery is carried out, the *Allen test* is performed to verify the presence of collateral circulation to the hand (Table 2–1). If arterial occlusion of the radial artery occurs after arterial puncture, the presence of collateral circulation protects the hand from ischemic damage. An alternative method of performing the Allen test is presented in Chapter 13.

Purpose of the Test

Arterial puncture is used to obtain a sample of arterial blood for analysis of blood gases and acid-base balance.

TABLE 2–1
THE ALLEN TEST

Purpose
In preparation for a radial artery puncture, the Allen test assesses the adequacy of collateral circulation to the hand.

Procedure
Elevate the hand to diminish the arterial blood flow.
Use one or two fingers to compress the radial artery at its pulse point on the wrist.
Observe for a color change in the hand. The hand should become blanched because of diminished blood flow.
Maintain the arterial compression, lower the hand, and observe for a color change. There should be a brisk return of pinkness to the hand, indicating effective collateral circulation from the ulnar artery.

Interpretation
When collateral circulation is adequate, the radial artery can be used for arterial puncture.
When there is a poor response to the Allen test, the other arm should be tested to search for a better site.
Abnormal results can be caused by a thrombus or arterial spasm that affects the radial artery or ulnar artery, or both. Poor collateral circulation bilaterally may be caused by a systemic problem, such as shock and poor cardiac output.

Procedure

A heparinized syringe and needle is used to collect 3 ml of arterial blood. For radial artery puncture, a 23- to 25-gauge needle is used. For brachial artery puncture, an 18- to 20-gauge needle is used. In many institutions, a prepackaged kit provides the equipment for blood gas studies.

Interfering Factors

- Poor collateral circulation to the extremities
- Inability to puncture the artery or withdraw blood
- Air mixed in with the blood specimen

Nursing Implementation

Pretest

Identify the patient by asking his or her name, checking the identification bracelet, and comparing the identification bracelet with the name on the requisition form.

When the radial artery is to be used, palpate the pulse of each wrist to select the site with the stronger circulation.

Perform the Allen test to assess the collateral circulation to the hand.

Position the hand so that the wrist is in slight dorsiflexion.

Explain to the patient that a sharp pain will be felt as the needle punctures the blood vessel. In some cases, a local anesthetic may be administered beforehand.

Critical Thinking: Why is the stronger pulse site selected? What are the risks of using the radial artery with the weaker pulse?

During the Test

The interior of the syringe and needle must be coated with heparin. The syringe in the blood gas kit may be heparinized already. If heparin must be added, 1 ml (1000 or 5000 U/ml) is drawn into a 10-ml syringe. After the syringe is rotated to coat the entire interior surface, the heparin is expelled. A small amount of heparin remains in the dead space and within the shaft of the needle.

Clean the skin over the pulse point with povidone-iodine, using sterile gauze. Remove this solution by wiping the skin with 70% alcohol. Allow the skin to dry.

With the bevel of the needle up and the syringe placed at a 45- to 60-degree angle, slowly insert the needle into the artery (Fig. 2–1). Blood will pulse into the syringe without your having to draw back on the plunger.

Once the required amount of blood is in the syringe, remove the needle. The amount is usually 3 ml, but the volume can vary according to the type of syringe and the test protocol (Henry, 1991).

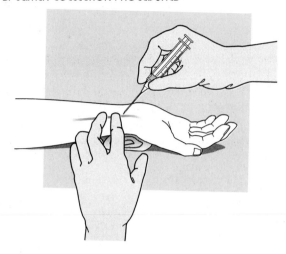

FIGURE 2–1. Technique for arterial puncture. Puncture of the radial artery can be performed only when both the radial and the ulnar arteries provide adequate circulation to the hand.

Posttest

Use a sterile gauze to apply immediate pressure to the puncture site for 5 minutes.

Remove the needle from the syringe. If there is air in the syringe, expel it.

QUALITY CONTROL

Any air in the syringe would be absorbed into the blood and alter the patient's blood gas values.

Place the airtight cap on the tip of the syringe.

Place the syringe on ice and arrange for immediate transport of the specimen to the laboratory.

Once the bleeding from the puncture site has stopped, apply a small sterile bandage.

Continue to assess the wrist and hand for signs of complications. It is common for the patient to complain of some temporary discomfort, such as aching, throbbing, or tenderness at the puncture site.

Complications

The three complications of arterial puncture are hemorrhage, infection, and thrombus formation, but the incidence is low. A summary of the complications of arterial puncture is presented in Table 13–2.

BLOOD COLLECTION: CAPILLARY PUNCTURE

(BLOOD)   ***Synonyms:***

capillary blood collection, skin puncture

Background Information

Capillary puncture is a technique whose use is likely to increase because of the changes in health care delivery. The trends of early patient discharge from the hospital and treatment in outpatient settings often require additional monitoring of the blood as part of the follow-up evaluation. Additionally, there is a growing trend to perform point-of-care testing, meaning that laboratory analysis of the blood is performed at the patient's bedside. This method is used particularly in high-volume areas when rapid results are required. The laboratory analyzer performs multiple tests on a small blood sample from a fingerstick or heelstick source (Matthews, 1992).

The traditional use of the capillary puncture is for patients with small or inaccessible veins. This method is useful in burn patients, those who are extremely obese, and patients in whom there is a tendency toward thrombus formation. It is the method of choice for obtaining blood samples from premature infants, neonates, and young babies. It may be used to preserve the total blood volume of the infant or small child, particularly when there is a need for multiple blood tests.

Because capillary blood is similar in composition to venous blood, capillary blood collection may be performed for a complete blood count, hematocrit determination, blood smear, coagulation studies, and most blood chemistry tests. The specimen source is always identified on the requisition slip because there may be differences between venous and capillary blood concentrations of calcium, glucose, potassium, and total protein.

Site of Collection

The available sites for collection of capillary blood include the finger, heel, and earlobe. The finger is often used for adults or older children. The most often used locations are the distal tips of the third and fourth fingers, slightly to the side (Fig. 2–2). There are few calluses on the sides of the fingers, and the lancet can puncture the skin more easily. The frontal tips or pads of the fingers are not used because there are many nerve endings and the puncture would be more painful.

The heel is used for premature infants, neonates, infants, small children, and special cases such as patients with thermal injury. With the heelstick technique, the medial or lateral plantar surface of the foot is used (Fig. 2–3). The heel and big toe are preferred. The central area of the plantar surface of the foot is never used. There is a risk of damage to the calcaneus bone, Achilles tendon, or other tendons, nerves, and cartilage that are located in the central area of the foot.

The earlobe may be used as the alternative puncture site of last resort in adults and older children, but it cannot be used for infants and neonates. It is a preferred site for obtaining arterialized blood for measurement of pH and P_{CO_2} because it is highly vascular tissue with few metabolic requirements. However, the blood values obtained from an earlobe site are unreliable in cases of low cardiac output and vasoconstriction. If the earlobe is used, the soft fleshy part is punctured, and the area of cartilaginous tissue avoided.

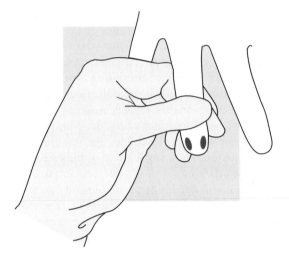

FIGURE 2–2. Capillary puncture site in the finger. In adults, the middle or ring finger is the preferred site for a capillary blood sample. The sterile lancet punctures the skin in the distal tip slightly to the side of the finger pad.

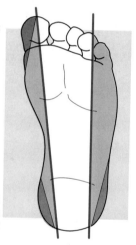

FIGURE 2–3. Heelstick sites for capillary puncture. The shaded areas are appropriate sites for neonates and infants, but the best sites are those of the heel and big toe, as indicated by areas of darker shading.

In the selection of the skin puncture site, the tissue should not be edematous, inflamed, or recently punctured. These factors cause increased interstitial fluid to mix with the blood, and they also increase the risk of an infection.

The heelstick method is preferred for sampling blood in the premature baby and infant. It is technically easier to perform and avoids the significant complications that can occur with arterial or venous puncture. There are some special considerations, however, because of the number of heelstick punctures performed and the small size of the patients.

Increasingly, infants are discharged from the nursery after a short stay. This means that additional blood tests for bilirubinemia, phenylalanine, hemoglobinopathy, and galactosemia as well as other screening tests are performed on an outpatient basis (Bender, 1992). Some of these tests are performed serially, meaning that multiple blood samples are taken over time. The nurse assesses the heels for signs of complications that can occur from repeated punctures.

The premature infant also needs special consideration when multiple blood samples are obtained by the heelstick technique. The premature infant may weigh as little as 500 gm. The heels are small and there is little depth to the tissue for the many punctures and tests that are needed. Additionally, blood flow is often inadequate, and two or three punctures may be needed to obtain the required amount of blood.

To help prevent injury to the calcaneus, the depth of the lancet must be controlled and careful selection of the tissue site must be carried out. To help prevent infection and hematoma, aseptic technique and gentle handling of the tissue are needed whenever blood is drawn. Because of repeated trauma to the heels of the premature infant, the nurse assesses this tissue for signs of localized complications. These complications can occur during the stay in the neonatal unit, or they can develop years later.

Critical Thinking: When the neonate requires multiple blood tests that use heelstick puncture, what posttest nursing measures can minimize the impairment to skin and tissue integrity?

Purpose of the Test

Capillary blood collection is used when a small amount of blood is sufficient or the venipuncture method is not feasible because of interfering factors arising from the patient's condition.

Procedure

A sterile lancet is used to collect capillary blood from a skin puncture site. The blood is blotted onto special filter paper (Fig. 2–4) or collected in a narrow-diameter glass tube. The tube is called a micropipette, microtube, or capillary tube.

Interfering Factors

• Reduced cardiac output
• Vasoconstriction

Nursing Implementation

Pretest

Identify the patient and check the requisition form with the patient's identification bracelet. Inform the patient that blood needs to be drawn from the designated site.

Particularly with small children, provide reassurance to help limit anxiety.

If pretest fasting or dietary restriction is required, verify that the instructions were followed for the correct period of time.

Assemble the equipment and put on a pair of gloves.

The patient may be seated or in the supine position.

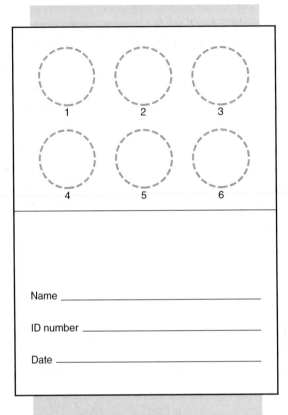

FIGURE 2–4. Capillary blood filter paper. Droplets of blood are blotted onto the filter paper at each circle. The nurse must saturate each circle before moving on to fill the next one. One must not *partially* fill some circles and then return to complete them later. To promote blood flow, the hand is kept lower than the heart and the finger is stroked in a distal direction.

During the Test

Assess the skin site for color and temperature and the absence of infection and edema. If the skin is cool or pale, the circulation may be diminished. Put the hand in warm water or apply a warm, moist compress to the site for a few minutes. This helps increase circulation to the skin.

Use a gauze and 70% alcohol to cleanse the skin site. Allow the skin to dry, because blood drops will not form on moist skin (Walters et al., 1990).

Holding the tissue between the thumb and the forefinger, use a firm, quick stroke to puncture the skin with the sterile lancet.

Wipe away the first drop of blood because it contains tissue fluids. Collect the subsequent drops of blood in capillary tubes or on the blotting paper.

Lower the hand or foot below heart level so that gravity can help promote blood flow. To obtain more blood, the tissue may be milked. The tissue near the puncture should not be squeezed because tissue fluids will mix with the blood.

The capillary tubes are held horizontally to prevent air bubbles. They should be filled two-thirds to three-quarters full and then sealed with clay.

Critical Thinking: After performing the fingerstick puncture, you obtain only a few drops of blood. What nursing measures can be used to increase the blood flow for an adequate test sample?

TABLE 2–2
COMPLICATIONS OF HEELSTICK PUNCTURE

Complication	Nursing Assessment
Infection	Localized redness and swelling Localized pain and tenderness Purulence or abscess formation Radiographic changes indicating osteomyelitis
Hematoma and bruising	Bruising and discoloration Firm swelling of the tissue Tenderness or pain Bleeding onto the skin

The circles on the filter paper are filled one at a time, until they are fully saturated. Allow the blood on the paper to air-dry for 10 minutes before it is placed in a collection envelope.

Posttest

Once the specimen collection is completed, wipe the puncture site with alcohol.

Instruct the patient to place a sterile gauze on the site and apply pressure until the bleeding stops.

If the infant or small child is crying, provide comfort.

Label all specimens and arrange for their prompt transport to the laboratory.

Complications

The most serious complication of heelstick puncture in infants is infection; fortunately, the incidence of this complication is low (Borris, 1992). The infection is usually localized in the soft tissue, and the most common causative organism is *Staphylococcus aureus*. Weeks later, however, the infection can develop into osteomyelitis. The source of the infection is poor aseptic technique, a contaminated lancet, or injury to the bone during the skin puncture.

Bruising and hematoma formation are more frequent complications. They occur from frequent skin punctures or excessive squeezing of the tissues during the collection of the blood samples (Fleishman, 1992).

The complications of heelstick puncture are presented in Table 2–2.

BLOOD COLLECTION: VENIPUNCTURE

(WHOLE BLOOD, SE-
RUM, PLASMA)

Synonyms:

phlebotomy, venous blood collection

Background Information

Venipuncture is performed by drawing and collecting a specimen of blood from a superficial vein. It is a quick method of obtaining a larger sample of blood, and the specimen can be used to perform many different laboratory analyses. Depending on the test to be performed, the analysis is carried out on whole blood, serum, or plasma.

Whole blood contains all the blood components. A centrifuge is used to separate the blood components and obtain either serum or plasma. If the blood has been collected in an anticoagulated tube, the centrifuge process produces plasma. If whole blood is collected in a tube without anticoagulant, the centrifuge process yields serum. Plasma is serum that contains fibrinogen.

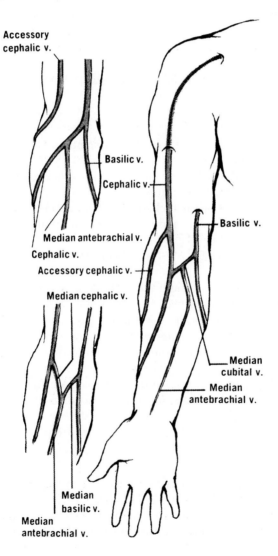

FIGURE 2–5. Veins of the arm. Diagram of some common patterns of the superficial veins of the upper limb. Only the larger channels at the elbow are shown: these are the ones most likely to be visible through the skin. The veins located in the antecubital fossa are preferred sites for venipuncture. (With permission from O'Rahilly, R. [1986]. *Anatomy* [p. 181]. Philadelphia: W.B. Saunders.)

Site of Collection

Critical Thinking: The patient is very obese, and the veins of the antecubital fossa are not visible or palpable. What modifications can be considered so that the venipuncture is successful?

The most common site for venipuncture is the antecubital fossa because there are several large superficial veins available. The most commonly used veins are the median cubital, the basilic, and the cephalic veins (Fig. 2–5). Veins of the wrists, hands, or ankles may also be used.

Intervening Variables

When there is an intravenous line, shunt, or other intravenous device in one arm, the other arm or another venous site must be selected. The reason for avoiding these sites is that the administration of intravenous fluids alters the composition of the blood specimen. Additionally, venous shunts are established for specific treatments, and they can be damaged by excessive punctures.

For a variety of physiologic and age-related reasons, locating a suitable vein is sometimes difficult. When the patient is severely dehydrated or hypotensive, or both, the veins have less fluid volume. They are less visible and less palpable and may be partially collapsed. Reduced cardiac output also diminishes the volume of blood in the peripheral veins.

Severe obesity can be a problem because the overlying layers of fat interfere with the location and palpation of a suitable vein. In the elderly, the superficial veins of the hands are highly visible and prominent, but it is difficult to use these sites. The veins are fragile, and venipuncture can cause a hematoma to form. Additionally, these veins move during the venipuncture process, making it difficult to enter the lumen of the vein. The excess movement is caused by the loss of supportive muscle and connective tissue associated with aging.

In the premature and newborn infant, the veins are small. Frequent venipuncture can cause severe complications, including damage to the veins and surrounding tissues.

If any of these interfering factors are present, causing difficulty with venipuncture, capillary puncture may be an acceptable alternative.

Purpose of the Test

Venipuncture is used to obtain a venous blood sample to be used for laboratory analysis. The serum component of the blood is used for most of the chemistry analyses.

Procedure

Either a vacuum tube system or a needle, syringe, and test tube containers are used to collect the blood sample. The selection of the color-coded specimen tube is based on the requirements of the specific test. Each laboratory blood test in this text lists the correct test tube to be used for that test.

Interfering Factors

- Dehydration
- Hypotension
- Obesity
- Fragility of veins
- Prematurity and infancy

Nursing Implementation

Pretest

Identify the patient, and check the requisition form with the patient's identification bracelet.

Inform the patient that blood needs to be drawn from the designated site. Provide reassurance to help limit anxiety (particularly with small children).

If pretest fasting or dietary restriction is required, verify that the instructions were followed for the correct period of time.

Assemble the equipment, and put on a pair of gloves.

The patient may be seated or in the supine position. The patient's arm is in extension, with easy access to the antecubital fossa.

During the Test

Inspect the antecubital fossae of both arms to select the best vein for the venipuncture. Ask the patient to open and close the hand a few times to help make the veins more visible.

Gently palpate the vein to determine its location, direction, width, and depth.

Cleanse the skin with 70% alcohol, and allow it to air-dry.

Apply the tourniquet about 2 to 3 in. above the antecubital fossa.

Using your fingertips, anchor the vein above and below the puncture site.

With the bevel up, insert the needle at a 15-degree angle along the pathway of the vein (Fig. 2–6).

Syringe Method

Once the needle is in the vein, gently aspirate blood into the syringe. Collect the volume of blood that is needed.

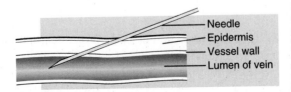

FIGURE 2–6. Needle placement during venipuncture. To obtain good blood flow, the needle is positioned correctly in the vein lumen. The needle should not rest against the upper wall of the vein or puncture through the vein wall on the opposite side.

Vacuum Tube System Method

Once the needle is in the vein, hold it firmly in place. Push the blood collection tube fully into the holder so that the blood flows through the needle and into the vacuum tube (Fig. 2–7). When multiple specimens are needed, remove each full tube and insert the next tube firmly into the holder.

After all blood has been collected, release the tourniquet.

Place a sterile gauze over the puncture site. Remove the needle. Use the gauze and your finger to compress the puncture site.

QUALITY CONTROL

When you draw blood by syringe or the vacuum tube system method, the tourniquet should not remain tied for more than 1 minute. The prolonged compression of the vein and stasis of the blood flow caused by the tourniquet results in clumping or hemolysis of the erythrocytes, which interferes with the laboratory analysis and alters some test results.

Posttest

Instruct the patient to continue compression of the puncture site for 2 to 5 minutes or until the bleeding stops.

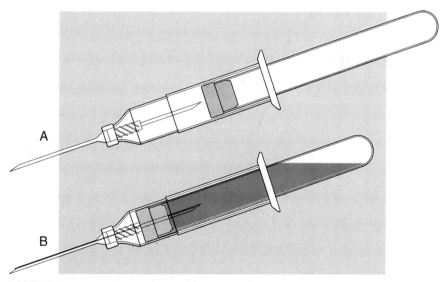

FIGURE 2–7. Function of the vacuum tube collection system. *A*, Prior to venipuncture, the vacuum tube is placed into the holder, resting on the tip of the sterile needle. *B*, Once the needle enters the vein, the tube is pushed to the front of the holder and the needle penetrates the stopper of the tube. Because of the negative pressure in the tube, the blood is pulled from the vein, through the needle, and into the vacuum tube.

When a syringe and needle were used, transfer the blood to the appropriate test tube containers.

Label every vial of blood with the patient's name and identification number, the time, and the date.

Perform any special measures that are needed to protect the specimen from deterioration. These measures are test-specific and are described throughout this text.

Assess the patient's arm to ensure that the bleeding has ceased. Apply an adhesive bandage as needed.

Remove gloves and wash your hands.

Arrange for prompt transport of the specimen to the laboratory.

Complications

Hematoma formation occurs when the vein continues to leak blood under the skin. The result is a large bruised area. The problem can be prevented by continued compression of the puncture site until clotting occurs. The patient can also elevate the arm and rest it on top of the head—this reduces pressure on the walls of the vein and the puncture site.

Dizziness or fainting can occur in some individuals. If the patient feels faint, a fall and possible injury can be prevented by helping him or her to a sitting or reclining position. First aid measures such as lowering the head between the knees or using smelling salts can help revive the patient.

STOOL COLLECTION

(FECES)

Synonym:

stool specimen

Background Information

The laboratory testing of fecal matter may involve chemical analysis that identifies the abnormal composition of the feces or may involve microbiologic analysis that identifies infectious organisms. Once the abnormality has been identified, there is often a need for additional diagnostic tests or procedures to determine the cause and location of the problem.

One group of abnormal fecal test results is caused by diseases that damage the intestinal mucosa, alter the integrity of the intestinal tissues, or interfere with the functions of digestion, absorption, and elimination. The fecal changes may include the presence of blood or an alteration in the composition of the feces. Examples of these diseases include malignancy of the stomach or colon, peptic ulcer, regional ileitis, celiac disease, or scleroderma.

A second group of abnormal fecal test results is caused by abnormality in the organs and ducts that secrete into the intestinal tract. These organs include the liver, pancreas, and gallbladder. The fecal changes can include excess fat in

Critical Thinking: Several children in the daycare center are positive for ova and parasites in the feces. To minimize the fecal-oral transmission of the parasites, develop a teaching plan for the child-care workers.

the stool or a lack of fecal urobilinogen. Examples of these conditions include cystic fibrosis, pancreatic cancer, hepatitis, and bile duct obstruction.

A third category of abnormal fecal test results is caused by infectious organisms that infect the intestinal tract. The organisms are discovered by microscopic examination of the stool or stool culture. The infection may be of bacterial, viral, parasitic, or other origin, often infecting the small or large intestine. Sometimes the infection causes damage to the intestinal mucosa or underlying tissue, resulting in blood in the stool. In this example, more than one abnormality can be detected in the analysis of fecal matter.

Purpose of the Test

Analysis of feces is used to screen for intestinal disease in an asymptomatic individual; to help identify abnormal intestinal function or abnormal function of the gallbladder, liver, or pancreas; and to help assess the patency of the biliary tree.

Procedure

A half-pint waterproof container that is clean and dry and has a wide mouth with a tight-fitting lid is used to collect approximately 1 to 2 oz of fecal matter.

Interfering Factors

- Improper specimen collection
- Contamination of the specimen with water or urine
- Delay in transport of the specimen
- Failure to follow pretest dietary instructions
- Pretest ingestion of antibiotics, cathartics, or barium, or administration of an enema

Nursing Implementation

Pretest

Ask the patient if he or she has had a recent barium x-ray study or recent treatment with oral antibiotics. Schedule the test accordingly.

QUALITY CONTROL

Barium sulfate interferes with the analysis of feces for approximately 2 weeks after ingestion. Stool culture is less likely to demonstrate the causative organism when antibiotics have been taken during the preceding 3 to 4 weeks (Proctor, 1991).

Instruct the patient about any dietary restrictions that are part of specific test preparations. For some of the tests, such as those looking for fecal fat and fecal occult blood, there are pretest dietary modifications.

Instruct the patient not to ingest castor oil, mineral oil, antacids, or antidiarrheal medications or to administer an enema before the test.

QUALITY CONTROL

These substances appear in the fecal matter and interfere with the chemical or microscopic analysis.

During the Test

Instruct the patient to evacuate directly into the container or a clean, dry bedpan. Tongue blades can be used to transfer a small amount of feces from the bedpan into the collection container.

Urine, water, or toilet paper must not be mixed in with the fecal specimen.

Once the specimen is obtained, place the lid on the container and wash your hands.

Posttest

Label the container with the patient's name and other appropriate data. Mark the time and date of the collection on the container and requisition slip.

Arrange for transport of the specimen within 30 minutes.

If there is a delay before transport, store the specimen in the refrigerator. The cool temperature preserves any microorganisms that may be present.

URINE COLLECTIONS

(URINE)

Synonyms:

Background Information

Urine provides a major source of data about the status and function of the urinary tract. In addition, because urine is an ultrafiltrate of the plasma, it is used to assess various homeostatic and metabolic processes of the body. Urine is easily collected, but the procedure must be performed completely and accurately. If there is an error in procedure, false or invalid test results can occur.

There are four basic urine collection procedures, which are based on the time or duration of the collection period: the first morning specimen, the random specimen, the fractional urine specimen, and the timed specimen. Since the purposes and methods vary, each of these procedures is discussed separately in subsequent sections of this chapter.

In addition to spontaneous voiding, there are several other possible methods of collection. A description of the special collection methods is presented here. When urine cannot be collected by normal voiding, these special methods are used for any of the basic collection procedures.

Special Collection Methods

CATHETERIZATION. A catheterized specimen is used when the patient cannot void or when an indwelling catheter is already in place. For straight catheterization, a sterile catheter is inserted through the urethra and into the bladder. The urine flows from the bladder, through the catheter, and into the specimen container. Once the bladder has been emptied, the catheter is removed.

With an indwelling catheter, fresh urine is collected directly from the catheter in all types of tests except the timed specimen. For the single urine specimen collection, the catheter is clamped below the port temporarily. After a short interval, a sterile needle and syringe are used to remove the urine sample through a special port in the catheter. Then the clamp is removed, and the urine flow to the collection bag resumes. A timed specimen has a much longer collection period and requires a larger volume of urine. At the start of the test, a new, empty collection bag is attached to the indwelling catheter and its tubing. The urine is removed from the collection bag at intervals and is added to the specimen collection container until the time period is completed.

PEDIATRIC SPECIMENS. If the child is toilet trained and can follow directions, the nurse can provide instructions to the parent or assist the child in the collection of the urine. For the infant or child who cannot control the release of urine voluntarily, a pediatric collection bag is used. The perineum is cleansed and dried, and then the bag is applied and fixed with an adhesive strip. For the male infant, the bag is placed over the penis. For the female infant, the bag is applied over the labia and perineum. In each gender, the rectum must be excluded to prevent the mixing of fecal matter with urine. Once the bag is in place, it is checked every 15 minutes until the urine is collected.

SUPRAPUBIC ASPIRATION. This method is used when an anaerobic culture is required or when there is a problem with external contamination of the urine culture, such as in infancy. With the use of sterile technique, the suprapubic aspiration is performed by the physician. A sterile needle is inserted through the abdominal wall above the symphysis pubis and then is advanced into the full bladder. A syringe is used to aspirate the urine specimen. The specimen is placed into a culture container, and the needle is removed. Complications with this procedure are rare (Henry, 1991).

FIRST MORNING SPECIMEN

(URINE)

Synonyms:

Background Information

The first morning specimen is the first urine to be voided after the patient awakens from sleep. This urine has been retained in the bladder for about 6 to 8 hours. Because of the lack of fluid intake or exercise during the period of sleep, the urine is concentrated and somewhat acidic. This type of specimen is preferred for routine screening. It is also preferred for the detection of specific substances, including nitrites, protein, and microorganisms. Concentrated urine or an incubation period is needed to readily detect these substances in the urine (Jones, 1992).

Purpose of the Test

The first morning specimen is used for routine urinalysis that includes chemical and microscopic analysis. This specimen is also used to identify orthostatic proteinuria.

Procedure

A clean, dry plastic or glass container with a lid is used to collect a midstream urine specimen.

Interfering Factors

- Menstrual secretions
- Delay in the analysis of the urine
- Inadequate labeling of the specimen

Nursing Implementation

Pretest

Provide a urine container with a lid.

Instruct the patient to collect a midstream voided specimen. A midstream void means that the patient begins to urinate, and about halfway through the process the specimen is collected. With this method, the initial urine flow washes the bacteria out of the distal urethra before the specimen is collected.

In some protocols, a midstream clean-catch method is used. If this is the case, provide the patient with the materials and instructions, as presented in Table 2–3.

Posttest

Seal the lid of the container completely to prevent leakage.

Label the container (not the lid) appropriately with the patient's name and other pertinent information, including the date and time of the collection.

TABLE 2–3
MIDSTREAM CLEAN-CATCH URINE PROCEDURE

Purpose

This method of urine collection reduces the external sources of contamination before the urine is collected. The contaminants are the bacteria and secretions of the skin that surround the urethra and also reside in the distal portion of the urethra.

Procedure

Cleansing Process: Male

The glans is exposed and cleansed, with the use of three sterile cotton balls or gauze squares moistened with a mild antiseptic solution.

The first cotton ball cleanses the tissue from the urethral meatus to the ring of the glans in a single stroke. The cotton ball is then discarded. The process is repeated with the other two cotton balls, cleansing the remaining areas of the glans.

If the male is uncircumcised, the foreskin must be retracted and the tissue under the foreskin cleansed thoroughly before the preceding steps are taken.

Cleansing Process: Female

The labia minora are separated to expose the urinary meatus. They must then remain separated throughout the cleansing process and urine collection phase.

The exterior mucous membranes and the meatus are cleansed, with the use of three sterile cotton balls or gauze squares moistened with a mild antiseptic.

The first moist cotton ball cleanses the tissue on one side of the urinary meatus, with a single stroke from front to back. The cotton ball is discarded. The second cotton ball cleanses the other side of the meatus, with the same motion and direction. The third cotton ball cleanses the center of the meatus, wiping in a single motion, also from front to back.

Midstream Collection

The patient begins to void into the toilet or bedpan.

The urine washes residual bacteria and secretions from the distal urethra.

At about the midpoint of voiding, the urine stream is interrupted. On release of the urine, 1 to 3 oz of urine is collected in the specimen container.

The container must not touch the perineal tissues or hair either during or after collection. The patient's fingers must not touch the inside of the container or lid.

Once there is sufficient urine in the container, the patient finishes voiding into the toilet or bedpan, and the remaining amount is discarded.

Ensure that the specimen is delivered to the laboratory immediately. If there is an anticipated delay, the specimen must be refrigerated or a preservative added to the urine container.

QUALITY CONTROL

With a delay of 2 hours or more before analysis is performed, the nonrefrigerated, unpreserved specimen can undergo a number of changes. The changes vary among the individual specimens, but almost every laboratory value can be altered. The causes of the changes are multiple and include oxidation, reduction, bacterial proliferation (White, 1992), solute precipitation, decomposition, and the disintegration of the cells and casts.

RANDOM SPECIMEN

(URINE)

Synonyms:

Background Information

The random urine specimen is one that can be collected at any time. It is easy and convenient for the patient because there is no need to plan or schedule the test. Even though the daytime activities of fluid intake and exercise alter the composition of the urine, there is no need to control these variables. The specimen is usually satisfactory for the purposes of screening or routine urinalysis.

Cytologic studies are also performed on random urine samples. For this test, the patient must drink extra fluids prior to each of several urine samples that are collected. The goal is to flush out an increased number of cells so that the detection of abnormal cells is enhanced. Random samples are also used for urine cultures, with the goal of identifying microbial growth and the presence of infection.

Purpose of the Test

The random specimen is used for routine urinalysis that includes chemical and microscopic examination. This method of collection is also used for bacterial culture and cytologic studies to help identify the cause of disease in the urinary tract.

Procedure

Critical Thinking: Ten days after the request, the female patient from a different cultural background has not yet produced the urine specimen. What are possible reasons for the failure to comply? How can the nurse resolve the problem?

For routine urinalysis or a random urine screen, a clean plastic or glass container with a lid is used to collect a urine sample at any time. A midstream clean-catch method is used (see Table 2–3).

For bacterial, fungal, or viral culture, a sterile plastic or glass container with a lid is used to collect the random urine sample. The midstream clean-catch method is used. In special cases, a catheter or suprapubic aspiration is used to obtain the random specimen.

For cytologic studies, the midstream clean-catch method is used to collect each specimen in a clean plastic or glass container with a lid. Daily specimens are collected for 3 to 5 consecutive days.

Interfering Factors

- Menstrual secretions
- Delay in the analysis of the urine
- Inadequate labeling of the specimen
- Contamination of the specimen

Nursing Implementation

Pretest

Provide written and verbal instructions regarding how to cleanse the urethral meatus and surrounding tissue and how to collect the specimen.

Provide the appropriate collection container or containers.

For cytologic studies, instruct the patient to drink 24 to 32 oz. of water each hour for 2 hours before voiding. In some laboratory protocols, the patient is also instructed to exercise for 5 minutes by skipping or jumping rope before voiding. The activity and fluid volume should increase the yield of cells needed for the study. This process is repeated daily for 3 to 5 days to provide for the analysis of three to five consecutive urine specimens (Brunzel, 1994).

Posttest

Seal the lid of the container completely to prevent leakage.

Label the container (not the lid) appropriately with the patient's name and other pertinent information, including the date and time of the collection.

Ensure that the specimen is delivered to the laboratory immediately. If there is an anticipated delay, the specimen must be refrigerated or a preservative added to the urine container.

QUALITY CONTROL

With a delay of 2 hours or more before analysis is performed, the nonrefrigerated, unpreserved specimen can undergo a number of changes. The changes vary among the individual specimens, but almost every laboratory value can be altered. The causes of the changes are multiple and include oxidation, reduction, bacterial proliferation, solute precipitation, decomposition, and the disintegration of the cells and casts.

FRACTIONAL COLLECTION

(URINE)

Synonym:

double-voided specimen

Background Information

A fractional collection of urine is a method used to compare a particular component of the urine with the serum level of that component. Blood samples and urine samples are collected at specific times, and the laboratory analysis measures the amount of the component found in each specimen.

The serum sample is measured for the blood level during controlled conditions such as a fasting state or after administration of a dye or solute. The urine samples are measured for the baseline and renal threshold values. One example of the fractional collection is the glucose tolerance test.

Purpose of the Test

Fractional collection is used to compare blood and urine values in screening for diabetes mellitus and in the diagnosis of some liver and kidney disorders.

Procedure

Generally, baseline blood and urine specimens are obtained first. The patient then receives a measured intravenous or oral substance such as food, dye, or glucose. Thereafter, timed blood and urine specimens are collected.

Interfering Factors

- Failure to complete the pretest preparation
- Failure to collect all urine specimens
- Failure to obtain all urine specimens at the correct times
- Failure to label all specimens accurately

Nursing Implementation

Pretest

Provide the patient with written and verbal instructions. Some of these tests require nothing by mouth (NPO) status for 6 to 8 hours before the test. Some have instructions to void and discard the first morning specimen.

During the Test

Administer the prescribed glucose solution, injectable dye, or other measured substance used in the test.

Collect each urine specimen in a separate container at the specific time interval required by the protocol.

Label each container (not the lid) with the patient's name and other appropriate identifying information. The time of each voided specimen is also recorded on the container (e.g., 1/2-hour specimen, 1-hour specimen).

Posttest

Send all specimens to the laboratory together without delay.

QUALITY CONTROL

If there is a delay of more than 2 hours, the specimens must be preserved by refrigeration. Many components of urine are altered when the specimen remains warm and there is a delay in performing the analysis. In particular, the level of urinary glucose becomes falsely decreased because of cellular and bacterial glycolysis.

TIMED COLLECTION

(URINE)

Synonyms:

Background Information

The timed collection is used for the quantitative analysis of a specific urinary component. Circadian rhythms, diurnal rhythms, metabolism, exercise, and hydration all affect the excretion rate of substances in the urine. At certain times during a 24-hour period, there is increased excretion of substances such as electrolytes, hormones, proteins, and urobilinogen, and at other times there is decreased excretion. By collecting the quantity of urine over a specified period, there is greater accuracy of measurement than there is with a random specimen.

Sometimes, an abnormal substance is not present in the urine at all times. Thus, the urine is collected for a longer period, in the hope of identifying small amounts of the component that are occasionally present. Urine cytologic testing requires a 2-hour collection period repeated over several days. The parasites *Schistosoma* and *Onchocerca* are detected in urine that is collected over a 24-hour period.

Time Intervals

The designated time period for a urine collection depends on the specific component to be tested. Some tests are for a *predetermined length of time*, such as a 2-hour, 12-hour, or 24-hour urine collection. Other tests are for a *specific time of day*, such as 12 PM to 4 PM. In these instances, the time frame reflects when the substance is maximally excreted in the urine each day.

Purpose of the Test

The timed collection is used to perform quantitative urine assays and clearance tests and to identify abnormal cytology, or ova and parasites in the urine.

Procedure

A large (3000-ml) clear or brown glass or plastic container with a lid is used to collect all urine within the designated period.

QUALITY CONTROL

To prevent changes in the quality of the urine over time, all timed specimen containers are kept cool in a basin of ice or in the refrigerator. Some tests require that a preservative be added to the container before the collections begin. Information about the additive is described by the written laboratory protocol.

Interfering Factors

- Failure to discard the first voided specimen before the procedure begins
- Failure to collect all the urine voided during the test period
- Failure to refrigerate or preserve the urine specimen
- Improper labeling

Nursing Implementation

Pretest

Provide both written and verbal instructions regarding the collection of the urine. These instructions must include the specific times for the collection period.

Advise the patient who works or is in school that it is easiest to collect the specimen on the weekend.

For a 24-hour urine collection, advise the patient to moderately limit the fluid intake during the collection period. Alcohol intake should be avoided for 24 hours before and during any timed collection of the urine.

Other restrictions are part of specific test protocols. Some tests have specific dietary restrictions, and some medications need to be withheld for a specific period. Special restrictions or modifications are included in the patient's pretest instructions.

During the Test

Critical Thinking: A 4-year-old child completed the 24-hour urine collection, but the mother states that the child "wet the bed during the night." What instructions do you give to the mother?

ALL TIMED COLLECTIONS

Maintain the specimen and container on ice or in the refrigerator during the collection period. Such measures prevent deterioration of the specimen.

During the time period, all urine is added to the collection container. If any urine spills or if a specimen is discarded accidentally, the test is invalid. The stored specimen is discarded, and a new collection period is started on the following day.

24-HOUR COLLECTION

The first void of the morning is discarded, and the urine collection period begins at 8 AM.

Place all urine for 24 hours into the container. This includes the first void specimen of the next morning.

Posttest

Label the container (not the lid) with the patient's name and other appropriate identifying data. Include the time and date of the start and the completion of the urine collection period.

Arrange for prompt delivery of the specimen to the laboratory.

REFERENCES

Bender, D. (1992). Comparative newborn screening studies. *Neonatal Intensive Care, 3*, 64–65.

Borris, L.C. (1992). Complications of heel pad punctures for blood sampling in the newborn. *Neonatal Intensive Care, 3*, 63–64.

Brunzel, N.A. (1994). *Fundamentals of urine and body fluid analysis.* Philadelphia: W.B. Saunders.

Collecting a 24-hour urine sample. (1990). *Patient Care, 24*, 99.

Fleishman, A.R. (1992). Critical considerations for infant heel blood sampling. *Neonatal Intensive Care, 3*, 62–63.

Henry, J.B. (1991). *Clinical diagnosis and management* (18th ed.) Philadelphia: W.B. Saunders.

Jones, E. (1992). Urine collection: In search of a fine specimen. *Nursing Times, 88*, 62–63.

Matthews, D. (1992). Comparative studies of time requirements and repeat sticks during heelstick. *Neonatal Intensive Care, 3*, 66–68.

Proctor, E.M. (1991). Laboratory diagnosis of amebiasis. *Clinics in Laboratory Medicine, 11*, 829–859.

Walters, N.J., et al. (1990). *Basic laboratory techniques,* (2nd ed.). Albany, NY: Delmar.

White, S. (1992). Urine collection: Choosing the right container. *Nursing Times, 88*, 64.

PART II

MULTISYSTEM LABORATORY TESTS

Urinalysis Screen

Urinalysis is one of the oldest and most common laboratory tests in existence. It produces a large amount of information about possible diseases of the kidneys and lower urinary tract as well as systemic diseases that alter the composition of the urine. Urinalysis is also valuable because normal results are used to exclude a number of possible alternative diagnoses.

Urinalysis has several additional advantages over more sophisticated alternatives, particularly in the initial stage of diagnosis. Urinalysis is economical, and the analysis can be performed rapidly. Furthermore, the specimen can be obtained easily, noninvasively, and without risk to the patient.

LABORATORY TESTS

Components of Urinalysis

URINALYSIS

(URINE)

Synonym:

UA

─────────────────── **NORMAL VALUES** ───────────────────

Color: yellow, clear	Occult blood: Negative
Specific gravity: 1.003–1.029	RBCs (male): 0–3 per HPF
pH: 4.5–7.8	RBCs (female): 0–5 per HPF
Protein: Negative	WBCs: 0–5 per HPF
Bilirubin: Negative	Bacteria: Negative
Urobilinogen: Normal	Leukocyte esterase: Negative
Glucose: Negative	Casts: 0–4 hyaline casts per LPF
Ketones: Negative	Crystals: Few

Background Information

Analysis of the urine consists of two parts: the macroscopic, or chemical, analysis and the microscopic analysis. Except for the observation of color and clarity, the macroscopic component is performed with the dipstick method. Some laboratories do not perform the microscopic component routinely unless there is an abnormal result in the chemical analysis or a specific request for the microscopic examination.

When microscopic analysis is performed, the initial phase is a scanning of the specimen under a low-power field (LPF). The purpose is to search for cells, casts, and crystals. If these components are located, the microscopic high-power field (HPF) is used to obtain greater detail about the findings.

COLOR AND CLARITY. Normal urine is yellow and clear. The yellow varies in tone from pale to stronger yellow, depending on the urine's concentration and specific gravity. There are many possible changes of color or clarity, some of which are presented in Table 3–1. In addition, some medications and chemicals are responsible for changes in urine color.

SPECIFIC GRAVITY. The specific gravity is a measurement of the ability of the kidneys to concentrate and excrete the urine. The measurement indicates the proportion of dissolved solid components to water. In the normal elderly population, the specific gravity decreases proportionately with advancing years.

Concentrated urine has a higher specific gravity because there is a greater proportion of components to water in its composition. For example, a specific gravity greater than 1.020 indicates concentrated urine with a composition of more solute or less water, or both. If glucose or protein is present in the urine, the specific gravity value also rises. The presence of these additional abnormal components must be considered in the evaluation of the findings.

Diluted urine has a lower specific gravity because there are fewer components in proportion to the amount of water in the urine. For example, a specific gravity less than 1.009 indicates diluted urine with a composition of less solute or more water, or both.

In the individual with healthy renal function and normal fluid intake, the specific gravity of the initial glomerular filtrate is 1.010. In normal physiology, as the filtrate passes through the tubule system, there is an ongoing exchange of

TABLE 3–1
CAUSES OF CHANGE IN URINE COLOR AND CLARITY

Characteristic	Cause
Clarity	
Cloudy, smoky, hazy	Pyuria
	Bacteriuria
	Phosphates in the urine
Color	
Colorless	Overhydration
	Diuretic therapy
	Diabetes mellitus
	Diabetes insipidus
Dark	Acute intermittent porphyria
Red or pink	Hematuria
	Ingestion of beets, berries, fava beans, red food coloring, rhubarb
Dark yellow or orange	Bile
Green	*Pseudomonas* bacteriuria
	Urinary bile pigments

solutes and water that alter the specific gravity of the filtrate and ultimately the urine. When the specific gravity of urine remains *fixed* (unvarying over time) at 1.010, that value is an indication of severe renal damage. When the specific gravity of the urine is the same as that of the glomerular filtrate, it indicates that the renal tubules cannot resorb water and effectively concentrate the urine.

pH. With an average dietary intake and normal metabolism, the body produces a continuous supply of hydrogen ions and acids. As part of the acid-base balance, the kidneys remove excess hydrogen ions from the blood and excrete them in the urine.

The urinary pH is affected by dietary intake. A large intake of acidic fruits or protein causes the urine to be more acidic, with a lower urinary pH value. A large intake of citrus fruits and vegetables causes the urine to be more alkaline, with a higher urinary pH value. A normal dietary intake produces slightly acidic urine, with an average pH value of 6.0.

In abnormal physiology, a urine pH greater than 6.5 indicates the presence of bicarbonate in the urine. Alkaline urine may occur because of systemic alkalosis (respiratory or metabolic). It also may occur because of a renal tubular disorder, with the decreased ability of the renal tubules to form ammonia and exchange hydrogen ions for cations such as sodium. Metabolic acidosis results from the tubular damage and the inability to regulate acid-base balance (Geyer, 1993). In urine with a pH greater than 7.0, calcium carbonate, calcium phosphate, or magnesium ammonium phosphate stones can form.

A urinary pH less than 5.5 indicates the absence of bicarbonate ions in the urine. The cause of the problem may be systemic acidosis (respiratory or metabolic), with the excess hydrogen ions of the extracellular fluids spilling into the urine. Xanthine, cystine, or uric acid stones can form in highly acidic urine.

PROTEIN. In normal physiology, minimal amounts of protein are excreted in the urine, mostly as albumin. The albumin is filtered out by glomeruli, with a greater amount released into the urine during the daytime or after strenuous exercise.

The presence of excess urinary albumin is an indicator of glomerular disease. The nephrotic syndrome produces a great loss of albumin in the urine. The renal loss may also be associated with systemic disease that causes glomerular damage.

The dipstick method may be used to detect protein in the random urine sample. This rapid assessment method is useful in detecting albumin, but it is less sensitive to globulins and other plasma proteins that enter the urine (Moore and Carome, 1993). It cannot detect the small amounts of protein that appear in the urine during the early stage of renal damage, and the dipstick method is not sensitive enough to detect low-molecular-weight proteins in the urine. (Additional discussion of urinary protein is presented in Chapter 20.)

BILIRUBIN. Bilirubinuria is an abnormal finding that results from an increase in the serum conjugated (direct) bilirubin. The level of urine bilirubin rises in some conditions of hepatocellular jaundice and liver disease. Bilirubinuria is frequently present in obstructive jaundice, with either intrahepatic or extrahepatic biliary obstruction. The test for bilirubin does not measure the unconjugated (indirect) bilirubin that is caused by hemolytic jaundice because these bilirubin molecules cannot pass through the glomeruli easily. (Additional discussion of bilirubin is presented in Chapter 18.)

UROBILINOGEN. This substance is normally excreted in the urine in small amounts. When the values are low or normal, the urobilinogen cannot be detected with the dipstick method and routine urinalysis. When urobilinogen levels are elevated, urinalysis indicates the need to follow up with a 2-hour urine urobilinogen test for specific measurement. The elevated level is an indicator of damage to the liver tissue, impaired liver function , or hemolytic anemia. (A discussion of the 2-hour urine urobilinogen test is presented in Chapter 18.)

GLUCOSE. Glycosuria is usually an indicator of significant hyperglycemia and diabetes mellitus. When a fasting specimen is obtained, it is highly specific and accurate in the detection of glucose in the urine. The nonfasting, random sample is much less specific.

The urine glucose test is best used as a screening test for the healthy population and in monitoring control of the type II diabetic patient. The dipstick method is not sensitive enough to be useful as a quantitative measure of glucose in the urine. Because of the poor sensitivity and inability to detect hypoglycemia, the urine glucose dipstick test also is not sufficient for the monitoring of the type I diabetic patient.

KETONES. In starvation or abnormal carbohydrate metabolism, large quantities of ketone bodies appear in the urine before the serum levels of ketones are elevated. Urinalysis is useful in monitoring known diabetics, particularly when they are ill, hyperglycemic, or pregnant.

Ketonuria is not limited to diabetics. In children, ketonuria can occur during febrile illness or as the result of severe diarrhea and vomiting. It may also occur during a normal pregnancy. Additionally, elderly individuals can experience ketonuria as the result of fasting.

Critical Thinking: The result of the urinary occult blood test is positive. Because he cannot see any blood, the patient does not think that the result is important. How can you respond effectively?

OCCULT BLOOD. A positive result from a dipstick test for occult blood in the urine occurs when intact erythrocytes, hemoglobin, or myoglobin is present. Like gross hematuria, microscopic hematuria is caused by diseases of the kidney or lower urinary tract or by a nonurinary problem of medical origin. When the occult blood test result is positive, a microscopic examination of the urine is performed to identify red blood cells (RBCs) and red cell casts. Additional laboratory or diagnostic tests are also indicated to diagnose and locate the cause of the bleeding.

Hematuria is a relatively common finding with many possible causes. It can be an indicator of serious disease. The bleeding can be intermittent and the blood loss minimal, but these patterns bear no relationship to the severity of the disease (Paola, 1990).

Myoglobin is released from injured skeletal or cardiac muscle into the blood. Myoglobin release has many possible causes related to muscle tissue damage, including damage of a toxic, traumatic, ischemic, or infectious origin. The myoglobin is then filtered from the blood by the glomeruli and excreted in the urine. Myoglobin is associated with renal failure, but the exact relationship is unknown.

RED BLOOD CELLS. Normal urine may exhibit a few RBCs without any significant pathologic cause. The presence of a few cells is considered acceptable under HPF microscopic visualization. Significant hematuria is indicated by one episode of gross hematuria or one episode of high-grade microhematuria, with an RBC count greater than 100 cells per HPF (Paola, 1990). Significant hematuria is an indicator for further diagnostic evaluation.

When accompanied by proteinuria, red cell casts, or renal tubular cells, the hematuria is usually of renal or lower urinary tract origin. When there are RBCs but no casts and only minimal proteinuria, the disorder is likely to be of urologic origin. Glomerular diseases often cause the RBCs to be misshapen, fragmented, hypochromic, and small. The cause of these RBC changes is unknown, but they may be due to the passage of RBCs through damaged glomeruli or to osmotic changes in the renal tubules.

WHITE BLOOD CELLS. There are few to no white blood cells (WBCs) in normal urine. An elevated WBC count indicates pyuria. When WBCs are clumped, it indicates severe urinary tract infection. The microscopic urinalysis finding of 5 to 10 WBCs per HPF (5 to 10 WBCs per mm^3) is a significant elevation that indicates the presence of urinary tract infection. The combination of an elevated WBC count and the presence of WBC casts is an indicator of infection of renal origin (Little et al., 1989).

BACTERIA. Most urinary tract infections are characterized by a significant number of bacteria in the urine. The bacteria are visualized during high-power microscopic examination of the centrifuged specimen. The bacteria can be characterized with a Gram stain. The finding of a bacteria count greater than 10^5 bacteria per ml is considered diagnostic of urinary tract infection (Pappas, 1991).

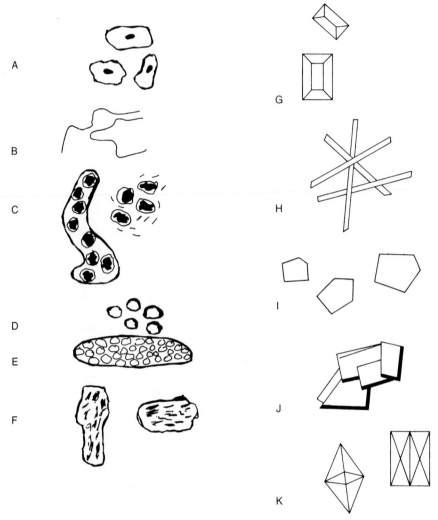

FIGURE 3–1. Elements of urinary sediment. *A,* Epithelial cells. *B,* Mucus-secreting cells. *C,* White blood cell cast, white blood cells, and bacteria. *D,* Red blood cells. *E,* Red blood cell cast. *F,* Waxy casts. *G,* Triple phosphate crystals. *H,* Calcium phosphate crystals. *I,* Cystine crystals. *J,* Uric acid crystals. *K,* Calcium oxalate crystals. (With permission from Little, D.N., Thompson, M.E., & Thompson, D.E. [1989]. The diagnostic evaluation, urinalysis and imaging. *Primary Care, 16,* 864.)

Bacteria can also be detected with the nitrite dipstick method. In the presence of most urinary bacteria, the dipstick turns pink (positive result) within 60 seconds. This method does not measure the severity of infection or identify the type of bacteria.

LEUKOCYTE ESTERASE. The leukocyte esterase test is an indirect method used to detect bacteria in the urine. The dipstick method identifies lysed or intact

WBCs (neutrophils). When these cells are present, the bacteria must also be present.

When leukocyte esterase is used as a screening test, it should be combined with the nitrite dipstick test to avoid false-negative results. When leukocytes or neutrophils are present in the urine, the leukocyte esterase dipstick turns blue in 1 minute. For greatest accuracy, the dipstick result is read in 5 minutes. Sometimes inaccuracies occur among examiners in reading the results of the dipstick test, particularly when the patient is asymptomatic (Lachs et al., 1992).

CASTS. Casts are globulin protein structures that are precipitated in the renal tubules. They are found in the urine sediment, and the different types are identified during microscopic examination (Fig. 3–1). The presence of a great number of casts is an indicator of renal parenchymal disease.

Granular casts are associated with glomerulonephritis and renal pathologic conditions. Fatty casts are produced in the nephrotic syndrome. Cellular casts can have RBCs, WBCs, or renal tubular cells, or a mix of these different cells. They are indicators of inflammation or infection of glomeruli, renal tubules, or renal interstitial tissue.

Hyaline casts are the most common type of cast, but their presence may or may not be significant. Hyaline casts can appear after strenuous exercise, with fever, or in congestive heart failure. Persistent large numbers of hyaline casts are an indication of renal disease.

CRYSTALS. Crystals are the end products of food metabolism and, when present, are found in urinary sediment. A variety of crystals can be identified by microscopic examination, based on their characteristic shapes (see Fig. 3–1). Crystals can be found in healthy urine, although most individuals have few or none present in urine.

Critical Thinking: As the child recovers from acute glomerulonephritis, how do particular urinalysis findings help evaluate the patient's response to treatment?

Crystals are seen commonly in patients with urolithiasis, toxic damage to the kidneys, or chronic renal failure. Uric acid, xanthine, and cystine crystals or their calculi are often present in acidic urine. Calcium carbonate, calcium phosphate, and magnesium ammonium phosphate crystals or their calculi are often present in alkaline urine. The presence of cellular elements or crystals, or both, causes the urine to become cloudy.

Purpose of the Test

Urinalysis is performed to screen for urinary tract disorders, kidney disorders, urinary neoplasms, and other medical conditions that produce changes in the urine. This test is also used to monitor the effects of treatment of known renal or urinary conditions.

Procedure

A clean container with a lid is used to collect 15 ml or more of urine. A random sample may be used, but the first-voided specimen of the morning is preferred.

Findings

ELEVATED VALUES

Specific Gravity

Dehydration
Fever
Profuse sweating
Vomiting, diarrhea, or both
Glycosuria
Proteinuria
Congestive heart failure
Adrenal insufficiency
Altered secretion of antidiuretic
  hormone

Protein

Nephrotic syndrome
Renal disorders associated with
  Hypertension
  Diabetes mellitus
  Systemic lupus erythem-
    atosus
  Amyloidosis

Urobilinogen

Hemolytic anemia
Hepatitis (infectious, toxic,
  chemical)
Cirrhosis
Congestive heart failure

Ketonuria

Acidosis
Alcoholic ketoacidosis
Diabetic ketoacidosis
Fasting or starvation
Increased protein intake

Casts

Glomerulonephritis
Chronic renal disease
Nephrotic syndrome
Bacterial pyelonephritis
Renal failure

Occult Blood

Glomerulonephritis
Urolithiasis
Urinary tract infection
Tumor, benign or malignant

pH

Metabolic alkalosis
Respiratory alkalosis
Bacteriuria (*Proteus* sp., *Pseudomonas*)
Vegetarian diet
Nasogastric suctioning
Prolonged vomiting
Falconi syndrome
Milkman syndrome
Alkali therapy

Bilirubin

Hepatitis (infectious, toxic,
  chemical)
Biliary obstruction (intrahepatic or
  extrahepatic)

Glucose

Hyperglycemia
Diabetes mellitus

Crystals

Uric Acid Crystals

Gout
Rapid nucleic acid turnover
Urolithiasis

Calcium Oxalate Crystals

Chronic renal failure
Ethylene glycol ingestion
Urolithiasis

Triple Phosphate Crystals

Obstructive uropathy
Urinary tract infection
Urolithiasis

Red Blood Cells

Benign tumor
Carcinoma
Urinary calculi
Glomerulonephritis

Polycystic kidney

Renal infarct

Lupus nephritis

Goodpasture syndrome

Benign prostatic hypertrophy

Blood dyscrasia, hemolysis
  of RBCs

Endocarditis

Leukemia

Poison (snake or spider bite)

Parasitic disease

Thermal or crush injury

Trauma

Severe exercise, jogging

IgA neuropathy

Lupus nephritis

Sclerosis

Urinary tract infection

Trauma from exercise

White Blood Cells

Urinary tract infection (cystitis,
  prostatitis, urethritis, pyelonephritis)

Bacteria

Chronic urinary tract infection

Pyelonephritis

Cystitis, acute or chronic

DECREASED VALUES

Specific Gravity

Overhydration

Diuresis

Hypotension

Pyelonephritis

Glomerulonephritis

Renal tubular dysfunction

Severe renal damage

Diabetes insipidus

pH

Metabolic acidosis

Respiratory acidosis

Diabetes mellitus

Diarrhea

Starvation

Emphysema

Renal failure

Interfering Factors

- Insufficient quantity of urine
- Contamination of the specimen
- Prolonged delay before analysis is performed
- Warming of the specimen

Nursing Implementation

Pretest

Instruct the patient to collect a sample of urine, preferably on arising in the morning. (The specimen must not be contaminated by toilet paper, toilet water, feces, or secretions. Women should not collect urine during menstruation, to prevent contamination with the bloody discharge.)

Posttest

Label the container with the patient's name, the time, and the date of the voiding.

Arrange for transport of the specimen to the laboratory within 30 minutes. If this cannot be accomplished, refrigerate the specimen.

QUALITY CONTROL

Refrigeration preserves the elements of the urine, but the delay can cause crystals to precipitate. If the specimen stands at room temperature, the warmth causes bacteria and WBCs to decompose.

REFERENCES

Ford, H. (1992). Feeling off-colour. . .colour of urine and faeces can indicate disease. *Nursing Times*, *88*, 64, 66, 68.

Geyer, S.J. (1993). Urinalysis and urinary sediment in patients with renal disease. *Laboratory Clinics of North America*, *13*, 13–20.

Henry, J.B. (Ed.). (1991). *Clinical diagnosis and management by laboratory methods* (18th ed.). Philadelphia: W.B. Saunders.

Hurlbut, T.A., et al. (1991). The diagnostic accuracy of rapid dipstick tests to predict urinary tract infection. *American Journal of Clinical Pathology*, *96*, 582–588.

Jones, E. (1992). Urine collection: In search of a fine specimen. *Nursing Times*, *8*, 62–63.

Lachs, M.S., et al. (1992). Spectrum bias in the evaluation of diagnostic tests: Lessons from the rapid dipstick test for urinary tract infection. *Annals of Internal Medicine*, *117*, 135–140.

Little, D.N., Thompson, M.E., & Thompson, D.E. (1989). The diagnostic evaluation, urinalysis, and imaging. *Primary Care*, *16*, 857–871.

Moore, J., Jr., & Carome, M.A. (1993). Proteinuria. *Clinics in Laboratory Medicine*, *13*, 21–31.

Paola, A.S. (1990). Hematuria: Essentials of diagnosis. *Hospital Practice*, *25*, 144–152.

Pappas, P.G. (1991). Laboratory in the diagnosis and management of UTIs. *Medical Clinics of North America*, *75*, 313–323.

Teitz, N.W. (Ed.). (1990). *Clinical guide to laboratory tests* (2nd ed.). Philadelphia: W.B. Saunders.

White, S. (1992). Urine collection: Choosing the right container. *Nursing Times*, *88*, 64.

CHAPTER 4

Hematology Screen

The total blood volume consists of 60% plasma and 40% cells. The blood performs the critical function of transporting oxygen, nutrients, hormones, and enzymes to the cells. It transports waste products and carbon dioxide from the cells to the lungs, kidneys, and biliary tract as organs of excretion. Blood also regulates the body pH and water balance and helps to regulate the body temperature.

Plasma is a clear yellowish fluid that contains proteins, fats, carbohydrates, iron, vitamins, and trace elements. It is the fluid medium in which the cells circulate. The largest protein component in plasma is albumin. The albumin serves to maintain blood volume, viscosity, and osmotic pressure. The other plasma proteins are the immunoglobulins, which provide the defense against microbes and foreign antigens, and the clotting factors, which are essential for coagulation and protection from blood loss (Alkire and Collingwood, 1990).

The *cells* of the blood consist of erythrocytes, leukocytes, platelets, and lymphocytes. The bone marrow is responsible for hematopoiesis and some lymphocytopoiesis (Table 4–1). The marrow responds to stimuli from the microenvironment for the initiation and continuation of hematopoiesis. The blood cells originate from hematopoietic stem cells, with formation, differentiation along specific lines, proliferation, and maturation occurring during hematopoiesis. When the cells are mature enough, they are released into the blood.

The process of hematopoiesis is supported by colony-stimulating factors. These hormone-like glycoproteins stimulate and regulate hematopoiesis so that sufficient numbers of specific cells are available in the blood. Under normal conditions, the number of circulating blood cells remains constant, with a balance between the rate of cell loss and the rate of cell production (Hays, 1990).

TABLE 4-1
HEMATOPOIESIS AND LYMPHOCYTOPOIESIS

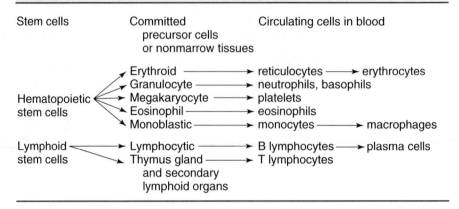

Stem cells	Committed precursor cells or nonmarrow tissues	Circulating cells in blood
Hematopoietic stem cells	Erythroid	reticulocytes → erythrocytes
	Granulocyte	neutrophils, basophils
	Megakaryocyte	platelets
	Eosinophil	eosinophils
	Monoblastic	monocytes → macrophages
Lymphoid stem cells	Lymphocytic	B lymphocytes → plasma cells
	Thymus gland and secondary lymphoid organs	T lymphocytes

The process of lymphocytopoiesis originates in the lymphoid stem cells. In response to signals from the lymphatic tissues, the lymphoid stem cells form lymphocytes along two different lines. In the bone marrow, B lymphocytes are formed and released into the blood and lymphatic fluids. With stimulation from antigens, the B lymphocytes become plasma cells and release antibodies. After the initial differentiation of the lymphoid stem cell in the marrow, the thymus gland and secondary lymphoid organs form the second line of lymphocytes—the T lymphocytes, which are released into lymphatic fluid and, ultimately, the blood.

This chapter focuses on the basic tests of blood cells, involving the number, concentration, and structure of the cells. (Chapter 6 focuses on coagulation tests and Chapter 16 addresses the diverse hematologic tests and procedures related to the blood cells and bone marrow.)

LABORATORY TESTS

COMPLETE BLOOD COUNT

(BLOOD)

Synonyms:

CBC, blood cell profile, hemogram

━━━━━━━━━━━━━━ **NORMAL VALUES** ━━━━━━━━━━━━━━

WHITE BLOOD CELL COUNT (WBC):	$4.5–11 \times 10^3/\mu l$ *or* SI $4.5–11 \times 10^9/L$
RED BLOOD CELL COUNT (RBC):	Male: $4.6–6.2 \times 10^6/\mu l$ *or* SI $4.6–6.2 \times 10^{12}/L$
	Female: $4.2–5.4 \times 10^6/\mu l$ *or* SI $4.2–5.4 \times 10^{12}/L$
HEMOGLOBIN:	Male: 13.5–18 g/dl *or* SI 135–180 g/L
	Female: 12–16 g/dl *or* SI 120–160 g/L
HEMATOCRIT:	Male: 40–54% *or* SI 0.4–0.59 (volume fraction)
	Female: 38–47% *or* SI 0.38–0.47 (volume fraction)
RED CELL INDICES:	Mean Corpuscular Volume (MCV): 80–96 μm^3 *or* SI 80–96 fL
	Mean Corpuscular Hemoglobin (MCH): 27–31 pg *or* SI 27–31 pg
	Mean Corpuscular Hemoglobin Concentration (MCHC): 32–36% *or* SI 0.32–0.36 (concentration fraction)
	Red Cell Distribution Width (RDW-CV): 13.1% (range: 11.6–14.6%) (Henry, 1990)
PLATELET COUNT:	Adult: 150,000–450,000 cells/μl *or* SI $150–450 \times 10^9/L$
	Newborn: 84,000–478,000 cells/μl *or* SI $84–478 \times 10^9/L$

Background Information

The basic hematology screen consists of a complete blood count (CBC) and a peripheral blood smear. The CBC provides the count of each type of blood cell in the circulation, measurements of the hemoglobin and hematocrit, and measurements of the parameters of the erythrocyte by red cell indices. The WBC differential provides the counts of each type of leukocyte. The peripheral blood smear provides a microscopic view of the blood cells to verify the count and to identify abnormalities of cellular shapes and structures.

AUTOMATED ANALYZERS. Today, the CBC is carried out by automated hematology analyzers. The definition of the "complete" blood count has changed with the increasing sophistication of automation. The CBC is often an "abbreviated" blood count based on the technical capability of the particular analyzer used (Koepke, 1993). Generally, automated analyzers include analysis of the hemoglobin, hematocrit, red cell count, red cell indices, white cell count, and platelet count. Some CBC findings include some or all parts of the WBC differential. Some of the CBC reports include platelet indices, although the interpretation and clinical use of this component is still undergoing scientific examination. In some institutions, the platelet count, the differential count, the reticulocyte count, and the peripheral smear are not part of the basic CBC and must be ordered separately.

TECHNOLOGY OF THE ANALYZERS. The different types of analyzers are based on the principles of either *electric impedance* or *light scattering*. Based on the characteristics of the cells, the analyzers are able to identify the different cells and count them (Ward et al., 1994).

In *electric impedance* methodology, the analyzer measures the difference in electric conductivity as each cell passes through a tiny opening in the electric field. The analyzer differentiates among the cells based on the cell size. For the differential count, reagents are used to alter the cell's nucleus and cytoplasm. The analyzer can then differentiate among some or all of the types of leukocytes and count them.

In *light scatter* methodology, each cell passes through a quartz flow cell in the analyzer. As the cells pass through in single file, they cross a beam of laser light. As the cell interrupts the beam, it results in a scattering of light in all directions. The patterns of light scattering are detected, and the computer recognizes the distinct pattern that is characteristic for each cell type. The computer analysis provides the count and cell sizing for the different types of cells. The structures inside each blood cell are also identified by the scattering pattern of laser light so that hemoglobin, cell nuclei, and the characteristics of cytoplasm are identified and classified.

REFERENCE VALUES. The common reference values of the CBC are those obtained by manual analysis procedures. The manual methods produce values that are usually higher because small amounts of plasma adhere to the walls of the collection tube as the fluid and cells are removed. This is particularly true when capillary tubes are used to collect the specimens.

The values of the automated analyzers are accurate and precise for most cell counts. Since there are many different types of analyzers and several methods of analysis, the interpretation of the values should be based on the reference values of the specific laboratory that performed the test.

This discussion of the CBC provides an overview of different parts of the test as performed for screening purposes. Each component is also presented further on as an individual test, with more depth of discussion. The patient may be monitored by repeated CBC testing or by the specific component tests that are pertinent to the health problem and its treatment.

Purpose of the Test

The CBC is used to assess the patient for anemia, infection, inflammation, polycythemia, hemolytic disease, the effects of ABO incompatibility, leukemia, and the status of dehydration. It is also used to identify the cellular characteristics of the peripheral blood.

Procedure

A purple-topped tube with ethylenediaminetetraacetic acid (EDTA) anticoagulant is used to collect 7 ml of venous blood. As an alternative, two purple-tipped capillary tubes can be used to collect blood from a heelstick, earlobe, or finger puncture.

For the peripheral blood smear, two slides are prepared immediately using drops of venous or capillary blood.

QUALITY CONTROL

With venipuncture, the tourniquet should be tied lightly for a brief time to prevent pooling of cells in the vein at the site of blood collection. The venipuncture technique must be smooth, with a blood flow that fills the vacuum tube readily. If the blood demonstrates excessive turbulence because of a flawed venipuncture technique, the hemolysis of the erythrocytes will alter the test results. After the blood is collected, the tube is gently inverted 5 to 10 times to mix the anticoagulant and prevent clotting.

Findings

Critical Thinking: The infant has severe diarrhea and fever, and you suspect a nursing diagnosis of fluid volume deficit. Which components of the CBC are pertinent in this case? Why would the results be elevated?

ELEVATED VALUES

White Cell Count
Infection
Inflammation
Leukemias

Hemoglobin
Polycythemia
Hemoconcentration

Red Cell Indices
MCV: Pernicious anemia
      Vitamin B_{12} or folate deficiency
MCH: Hereditary spherocytosis
MCHC: Hereditary spherocytosis
RDW: Microcytic anemias

Red Cell Count
Polycythemia
Renal tumor
Hemoconcentration

Hematocrit
Polycythemia
Hemoconcentration

Platelets
Myeloproliferative diseases
Multiple myeloma
Iron deficiency anemia
Postsplenectomy response
Hodgkin disease
Lymphomas
Renal disease
Infection or inflammation

DECREASED VALUES

White Blood Cells
Aplastic anemia
Bone marrow depression
Pernicious anemia
Some infectious or parasitic diseases

Red Blood Cells
Hemorrhage
Hemodilution
Anemia
Aplastic anemia
Bone marrow depression
Hemolysis of erythrocytes

Hemoglobin
Hemorrhage
Anemia

Hematocrit
Hemorrhage
Anemia

Hemolysis of erythrocytes
Hemodilution
Red Cell Indices
MCV: Iron deficiency anemia
      Chronic inflammation
MCH: Iron deficiency anemia
MCHC: Iron deficiency anemia

Hemolysis of erythrocytes
Hemodilution
Platelets
Idiopathic thrombocytopenic
  purpura
Aplastic anemia
Anemias
Malignancy of the spleen
Disseminated intravascular
  coagulation
Bone marrow depression
Systemic lupus erythematosus
Uremia
Liver disease

Interfering Factors

- Hemolysis
- Coagulation of the specimen
- Hemodilution

Nursing Implementation

During the Test

Ensure that the blood is not taken from the hand or arm that has an intravenous line. Hemodilution with intravenous fluids causes a false decrease in the values of some tests.

Posttest

Arrange for prompt transport of the specimen. If there is an anticipated delay, refrigerate the specimen.

HEMATOCRIT

(BLOOD)

Synonyms:

Hct, microhematocrit, packed cell volume, PCV

NORMAL VALUES

Male: 40–54% *or* SI 0.4–0.59 (volume fraction)
Female: 38–47% *or* SI 0.38–0.47 (volume fraction)

Background Information

The hematocrit is a measurement of the proportion of whole blood volume occupied by erythrocytes. The value is expressed as a percentage or fraction of cells to whole blood. For example, a hematocrit value of 40% means that there are 40 ml of erythrocytes in 1 dl of blood.

VARIATIONS OF NORMAL VALUES. In laboratory analysis performed by the manual method, the normal value is slightly higher than that performed by the automated method. Additionally, regardless of the test methodology, the normal value for males is slightly higher than that for females. The pregnant female has a slightly lower normal value than that of the nonpregnant female because of the greater blood volume during pregnancy. In men older than 65 years of age, the normal value is slightly lower than for younger males. For all individuals, the normal value can be 5 to 6% lower when blood is drawn with the patient in a recumbent position as opposed to an upright position.

ELEVATED VALUES

The hematocrit rises when there is an increase in the number of erythrocytes, as in polycythemia vera, or a reduction in the plasma fluid volume, as in dehydration. When the fluid volume is decreased, the blood becomes concentrated, with increased viscosity. The possible panic value is a hematocrit reading of greater than 60% (SI: >0.6 [volume fraction]).

DECREASED VALUES

The hematocrit falls to less than normal when there is an excessive loss of erythrocytes, as in anemia or after excessive bleeding. It can also decrease because of excessive intravenous fluids that exert a dilutional effect.

In bleeding or hemorrhage, the hematocrit drops several hours after the bleeding episode. The severity of the drop in value correlates directly with the amount of blood lost. The possible panic value is a hematocrit reading of less than 18% (SI: <0.18 [volume fraction]).

Critical Thinking: The patient has a bleeding duodenal ulcer, and the latest hematocrit result is 20% (SI: 0.20). What nursing actions are indicated?

Purpose of the Test

The hematocrit is useful in the evaluation of blood loss, anemia, hemolytic anemia, polycythemia, and dehydration.

Procedure

A purple-topped tube with EDTA is used to collect 7 ml of venous blood. As an alternative, two purple-tipped capillary tubes can be used to collect blood from a heelstick, earlobe, or finger puncture.

QUALITY CONTROL

With venipuncture, the tourniquet should be tied lightly for a brief time to prevent pooling of cells in the vein at the site of blood collection. Venipuncture technique must be smooth, with a blood flow that fills the vacuum tube readily. If the blood shows excessive turbulence because of flawed venipuncture technique, the hemolysis of the erythrocytes will alter the test results. After the blood is collected, the tube is inverted gently 5 to 10 times to mix the anticoagulant and prevent clotting.

Findings

ELEVATED VALUES

Polycythemia vera
Secondary polycythemia
Dehydration

Extreme physical exertion
Hemoconcentration

DECREASED VALUES

Recent hemorrhage
Anemia

Hemolytic anemia
Hemodilution

Interfering Factors

- Hemolysis
- Coagulation of the specimen
- Hemodilution

Nursing Implementation

Pretest

When the patient is hemorrhaging or has just had a severe bleeding episode, both hemoglobin and hematocrit values are monitored at regular intervals. The results indicate the severity of the blood loss. Likewise, after transfusion replacement of packed cells or whole blood, the same tests are used to evaluate the effectiveness of treatment. Ensure that the tests are performed at the indicated times.

During the Test

Ensure that the blood sample is not taken from a vein in the hand or arm with an intravenous line. Hemodilution with intravenous fluids or plasma will lower the hematocrit value falsely.

Posttest

Arrange for the prompt transport of the specimen to the laboratory. If there is an anticipated delay, refrigerate the specimen to prevent the deterioration of cells.

HEMOGLOBIN

(BLOOD)

Synonyms:

Hgb, Hb, total hemoglobin

NORMAL VALUES

Male:	13.5–18 g/dl *or* SI 135–180 g/L
Female:	12–16 g/dl *or* SI 120–160 g/L
Child:	11–16 g/dl *or* SI 110–160 g/L
Infant:	10–15 g/dl *or* SI 100–150 g/L
Newborn:	14–24 g/dl *or* SI 140–240 g/L

Background Information

Hemoglobin is the oxygen-carrying compound contained in each erythrocyte. The large amount of hemoglobin and the broad surface area of each erythrocyte enables the RBCs to have a large oxygen-carrying capacity and to function with marvelous efficiency.

Each hemoglobin molecule consists of the protein *globin* and the iron-containing pigment *heme*. At the lungs, the heme molecules combine with oxygen for transport to the cells. At the cell level, oxygen is released and the globin molecule combines with a molecule of carbon dioxide for the return trip to the lungs.

VARIATION IN NORMAL VALUES. The normal value of hemoglobin varies among individuals of different age, gender, race, and geographic location. The normal hemoglobin value is higher in males than in females. It is usually lower in the premature infant than in the full-term infant at birth. After age 10 years, the hemoglobin value is slightly lower in blacks than in whites. Men older than 65 years of age have a slightly lower value than do those who are younger. The normal value is slightly higher in individuals who live in high-altitude areas. The value is 5 to 6% lower in patients who have their blood drawn when in a recumbent position as opposed to an erect position.

ELEVATED VALUES

An elevated hemoglobin value may be due to an excess production of erythrocytes or dehydration.

DECREASED VALUES

An individual generally is considered anemic when the hemoglobin value is less than 13 g/dl (SI: <130 g/L) for the male and less than 11 g/dl (SI: <110 g/L) for the female. The possible panic value is less than 6 g/dl (SI: <60 g/L). The low value can be caused by a low RBC count, a lack of hemoglobin in each erythrocyte, or fluid retention. In fluid retention, there is a *relative* low RBC count and hemoglobin value because of the disproportionate amount of water in the blood.

Critical Thinking: At the nursing health center, a routine CBC for a 3-year-old child reveals a hemoglobin value of 10.6 g/dl (SI: 106 g/L). To help validate the suspected nursing diagnosis of nutrition alteration: less than body requirements, what additional assessment data are needed?

Purpose of the Test

The hemoglobin is used to measure the severity of anemia or polycythemia, and it monitors the response to treatment of anemia. It is also used to calculate the MCH and MCHC values.

Procedure

A purple-topped tube with EDTA is used to collect 7 ml of venous blood. As an alternative, two purple-tipped capillary tubes can be used to collect blood from a heelstick, earlobe, or finger puncture.

QUALITY CONTROL

With venipuncture, the tourniquet should be tied lightly for a brief time to prevent pooling of cells in the vein at the site of blood collection. A smooth venipuncture technique will produce a blood flow that fills the vacuum tube readily. If the blood has excessive turbulence because of flawed venipuncture technique, the hemolysis of the erythrocytes will alter the test results. After the blood is collected, the tube is inverted gently 5 to 10 times to mix the anticoagulant and prevent clotting.

Findings

ELEVATED VALUES

Polycythemia vera   Dehydration
Secondary polycythemia   Hemoconcentration

DECREASED VALUES

Recent bleeding   Hemorrhage
Fluid retention   Anemia
                           Hemolysis of red cells

Interfering Factors

- Hemolysis
- Coagulation of the specimen
- Lipemia
- WBC count greater than $50 \times 10^3/\mu l$ (SI: $>50 \times 10^9/L$)

Nursing Implementation

Pretest

When the patient is hemorrhaging or has just had a severe bleeding episode, both hemoglobin and hematocrit measurements are taken at regular intervals. The results indicate the severity of the blood loss. Likewise, after transfusion replacement of packed cells or whole blood, the same tests are used to evaluate the effectiveness of treatment. Ensure that the tests are performed at the indicated times.

During the Test

Ensure that the blood sample is not taken from the hand or arm that has an intravenous line in the vein because of the dilutional effect on RBC concentration.

Posttest

Arrange for prompt transport of the specimen to the laboratory. If there is an anticipated delay, refrigerate the specimen to prevent deterioration of the cells. Without refrigeration, the specimen must be analyzed within 4 hours.

PERIPHERAL BLOOD SMEAR

(BLOOD)

Synonyms:

blood smear morphology, morphologic examination of the blood, peripheral smear

─────────────────────────── **NORMAL VALUES** ───────────────────

Normal cell morphology

Background Information

The peripheral blood smear is a visual microscopic examination of stained blood cells. In most hematologic diseases, characteristic changes can be seen in the blood cells. There may be changes in the size, structure, and shape of the cells or changes in the number and distribution of the cells, or a combination of these changes may be seen. The microscopic visualization of these changes helps diagnose or confirm the hematologic diagnosis. The three hematologic lines of leukocytes, erythrocytes, and platelets can be examined in the peripheral blood smear.

For quality assurance or total quality management, a microscopic examination of slides is performed manually to check the accuracy of the cell counts performed by automated technology. The manual examination is also performed to visually identify abnormal cells that are flagged during the automated cell count. Lastly, the slides provide additional information when the patient's condition indicates unexplained or suspicious findings.

Digital image processing may also be used to perform some automated aspects of the examination. Slides are prepared, and the equipment performs the microscopic examination. The characteristics of the cells are compared with the cells in the computer memory. The normal cells match the computer software categories. They are identified, differentiated, and counted. Abnormal cells or unknown cells do not have a match in the computer data. The computer marks these cells and indicates their location on the slide. The technician or pathologist investigates the abnormalities in a second review.

MORPHOLOGIC FEATURES OF RED CELLS. Normal erythrocytes are circular, nonnucleated discs of uniform size, color, shape, and cytoplasmic appearance. The cells are paler in the center than in the periphery. They are described as normocytic (size) and normochromic (color). The patient can be anemic despite these normal characteristics. A normocytic, normochromic anemia is one that is caused by hemolysis of erythrocytes or blood loss. The cells are normal, but there are too few of them.

Abnormal erythrocytes vary in size, color, hemoglobin content, shape, staining properties, and structure. The altered size is due to a defect in erythropoiesis. The bone marrow can be adversely affected by genetics, poor nutrition, changes in bone marrow cells, or changes in bone marrow function.

Abnormal color is due to an alteration in hemoglobin content. Too little hemoglobin causes a pale color. The problem may be due to iron deficiency or abnormal hemoglobin synthesis.

Poikilocytosis refers to abnormally shaped red cells. Abnormal erythrocyte structure includes the presence of a nucleus that identifies these cells as normoblasts, basophilic stippling, Howell-Jolly bodies, or Heinz bodies. The variations of some of the characteristics of erythrocytes and their relationships to hematologic disease are presented in Table 4–2.

MORPHOLOGIC FEATURES OF WHITE CELLS. The microscopic evaluation of leukocytes is the same as the differential count. There are five types of leukocytes: neutrophils, eosinophils, basophils, monocytes, and lymphocytes. These cells should be within a normal range in number, concentration, and stage of maturity. A complete discussion of these cells is presented further on under White Blood Cell Differential.

MORPHOLOGIC FEATURES OF PLATELETS. The microscopic evaluation of platelets provides an estimate of the platelet count, with an evaluation of the size and structure of the cytoplasm of the cell. The increased concentration of large cells occurs in myeloproliferative diseases and immune thrombocytopenia.

Purpose of the Test

The cells of the blood are examined microscopically to help identify causes of anemia and to evaluate the function of the bone marrow. Abnormal cell counts, concentrations, or morphologic features are investigated and the accuracy of cell counts performed by automated technology are also assessed.

TABLE 4–2
CHARACTERISTICS OF ERYTHROCYTES—RELATIONSHIPS TO HEMATOLOGIC DISEASES

Characteristics	Interpretation	Pathophysiology	Associated Disorders
Size			
Normocytic	Normal cell size	Adequate response by the bone marrow	None
		Shortened life span of the erythrocytes—increased hemolysis	Acute blood loss Hemolytic anemia
		Impaired release of iron from reticuloendothelial system	Anemia of chronic disease
Macrocytic or megalocytic	Larger than normal cell size	Marrow disorder with defective DNA that affects cell development during erythropoiesis	Deficiency of vitamin B_{12} or folic acid Megaloblastic anemias
		Uptake of cholesterol and bile salts by the erythrocyte membranes	Liver disease and obstructive jaundice
Microcytic	Smaller than normal cell size	Deficiency of heme, a lack of iron, or impaired hemoglobin synthesis	Iron deficiency anemia, thalassemia, sideroblastic anemia, lead poisoning, vitamin B_6 deficiency
Color			
Normochromic	Normal hemoglobin content	Normal iron stores, normal hemoglobin synthesis	Anemia due to hemorrhage, with loss of erythrocytes
Hyperchromic	Erythrocyte saturated with hemoglobin	A relative increase of hemoglobin within the erythrocyte that has a small diameter and small cell membrane; the cell is spherical	Spherocytosis

Table continued on following page

TABLE 4–2
CHARACTERISTICS OF ERYTHROCYTES—RELATIONSHIPS TO HEMATOLOGIC DISEASES *Continued*

Characteristics	Interpretation	Pathophysiology	Associated Disorders
Hypochromic	Erythrocyte with diminished hemoglobin	Iron deficiency in proportion to erythropoiesis Defective hemoglobin synthesis	Iron deficiency anemia Thalassemia, lead poisoning, sideroblastic anemia
Shape Elliptocyte	Elliptical or oval shape	Cytoplasm and cholesterol in the cell membrane are polarized in areas of convexity; increased hemolysis can occur	Hereditary elliptocytosis, thalassemia, iron deficiency, sickle cell disease, other hemolytic diseases
Spherocyte	Sphere-shaped cell	Genetic disease of the bone marrow; the abnormal cells have a shorter life span	Hereditary spherocytosis, immune disease, and other hemolytic anemias
Target cell	Hemoglobin is distributed on the perimeter and in the center, giving "target" appearance	Deficient hemoglobin for the normal cell size	Hemoglobin C, D, S diseases, thalassemia, iron deficiency
		Too large a cell membrane and cell size for a normal amount of hemoglobin	Obstructive, jaundice, liver disease
Sickle cell	Crescent-shaped cells	In conditions of deoxygenation, the hemoglobin S becomes elongated and rigid; cell membranes also become sickle-shaped	Sickle cell trait, sickle cell disease, other sickling hemoglobinopathies
Poikilocytosis	Varied, irregular shapes of cells (teardrop, tennis racket, horned, helmet shapes)	Irreversible alterations of cell membrane from rapid erythropoiesis or extramedullary erythropoiesis	Megaloblastic anemia, hemolytic anemia, uremia, liver disease, metastatic cancer, toxicity, idiopathic myelofibrosis

Table continued on following page

TABLE 4–2
CHARACTERISTICS OF ERYTHROCYTES—RELATIONSHIPS TO HEMATOLOGIC DISEASES *Continued*

Characteristics	Interpretation	Pathophysiology	Associated Disorders
Schistocyte	Red cell fragments	Partial splitting or phagocytosis of the cell, without loss of hemoglobin	Hemolytic anemia, disseminated intravascular coagulation, malignant hypertension, cancer, cardiac valve prosthesis, burns, uremia
Structure			
Nucleated	Normoblasts are immature red cells with nuclei	Normal in fetus or infant, but not in adults; extreme demand on bone marrow to produce cells rapidly	Erythroblastosis fetalis, thalassemia major
		Extramedullary erythropoiesis	Idiopathic myelofibrosis
		With neutrophilia, the bone marrow cells are altered	Leukemias, metastatic cancer of the bone marrow, multiple myeloma, Gaucher disease
Basophilic stippling	Basophilic granules in cells	Abnormal hemoglobin synthesis and increased erythropoiesis	Lead poisoning, megaloblastic anemia
Howell-Jolly bodies	Remnants of nuclear material in cells	Abnormal erythropoiesis	Postsplenectomy, megaloblastic anemia, hemolytic anemia
Heinz bodies	Irregular patches of hemoglobin in the cells	Genetic abnormality of hemoglobin formation; hemoglobin is oxidized and nonfunctional	Cell injury, hemoglobinopathy, hemolytic anemia

Procedure

A purple-topped tube with EDTA is used to collect 7 ml of venous blood. As an alternative, two purple-tipped capillary tubes can be used to collect blood from a heelstick, earlobe, or finger puncture.

For the peripheral blood smear, two slides are prepared immediately using drops of venous or capillary blood.

QUALITY CONTROL

With venipuncture, the tourniquet should be tied lightly for a brief time to prevent pooling of cells in the vein at the site of blood collection. A smooth venipuncture technique will allow the blood to flow into the vacuum tube readily. Flawed venipuncture technique will produce excessive turbulence, causing hemolysis of the erythrocytes and altering the test results. The tube is gently inverted 5 to 10 times after the blood is collected to mix the anticoagulant and prevent clotting.

Findings

See Table 4–2 for abnormal values.

Interfering Factors

- Hemolysis
- Coagulation
- Inadequate slide preparation technique

Nursing Implementation

During the Test

When collecting venous blood, the tube must be filled. This prevents degenerative changes in the cells because of too much EDTA.

When heelstick, finger, or earlobe puncture is used, do not use the first drop of blood or squeeze the tissue. This helps limit the presence of endothelial cells and damaged blood cells.

Posttest

Arrange for prompt transport of the specimen to the laboratory.

QUALITY CONTROL

Degenerative changes in neutrophils occurs within 30 minutes. Enlargement of platelets occurs after 3 hours. If there is a delay before the blood is analyzed, the specimen must be refrigerated.

PLATELET COUNT

(BLOOD)

Synonym:

thrombocyte count

NORMAL VALUES

Adult: 150,000–450,000 cells/µl *or* SI 150–450 × 10^9/L
Newborn: 84,000–478,000 cells/µl *or* SI 84–478 × 10^9/L

Background Information

Platelets are the product of erythropoiesis of the bone marrow. After activity by the pluripotential and hematopoietic stem cells in the marrow, the line develops further through megakaryocyte cell division and the formation of the promegakaryocyte cell. During the next 7 to 10 days, a megakaryocyte matures, and fragments of its cytoplasm break off and enter the circulation as platelets. About 2000 to 7000 platelets are formed from one megakaryocyte. Two thirds of the total platelets are present in the circulation, and the remainder are stored in the spleen. The life span of the platelet is 7 to 10 days, with ultimate splenic destruction of senescent or damaged cells (Hays, 1990).

Platelets function to initiate the process of coagulation. When there is a nick or opening in a blood vessel, platelets quickly aggregate, adhere to the endothelial surface of the blood vessel, and plug the opening. As additional platelets and clotting factors arrive, the clot becomes firm and seals off the opening effectively.

VARIATION IN NORMAL VALUES. In laboratory testing, there is a considerable variation in the normal platelet count reference range. Newborns have a wider range of normal values than do adults. The normal value is slightly decreased during menstruation and pregnancy. The platelet count is also reduced relative to the excess fluid in the blood. This dilutional effect occurs with the administration of nonplatelet fluids, including intravenous fluids and packed red cell transfusions. When the platelets are counted, there is a variation between the reference range performed by manual counting and that carried out by an automated counter. Analysis of the test results is based on the reference value provided by the laboratory that performs the cell count.

ELEVATED VALUES

An excess number of platelets is called *thrombocytosis.* A platelet count greater than 1 million cells/µl is considered the possible panic range because of the risk of hemorrhage or thrombosis. The potential for hemorrhage probably results from defects in the platelets and the inability to form a clot. Thrombosis in either veins or arteries can occur as platelets aggregate and trap erythrocytes in the microcirculation. Common sites of vascular occlusion include the splenic, hepatic, and pulmonary veins; the mesenteric and axillary arteries; and the fingers and toes.

DECREASED VALUES

Critical Thinking: Your patient's platelet count is 47,000 cells/µL (SI: 47 × 10⁹ cells/L). What nursing actions should be implemented immediately?

A decreased number of platelets is called *thrombocytopenia.* A platelet count less than 100,000 cells/µl (SI: $<100 \times 10^9$/L) causes a prolonged bleeding time. The decrease in the number of platelets may coexist with platelet dysfunction, causing an even longer time needed to form a clot (Burns, 1990). If the platelet count drops to less than 50,000 cells/µl (SI: $<50 \times 10^9$/L), the patient's clotting ability is seriously compromised. There is a high risk of the development of spontaneous hemorrhage, particularly in the brain (Schneiderman, 1990).

The decrease in platelets is caused by three possible categories of pathophysiologic change: (1) deficient platelet production, (2) rapid platelet destruction, and (3) abnormal pooling of the platelets (Table 4–3). The most common cause is the accelerated destruction of platelets. The bone marrow responds with

TABLE 4–3
PATHOPHYSIOLOGIC CAUSES OF THROMBOCYTOPENIA

Category	Pathophysiology	Cause
Deficient platelet production	Impairment of bone marrow with reduced numbers of stem cells or megakaryocytes	Drugs, aplastic anemia, radiation chemotherapy, malignancy of the bone marrow
	Ineffective thrombopoiesis	Deficiency of iron, vitamin B_{12}, folic acid
	Defective production or regulation of thrombopoietin	Inherited genetic disorder
Platelet destruction	*Intracorpuscular destruction* Defects in platelet structure with short platelet life span	Inherited genetic disorder
	Extracorpuscular destruction Immunologic destruction of platelets by IgG antibodies	Autoimmune processes Infection
	Excess clotting or mechanical damage to platelets	Disseminated intravascular coagulation Infection Cardiac valve replacement Microvascular clotting disorder
Abnormal distribution or pooling	Splenic disorder with hypersplenism	Malignancy, infection infiltrates, congestion

accelerated production of new cells, but when the platelet destruction is rapid and extensive, the response of the marrow is inadequate.

Purpose of the Test

The platelet count is used to assess the ability of the bone marrow to produce platelets and to identify the destruction or loss of platelets in the circulation. It is also used to evaluate the untoward effects of chemotherapy or radiation treatment.

Procedure

A purple-topped tube with EDTA is used to collect 7 ml of venous blood. As an alternative, two purple-tipped capillary tubes are used to collect blood from a heelstick, earlobe, or finger puncture.

QUALITY CONTROL

When venipuncture is performed, the tourniquet should be tied lightly for a brief time to prevent pooling of cells in the vein at the site of blood collection. Venipuncture technique must be smooth, with a blood flow that fills the vacuum tube readily. If excessive turbulence of the blood results from flawed venipuncture technique, the erythrocytes will undergo hemolysis, altering test results. After the blood is collected, the tube is gently inverted 5 to 10 times to mix the anticoagulant and prevent clotting.

Findings

ELEVATED VALUES

Myeloproliferative diseases
  Polycythemia vera
  Myelofibrosis
  Chronic myelocytic
    leukemia
  Thrombocythemia
Posthemorrhage regeneration
Iron deficiency anemia

Multiple myeloma
Postsplenectomy response
Acute or chronic infection
Inflammatory diseases
Hodgkin disease
Lymphoma
Chronic renal disease
Renal cysts

DECREASED VALUES

Idiopathic thrombocytopenic
  purpura
Systemic lupus erythematosus
Aplastic anemia
Megaloblastic anemia
Severe iron deficiency anemia

Liver disease
Uremia
Infection
Parasitic diseases (malaria,
  toxoplasmosis, histoplasmosis)
Massive blood transfusion

Malignancy of the spleen
Radiation-chemotherapy
Disseminated intravascular
    coagulation
Fanconi syndrome
Wiskott-Aldrich syndrome

Thyroid disease
Uremia
Eclampsia

Interfering Factors

- Platelet clumping
- Multiple transfusions

Nursing Implementation

Pretest

Instruct the patient to avoid strenuous exercise prior to the test because exertion and stress elevate the test results temporarily.

Posttest

Assess the puncture site for signs of bleeding or lack of clot formation.
Using sterile gauze, apply pressure to the site or raise the arm above the head while maintaining pressure on the site.
When the platelet count is decreased, institute measures to protect the patient from trauma, bruising, or cuts. Do not advocate the use of aspirin for any reason because this medication interferes with the platelets' ability to adhere in the clotting process.

RED BLOOD CELL COUNT

(BLOOD)

Synonyms:
RBC, red cell count, erythrocyte count

NORMAL VALUES

Male: 4.6–6.2×10^6 μl *or* SI 4.6–6.2×10^{12}/L
Female: 4.2–5.4×10^6/μl *or* SI 4.2–5.4×10^{12}/L

Background Information

Erythropoiesis, the formation of erythrocytes, occurs in the bone marrow. The red cell production begins with the division and maturation of the pluripotential and hematopoietic stem cells. In response to decreased oxygen tension and the stimulus of erythropoietin, the ongoing cell division, differentiation, and maturation proceed along the erythrocyte line until reticulocytes are produced. After remaining in the marrow for 1 to 2 days, the reticulocytes are released into the blood. The reticulocytes reach the final stage of maturity in 1 to 2 additional days in the blood. The erythrocytes function to transport oxygen from the lungs to the cells and to transport carbon dioxide from the cells to the lungs.

The maintenance of a normal number of erythrocytes in the blood is dependent on the ability of the bone marrow to continuously replace the erythrocytes that are lost or destroyed. Because of the fragility of the cell membrane, the life span of the RBC is approximately 120 days. The bone marrow must produce approximately 1 million new erythrocytes per second to maintain adequate replacement.

The stimulus for additional production of erythrocytes is cellular oxygen deficiency that triggers the flow of erythropoietin by the kidneys. Erythropoietin is a colony-stimulating factor that promotes erythropoiesis at various stages of differentiation in the bone marrow.

There are numerous factors that can create an imbalance between erythrocyte production and destruction. With excess production and a normal rate of destruction, the RBC count is elevated. With either diminished production or excess destruction of red cells in the blood, their number is decreased.

VARIATION IN NORMAL VALUES. The normal red cell count is higher in men than in women and it is higher in individuals who live at high altitudes. The normal value is lower in men older than 65 years old when compared with younger men. The red cell count is 5 to 6% lower when the blood is drawn from a recumbent patient than one in an upright position.

ELEVATED VALUES

Increases in the red cell count may be due to hyperactivity of the bone marrow cells or an increase in erythropoietin from renal disease. Relative polycythemia may also produce an increased red cell count. When this problem is caused by dehydration, there are a normal number of erythrocytes, but they are concentrated in the diminished fluid volume of the plasma.

DECREASED VALUES

Decreases in the red cell count can occur from an excessive loss of cells, as in hemorrhage. It can also occur because of rapid or accelerated hemolysis of the red cells. When the bone marrow tissue is damaged by excess radiation or chemotherapy, or when there is a lack of erythropoietin from renal disease, too few red cells are produced and the blood count is low.

Critical Thinking: The patient on hemodialysis asks why he always has a low number of red blood cells. How can you explain the physiologic basis for this anemia to a patient with a limited education?

Purpose of the Test

The red cell count is used to evaluate anemia and polycythemia.

Procedure

A purple-topped tube with EDTA is used to collect 7 ml of venous blood. As an alternative, two purple-tipped capillary tubes can be used to collect blood from a heelstick, earlobe, or finger puncture.

QUALITY CONTROL

With venipuncture, the tourniquet should be tied lightly for a brief time to prevent pooling of cells at the site of blood collection. A smooth venipuncture technique produces a blood flow that fills the vacuum tube readily. If the blood demonstrates excessive turbulence because of flawed venipuncture technique, the hemolysis of the erythrocytes will alter the test results. After the blood is collected, the tube is gently inverted 5 to 10 times to mix the anticoagulant and prevent clotting.

Findings

ELEVATED VALUES

Polycythemia vera
Secondary polycythemia
Hemoconcentration

Renal carcinoma
Cerebral hemangioblastoma
Renal cyst

DECREASED VALUES

Anemia
Aplastic anemia
Immune response with hemolysis

Recent hemorrhage or blood loss
Hemodilution or excess intravenous fluids
Bone marrow failure
Glucose-6-phosphate dehydrogenase deficiency

Interfering Factors

- Hemolysis
- Coagulation of the specimen
- Hemodilution
- Cold agglutinins

Nursing Implementation

Pretest

Plan to obtain the specimen when the patient is calm and rested. Exercise, exertion, and fear all increase the red cell count.

During the Test

Ensure that the arm or hand that has an intravenous line is not used to obtain the specimen. Intravenous fluid dilutes the blood and falsely decreases the cell count.

RED CELL INDICES

(BLOOD)

Synonyms:

erythrocyte indices, indices, blood indices

─────────────────────── **NORMAL VALUES** ───────────────────────

MCV:	80–96 µm^3 *or* SI 80–96 fL
MCH:	27–31 pg *or* SI 27–31 pg
MCHC:	32–36% *or* SI 0.32–0.36 (concentration fraction)
RDW-CV:	13.1% (range 11.6–14.6%) (Henry, 1990)

Background Information

The red cell indices are a measure of the quality and characteristics of the erythrocyte and hemoglobin concentration. The abnormalities of the erythrocyte are used in the classification and evaluation of the different anemias. The indices consist of the MCV, MCH, and MCHC.

The values may be arithmetically calculated by using the values of the red cell count, the hemoglobin concentration, and the hematocrit. Today, however, most laboratories use automated blood analyzers, and the indices are automatically included in the CBC. In the automated count, a fourth category—the RDW—is also included. The reference values vary somewhat, depending on the method of analysis and the equipment used. To avoid misinterpretation, the evaluation of the test results should be based on the reference values of the laboratory that performs the procedure.

MEAN CORPUSCULAR VOLUME. The MCV calculates the average erythrocyte size based on a formula that uses the values of the hematocrit and RBC count. The unit value may be expressed in femtoliters (fl) or cubic micrometers (µm^3). The measurements are equivalent (1 fl = 1 µm^3). If the MCV value is elevated, the erythrocytes are large or macrocytic. If the MCV value is decreased, the erythrocytes are small or microcytic.

MEAN CORPUSCULAR HEMOGLOBIN. The MCH calculates the weight of the hemoglobin in the average erythrocyte based on a formula that uses the values of hemoglobin and the RBC count. The hemoglobin weight is expressed in picograms (pg). One picogram is equivalent to 1 micromicrogram (µµg) (1 pg = 1 µµg). The MCH value is elevated when the erythrocyte is large or macrocytic. The average concentration or percentage of hemoglobin in the average erythrocyte is based on a formula that uses the values of hemoglobin and the hematocrit. When the MCHC value is elevated, there is a high concentration of hemoglobin in the erythrocyte, and the cell is described as hyperchromic. When the value is in a normal range, the RBC is described as normochromic. When the MCHC value is decreased, there is a lower concentration of hemoglobin, and the erythrocyte is described as hypochromic.

RED CELL DISTRIBUTION WIDTH. The RDW is a numeric calculation of the range of sizes or widths of the erythrocytes. It is proposed that the elevated value of the RDW indicates an early sign of microcytic anemia, but this single test measurement is not sufficient for diagnosis. Research efforts have attempted to use this value to differentiate among the different types of microcytic anemia, particularly the anemias of iron deficiency and thalassemia. Although the automated analyzer is accurate in the measurement, the RDW is not sensitive enough to distinguish among the microcytic anemias (Savage, 1993).

Purpose of the Test

The red cell indices are used to help diagnose and classify anemias by measurement of size, hemoglobin weight, and hemoglobin concentration of the average erythrocyte.

Procedure

A purple-topped tube with EDTA is used to collect 7 ml of venous blood. As an alternative, two purple-tipped capillary tubes can be used to collect blood from a heelstick, earlobe, or finger puncture.

QUALITY CONTROL

With venipuncture, the tourniquet should be tied lightly for a brief time to prevent pooling of cells at the site of blood collection. The tube must be nearly filled. Venipuncture technique must be smooth so that the blood flow fills the vacuum tube readily. If the blood is excessively turbulent because of flawed venipuncture technique, erythrocyte hemolysis will alter the test results. After the blood is collected, the tube is inverted gently 5 to 10 times to mix the anticoagulant and prevent clotting.

Findings

ELEVATED VALUES

MCV:	Pernicious anemia	Diabetic ketoacidosis
	Vitamin B_{12} or folate deficiency	Macrocytic anemia
MCH:	Hereditary spherocytosis	
MCHC:	Hereditary spherocytosis	
RDW:	Microcytic anemia	

DECREASED VALUES

MCV:	Iron deficiency anemia	Anemia of chronic disease
	Lead poisoning	Microcytic anemia
	Thalassemia minor	
MCH:	Iron deficiency anemia	
MCHC:	Iron deficiency anemia	
RDW:	None	

Interfering Factors

- Hemolysis
- Coagulation of the specimen
- Autoagglutination
- Time delay in analysis of the blood

Nursing Implementation

Pretest

Vitamins should be discontinued for 2 weeks before the test, if possible. Folic acid, pyridoxine, and vitamin B_{12} alter the test results.

Posttest

Arrange for prompt transport of the specimen to the laboratory.

QUALITY CONTROL

The blood must be analyzed promptly. It cannot be used if it stands at room temperature for more than 10 hours or, if it is refrigerated, for more than 18 hours. The specimen cannot be frozen.

RETICULOCYTE COUNT

(BLOOD)

Synonym:

retic count

NORMAL VALUES

Adults:
Percentage of Cells: 0.5–1.5% *or* SI 0.005–0.015 (number fraction)
Cell Count: 25,000–75,000/µl *or* SI 25–75 × 10^9/L
Newborn: 1.1–4.5% *or* SI 0.011–0.045 (number fraction)

Background Information

Critical Thinking: Your patient receives iron replacement to correct the problem of iron deficiency anemia. To evaluate the response to the therapy, what changes in the red cell indices should occur?

Reticulocytes are immature erythrocytes. They are derived from pronormoblasts and their precursors in the bone marrow. Once they are formed, they remain in the marrow for 1 to 2 days to gain additional maturity. As the reticulocytes enter the blood, they still contain a bit of RNA and less than the full complement of hemoglobin. In the next 1 to 2 days in circulation, the reticulocytes complete their maturation and synthesis of hemoglobin.

Generally, there are few reticulocytes in the circulation in proportion to the number of erythrocytes. The normal reticulocyte count is expressed as a percentage of the erythrocyte count. Infants have higher reticulocyte counts at birth, but the count steadily decreases thereafter. By the second week of life, the normal value for the infant is the same as that of the adult.

The measurement of reticulocytes can be performed by manual counting of the cells, microscopic examination of stained slides, automated differential counts, or flow cytometry. The flow cytometry method can estimate the amount of RNA in the reticulocyte and thereby distinguish between immature and older reticulocytes. The term "left shift" means that there are more immature cells that contain greater amounts of RNA released from the bone marrow. This is an indicator of bone marrow "stress" and an early response to anemia (Johnson, 1993).

ELEVATED VALUES

An increase in reticulocytes indicates the ability of the bone marrow to produce erythrocytes. The elevated value is considered a healthy response after there is a loss of erythrocytes from hemorrhage or hemolysis. It is also a healthy response to anemia or a reduced amount of hemoglobin in the RBCs. The reticulocyte count may also rise after treatment for anemia. When there is a high demand for erythrocytes, the marrow releases very immature reticulocytes into the blood rather than allow these blood cells to mature for the full time in the marrow.

DECREASED VALUES

Critical Thinking: The patient experienced a continued loss of small amounts of blood from chronic gastritis. Which parts of the CBC help measure the severity of the problem and the body's physiologic response to the blood loss?

The reduced number of reticulocytes indicates that there is diminished erythropoiesis by the bone marrow. The cause may be a lack of stimulation by erythropoietin, disease that affects the bone marrow cells, or a faulty maturation process in the bone marrow.

Purpose of the Test

The reticulocyte count is used to evaluate erythropoiesis, distinguish among different types of anemia, assess the severity of blood loss, and evaluate the bone marrow response to treatment of anemia.

Procedure

A purple-topped tube with EDTA or a green-topped tube with heparin is used to collect 7 ml of venous blood. As an alternative, two purple-tipped capillary tubes can be used to collect blood from a heelstick, earlobe, or finger puncture.

> **QUALITY CONTROL**
>
> With venipuncture, the tourniquet should be tied lightly for a brief time to prevent pooling of cells in the vein at the site of blood collection. Venipuncture technique must be smooth, with a blood flow that fills the vacuum tube readily. If there is excessive turbulence in the blood because of flawed venipuncture technique, the hemolysis of the erythrocytes will alter the test results. After the blood is collected, the tube is inverted 5 to 10 times to mix the anticoagulant and prevent clotting.

Findings

ELEVATED VALUES

Iron deficiency anemia treatment Hemorrhage
Pernicious anemia treatment Chronic blood loss
Hemolytic anemia

DECREASED VALUES

Aplastic anemia Red cell aplasia
Iron deficiency anemia Renal disease
Anemia of chronic disease Endocrine disease
Sideroblastic anemia Pernicious anemia

Interfering Factors

- Multiple blood transfusions
- Coagulation of the specimen
- Hemolysis

Nursing Implementation

Pretest

If possible, schedule this test before a blood transfusion is started. Once blood is administered, there is dilution of the cells, and the reticulocyte count is decreased in proportion to the fluid volume. If multiple transfusions were already given, the results of this test are invalid. The reticulocytes are from the transfused blood and do not indicate the current status of the patient's bone marrow function.

During the Test

Do not permit the blood sample to be taken from the arm in which there is intravenous tubing. The fluid administration dilutes the blood and causes a low cell count.

WHITE BLOOD CELL COUNT

(BLOOD)

Synonyms:

white blood count, WBC, leukocyte count, white count

─────────────── **NORMAL VALUES** ───────────────

Adult:	$4.5–11 \times 10^3/\mu l$ *or* SI $4.5–11 \times 10^9$/L
Newborn:	$9000–30{,}000/\mu l$ *or* SI $9–30 \times 10^9$/L

Background Information

Leukocytes maintain the general functions of combating infection and inflammation. There are five types of leukocytes classified into two major groups: granular and nongranular. The granular leukocytes, consisting of neutrophils, eosinophils, and basophils, are formed by their precursor cells in the bone marrow. The nongranular lymphocytes, including some lymphocytes and all monocytes, are also formed by their precursor cells in the bone marrow. Some of the lymphocytes are formed by the thymus gland and lymph glands (Fig. 4–1).

Many of the leukocytes are phagocytic in their action. They are capable of rapid mobility to an area of infection or tissue damage, where they ingest many types of foreign cells, dead cells, or microorganisms. Each leukocyte capable of phagocytosis can ingest only some of this matter before its own metabolism is interfered with and it self-destructs. Other leukocytes function in allergy, hypersensitivity, or antigen-antibody responses. Each type of cell functions in specific ways, including vasodilation or the release of toxins or secretions that assist in the protective responses against foreign matter within the body.

The normal life span of these cells varies according to the type of leukocyte and the condition of the body at the time. In normal health, the life span is a bit longer than when infection or inflammation is present. Most neutrophils have a life span of only days or hours in the presence of infection. Nongranular leukocytes appear to have a much longer life span. The bone marrow must continuously replace destroyed leukocytes to maintain the normal complement of each type of cell. In the presence of infection or inflammation, the bone marrow activity increases greatly, and many leukocytes are produced to counteract the invasion by foreign cells or substances.

WHITE BLOOD CELL COUNT. The leukocyte count is the total number of the five types of leukocytes present in 1 mm^3 of blood. The leukocyte count is a general indicator of infection, tissue necrosis, inflammation, or bone marrow activity. More specific diagnostic information is obtained by the differential count that identifies the numbers of each type of WBC.

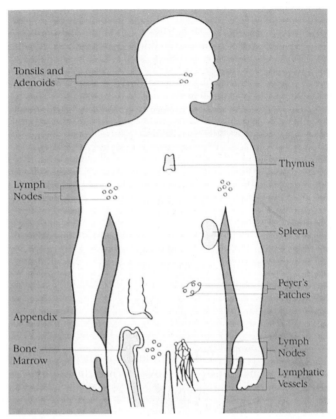

FIGURE 4–1. Organs of the immune system. The lymphocytes are produced in the bone marrow, thymus, and secondary lymphoid tissues. Some lymphocytes circulate in the blood, and others remain stored or are active in various parts of the immune system throughout the body. (With permission from Schindler, L.W. [1988]. *Understanding the immune system*, [NIH publication No. 88-529, p. 3]. Washington, D.C.: U.S. Department of Health and Human Services, Public Health Service, National Institutes of Health.)

VARIATION IN NORMAL VALUES. The leukocyte count can become falsely elevated with stress or exercise or after eating a heavy meal. The normal value is lower in children younger than age 15 years and also between the ages of 20 and 30 years. After age 30 years, men have a somewhat higher value than do women. The normal leukocyte count is lower in blacks than in whites.

ELEVATED VALUES

When the WBC count rises, it is called *leukocytosis*. This occurs in response to infection and is usually directly proportionate to the degree of bacterial invasion. The elevated value may also be caused by necrosis of tissue or malignancy of the bone marrow. A WBC count of 11,000 to 17,000 cells (11 to 17×10^3/μl *or* SI 11 to 17×10^9/L) is considered to be a mild to moderate leukocytosis. A WBC count of greater than 30,000 cells ($>30 \times 10^3/\mu l$ *or* SI $>30 \times 10^9/L$) is considered a possible panic value. *Hyperleukocytosis* is an extreme elevation of the WBC count and is a potential medical emergency. It is defined as a value greater than 100,000 cells ($>100 \times 10^3/\mu l$ *or* SI $100 \times 10^9/L$). This extreme elevation can cause a fatal hemorrhage in the lung or brain as the leukocytes clump or aggregate in the microvasculature. This high value is usually the result of acute myelogenous leukemia or chronic myelogenous leukemia in blast crisis (Cambell, 1991).

DECREASED VALUES

Critical Thinking: When the WBC count shows a result of 2.3×10^3 cells/μl (SI: 2.3×10^9 cells/L), how should the nursing plan be modified to protect the patient?

When the WBC count falls to less than normal limits, it is called *leukopenia*. Mild leukopenia is indicated by a WBC count of 3000 to 5000 cells (3 to 5 × $10^3/\mu l$ *or* SI 3 to 5 × $10^9/L$). Severe leukopenia and a possible panic value occurs with a WBC count less than 2500 cells ($<2.5 \times 10^3/\mu l$ *or* SI $<2.5 \times 10^9/L$). The marked decrease is usually in neutrophils, although all five forms of leukocytes may be decreased. With such a decreased value, the patient is at risk because there is little defense against infection. Decreases in the leukocyte count are usually due to bone marrow depression or particular infection that has exhausted the supply of neutrophils and bone marrow reserves.

Purpose of the Test

The WBC count indicates the possible presence and severity of infection or inflammatory response. When the results are abnormal, it may indicate the need for additional tests such as a WBC differential or a bone marrow biopsy. The WBC count is used to monitor the bone marrow's response to chemotherapy, radiation treatment, toxic exposure to heavy metals, chemical poisons, or the untoward effects of some medications.

Procedure

A purple-topped tube with EDTA is used to collect 7 ml of venous blood. As an alternative, two purple-tipped capillary tubes can be used to collect blood from a heelstick, earlobe, or finger puncture.

QUALITY CONTROL

With venipuncture, the tourniquet should be tied lightly for a brief time to prevent pooling of cells at the site of blood collection. Venipuncture technique must be smooth, with a blood flow that fills the vacuum tube readily. If there is excessive turbulence in the blood because of flawed venipuncture technique, the hemolysis of the erythrocytes will alter the test results. After the blood is collected, the tube is inverted gently 5 to 10 times to mix the anticoagulant and prevent clotting.

Findings

ELEVATED VALUES

Bacterial infection
Tissue necrosis (burns, gangrene,
　myocardial infarction)
Lymphoma
Leukemia

Chronic infection
Varicella
Mumps
Rubeola
Cancer (liver, intestine)
Leukemoid reaction

DECREASED VALUES

Brucellosis
Typhoid fever
Viral infections (influenza,
　rubella, hepatitis)
Typhus
Dengue
Malaria
Systemic lupus erythematosus

Pernicious anemia
Aplastic anemia
Radiation
Antineoplastic drugs
Toxic ingestion of heavy
　metals or chemical
　poisons
Gaucher disease
Felty syndrome

Interfering Factors

• Hemolysis
• Coagulation of the specimen
• Strenuous exercise
• Digestion of a heavy meal

Nursing Implementation

Pretest

Plan to obtain the specimen when the patient is calm and physically quiet.
When the test is planned in advance, instruct the patient to avoid strenuous
　exercise for 24 hours before the test.
Comfort the crying infant or child.

QUALITY CONTROL

With stress or distress, the adrenaline causes a rise in the WBC
count within 30 minutes.

Instruct the patient to avoid a heavy meal before the test because the
　digestion process causes a temporary rise in the WBC count.

Posttest

In evaluating the WBC count of a newborn, plan for repeat testing several times. The same vascular source (vein, capillary) should be used. This repetition helps provide accurate data and limits variations due to extraneous sources.

With a severe decrease in the WBC value, initiate measures to protect the patient from exposure to infection.

WHITE BLOOD CELL DIFFERENTIAL

(BLOOD)

Synonyms:

differential leukocyte count, peripheral differential, white blood cell morphology, WBC differential

—————————————— **NORMAL VALUES** ——————————————

NEUTROPHILS
Segmented Neutrophils
Mean percent: 56% *or* SI 0.56 (mean number fraction)
Cell count (range): 1800–7800/µl *or* SI 1.8–7.8 × 10^9/L
Bands
Mean percent: 3% *or* SI 0.03 (mean number fraction)
Cell count (range): 0–700/µl *or* SI 0–0.07 × 10^9/L
Eosinophils
Mean percent: 2.7% *or* SI 0.027 (mean number fraction)
Cell count (range): 0–450/µl *or* SI 0–0.45 × 10^9/L
Basophils
Mean percent: 0.3% *or* SI 0.003 (mean number fraction)
Cell count (range): 0–200/µl *or* SI 0–0.2 × 10^9/L
Lymphocytes
Mean percent: 34% *or* SI 0.34 (mean number fraction)
Cell count (range): 1000–4800/µl *or* SI 1–4.8 × 10^9/L
Monocytes
Mean percent: 4% *or* SI 0.04 (mean number fraction)
Cell count (range): 0–800/µl *or* SI 0–0.8 × 10^9/L

Background Information

The differential count identifies the five different types of leukocytes by microscopic visualization of the peripheral blood smear or by use of an automated analyzer that differentiates and counts the cells. The results indicate the percentage of each type of cell, and the cell counts indicate the number of each type of cell per measured volume of blood.

The leukocytes originate in the bone marrow, beginning with the division of the pluripotential stem cell. The subdivisions are the hematopoietic stem cell, the colony-forming units-granulocyte, erythrocyte, macrophage, and megakaryocyte, and the lymphoid stem cell colony-forming unit-lymphocyte.

Through increasing formation, maturation, and differentiation along specific cell lines, the hematopoietic stem cell ultimately produces monocytes and macrophages, neutrophils, eosinophils, and basophils. The lymphoid stem cell produces B cells from the bone marrow and T cells from the thymus and other lymphoid tissues.

NEUTROPHILS. These are the most active cells responding to tissue damage or infection. They are phagocytes that provide an early, rapid removal of cellular debris and a large number of bacteria. Of all the leukocytes, the neutrophils are the largest group. In normal health, only a small number circulate in the blood, with an additional supply in pools that are attached to the vascular endothelium. The largest supply is stored in the bone marrow and is released on demand. The circulating neutrophils have a life span of only 3 to 6 hours.

With increased demand, the first phase of response is the release of the pools of neutrophils attached to the vascular endothelium. This is a rapid but brief response that occurs in minutes to hours. When the demand continues, the bone marrow releases greater numbers of neutrophils 4 to 24 hours following stimulation. If demand persists, the bone marrow responds with sustained neutrophil production and release of cells (Peterson and Hrisinko, 1993).

ELEVATED VALUES

Neutrophilia occurs in response to bacterial infection, particularly that caused by staphylococci or streptococci. It also arises in response to inflammatory disease or conditions that cause tissue necrosis. Severe neutrophilia, particularly with a shift toward releasing immature neutrophils or even precursor marrow cells, may be caused by malignancy of the bone marrow, especially chronic myeloid leukemia.

DECREASED VALUES

Neutropenia may be caused by the depletion of the available pool of neutrophils during severe infection, damage to the circulating neutrophils, or damage to the bone marrow cells. Other conditions destroy not only neutrophils but also other types of blood cells and their precursor cells in the bone marrow. As a result, cytopenia or pancytopenia develops (Foucar et al., 1993).

BANDS. Band neutrophils are the more immature form of a segmented neutrophil. An increase in bands is equivalent to a "left shift," meaning that the marrow is releasing immature cells instead of neutrophils. It is believed that bandemia is an early indicator of sepsis. Although the bands are counted by an automated analyzer, the clinical usefulness of this part of the differential count is still in a research stage. The identification of the band cell is not adequately defined with a clear distinction among the more immature precursor, the metamyelocyte, the band neutrophil, and the more mature segmented neutrophil. Additionally, the reference ranges require further study (Novak, 1993).

EOSINOPHILS. These are granulocytes that contain toxic substances used to kill foreign cells in the blood. They also participate in the inflammatory response by phagocytosis. They digest the antigen-antibody complexes and clean up the late stages of inflammation.

ELEVATED VALUES

Eosinophilia occurs in response to allergic disorders, inflammation of the skin, parasitic infection in the tissues, some other infections and inflammations, metastatic malignancy, tissue necrosis, and in some hematologic disorders that cause a change in the bone marrow.

DECREASED VALUES

Eosinopenia occurs with most infections that produce purulence.

BASOPHILS. These are granulocytes involved in modifying or calming systemic allergic reactions and anaphylaxis. Mast cells are sometimes called tissue basophils. Mast cells and basophils are produced by the same precursor cells. The basophils release histamine, heparin, and serotonin into the circulation during an episode of inflammation.

ELEVATED VALUES

Basophilia occurs during the healing phase of inflammation and in chronic inflammation. It occurs in the presence of hypersensitivity reactions to foods, pollens, and injected protein substances. It also occurs after radiation therapy and in myeloproliferative disorders, including myeloid leukemia.

DECREASED VALUES

Basopenia occurs during acute infection, hyperthyroidism, and stress.

LYMPHOCYTES. These are nongranulocytes produced in the bone marrow, thymus, and lymphoid organs. The two classes of lymphocytes are the B cells and the T cells. There are about 1 trillion lymphocytes in the body, and they are responsible for the activities of the immune system. All lymphocytes recognize foreign antigens in the circulation. Some of these antigens are attacked and destroyed by the lymphocytes in the blood. Other antigens are carried to the lymph glands via the lymphatic fluid. In the lymph nodes, the antigens become enmeshed with the immune cells, and the antigens are destroyed.

B cells are genetically programmed to make antibodies. Each cell is individualized for the manufacture of a specific antibody against a specific antigen. For example, one B cell makes antibodies against a respiratory bacillus and another makes antibodies against an influenza virus. When the B cell encounters a specific antigen, it engulfs the antigen. With the help of a T cell and interleukins, the B cell complex gives rise to plasma cells that manufacture and release many antigen-specific antibodies (Fig. 4–2). The circulating antibodies are called immunoglobulins. Antibodies act in different ways to destroy antigens. Some release toxins on the antigens or coat them so that scavenger cells will engulf and destroy them. Other antibodies initiate the complement cascade to kill the antigen.

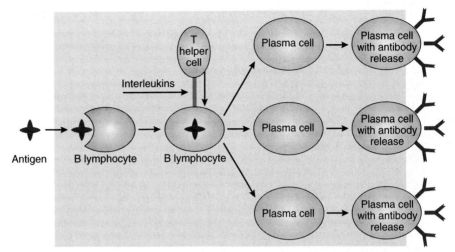

FIGURE 4–2. The process of antibody formation. The activation of B lymphocytes and T-helper cells produces plasma cells and antigen-specific antibodies.

T cells of different kinds act to regulate the immune response. Helper-inducer T cells activate the B cells and assist in the production of antibodies. Cytotoxic T cells are killer cells that destroy cells infected by virus, malignant cells, and foreign tissue cells, such as those of an organ graft. Suppressor T cells act to discontinue or reduce the manufacture of antibodies and suppress the immune response. In human immunodeficiency virus infection, helper T cells are destroyed by the virus. This activator of the immune response system is lost and only suppressor T cells remain. The regulatory balance is gone, and the immune system remains suppressed.

ELEVATED VALUES

Lymphocytosis occurs in response to bacterial, viral, and other causes of infection. It also occurs in some hematologic disorders, including lymphocytic leukemia.

DECREASED VALUES

Lymphopenia occurs with impaired lymphatic drainage, some advanced cancers, bone marrow failure, and immunologic deficiency that decreases the T lymphocytes.

MONOCYTES. These are nongranulocytes that are released from the bone marrow while still in an immature form. Once in the circulation, the monocytes become macrophages capable of phagocytosis. Monocytes are long-lived cells unless they are destroyed by phagocytosis. In the tissues, the monocytes are the cells of the reticuloendothelial system. In the blood, they remove debris or foreign particles from the circulation. In phagocytosis, they perform the same work as neutrophils, but their numbers are greater and they are capable of more work. They also participate in the immune response.

ELEVATED VALUES

Monocytosis occurs in response to infection of all kinds as well as in granulomatosis, collagen disease, and some hematologic disorders.

DECREASED VALUES

Monopenia occurs because of bone marrow injury or failure and in some forms of leukemia.

Purpose of the Test

The WBC differential assesses the ability of the body to respond to and eliminate infection. It also detects the severity of infection, allergic reactions, and parasitic infection and identifies various stages of leukemia.

Procedure

A purple-topped tube with EDTA is used to collect 7 ml of venous blood. As an alternative, two purple-tipped capillary tubes can be used to collect blood from a heelstick, earlobe, or finger puncture.

For the peripheral blood smear, two slides with coverslips are prepared immediately using drops of venous or capillary blood.

QUALITY CONTROL
With venipuncture, the tourniquet should be tied lightly for a brief time to prevent pooling of cells in the vein at the site of blood collection. Venipuncture technique must be smooth, with a blood flow that fills the vacuum tube readily. If the blood has excessive turbulence because of flawed venipuncture technique, the hemolysis of the erythrocytes will alter the test results. After the blood is collected, the tube is inverted gently 5 to 10 times to mix the anticoagulant and prevent clotting.

Findings

Critical Thinking: The differential count shows an elevation of several types of leukocytes, and the physician informs the patient of the need for a bone marrow examination. Later, you notice that the patient appears quiet and tense. How can you help the patient cope?

ELEVATED VALUES

Neutrophils	Eosinophils
Chronic myelogenous leukemia	Skin diseases (pemphigus, eczema, exfoliative dermatitis)
Bacterial infection	
Rheumatic fever	
Severe burns	Trichinosis, *Echinococcus* disease
Ketoacidosis	
Carcinoma or sarcoma	Scarlet fever
Myeloproliferative diseases	Chronic myelogenous leukemia
Down syndrome	Myeloproliferative diseases
	Hodgkin disease

Malignancy
Rheumatoid arthritis
Sarcoidosis
Allergic reaction to drugs
Allergies (hay fever, hives, asthma)

Basophils

Hypersensitivity reactions
Ulcerative colitis
Chronic hemolytic anemia
Hodgkin disease
Myxedema
Chronic myelogenous leukemia
Polycythemia vera

Lymphocytes

Infectious mononucleosis
Infectious hepatitis
Cytomegalovirus infection
Pertussis
Brucellosis
Tuberculosis
Syphilis
Lymphocytic leukemia
Lymphosarcoma cell leukemia

Monocytes

Acute infection (bacterial, viral,
   mycotic, rickettsial, protozoan)
Tuberculosis
Syphilis
Brucellosis
Sarcoidosis
Ulcerative colitis
Chronic myeloid leukemia
Myeloproliferative diseases
Multiple myeloma
Hodgkin disease
Non-Hodgkin lymphomas
Acute monocytic leukemia
Myelomonocytic leukemia
Lupus erythematosus
Polyarteritis nodosa
Rheumatoid arthritis

DECREASED VALUES

Neutrophils

Infection
Drug reaction
Autoimmune neutropenia
Maternal antibody production
Aplastic anemia
Radiation or chemotherapy
Megaloblastic anemia
Hypersplenism
Cancer of the bone marrow

Eosinophils

Allergies
Pyogenic infection
Shock
Postsurgical response

Basophils

Hyperthyroidism
Pregnancy
Stress
Cushing syndrome

Lymphocytes

Thoracic duct drainage
Severe right-sided heart failure
Hodgkin disease
Systemic lupus erythematosus
Aplastic anemia
Human immunodeficiency virus infection
Miliary tuberculosis
Renal failure
Terminal cancer

Monocytes

Hairy cell leukemia
Bone marrow failure
Aplastic anemia

Interfering Factors

- Temperature changes
- Exercise
- Pregnancy
- Pain
- Mental or physical stress
- Heightened emotion

Nursing Implementation

Pretest

Since the differential count rises falsely in conditions of mental and physical stress, prepare the patient as follows:

Instruct the physically active patient to avoid strenuous activity for 24 hours before the test. The false rise is due to the release of pooled neutrophils attached to vascular walls and an increase in circulating lymphocytes.

Calm the crying infant and relieve the pain or distress experienced by the patient.

To avoid an increase in apprehension, reassure the patient about the simplicity of the procedure.

Posttest

Arrange for prompt transport of the blood to the laboratory.

QUALITY CONTROL

If the blood remains standing in the tube, deterioration of the cells begins within 30 minutes. Different cells are affected at different rates, but the deterioration affects the nuclei and cytoplasm of the leukocytes.

REFERENCES

Alkire, K., & Collingwood, J. (1990). Physiology of the blood and bone marrow. *Seminars in Oncology Nursing, 6,* 99–108.

Brown, S. (1990). Behind the numbers on the CBC...complete blood count. *RN, 53,* 46–48, 50–51.

Burns, E.R. (1990). When to suspect a bleeding disorder. *Emergency Medicine, 22,* 67–73.

Cambell, T.M. (1991). Hyperleukocytosis in leukemia. *Dimensions in Oncology Nursing, V,* 11–14.

Foucar, K., Duncan, M.H., & Smith, K.J. (1993). Practical approach to the investigation of neutropenia. *Clinics in Laboratory Medicine, 13,* 879–893.

Hays, K. (1990). Physiology of normal bone marrow. *Seminars in Oncology Nursing, 6,* 3–8.

Henry, J.B. (Ed.). (1990). *Clinical diagnosis and management by laboratory methods* (18th ed.). Philadelphia: W.B. Saunders.

Jacobs, D.S., et al. (Eds.). (1988). *Laboratory test handbook* (2nd ed.). Baltimore: Williams & Wilkins.

Johnson, R.L. (1993). Flow cytometry from research to clinical laboratory practice. *Clinics in Laboratory Medicine, 13,* 831–852.

Koepke, J.A. (1993). Fitting the cell counter to the bed count. *Clinics in Laboratory Medicine, 13,* 817–829.

Koepke, J.A. (1992). Reference values for reticulocyte. *Medical Laboratory Observer, 24,* 16.

Novak, R.W. (1993). The beleaguered band count. *Clinics in Laboratory Medicine, 13,* 895–903.

Peterson, L.A., & Hrisinko, M.A. (1993). Benign lymphocytosis and reactive neutrophilia. *Clinics in Laboratory Medicine, 13,* 863–877.

Savage, R.A. (1993). The red cell indices. *Clinics in Laboratory Medicine, 13,* 773–785.

Schneiderman, E. (1990). Thrombocytopenia in the critically ill patient. *Critical Care Nursing Quarterly, 13,* 1–6.

Teitz, N.W. (Ed.). (1990). *Clinical guide to laboratory tests* (2nd ed.). Philadelphia: W.B. Saunders.

Threatte, G.A. (1993). Usefulness of the mean platelet volume. *Clinics in Laboratory Medicine, 13,* 937–950.

Ward, K.M., Lehman, C.A., & Leiken, A.M. (1994). *Clinical laboratory instrumentation and automation. Principles, application and selection.* Philadelphia: W.B. Saunders.

CHAPTER 5

Blood Chemistry Screen

The sequential multiple analyzer computer (SMA or SMAC) is a laboratory instrument that uses a single blood, serum, or plasma specimen to provide rapid automated analysis of multiple clinical chemistry tests. SMA 6/60 means that the SMA is used to analyze the blood for six chemistry tests in 60 minutes. When requested, the blood chemistry panel can include 7, 12, or 20 chemistry tests in 60 minutes.

With current technologic advances, the newest equipment can analyze whole blood instead of plasma or serum. The process is more automated, producing faster results. With changes in the software and disposable parts of the equipment, the menu of tests can be expanded (Schembri et al., 1992).

For any of the SMA chemistry panels, a single 10-ml sample of venous blood is collected in a red-topped tube.

This chapter includes the six tests of the basic chemistry panel. The testing may be performed as a multiple chemistry screen or as individual tests. The basic chemistry screen is used to evaluate electrolyte balance, acid-base balance, osmolarity, and renal function. Additional blood chemistry tests are presented in the appropriate chapters of Part IV of this text.

LABORATORY TESTS

CARBON DIOXIDE, TOTAL

(SERUM)

Synonyms:

carbon dioxide content, T_{CO_2}

--- NORMAL VALUES ---

Adult (Venous): 22–26 mEq/L *or* SI 22–26 mmol/L
Adult (Arterial): 19–24 mEq/L *or* SI 19–24 mmol/L
Infant (Capillary): 20–28 mEq/L *or* SI 20–28 mmol/L

Background Information

Total carbon dioxide measures the combined forms of carbon dioxide transported in the blood. Some of the total carbon dioxide is dissolved in plasma and some is combined with amino groups on hemoglobin molecules. The largest component is bicarbonate ion, composing 90% of the total carbon dioxide content in the blood. The total carbon dioxide content provides the principal extracellular buffer system, which is called the bicarbonate–carbonic acid buffer. Buffer systems are needed in the regulation of acid-base balance. The concentration of carbon dioxide is controlled by the lungs, and the concentration of bicarbonate is controlled by the kidneys.

HYPOCAPNIA. This is a low serum level of carbon dioxide. The possible panic value of total carbon dioxide is a serum level less than 15 mEq/L (SI: <15 mmol/L). Hypocapnia is caused by excess elimination of carbon dioxide, excess elimination of bicarbonate, excess accumulation of hydrogen ions in the blood, or a combination of these conditions.

HYPERCAPNIA. This is an elevated serum level of carbon dioxide. The possible panic value of total carbon dioxide is a serum level greater than 50 mEq/L (SI: >50 mmol/L). Hypercapnia often is caused by poor carbon dioxide excretion by the lungs or an inadequate respiratory drive.

To fully evaluate acid-base disturbance, a total carbon dioxide determination is usually performed with pH and P_{CO_2} monitoring. (These additional tests and the discussion of acid-base balance are presented in Chapter 13.)

Critical Thinking: When the adult patient with emphysema has a venous carbon dioxide value of 46 mEq/L (SI: 46 mmol/L), which nursing measures can help improve the ventilatory ability?

Purpose of the Test

The total carbon dioxide determination is used to help evaluate acid-base balance and the bicarbonate buffer system.

Procedure

For venous blood testing, a red-capped tube is used to collect 10 ml of venous blood.

For arterial blood testing, a green-topped tube with heparin is used to obtain 5 ml of arterial blood.

For capillary blood testing, a puncture of the heel, earlobe, or finger and a capillary tube are used to collect capillary blood.

QUALITY CONTROL
The rubber stopper must remain firmly in place so that the carbon dioxide cannot diffuse out and result in a falsely lowered value.

Findings

ELEVATED VALUES

Respiratory acidosis
Emphysema
Pneumonia
Cystic fibrosis
Congestive heart failure
Pulmonary edema

Metabolic alkalosis
Hypokalemia
Excessive intake of antacids
Severe, prolonged vomiting
Cushing syndrome
Primary aldosteronism

DECREASED VALUES

Respiratory alkalosis
Hyperventilation
Metabolic acidosis
Diabetes mellitus

Renal tubular acidosis
Renal failure
Dehydration
Hypovolemia
Severe diarrhea

Interfering Factors

• None

Nursing Implementation

No specific patient instruction or intervention is needed.

CHLORIDE, SERUM

(SERUM)

Synonym:
Cl⁻

Background Information

Sodium (Na⁺), potassium (K⁺), bicarbonate (HCO_3^-), and chloride (Cl⁻) are electrolytes with positive or negative charges. The positively charged electrolytes

━━━━━━━━━━━━━ **NORMAL VALUES** ━━━━━━━━━━━━━

Adult and Child: 98–107 mEq/L *or* SI 98–107 mmol/L
Newborn: 98–113 mEq/L *or* SI 98–113 mmol/L
Premature: 95–110 mEq/L *or* SI 95–110 mmol/L

or ions are called cations and the negatively charged electrolytes are called anions. In combination, the electrolytes determine the osmolarity, pH, and hydration status in intracellular and extracellular fluids. Chloride is a major extracellular anion.

Chloride generally increases or decreases in direct relationship to sodium. This means that as the concentration of sodium rises, chloride also rises, and as the concentration of sodium falls, chloride also falls. The concentration of chloride increases or decreases inversely with bicarbonate. This means that as the concentration of chloride increases, the bicarbonate level decreases, and as the concentration of chloride decreases, bicarbonate increases.

Chloride is ingested in food, and most of it is absorbed by the gastro-intestinal tract. The glomeruli of the kidneys filter chloride out of the extra-cellular fluids, and the renal tubules resorb the amount of chloride needed to maintain homeostasis. The excess of this anion is excreted in urine. The normal serum level remains in a steady range, with a slight drop after meals. The postprandial decrease occurs as hydrochloric acid (HCl) is produced for digestion.

HYPERCHLOREMIA. This is an elevated level of chloride in the blood and extracellular fluid. The possible panic level is greater than 115 mEq/L (SI: >115 mmol/L). Hyperchloremia occurs during metabolic acidosis, with the rise in chloride caused by the excessive loss of bicarbonate. Loss of bicarbonate occurs in loss of fluid and electrolytes from the small or large intestine, renal tubular acidosis, and mineralocorticoid deficiency. The chloride concentration may also rise with dehydration.

HYPOCHLOREMIA. This is a decreased level of chloride in the blood and extracellular fluid. The possible panic value is less than 80 mEq/L (SI: <80 mmol/L). Hypochloremia is a loss of chloride from the body. It occurs during a loss of hydrochloric acid from the upper gastrointestinal tract as well as from mineralocorticoid excess, salt-losing renal disease, or diabetic acidosis. The low level of chloride may also occur in conditions that cause a rise in bicar-bonate or a decreased sodium concentration. Hypochloremia may occur with overhydration.

Critical Thinking: How does the nurse act as an advocate when the dying patient refuses hydration to correct electrolyte imbalance? Does the age of the patient make a difference in the nurse's response?

Purpose of the Test

Serum chloride measurements are obtained in the evaluation of electrolyte levels, water balance, and acid-base balance and in the measurement of the cation-anion balance (anion gap).

Procedure

A red-topped tube is used to collect 7 ml of venous blood. In infants, a heelstick, finger, or earlobe puncture and a capillary tube may be used to collect capillary blood.

QUALITY CONTROL
Venipuncture technique must be smooth, with a blood flow that fills the vacuum tube readily. If there is excessive turbulence because of poor technique, the hemolysis of the erythrocytes will alter the test results.

Findings

ELEVATED VALUES

Dehydration
Renal tubular acidosis
Prolonged diarrhea
Acute renal failure

Diabetes insipidus
Respiratory alkalosis
Hyperparathyroidism
Adrenocortical hyperfunction

DECREASED VALUES

Prolonged vomiting
Nasogastric drainage
Salt-losing nephritis
Chronic renal failure
Metabolic alkalosis
Chronic respiratory acidosis

Addison disease
Congestive heart failure
Intestinal fistula
Overhydration
Syndrome of inappropriate
    antidiuretic hormone
Diuretic therapy

Interfering Factors

• Hemolysis
• Warming of the specimen

Nursing Implementation

Pretest

For a routine test, instruct the patient to discontinue all food and fluids for 8 hours before the test. This prevents the normal drop in value after eating. For tests performed on an urgent or emergency basis, the fasting status is omitted.

Posttest

Arrange for prompt transport of the blood to the laboratory. The serum or plasma will require refrigeration until the analysis can be performed.

CREATININE

(SERUM)

Synonyms:

plasma creatinine, Pcr

NORMAL VALUES

Adult Male:	0.7–1.3 mg/dl *or* SI 62–115 μmol/L
Adult Female:	0.6–1.1 mg/dl *or* SI 53–97 μmol/L
Adolescent:	0.5–1 mg/dl *or* SI 44–88 μmol/L
Child:	0.3–0.7 mg/dl *or* SI 27–62 μmol/L
Infant:	0.2–0.4 mg/dl *or* SI 18–35 μmol/L
Newborn:	0.3–1 mg/dl *or* SI 27–88 μmol/L

Background Information

Creatinine is an amino acid and waste product derived from creatine, which is an intermediate product of protein metabolism. Creatine is synthesized in the liver, kidneys, and pancreas and is stored in muscle tissue. As creatine is metabolized in muscle tissue, creatinine is the end product. Creatinine is released into extracellular fluids, including the blood, and is excreted in urine.

In the kidneys, creatinine is filtered out of the blood by glomeruli and is usually not resorbed. Additional creatinine is secreted by the renal tubules, and the waste product becomes a component of urine. When the kidneys are functional, they maintain the serum creatinine level at a minimally low value. When renal function is impaired, the serum creatinine level rises.

In the early phase of renal disease, the kidneys are able to compensate and maintain the normally low serum level of creatinine. When the glomerular filtration rate decreases, the renal tubules compensate by secreting greater amounts of creatinine. Additionally, excess serum creatinine can be eliminated by nonrenal mechanisms when the kidneys are not functioning well. It is suspected that the intestines also compensate and remove some excess creatinine from the extracellular fluids. Because of these compensatory abilities, the serum creatinine level is not a sensitive indicator of early renal disease.

When glomerular filtration decreases to half of its normal rate, and only about half the nephrons are functioning, the serum creatinine level rises to about double the normal value. As renal failure progressively worsens, the serum creatinine level continues to rise in proportion to the severity of the disease (Duarte and Preuss, 1993).

Critical Thinking: Why is serum creatinine more specific than urea nitrogen in the diagnosis of renal failure?

The serum creatinine level also rises in prerenal failure, as the blood flow to the kidneys is diminished. The serum levels are decreased in conditions that result in decreased muscle mass, in muscle wasting diseases, or in liver disease. In these disorders, there is less creatine synthesis and storage and less creatinine production.

Purpose of the Test

A serum creatinine determination is the most common laboratory test used to evaluate renal function and to estimate the effectiveness of glomerular filtration.

Procedure

A red-topped tube is used to collect 7 to 10 ml of venous blood. For infants and small children, a heelstick, earlobe, or finger prick is used to fill a capillary pipette.

QUALITY CONTROL
Venipuncture technique must be smooth, with a blood flow that fills the vacuum tube readily. If the blood has excessive turbulence because of flawed technique, the hemolysis of the erythrocytes will alter the results.

Findings

ELEVATED VALUES

Acute or chronic renal failure
Renal artery stenosis
Shock
Urinary tract obstruction
Rhabdomyolysis

Uremia or azotemia
Congestive heart failure
Dehydration
Acromegaly or gigantism

DECREASED VALUES

Advanced liver disease
Hyperthyroidism
Muscular dystrophy
Dermatomyositis

Long-term corticosteroid
  therapy
Paralysis
Polymyositis

Interfering Factors

- Hemolysis
- Warming of the specimen

Nursing Implementation

Pretest

Instruct the patient to fast from food and fluids for 8 hours before the test when indicated by the laboratory protocol. In some methods of analysis, lipemia causes a false elevation. Recent meat ingestion can also cause a false elevation.

Posttest

Arrange for prompt transport of the specimen to the laboratory.

QUALITY CONTROL

In the laboratory, the serum must be separated from the cells promptly to avoid the formation of ammonia. The serum must be refrigerated until it is analyzed. Warming to greater than 30° C causes the creatinine level to falsely become elevated.

POTASSIUM

(SERUM)

Synonym:

K⁺

NORMAL VALUES	
Adult:	3.5–5.1 mEq/L *or* SI 3.5–5.1 mmol/L
Child:	3.4–4.7 mEq/L *or* SI 3.4–4.7 mmol/L
Infant:	4.1–5.3 mEq/L *or* SI 4.1–5.3 mmol/L
Newborn:	3.7–5.9 mEq/L *or* SI 3.7–5.9 mmol/L
Premature (48 hours):	3.0–6.0 mEq/L *or* SI 3.0–6.0 mmol/L

Background Information

Potassium is an electrolyte that is present in all body fluids. Most of the potassium is concentrated in the intracellular fluids, with a small portion concentrated in the extracellular fluids, including the blood. The intracellular amount of potassium is usually 30 to 40 times greater than the amount of potassium present in the extracellular fluid (Latta et al., 1993).

The renewable source of potassium comes from the daily food intake. About 90% of the potassium intake is absorbed by the intestinal tract, and the unabsorbed portion is excreted in the feces. Once the absorbed portion enters the blood and extracellular fluids, it is distributed throughout the body, primarily within the cells (Fig. 5–1).

The regulation of the extracellular potassium concentration is performed by the kidney, with excretion of excess potassium in the urine (Latta et al., 1993). In normal physiology, the extracellular potassium remains in a relatively narrow range. There is, however, a variation of the normal range in individuals of different geographic regions, probably based on environmental rather than genetic factors (Reidenberg et al., 1993).

There is considerable danger associated with either a depletion or an excess of potassium. The abnormal potassium concentration causes disturbances in the membrane potential and altered function of neuromuscular tissue, including the

Critical Thinking: What ECG manifestations indicate the need for serum potassium levels?

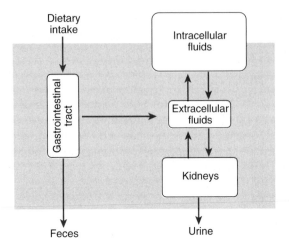

FIGURE 5–1. Homeostatic balance of potassium. Through the functions of resorption and excretion, the kidneys are the best regulator of potassium balance in the extracellular fluids.

loss of cardiac contractility. With depletion or excess of this cation, the patient is at risk for the development of shock, respiratory failure, or cardiac arrhythmias, including ventricular fibrillation.

HYPOKALEMIA. This is a decreased amount of potassium in the extracellular fluid. A possible panic value is less than 2.5 mEq/L (SI: <2.5 mmol/L) for all age groups. Hypokalemia can occur with fluid losses from the gastrointestinal tract, skin, or kidneys.

The injury to the gastrointestinal tissue can cause large losses of extracellular fluid, and it can also prevent the absorption of potassium from dietary intake. Potassium can be lost in sweat from the skin or from the secretion of extracellular fluid in areas denuded of skin. When the kidneys excrete high volumes of fluid, the potassium is washed out without opportunity for the renal tubules to resorb the needed electrolyte. Diuretic therapy is the most common cause of urinary potassium loss. Potassium can also be lost in conditions that cause renal tubular acidosis and excessive mineralocorticoid hormone levels.

Hypokalemia can also result from a decreased dietary intake or from alkalosis. In alkalosis, the potassium has increased entry into the cells, and there is a rise in the intracellular concentration of the cation.

HYPERKALEMIA. This is an elevated level of potassium in the extracellular fluid and blood. In adults, the possible panic value is greater than 6.5 mEq/L (SI: >6.5 mmol/L); in newborns it is greater than 8 mEq/L (SI: >8 mmol/L).

The most common source of hyperkalemia is renal disease. The potassium value also will rise with mineralocorticoid deficiency or metabolic acidosis. Additionally, the damage to tissue and cells causes a release of intracellular potassium into the extracellular fluids.

In renal disease, the glomeruli may be unable to filter the blood, causing a rise in the serum value and a decrease in the excretion of potassium in the urine. In acute renal failure, the potassium level begins to rise with the onset of oliguria. In chronic renal failure, the potassium level does not begin to rise until there is a 75% reduction in the glomerular filtration rate.

With the slower onset of chronic renal failure, the body is able to adapt its control of the potassium level. In the compensation, the renal tubules do not resorb potassium, and so there is greater excretion of potassium in the urine. Additionally, the intestinal tract absorbs less dietary potassium and excretes more of the cation in the feces.

Purpose of the Test

Serum potassium is used to evaluate electrolyte balance, acid-base balance, hypertension, renal disease or renal failure, and endocrine disease. It is used to monitor the patient receiving treatment for ketoacidosis as well as those receiving hyperalimentation, dialysis, diuretic therapy, and intravenous therapy.

Procedure

A red- or green-topped tube is used to collect 5 to 7 ml of venous blood.

QUALITY CONTROL
Venipuncture technique must be smooth, with a blood flow that fills the tube readily. If the blood has excessive turbulence because of flawed technique, hemolysis of erythrocytes causes a false rise in the serum value.

Findings

ELEVATED VALUES

Rapid or excessive intravenous potassium replacement
Dehydration
Acute renal failure
Chronic renal failure
Potassium-sparing diuretics

Massive hemolysis
Acidosis
Diabetic ketoacidosis
Traumatic crush injury
Severe burns
Addison disease

DECREASED VALUES

Diuretic therapy
Intravenous fluid therapy without potassium replacement
Vomiting or diarrhea
Severe burns
Renal tubular acidosis

Excessive sweating
Fistula drainage
Bartter syndrome
Alkalosis
Primary aldosteronism
Secondary aldosteronism

Interfering Factors

• Hemolysis

Nursing Implementation

Pretest

In drawing the blood, it is preferable to avoid the use of a tourniquet. If the tourniquet is applied loosely, the fist should not be clenched. These measures prevent hemolysis of erythrocytes and a false elevation of the potassium value.

Posttest

Arrange for transport of the specimen to the laboratory as quickly as possible.

QUALITY CONTROL

A clotted specimen causes a false elevation of the serum value when intracellular potassium is released into the extracellular serum.

SODIUM

(SERUM)

Synonym:

Na$^+$

NORMAL VALUES

Adult:	136–145 mEq/L *or* SI 136–145 mmol/L
Child:	138–145 mEq/L *or* SI 136–145 mmol/L
Infant:	139–146 mEq/L *or* SI 139–146 mmol/L
Newborn:	133–146 mEq/L *or* SI 133–146 mmol/L
Premature (48 hours):	128–148 mEq/L *or* SI 128–148 mmol/L

Background Information

Sodium is an electrolyte found in all body fluids. About 85% of the total sodium is present in the extracellular fluid, and the remainder is intracellular (DeVita and Michelis, 1993). As the major extracellular cation, sodium is responsible for osmolarity and the intravascular osmotic pressure.

With the change of sodium concentration in the blood, there are resultant changes in the water content into or out of cells. Thus, the alteration of sodium content is responsible for dehydration or overhydration within cells or in extracellular fluids. The measurement of serum sodium is reflective of sodium content in serum or extracellular fluids.

In normal physiology, the level of serum sodium remains in a relatively narrow range. The homeostatic balance of sodium, water, and osmolarity is regulated by renal, posterior pituitary, and hypothalamic functions.

The daily intake of sodium is balanced by an equivalent amount of sodium excretion. The glomeruli of the kidneys filter the sodium from the extracellular fluids freely, with renal tubular resorption of isotonic concentrations of the electrolyte. The excess sodium is excreted in the urine. The amount of urinary excretion depends on the daily intake of sodium and the hydration status of the individual.

HYPONATREMIA. This is a low level of serum sodium. When serum values are less than 120 mEq/L (SI: <120 mmol/L), the hyponatremia is severe. One source of hyponatremia is sodium loss. The origin of the problem is usually renal, incuding renal tubular defects, advanced renal failure, or loop diuretic therapy. Each of these conditions alters the excretion of sodium and water in the proper concentrations. Metabolic alkalosis, ketonuria, or endocrine deficiency may also cause hyponatremia. In all these conditions, there is excessive loss of sodium or excessive resorption of water by the kidney.

Nonrenal causes of sodium loss include fluid and electrolyte losses from the gastrointestinal tract, "third space" losses, and severe thermal injury. The hyponatremia may also be due to an increase in total body water, such as in conditions that cause edema. Although there is also some sodium retention in the extracellular fluids, the amount of water retention is much greater and the serum is diluted.

HYPERNATREMIA. This is an elevation of serum sodium that usually occurs in patients who have little or no fluid intake or who have an inadequate regulation of thirst. A serum value greater than 160 mEq/L (SI: >160 mmol/L) is a serious elevation. The loss of total body water increases the concentration of sodium and the osmolarity of the blood.

In nonrenal causes of hypernatremia, there is a loss of body fluid without adequate replacement. This can occur in diuresis, profuse sweating, diarrhea, burns, and respiratory infection. Renal losses of fluid may result from advanced renal failure.

The fluid loss can also be due to the failure of the kidney to secrete antidiuretic hormone because of a central nervous system disturbance. In some cases, the kidneys do not respond to antidiuretic hormone because of disease that affects the renal tubules. In the case of a lack of antidiuretic hormone, the tubules cannot resorb water. The urine is diluted and of high volume as the water is excreted.

Critical Thinking: The adult patient has a serum sodium level of 155 mEq/L (SI: 155 mmol/L) and a nursing diagnosis of fluid volume excess. As treatment to restore a fluid and electrolyte balance progresses, how does the nurse evaluate the patient's outcome?

Purpose of the Test

Serum sodium levels are used to monitor electrolyte balance, water balance, and acid-base balance. They are also used in the evaluation of disorders of the central nervous system, musculoskeletal disorders, or diseases of the kidneys or adrenal glands.

Procedure

A red- or green-topped tube is used to obtain 5 to 7 ml of venous blood. For infants and small children, a heelstick, earlobe, or finger puncture and a capillary tube are used to obtain capillary blood.

QUALITY CONTROL

Venipuncture technique must be smooth, with a blood flow that fills the tube readily. If the blood has excessive turbulence because of poor technique, the hemolysis of the erythrocytes will falsely elevate the test results.

Findings

ELEVATED VALUES

Dehydration
Cushing syndrome
Primary aldosteronism
Secondary aldosteronism
Inadequate thirst

Diabetic acidosis
Azotemia
Excessive saline infusion
Profuse sweating
Vomiting or diarrhea

DECREASED VALUES

Addison disease
Hypopituitarism
Vomiting or diarrhea
Burns
Acute water intoxication
Cirrhosis
Congestive heart failure
Central nervous system disturbance (trauma, tumor)

Diuretic therapy
Salt-wasting nephritis
Hypothyroidism
Glucorticoid deficiency
Syndrome of inappropriate antidiuretic hormone
Acute or chronic renal failure
Nephrotic syndrome
Ketonuria
Bicarbonaturia

Interfering Factors

- Hemolysis

Nursing Implementation

Pretest

The blood should be drawn without a tourniquet to avoid clotting and hemolysis.

Posttest

Arrange for prompt transport of the specimen to the laboratory.

QUALITY CONTROL

In the laboratory, the serum must be separated from the cells by centrifuge as soon as possible. This prevents clotting and hemolysis.

UREA NITROGEN

(SERUM)

Synonyms:

blood urea nitrogen, BUN

-- **NORMAL VALUES** --

Older adult (>60 years):	8–21 mg/dl *or* SI 2.9–7.5 mmol/L
Child to adult (1–40 years):	5–20 mg/dl *or* SI 1.8–7.1 mmol/L
Infant (birth–1 year):	4–16 mg/dl *or* SI 1.4–5.7 mmol/L

Background Information

Urea nitrogen is the major nitrogenous end product of protein and amino acid catabolism. It is manufactured in the liver, diffuses across cell membranes, and is distributed throughout intracellular and extracellular fluids. Urea nitrogen is excreted from the body primarily by the kidneys, with lesser amounts excreted in sweat or degraded by intestinal bacteria.

In the kidneys, almost all urea is filtered out of the blood by glomerular function. Some urea is resorbed with water in the renal tubules, but the larger remainder is removed from the body in urine. The amount of urea that is excreted is dependent on the state of hydration and the flow of the urine in the kidneys. If the patient is dehydrated and there is a low tubular flow of urine, more urea is resorbed, and the serum level rises. If there is overhydration and a high rate of tubular flow of urine, there is less urea resorbed, and a lower serum level results (Duarte and Preuss, 1993).

ELEVATED LEVELS. In addition to dehydration, the urea nitrogen level can rise because of other, nonrenal factors, including increased urea production associated with increased dietary protein intake and increased catabolism such as with corticosteroid therapy or muscle-wasting diseases. When there is excess production of urea, the serum level rarely rises to greater than 40 mg/dl (SI: >14.2 mmol/L).

In renal causes of an elevated blood urea nitrogen (BUN) level, the problem may be a prerenal, intrarenal, or postrenal pathologic condition. Prerenal disease includes poor renal blood flow as in shock or renal artery stenosis. The impaired circulation slows the glomerular filtration rate and limits renal function. Intrarenal disease includes damage to the renal parenchyma, with resultant acute or chronic renal failure. Generally, the urea nitrogen level does not begin to rise

Critical Thinking: In light of rising health care costs and managed care initiatives to contain the costs, should all patients have the right to hemodialysis treatment?

until there is a loss of at least 50% of glomerular function (Henry, 1991). Postrenal problems are related to obstruction in the kidney or in the urinary tract. They cause increased tubular resorption of the urea.

Renal causes of azotemia result in a dramatic rise in the BUN level. A BUN level of 100 mg/dl or higher (SI: ≥35.7 mmol/L) is extremely elevated and defines the condition of uremia. The patient will become stuporous or comatose because of the advancing renal failure.

Purpose of the Test

The BUN level is used to evaluate renal function. With serum creatinine, it is used to monitor patients in renal failure or those receiving dialysis therapy.

Procedure

A red-topped tube is used to obtain 7 ml of venous blood.

Findings

ELEVATED VALUES

Acute or chronic renal failure   Shock
Renal artery stenosis   Hemorrhage
Postrenal obstruction   Stress
Congestive heart failure   Burns
Increased protein intake   Dehydration
Hyperalimentation   Ketoacidosis
Long-term steroid therapy   Diabetes mellitus

DECREASED VALUES

Overhydration   Starvation
Intravenous therapy   Low-protein diet
Acromegaly   Severe liver damage

Interfering Factors

• None

Nursing Implementation

No specific patient instruction or nursing intervention is needed.

REFERENCES

1. Dennison, R.D., et al. (1992). Myths and facts . . .about electrolyte imbalance: Part 2. *Nursing, 22*, 26.

2. DeVita, M.V., & Michelis, M.F. (1993). Perturbations in sodium balance: Hyponatremia and hypernatremia. *Clinics in Laboratory Medicine, 13,* 135–148.
3. Duarte, C.G., & Preuss, H.G. (1993). Assessment of renal function—Glomerular and tubular. *Clinics in Laboratory Medicine, 13,* 33–52.
4. Henry, J.B. (Ed.). (1991). *Clinical diagnosis and management by laboratory methods* (18th ed.). Philadelphia: W.B. Saunders.
5. Hurley, R.M. (1993). Assessment of renal function in the young: Special considerations. *Clinics in Laboratory Medicine, 13,* 257–268.
6. Jacobs, D.S., et al. (Eds.). (1990). *Laboratory test handbook.* Baltimore: Williams & Wilkins.
7. Latta, K., Hisano, S., & Chan, J.C.M. (1993). Perturbations in potassium balance. *Clinics in Laboratory Medicine, 13,* 149–156.
8. Melillo, K.D. (1993a). Interpretation of abnormal laboratory values in older adults: Part 1. *Journal of Gerontological Nursing, 19,* 39–45.
9. Melillo, K.D. (1993b). Interpretation of abnormal laboratory values in older patients: Part 2. *Journal of Gerontological Nursing, 19,* 35–40.
10. Quiles, R., et al. (1993). Automated enzymatic determination of serum sodium. *Clinical Chemistry, 39,* 500–503.
11. Reidenberg, M.M., et al. (1993). Differences in serum potassium concentrations in normal men in different geographic locations. *Clinical Chemistry, 39,* 72–75.
12. Ruttimann, S., et al. (1993). Multiple biochemical blood testing as a case-finding tool in ambulatory medical patients. *American Journal of Medicine, 94,* 141–148.
13. Schembri, C.T., et al. (1992). Portable simultaneous multiple analyte whole-blood analyzer for point-of-care testing. *Clinical Chemistry, 38,* 1665–1670.
14. Teitz, N.W. (Ed.). (1990). *Clinical guide to laboratory tests* (2nd ed.). Philadelphia: W.B. Saunders.

CHAPTER 6

Coagulation Screen

This chapter addresses the laboratory tests and diagnostic procedures that evaluate the coagulation processes. These processes include clot formation and clot lysis or the degradation of thrombus.

When bleeding occurs, the coagulation process involves the activation and function of platelets and the activation and interaction of coagulation factors to seal the injured blood vessel with a thrombus. Once the vascular tissue heals, the fibrinolytic response dissolves the thrombus so that blood flow can resume.

Some of the blood tests and procedures measure the time that it takes for a clot to form. Others measure the presence or function of the components of coagulation and fibrinolysis. Disorders of coagulation can result in bleeding or hemorrhage because of an inability or a delayed ability to form a clot. Excessive or rapid formation of a thrombus can also occur because of abnormal coagulation processes.

The disorders that affect coagulation ability can be congenital, as in hemophilia, or acquired, as in malignancy or pregnancy (Peric-Knowlton, 1992). Some diseases affect the coagulation system directly, for example, through the loss of platelets or abnormal platelet function. A number of other systemic illnesses affect a primary organ, such as the liver or kidney, with an alteration in coagulation as a secondary effect.

LABORATORY TESTS

The laboratory tests and diagnostic procedures identify the existence of a coagulation disorder and also determine the part of the coagulation system that is affected. In this way, the treatment is specific and more likely to restore clotting ability.

ACTIVATED PARTIAL THROMBOPLASTIN TIME

(BLOOD)

Synonyms:

aPTT, partial thromboplastin time, PTT

--- NORMAL VALUES ---

Average Value:	25–35 seconds
Newborns:	<90 seconds
Premature Infants:	<120 seconds

Background Information

The activated partial thromboplastin time (aPTT) measures the number of seconds needed for a clot to form. In the laboratory, the patient's plasma is mixed with a reagent that includes excess calcium. If the plasma has all the intrinsic coagulation factors present, all the extrinsic factors present, and a normal component of inhibitors of coagulation present (Table 6–1), the aPTT is within normal limits. The aPTT time is shortened when the patient's coagulation system is already activated. The test value is prolonged, and clotting ability is also impaired when there is a 30 to 40% deficiency of one or more clotting factors or when inhibitors of these factors are active.

The test results include the patient's value and the control value. The control value varies according to the reagent used, and it varies from test to test. To correct for the variation, the control value of the test is the reference or normal value that is used to evaluate the patient's test result.

Critical Thinking: The patient must receive a prescribed dose of heparin every 8 hours. Prior to administration of the medication, what nursing assessments must be done?

The aPTT is used to monitor the results of anticoagulation therapy with heparin. The dosage of heparin is adjusted to maintain a therapeutic result, with the aPTT at about 1½ to 2 times the normal value. In this elevated range, the patient takes longer to make a clot and a thrombus or embolus is less likely to develop.

If there is an impairment of the coagulation system or an excessive dose of heparin has been administered, the aPTT result will demonstrate severe elevation beyond the therapeutic range. The possible panic value is greater than 70 seconds, indicating hyperanticoagulation with the threat of hemorrhage. In addition, the patient may also experience thrombocytopenia and a new onset of thromboembolic problems (Jacobs et al., 1990).

TABLE 6–1
COAGULATION FACTORS—ACTIVATORS AND INHIBITORS

Category	Factor	Synonym
Activators		
	I	Fibrinogen
	II	Prothrombin
	III	Tissue thromboplastin
	IV	Calcium
	V	Proaccelerin
	VII	Prothrombin, proconvertin accelerator, stable factor
	VIII	Antihemophilic factor
	IX	Christmas factor, plasma thromboplastin component (PTC)
	X	Stuart-Prower factor
	XI	Plasma thromboplastin antecedent (PTA)
	XII	Hageman factor
	XIII	Fibrin stabilizing factor
	Prekallikrein	—
	HMWK	High-molecular-weight kininogen
Inhibitors		
	Antithrombin III	AT-III
	Protein C	PC
	Protein S	PS

Purpose of the Test

The aPTT is used to evaluate the coagulation system and to help identify congenital and acquired deficiencies of the intrinsic and extrinsic pathways of the coagulation system and inhibitors of the coagulation system. It is used to monitor the effect of heparin anticoagulant therapy and to adjust the next dose of the drug based on the test results.

Procedure

A blue-topped tube with sodium citrate is used to obtain 4.5 ml of venous blood. As an alternative, a heelstick, earlobe, or finger puncture may be used to collect capillary blood in siliconized sodium citrate micropipettes.

QUALITY CONTROL

The tube must be filled with blood. If there is too little blood, the proportion of sodium citrate to blood will be greater than it should be and will result in a false elevation of the test results.

To mix the anticoagulant with the blood, the specimen tube is tilted gently from side to side 5 to 10 times.

When multiple specimens are drawn, the aPTT test specimen is obtained last. When this is the only test specimen taken, a double-tube technique must be used to prevent specimen contamination with tissue thromboplastin. In the double-tube technique, a 1- to 2-ml blood sample is obtained and discarded; the blue-topped tube is then used to collect the test sample.

Venipuncture technique must be smooth, with a blood flow that fills the vacuum tube readily. If the blood has excessive turbulence because of flawed venipuncture technique, the hemolysis greatly shortens the aPTT result in normal individuals.

Findings

ELEVATED VALUES

Excess administration of heparin
Deficiency of one or more coagulation factors
Excessive inhibition of the coagulation system
Disseminated intravascular coagulation (DIC)
Specific and nonspecific circulatory anticoagulants such as lupus anticoagulant
Liver failure
Vitamin K deficiency

DECREASED VALUES

Hypercoagulable states (with arterial or venous thrombus formation)

Interfering Factors

- Hemolysis
- Inadequate blood sample
- Prolonged delay before analysis is performed

Nursing Implementation

Pretest

When heparin is given in intermittent doses, ensure that the specimen is drawn 1 hour before the next dose. When the specimen is obtained less than 3 hours after a heparin dose is given, the aPTT result will be excessively elevated.

When heparin is given in a continuous infusion, special timing of the test is unnecessary.

During the Test

Ensure that the heparin lock or the heparinized tube is not used to obtain the blood specimen.

Posttest

Arrange for prompt transport of the specimen to the laboratory.

QUALITY CONTROL

Specimens received more than 2 hours after collection must be rejected. The plasma must be separated from the cells as soon as possible. The plasma is then refrigerated until the test can be performed.

When the patient receives heparin anticoagulation therapy, monitor each aPTT result for a value in the therapeutic range. If the result is very elevated, notify the physician. Protamine sulfate is kept available to be used as prescribed. It is given intramuscularly as an antidote to heparin to reduce the potential for spontaneous bleeding or hemorrhage.

CLOT RETRACTION TIME

(BLOOD)

Synonyms:

──────────── **NORMAL VALUES** ────────────

Retraction of the clot starts in 1 hour and is complete in 24 hours.

Background Information

There is no single test that fully reflects the complex activities of platelets. Clot retraction is one of the tests of coagulation that is used to study the function of platelets in clot formation.

Following a vascular injury, platelets adhere to the vascular endothelium and aggregate. With the activation of the coagulation system, fibrin is formed to reinforce the platelet aggregation. A clot or thrombus is formed to provide a firm seal at the injury site. Once the clot has formed, the normal process of clot retraction or clot contraction begins within 1 hour and is completed in 24 hours.

In the testing procedure, the clot forms in a test tube and retracts from the sides of the tube, changing its characteristics over a measured period of time. As the serum and some red blood cells leak out of the clot, the clot should retract by 40 to 50%. With this consolidation, the clot should finally appear to be dry, firm, and intact, with only 5% of the serum remaining within the clot.

Clot retraction is dependent on a normal platelet count and normal platelet function. In addition, the blood must have a normal hematocrit and fibrinogen level. In thrombocytopenia, there are a reduced number of platelets. With thrombasthenia, also known as Glanzmann disease, there is poor or abnormal platelet function. The inadequate platelet count and platelet function affect the ability to form a clot. The clot retraction is described as delayed, incomplete, or poor. In the test, the clot remains soft, soggy, and friable, with an excess retention of serum.

Abnormal clot retraction that is not related to platelets can also occur. If no clot formation occurs, as in DIC and hemophilia, no clot retraction can occur. With excess fibrinolysis, the clot forms initially but then dissolves. In a third example of abnormality, a decrease in fibrinogen inhibits both clot formation and clot retraction.

Purpose of the Test

The clot retraction time investigates the function of platelets, particularly in the diagnosis of Glanzmann disease, which is an inherited condition.

Procedure

A red-topped tube is used to collect 10 ml of venous blood. The tube must be filled. In some laboratories, the blood is drawn with a syringe and then transferred into a graduated centrifuge tube immediately.

QUALITY CONTROL

With venipuncture, the tourniquet should be tied lightly for a brief time to prevent pooling of cells in the vein at the site of blood collection. Venipuncture technique must be smooth, with a blood flow that fills the vacuum tube or syringe readily. If the blood has excessive turbulence because of flawed venipuncture technique, the hemolysis of the erythrocytes will alter the test results.

Findings

ABNORMAL VALUES

Thrombocytopenia	Thrombasthenia
Anemia	DIC
Hyperfibrinogenemia	Secondary fibrinolysis

Interfering Factors

- Aspirin therapy
- Hemolysis
- Coagulated specimen

Nursing Implementation

Posttest

Ensure that the specimen tube is labeled correctly. Arrange for prompt transport of the specimen to the laboratory.

QUALITY CONTROL
The blood must arrive at the laboratory and be prepared for the test within 1 hour. The blood is placed in a graduated centrifuge tube and immersed in a water bath to keep the blood temperature steady at 37° C.

CLOTTING TIME

(BLOOD)

Synonyms:

Lee-White clotting time, Lee-White, L-W, Lee-White coagulation time, whole blood clotting time

——— NORMAL VALUES ———

8–15 minutes

Background Information

The clotting time is used to monitor the effect of heparin therapy. In normal health, it takes 8 to 15 minutes for a clot to form in a specimen of whole blood. When the patient undergoes anticoagulation with heparin, the clotting time is prolonged.

Blood coagulation is based on an adequate number of platelets, their ability to function effectively, the presence of adequate fibrinogen, a normal hematocrit level, and the activity of the coagulation factors in the intrinsic pathway of coagulation. Heparin activates antithrombin III, which is a major inhibitor of the coagulation cascade. Antithrombin III binds with thrombin and helps limit the formation of a thrombus and the extension of the size of the thrombus (Berg, 1992). Thus, the effect of heparin is to prolong the clotting time.

The clotting time test is imprecise because of the variation in the standards and among technologists and laboratories. The test also can be inaccurate and somewhat unreliable, particularly when heparin therapy is administered. Because of problems of reliability, the clotting time is not used much and may not be performed by some laboratories. The aPTT has replaced the clotting time test in most institutions.

Purpose of the Test

The clotting time may be used to monitor the effectiveness of heparin therapy and assess the intrinsic pathway of coagulation.

Procedure

Using a plastic syringe to draw 3 ml of venous blood, 1 ml of blood is placed in each of three glass test tubes. A stopwatch is used to measure the time needed for a clot to form. The watch is started after the third tube is filled, and it is stopped when the clot is formed in the third tube.

QUALITY CONTROL
With venipuncture, the tourniquet should be tied lightly for a brief time to prevent pooling of cells in the vein at the site of blood collection. Venipuncture technique must be smooth, with the blood filling the syringe readily. If there is excessive turbulence because of flawed venipuncture technique, hemolysis of the erythrocytes will alter the test results.

Findings

ELEVATED VALUES
Severe deficiency of clotting factors
Presence of heparin anticoagulant

Interfering Factors

- Recent administration of heparin
- Hemolysis

Nursing Implementation

Pretest

When heparin is given in intermittent doses, ensure that the specimen is drawn at least 3 hours after the last dose of heparin. When the specimen is obtained less than 3 hours after a heparin dose is given, the test result will be excessively elevated. Record the time of the most recent dose on the requisition slip.

When heparin is given in a continuous infusion, special timing of the test is unnecessary.

During the Test

Ensure that the heparin lock or the heparinized tube is not used to obtain the blood specimen.

Posttest

Ensure that the venipuncture site has sealed and that the patient is not bleeding. Use a sterile gauze to apply pressure to the puncture site as needed. Keeping pressure on the site, instruct the patient to raise the arm over the head. The combination of pressure and elevation should help the process of coagulation and stop the bleeding.

Ensure that the test tubes are labeled correctly and arrange for prompt transport of the specimen to the laboratory.

QUALITY CONTROL

The specimen tubes must be maintained in a water bath at 37° C to control the temperature of the blood during coagulation.

COAGULATION FACTOR ASSAY

(PLASMA)

Synonym:

factor assay

NORMAL VALUES

General Values:	50–150% of normal activity *or* SI 50–150 AU
Factor II:	0.5–1.5 U/ml or 0.5–1.5 kU/L
	60–150% of normal activity *or* SI 60–150 AU
Factor V:	0.5–2 U/ml or 0.5–2 kU/L
	60–150% of normal activity *or* SI 60–150 AU
Factor VII:	65–135% *or* SI 65–135 AU
Factor VIII:	60–145% *or* SI 60–145 AU
Factor IX:	60–140% *or* SI 60–140 AU
Factor X:	60–130% *or* SI 60–130 AU
Factor XI:	60–135% *or* SI 60–135 AU
Factor XII:	60–150% *or* SI 60–150 AU
Factor XIII:	Clot is stable in 5 mol of urea for 24 hours at 37° C

Background Information

To achieve hemostasis, with the formation of a clot to arrest the bleeding, a series of highly ordered and complex chemical interactions occurs. The process of coagulation consists of three interacting components: platelet aggregation, the activation of the intrinsic pathway, and the activation of the extrinsic pathway.

Platelets form the initial plug and then aggregate to seal the bleeding vessel.

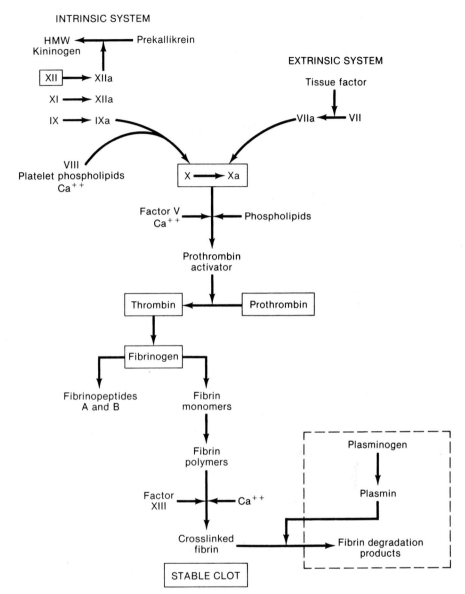

FIGURE 6–1. The coagulation pathways. Two interdependent pathways form a common pathway for clot formation. Once plasminogen is activated, the process of fibrinolysis or the dissolving of the clot begins. (With permission from Clochesy, J.M., et al. [1993]. *Critical care nursing* [p. 1052]. Philadelphia: W.B. Saunders.)

Simultaneously, coagulation factors are activated via the intrinsic and extrinsic pathways and ultimately form fibrin (Fig. 6–1). Once fibrin fibers are integrated into the clot, the clot becomes stable and firm. This seals off the injured blood vessel so that no more blood is lost. Beneath the clot, the injured wall of the blood vessel can heal.

The extrinsic pathway is activated by tissue trauma and the release of factor III—tissue thromboplastin. This factor then activates factor VII—prothrombin. Prothrombin stimulates the intrinsic pathway by activation of factors IX and X.

The intrinsic pathway is activated by vascular trauma, with the contact of collagen, prekallikrein, and high-molecular-weight kininogen at the site of injury. These contact factors initiate the conversion of factor XII. The intrinsic pathway proceeds by activation of additional coagulation factors in a series of events until fibrin is formed.

Although the activation of coagulation factors is in a cascade pattern for both the extrinsic and the intrinsic pathways, the coagulation response is not totally linear. There are additional crossover reactions and feedback loops that also occur at multiple levels of the cascade. These actions produce interdependence between the pathways, further enhancing the response of the coagulation system (Henry, 1991).

The coagulation factors are circulating plasma proteins (see Table 6–1). Once they become activated, each has a specific function in the coagulation process. The coagulation factor assay identifies one or more of the factors that are responsible for impaired coagulation ability. The coagulation factors that are part of the assay are factors II, V, VII, VIII, IX, X, XI, XII, and XIII.

Purpose of the Test

This test is used to detect the deficiency of one or more coagulation factors in coagulation disorders that are of congenital or acquired origin.

Procedure

Critical Thinking: When a Chinese patient has his blood drawn, he becomes very upset. He believes that once the blood is removed, it cannot be replaced. How do you respond to his cultural belief?

A blue-topped tube with sodium citrate is used to obtain 4.5 ml of venous blood. As an alternative, a heelstick, earlobe, or finger puncture may be used to collect capillary blood in siliconized sodium citrate micropipettes.

QUALITY CONTROL

The tube must be filled with blood. If there is too little blood, the proportion of sodium citrate will be greater than that of blood and result in a false elevation of the test results.

To mix the anticoagulant with the blood, the specimen tube is gently tilted from side to side 5 to 10 times.

When multiple specimens are drawn, the coagulation factor assay specimen is obtained last. When this is the only test specimen, a double-tube technique must be used to prevent specimen contamination with tissue thromboplastin. In the double-tube technique, a 1- to 2-ml blood sample is obtained and discarded and the blue-topped tube is then used to collect the test sample.

Findings

ELEVATED VALUES

Oral contraceptive therapy (elevation of factors II, VII, IX, X, and XII)

DIC (elevation of factor VIII)

DECREASED VALUES

Hemophilia A (deficiency of factor VIII)
Hemophilia B (deficiency of factor IX)
Hemophilia C (deficiency of factor XI)
Parahemophilia (deficiency of factor V)
von Willebrand disease (elevation of factor VIII)
Lupus erythematosus (deficiency of factor II)
Liver disease (deficiencies of factors II, V, IX, X, XIII)
Vitamin K deficiency (deficiencies of factors II, IX, X)
DIC (deficiencies of factors V, VIII)
Factor V inhibitors
Gaucher disease (deficiency of factor IX)
Nephrotic syndrome (deficiency of factor IX)
Amyloidosis (deficiency of factor X)
Renal or adrenocortical malignancy (deficiency of factor X)

Interfering Factors

- Anticoagulant therapy
- Inadequate blood sample
- Hemolysis
- Coagulation
- Pregnancy
- Time delay before analysis
- Warming of the specimen

Nursing Implementation

Pretest

Schedule this test 2 weeks after coumarin therapy is discontinued or 2 days after heparin therapy is discontinued.

A specialized coagulation laboratory may be needed to perform the test. Coordinate with the local laboratory facility regarding the scheduling and transport of the specimen.

On the requisition slip, list any history of medication that interferes with coagulation, including a history of oral contraceptive use or anticoagulant therapy.

Posttest

Ensure that the venipuncture site has sealed and that the patient is not bleeding. Use a sterile gauze to apply pressure to the puncture site as needed. Keeping pressure on the site, instruct the patient to raise the arm over the head. The combination of pressure and elevation should help coagulation to occur and stop the bleeding.

Place the specimen in a cup of iced water immediately after the blood is drawn.

Arrange for prompt transport of the chilled specimen to the laboratory.

QUALITY CONTROL

With refrigeration, the coagulation factors are stable for about 2 hours. If there is a delay of more than 2 hours before analysis, the plasma must be frozen.

COAGULATION INHIBITORS

(SERUM, PLASMA)

Synonyms:

antithrombin III, protein C, protein S

NORMAL VALUES

ANTITHROMBIN III	**Plasma:** 21–30 mg/dl *or* SI 210–300 mg/dL
	Plasma, Bioassay Method: 86–113% of normal activity *or* SI 86–113 AU
PROTEIN C	**Plasma:** 71–142% of normal activity *or* SI 0.71–1.42 (fraction of whole)
	2.82–5.65 g/ml or SI 2.82–5.65 mg/L
PROTEIN S	**Plasma:** 61–130% of normal activity *or* SI 0.61–1.30 (fraction of whole)

Background Information

The process of coagulation is complex and involves many components and interactions. The regulation or control of the coagulation cascade consists of a balance between the activation and inhibition of the coagulation factors. Antithrombin III, protein C, and protein S all are natural inhibitors of coagulation. By neutralizing the actions of the coagulation factors, the formation of a thrombus or blood clot is inhibited. A patient may have deficiencies of one or more of these coagulation factors. Since there is more than one method of analysis, the reference values vary according to the method used.

ANTITHROMBIN III. This is the primary inhibitor of the activated form of factor X (factor Xa) and thrombin (factor IIa). It also inhibits the activity of factors XII, XI, and IX. In the presence of adequate antithrombin III, heparin is greatly enhanced in its anticoagulant action. With low or inadequate levels of antithrombin III, patients can experience a resistance to heparin, but they respond to anticoagulant therapy with coumarin. The deficiency of antithrombin III results in the formation of recurrent or extensive thrombus formation or a thromboembolic disorder.

The deficiency of antithrombin III can be hereditary or acquired. The protein can also be decreased because of excessive consumption, as in DIC (Esparaz and Green, 1990).

PROTEIN C. This is synthesized by the liver and is a natural inhibitor of coagulation. It is activated by thrombin. It functions to inhibit activated factors V and VIII and prolongs the conversion of prothrombin to thrombin. These activities delay or reduce thrombus formation. In addition, protein C enhances the activity of tissue plasminogen activator (t-PA) in the lysis or dissolving of the thrombus.

Reduced levels of protein C cause recurrent or extensive thrombus formation. When the cause is hereditary, homozygous protein C deficiency usually results in death in infancy. Heterozygous protein C deficiency is less severe. There is either too little of the protein or it is not completely functional. These patients often experience thrombus formation in adulthood in the form of a deep vein thrombosis, thrombophlebitis, pulmonary embolus, or a hypercoagulable state (Bachman, 1991). Acquired deficiency is associated with the decreased synthesis of protein C in liver disease.

PROTEIN S. Like protein C, protein S is a vitamin K–dependent coagulation protein that is synthesized by the liver. It is a cofactor of protein C, accelerating and enhancing the effect of protein C. In combination, proteins C and S inhibit the formation of a thrombus. The patient who has a deficiency of protein S also has the tendency to form recurrent thrombi in the form of a deep vein thrombosis, thrombus, embolus, or hypercoagulable state. The condition may be of hereditary or acquired origin.

Purpose of the Tests

The three tests are used to investigate the underlying cause of a thrombus, particularly in young adults or in patients who have a family history of thrombus formation. These tests are also used to assess the cause of a hypercoagulable state and fibrinolytic state. Antithrombin III is used to evaluate the response to heparin or to investigate the cause of heparin failure.

Procedure

Antithrombin III: Two blue-topped tubes with sodium citrate are used to collect 4.5 ml of blood in each tube.

Protein C: One blue-topped tube with sodium citrate is used to collect 4.5 ml of venous blood.

Protein S: One blue-topped tube with sodium citrate is used to collect 4.5 ml of venous blood.

As an alternative, a heelstick, earlobe, or finger puncture may be used to collect capillary blood in siliconized sodium citrate micropipettes.

QUALITY CONTROL

The tube must be filled with blood. If there is too little blood, the proportion of sodium citrate will be greater than that of blood and a false elevation of the test results will occur.

To mix the anticoagulant with the blood, the specimen tube is tilted gently from side to side 5 to 10 times.

When multiple specimens are drawn, the coagulation inhibitor specimen is obtained last. When this is the only test specimen, a double-tube technique must be used to prevent specimen contamination with tissue thromboplastin. In the double-tube technique, a 1- to 2-ml blood sample is obtained and discarded and the blue-topped tube is then used to collect the test sample.

Venipuncture technique must be smooth, with a blood flow that fills the vacuum tube readily. If the blood has excessive turbulence because of flawed venipuncture technique, the hemolysis alters the test results.

Findings

ELEVATED VALUES

Antithrombin III

Acute hepatitis
Renal transplant

Vitamin K deficiency
Inflammatory disorder

DECREASED VALUES

Antithrombin III

Congenital deficiency
DIC
Nephrotic syndrome
Pregnancy or postpartum condition

Liver transplant
Hepatectomy
Cirrhosis
Chronic liver failure

Proteins C and S

Congenital deficiency
DIC

Cirrhosis

Interfering Factors

• Hemolysis
• Coagulation of the specimen

- Warming of the specimen
- Heparin
- Time delay in analysis of the specimen

Nursing Implementation

Pretest

Schedule the test 2 to 4 weeks after anticoagulation therapy has been discontinued. The test results can be altered because of thrombus, anticoagulant therapy, or inflammatory disease processes (Schenk and Goodnight, 1992).

If the patient is currently receiving anticoagulant therapy, include the name and dosage of the drug on the requisition slip. Coumarin therapy lowers the patient's test values, and heparin invalidates the test results for antithrombin III and protein C.

During the Test

Do not allow the blood to be collected from the arm with an intravenous line or a heparin lock device.

Posttest

Place the antithrombin III tubes on ice immediately and arrange for prompt transport of all speciments to the laboratory.

QUALITY CONTROL

These three tests become invalid if there is a delay of more than 2 to 4 hours before the blood is prepared for analysis. The coagulation inhibitors are more stable in cold temperatures.

D-DIMER TEST

(PLASMA)

Synonym:
fibrin degradation fragment

―――――――――――――――― **NORMAL VALUES** ――――――

Latex Beads: <250 ng/ml *or* SI <250 µg/L
Enzyme-Linked Immunosorbent Assay (ELISA): No D-dimer fragments are present

Background Information

Critical Thinking: Your patient with DIC experiences tissue perfusion alterations that are related to hemorrhage and thrombosis. Develop a comprehensive assessment plan that includes the monitoring of specific coagulation tests.

D-dimer is a fragment of fibrin that is formed as a result of fibrin degradation and clot lysis. The ELISA method is a highly specific method that is used for emergency screening to exclude the presence of a deep vein thrombus. There is no deep vein thrombus present when the results are less than normal by latex bead method or absent by the ELISA method.

Elevated test results or the presence of D-dimer fragments is evidence that there was thrombus formation and lysis of the thrombus by the enzyme activity of plasmin. The combination of elevated levels of fibrin split-products and D-dimer fragments is highly predictive of DIC.

Purpose of the Test

The D-dimer test is used as a screening test for deep vein thrombosis. It helps determine whether a clot is present in the diagnosis of DIC, an acute myocardial infarction, and unstable angina. It is also used in the diagnosis of hypercoagulable conditions that cause recurrent thrombosis.

Procedure

A plastic syringe and a special plastic tube with sodium citrate and aprotinin additives are used to collect 4.5 ml of venous blood.

Findings

ELEVATED (POSITIVE) VALUES

Thrombotic disease
    Deep vein thrombosis
    Pulmonary embolism
    Arterial thromboembolism
    Thrombolytic-defibrination therapy

DIC
Sickle cell anemia crisis
Pregnancy (postpartum)
Malignancy
Surgery

Interfering Factors

- None

Nursing Implementation

Posttest

Arrange for immediate transport of the specimen to the laboratory. The patient is acutely ill and the test results are needed as quickly as possible.

EUGLOBULIN CLOT LYSIS

(BLOOD)

Synonyms:

euglobulin lysis time, fibrinolysis time, euglobulin clot lysis time

═══════════════════ **NORMAL VALUES** ═══════════════════

Lysis Time: 1.5–4 hours

Background Information

Fibrinolysis is the dissolution of a formed clot. Once the injured blood vessel is sealed, the clot or thrombus begins to dissolve as a normal process that permits the blood flow to resume. In the function of the fibrinolytic system (Fig. 6–2), plasminogen is converted to the enzyme plasmin. The activation of plasminogen and its conversion to plasmin is aided or accelerated by t-PA, urokinase, and streptokinase. Plasmin degrades the bonds of fibrin, and clot lysis occurs. In normal fibrinolytic activity, it takes 1½ to 4 hours to achieve euglobulin clot lysis, with the release of fibrin degradation products.

When the euglobulin clot lysis time is shortened, there is increased fibrinolysis. This problem is usually associated with increased activity of the plasminogen activators. Clot lysis time can be as short as 5 to 10 minutes. If there is 100% clot lysis in less than 1 hour, the patient is at great risk for bleeding.

Purpose of the Test

The euglobulin clot lysis test assesses systemic fibrinolysis and abnormality that result in the rapid dissolution of a thrombus. It may be used to monitor fibrinolytic therapy with urokinase, streptokinase, or t-PA to dissolve a thrombus.

Procedure

A blue-topped tube with sodium citrate is used to obtain 4.5 ml of venous blood. As an alternative, a heelstick, earlobe, or finger puncture may be used to collect capillary blood in siliconized sodium citrate micropipettes.

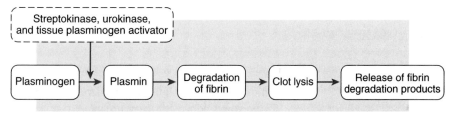

FIGURE 6–2. Simplified diagram of the process of fibrinolysis.

QUALITY CONTROL

The tube must be filled with blood. If there is too little blood, the proportion of sodium citrate will be greater than that of blood and will result in a false elevation of the test results.

To mix the anticoagulant with the blood, the specimen tube is tilted gently from side to side 5 to 10 times.

When multiple specimens are drawn, the euglobulin lysis test specimen is obtained last. When this is the only test specimen, a double-tube technique must be used to prevent specimen contamination with tissue thromboplastin. In the double-tube technique, a 1- to 2-ml blood sample is obtained and discarded and the blue-topped tube is then used to collect the test sample.

Venipuncture technique must be smooth, with a blood flow that fills the vacuum tube readily. If the blood has excessive turbulence because of flawed venipuncture technique, the hemolysis alters the test results.

Findings

DECREASED VALUES (SHORTENED LYSIS TIME)
Circulatory collapse, shock
Pulmonary or pancreatic surgery
Pyogenic reactions
Epinephrine injection
Obstetric complications
DIC

Interfering Factors

- Hemolysis
- Coagulation of the specimen
- Flawed venipuncture technique
- Inadequate amount of specimen
- Hemodilution
- Warming of the specimen
- Exercise

Nursing Implementation

Pretest

For the patient who is physically active, exercise is avoided for 1 hour prior to the collection of the specimen.

During the Test

Ensure that the specimen is not collected from the arm that has a catheter or intravenous line. The intravenous solution would dilute the specimen of blood.

After the tourniquet is applied, instruct the patient to relax the hand and refrain from clenching the fist. This will help prevent hemolysis of red blood cells.

Posttest

Immediately place the specimen on ice.

Arrange for immediate transport of the chilled specimen to the laboratory.

QUALITY CONTROL

The specimen must be delivered to the laboratory within 15 to 20 minutes. The specimen must be centrifuged and the plasma placed on ice. The plasma is tested within 30 minutes after obtaining the specimen.

FIBRINOGEN

(PLASMA)

Synonyms:

factor I, fibrinogen level

--- **NORMAL VALUES** ---

Adult:	200–400 mg/dl *or* SI 2–4 g/L
Newborn:	125–300 mg/dl *or* SI 1.25–3 g/L

Background Information

Fibrinogen is a coagulation protein that is manufactured by the liver. It is a precursor of fibrin and a vital contributor to the meshwork that binds platelets into an aggregation and ultimately clot formation. When there is an acute vascular injury or tissue injury with inflammation or necrosis, fibrinogen levels increase in the early phase of coagulation. Within 24 hours of the injury, the fibrinogen level rises dramatically.

At the site of vascular disruption, adhesive proteins and fibrinogen bind the platelets together and plug the break in the vascular wall (Fig. 6–3). As the clotting process progresses, the fibrinogen releases two pairs of peptide and converts to fibrin. The fibrin threads provide stability for the clot.

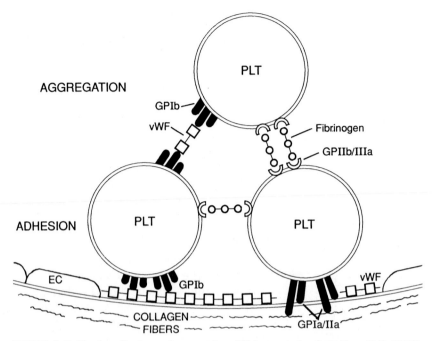

FIGURE 6-3. Platelet adhesion and aggregation. (With permission from Berg, D.E. [1992]. Components and defects of the coagulation system. *Nurse Practitioner Forum*, 3, 65.)

ELEVATED LEVELS

Elevated levels of fibrinogen normally occur during acute injury, but in other abnormal conditions, the fibrinogen level rises and an unwanted thrombus or embolus can occur. The fibrinogen level also rises in pregnancy.

DECREASED LEVELS

Decreased levels of fibrinogen result in a prolonged time for conversion of fibrinogen to fibrin. Excess bleeding occurs until the clot is formed. Newborns have a different form of fibrinogen that requires a longer time to form a clot. The fibrinogen of the newborn converts to the adult form during the first few months of life. Thereafter, the infant has the same reference value as that of the adult.

Purpose of the Test

The fibrinogen test is used to help diagnose bleeding disorders, including afibrinogenemia, DIC, and fibrinolysis.

Procedure

A blue-topped tube with sodium citrate is used to obtain 4.5 ml of venous blood. As an alternative, a heelstick, earlobe, or finger puncture may be used to collect capillary blood in siliconized sodium citrate micropipettes.

The tube must be filled with blood. If there is too little blood, the proportion of sodium citrate will be greater than that of blood and will result in a false elevation of the test results.

To mix the anticoagulant with the blood, the specimen tube is tilted gently from side to side 5 to 10 times.

When multiple specimens are drawn, the fibrinogen test specimen is obtained last. When this is the only test specimen obtained, a double-tube technique must be used to prevent specimen contamination with tissue thromboplastin. In the double-tube technique, a 1- to 2-ml blood sample is obtained and discarded and the blue-topped tube is then used to collect the test sample.

Venipuncture technique must be smooth, with a blood flow that fills the vacuum tube readily. If the blood has excessive turbulence because of flawed venipuncture technique, hemolysis alters the test results.

Findings

ELEVATED VALUES

Sepsis-infection   Malignancy
Inflammation   Traumatic injury

DECREASED VALUES

Hereditary afibrinogenemia   Severe liver disease
Hypofibrinogenemia   DIC

Interfering Factors

- Heparinization
- Pregnancy (third trimester)
- Recent surgery
- Inadequate amount of specimen
- Hemolysis
- Coagulation of the specimen

Nursing Implementation

Pretest

For the patient who receives intermittent doses of heparin, schedule the test at least 1 hour after the heparin dose is administered. In some methods of analysis, a recent heparin dose alters the test result.

Posttest

Arrange for prompt transport of the specimen to the laboratory.

QUALITY CONTROL
The results are invalid with a clotted specimen or a time delay of greater than 1 hour before the cells are separated from the plasma.

FIBRIN SPLIT-PRODUCTS

(SERUM, URINE)

Synonyms:

FSP, fibrin breakdown products, FBP, fibrin degradation products, FDP

─────────── **NORMAL VALUES** ───────────

Serum: <10 μg/ml *or* SI <10 mg/L
Urine: <0.25 μg/ml *or* SI <0.25 mg/L

Background Information

Fibrinolysis is the normal body process that breaks down and dissolves a formed clot. In this process, the fibrin bonds are split and fragments called fibrin split-products or fibrinogen degradation products are released. As fibrinolysis occurs, the blood level of fibrin split-products rises in proportion to the amount of activity. When the serum concentration reaches the possible panic level of greater than 40 μg/ml, the cause is likely to be DIC.

The level of urinary fibrin split-products does not correlate with the serum values. When proteinuria is present, the elevation of fibrin split-products is an indicator for clotting and lysis in the renal tissues. After renal transplantation, the elevated urinary level can be a predictor of rejection of the transplant.

Purpose of the Test

This test is used to help diagnose DIC and may be used in the study of disorders that produce clot formation and lysis of the clot.

Procedure

Blood: A special tube for fibrin split-products is used to collect 2 ml of venous blood. The tube is obtained from the coagulation laboratory and contains thrombin and an antifibrinolytic agent.

QUALITY CONTROL

The tube must not be overfilled. Once the blood is drawn, the tube is tilted from side to side 5 to 10 times to mix the blood with the clotting agents. The blood will coagulate.

Urine: A special tube for fibrin split-products is used to collect 2 ml of urine.

Findings

ELEVATED VALUES

Serum

DIC	Primary fibrinolysis
Myocardial infarction	Secondary fibrinolysis
Pulmonary embolus	Malignancy
Liver disease	Infection or inflammation

Urine

Kidney disease	Renal transplant rejection

Interfering Factors

SERUM

- Improper collection procedure
- Improper storage procedure

URINE

- Menstruation
- Hematuria

Nursing Implementation

Pretest

SERUM

No specific patient instruction or intervention is needed.

URINE

The presence of hematuria, particularly from menstrual flow, invalidates test results. If blood is present, postpone the test and notify the physician.

Posttest

Arrange for prompt transport of the specimen to the laboratory.

QUALITY CONTROL

For the serum analysis, the blood must clot in the tube for 30 minutes; the sample is then centrifuged to separate the cells from the serum.

PLATELET AGGREGATION

(PLASMA)

Synonyms:

aggregometer test, platelet function studies

NORMAL VALUES

Platelet aggregation occurs in 3–5 minutes.

Background Information

After an injury to a blood vessel, platelets initiate action in a coagulation response. The platelets adhere to the vascular endothelium and form a plug that prevents additional blood loss. At the same time that the coagulation system is activated, the platelets are stimulated in a second wave of activity to continue the coagulation process. The platelets change shape, develop pseudopods, contract, and release substances from their cytoplasmic granules. Ultimately, the platelets become sticky and are capable of binding plasma proteins, including fibrinogen. The platelets adhere to each other in platelet aggregation (Fig. 6–4).

In the patient with a coagulation disorder, platelet function is studied to help determine the cause of the problem. This test uses platelet-rich plasma and several chemical reagents to stimulate the platelets' ability to aggregate. In the presence of each of the chemical reagents, normal plasma specimens demonstrate rapid aggregation of the platelets. In patients who have thrombocytopathy (the abnormal function of platelets), platelet aggregation is decreased or absent. The cause of the disorder can be inherited or acquired.

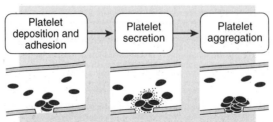

FIGURE 6–4. Platelet response to vascular injury.

Purpose of the Test

The platelet aggregation test is used to evaluate platelet function and detect a congenital or acquired platelet bleeding disorder.

Procedure

A plastic or glass syringe and a tube with sodium citrate are used to obtain 10 ml of venous blood.

Critical Thinking: The patient with advanced cirrhosis of the liver has disorders of platelets and platelet function. In your teaching plan, identify safety measures that help protect the patient from bleeding episodes.

QUALITY CONTROL

During venipuncture, the tourniquet should be tied lightly for a brief time to prevent pooling of the platelets in the vein at the site of blood collection. Venipuncture technique must be smooth, with a blood flow that fills the syringe readily. If there is excessive turbulence because of flawed venipuncture technique, the hemolysis of the erythrocytes will alter the test results. After the blood is put in the tube, the tube is gently tilted 5 to 10 times to mix the anticoagulant and prevent clotting.

Findings

ELEVATED VALUES

Raynaud phenomenon

DECREASED VALUES

Uremia
Liver disease
Leukemia

Macroglobulinemia
Myeloproliferative disorder
Hypothyroidism

Interfering Factors

- Clotting of the specimen
- Hemolysis
- Chilling of the specimen
- Lipemia
- Caffeine
- Thrombocytopenia

Nursing Implementation

Pretest

Schedule this test 10 days after medications that disrupt platelet function have been discontinued. Aspirin, antihistamines, and antiinflammatory and psychotropic drugs all interfere with platelet aggregation and can cause a bleeding disorder.

Instruct the patient to fast from food or to only eat low-fat foods for 8 hours before the test. Caffeine intake must be avoided on the day of the test.

Posttest

Ensure that the venipuncture site has sealed and that the patient is not bleeding. Use a sterile gauze to apply pressure to the puncture site as needed. Keeping pressure on the site, instruct the patient to raise the arm over the head. The combination of pressure and elevation should help the process of coagulation and stop the bleeding.

Arrange for immediate transport of the specimen to the laboratory.

QUALITY CONTROL

After the blood is drawn, the platelets are stable at room temperature for a limited time only. The test must be performed within 2 hours. The specimen cannot be chilled because platelets are activated at low temperatures.

PROTHROMBIN TIME

(PLASMA)

Synonyms:
PT, protime

--- **NORMAL VALUES** ---

Average: 10–13 seconds
Newborn to 6 months: 13–18 seconds

Background Information

The prothrombin time measures the amount of time needed to form a clot. The plasma specimen is mixed with a reagent that contains calcium and excess thromboplastin. The clot formation is dependent on the presence and activity of coagulation factors I, II, V, VII, and X. A deficiency of any of these factors prolongs the prothrombin time by 3 to 4 seconds.

Each test includes the control time in the report of the patient's value. The control time is the normal reference value to be used in the evaluation of the patient's test result. There is always some variation in the control value from test to test, depending on the type of reagent and test method used.

Healthy newborns and healthy premature newborns have normal values that are 2 to 3 seconds longer than the adult value. Once the infant reaches about 6 months of age, the reference value is the same as that of an adult.

One use of the prothrombin time is to monitor the anticoagulant effect of coumarin or warfarin therapy. These anticoagulants prolong the prothrombin time. The therapeutic range is 1¼ to 1½ times the normal value, a slightly lower level of anticoagulation than was recommended in the past. For the patient with a mechanical heart valve or repeated embolism, or both, the therapeutic range is 1½ to 2 times the normal value (Jacobs, 1990). Excessive anticoagulant therapy greatly prolongs the prothrombin time and introduces the threat of hemorrhage. The possible panic value is three times the normal value or more. For the patient who does not receive anticoagulant therapy, the possible panic value is greater than 20 seconds.

Critical Thinking: How do you teach the anti-coagulated patient to evaluate for and avoid nonprescription drugs that contain aspirin?

Purpose of the Test

The prothrombin time is used to evaluate the extrinsic coagulation system; to help screen for coagulation deficiency of factors II, V, VII, and X; and to monitor oral anticoagulant therapy. It is also used to investigate the effects of liver failure and DIC and to screen for vitamin K deficiency.

Procedure

A blue-topped tube with sodium citrate is used to obtain 4.5 ml of venous blood. As an alternative, a heelstick, earlobe, or finger puncture may be used to collect capillary blood in siliconized sodium citrate micropipettes.

QUALITY CONTROL

The tube must be filled with blood. If there is too little blood, the proportion of sodium citrate will be greater than that of blood and will result in a false elevation of the test results.

To mix the anticoagulant with the blood, the specimen tube is tilted gently from side to side 5 to 10 times.

When multiple samples are drawn, this test specimen is obtained last. When this is the only test specimen, a double-tube technique must be used to prevent specimen contamination with tissue thromboplastin. In the double-tube technique, a 1- to 2-ml blood sample is obtained and discarded and the blue-topped tube is then used to collect the test sample.

Venipuncture technique must be smooth, with a blood flow that fills the vacuum tube readily. If the blood has excessive turbulence because of flawed venipuncture technique, the hemolysis alters the test result.

Findings

ELEVATED VALUES

Fibrinogen deficiency
Prothrombin deficiency
Liver disease
Abnormal bleeding

Excess anticoagulant therapy
Deficiency of factor V, VI, or X
Vitamin K deficiency
DIC

Interfering Factors

- Lipemia
- Hemolysis
- Inadequate blood sample
- Prolonged delay before analysis is performed

Nursing Implementation

Pretest

Instruct the patient to discontinue intake of alcohol and caffeine for 24 hours before the test. Lipemia from these substances interferes with the accuracy of the test.

If the patient receives intermittent doses of heparin, ensure that the blood is drawn at least 2 hours after the last dose. Recent heparin administration prolongs the prothrombin time excessively.

Posttest

Ensure that the venipuncture site has sealed and that the patient is not bleeding. Use a sterile gauze to apply pressure to the puncture site as needed. Keeping pressure on the site, instruct the patient to raise the arm over the head. The combination of pressure and elevation should help coagulation and stop the bleeding.

Arrange for prompt transport of the specimen to the laboratory. Any prothrombin time specimen received more than 2 hours after the blood is drawn is rejected.

QUALITY CONTROL

The plasma must be separated from the cells as soon as possible and refrigerated until the test can be performed.

DIAGNOSTIC PROCEDURES

BLEEDING TIME

(BLOOD)

Synonyms:

-- NORMAL VALUES --

Bleeding time (Mielke): <10 minutes
Bleeding time (Ivy):   2–7 minutes
Bleeding time (Duke):   1–3 minutes

Background Information

The bleeding time is used for the patient who is suspected of having a clotting abnormality, particularly one that involves capillaries or platelet function. The bleeding time can be performed by one of three methods: the Mielke, Ivy, or Duke bleeding time. Each of these tests involves a skin puncture or cut, followed by a blotting of the drops of blood until the bleeding stops. The test is measured in the time (minutes) it takes a clot to form. The elevated level or prolonged time needed for clot formation indicates a vascular problem or disorder of platelet function. In this test, the result is usually normal for other causes of coagulation disorder.

The Mielke test is the preferred method because the length and depth of the incision are standardized by the use of a template. The Duke method is used with patients who cannot have an incision on either arm, for example, if bilateral casts or skin eruptions are present. In all three methods, the timing starts with the cut of the skin and stops when the bleeding ceases.

Purpose of the Test

The bleeding time test is used to screen for platelet malfunction or for a vascular defect that interferes with clotting.

Procedure

MIELKE BLEEDING TIME. A blood pressure cuff is applied to the arm and inflated to 40 mm Hg of pressure. This compresses the capillary circulation. Once the skin is cleansed with alcohol, a template is applied to the volar aspect of the forearm and a horizontal cut in the skin is completed. Filter paper is used to blot the drops of blood every 30 seconds until the bleeding ceases.

IVY BLEEDING TIME. A blood pressure cuff is applied to the arm and inflated to 40 mm Hg of pressure. Once the skin is cleansed with alcohol, two puncture wounds, 3 mm deep, are made on the volar aspect of the forearm. The blood drops are blotted with filter paper every 30 seconds until the bleeding ceases.

DUKE BLEEDING TIME. Once the skin is cleansed with alcohol, a sterile lancet is used to puncture the earlobe. The blotting procedure is the same as for the other two methods.

Findings

ELEVATED VALUES

Thrombocytopenia	von Willebrand disease
Glanzmann thrombasthenia	Gray platelet syndrome
DIC	Uremia, renal failure
Severe metabolic acidosis	Hereditary afibrinogenemia

Interfering Factors

- Laceration of a small vein
- Recent aspirin ingestion
- History of keloid formation

Nursing Implementation

Pretest

Schedule this test at least 7 days after the last dose of aspirin has been taken.
Explain the procedure to the patient. The patient should understand that a small scar can result from the puncture or incision. Some laboratories require a written consent.
For the Mielke or Ivy method, inspect the volar aspect of the forearm for rash, infection, or skin eruption. There should be none.

During the Test

Cleanse the site with alcohol and allow it to dry. When blotting the drops of blood, do not compress the skin.

QUALITY CONTROL

Compression promotes rapid coagulation and falsely alters the test result.

Measure the period of bleeding precisely.

Posttest

For the Mielke method, apply a butterfly dressing to the skin site.
As it heals, inspect the skin site daily for signs of infection.

CAPILLARY FRAGILITY TEST

(PRESSURE
MEASUREMENT)

Synonyms:

Rumpel-Leede test, tourniquet test, negative pressure suction cup capillary fragility test

———————————————— NORMAL VALUES ————————————————

Male: Less than 5 petechiae within a 2-in. circle
Female and Child: Less than 10 petechiae within a 2-in. circle

Background Information

The capillary fragility test is a procedure that gives a general estimate of the integrity or fragility of the capillary vascular tissue. When capillaries are healthy, they have effective capillary resistance. In abnormal conditions, the capillaries have increased vascular permeability and are described as fragile.

The test applies pressure on the tissue. The blood pressure cuff method applies positive pressure and the suction cup method applies negative pressure. With the application of pressure, healthy capillaries produce few petechiae or bruises. Fragile capillaries produce many petechiae or a bruise as the capillaries bleed or leak small amounts of blood.

Generally, the number of petechiae is an indicator of the severity of the vascular permeability. A large number of petechiae or a large bruise is associated with thrombocytopenia, a clotting disorder caused by too few platelets. A petechiae count of greater than 50 indicates a severe abnormality. A petechiae count of up to 20 indicates a mild to moderate abnormality.

Positive results can occur after menstruation or in postmenopausal women because of the lower estrogen level. The normal value is higher in women and children than in men. This test should not be performed on a patient with known DIC or a known bleeding disorder.

Purpose of the Test

The capillary fragility test is used to assess the fragility of the capillary walls, to evaluate spontaneous bruising or bleeding, and to identify one of the symptoms of thrombocytopenia.

Procedure

Positive Pressure Method: A sphygmomanometer cuff is placed on the upper arm and inflated to a predetermined pressure for 5 minutes. On deflation, the skin is inspected for petechiae or bruises.

Negative Pressure Method: A special suction cup is applied to the skin of the arm for 1 minute. On removal of the device, the skin is inspected for petechiae or bruises.

Findings

POSITIVE VALUES

Thrombocytopenia	Hereditary vascular abnormality
Polycythemia vera	Vitamin C deficiency
Purpura senilis	Vitamin K deficiency
DIC	von Willebrand disease
Factor VII deficiency	

Interfering Factors

- Skin that already has petechiae or bruising
- Known, active bleeding disorder

Nursing Implementation

Pretest

Ensure that the patient does not have a diagnosis of DIC or an active bleeding disorder because these conditions can result in severe bruising.

Explain the procedure to the patient.

Inspect the skin of the arms and hands for petechiae or bruises. Select the extremity that has none. There cannot be an intravenous line in this extremity.

During the Test

Apply the sphygmomanometer cuff to the upper arm. Inflate it to a pressure that is halfway between the systolic and diastolic pressures but no more than 100 mm Hg. For example, when the patient's blood pressure is 110/70, the cuff pressure is set at 90 mm Hg.

Maintain the pressure for 5 minutes and then deflate the cuff.

With the suction cup technique, apply the cup to the volar aspect of the forearm for 1 minute and then release the suction.

Posttest

After releasing the pressure, instruct the patient to open and close the hand several times to restore the circulation.

With the blood pressure method, inspect the skin for petechiae and bruises. They can cover the entire forearm and hand.

For either method, count the petechiae within a 2-in. diameter circle.

Describe the size and location of any bruises.

Record the findings in the patient's chart.

If the test is to be repeated, it should not be performed on the same arm within a 7-day period.

REFERENCES

Alvino, B.M. (1993). The hypercoagulable states. *Hospital Practice, 28,* 109–114, 119–121.

Bachman, J.A. (1991). Congenital antithrombin III, protein C and protein S deficiency: A literature review with nursing implementations. *Journal of Vascular Nursing, 9,* 17–20.

Bailes, B.K. (1992). Disseminated intravascular coagulation: Principles, treatment, nursing management. *AORN Journal, 55,* 515, 517–520, 522–529.

Berg, D.E. (1992). Components and defects of the coagulation system. *Nurse Practioner Forum, 3,* 62–71.

Burns E.R. (1990). When to suspect a bleeding disorder. *Emergency Medicine, 22,* 67–68, 70, 73.

Esparaz, B., & Green, D. (1990). Disseminated intravascular coagulation. *Critical Care Nursing Quarterly, 13,* 7–13.

Henry, J.B. (Ed.). (1991). *Clinical diagnosis and management by laboratory methods* (18th ed.). Philadelphia: W.B. Saunders.

Jacobs, D.S., et al. (Eds.). (1990). *Laboratory test handbook* (2nd ed.). Baltimore: Williams & Wilkins.

Litwack, K. (1991). Bleeding and coagulation in the PACU. *Critical Care Nursing Clinics of North America, 3,* 121–127.

Norris, M.K.G. (1992). Assessing fibrin split products. *Nursing, 22,* 29.

Peric-Knowlton, W. (1992). Acquired hypercoagulable states. *Nurse Practitioner Forum, 3,* 72–81.

Schenck, S., & Goodnight, S. (1992). Inherited hypercoagulable states: Questions and controversies. *Nurse Practitioner Forum, 3,* 82–85.

Teitz, N.W. (Ed.). (1990). *Clinical guide to laboratory tests* (2nd ed). Philadelphia: W.B. Saunders.

CHAPTER 7

Microbiologic Tests

There are numerous microorganisms that cause infection in an individual, including bacteria, viruses, fungi, and parasites. Most infectious agents are transmitted from person to person or from an environmental source to a person via an intermediate vector, such as an insect or a rodent. Additionally, many microorganisms normally reside on the skin or mucous membranes of the individual. They are considered the "normal flora" of the body. If these bacteria and other organisms enter tissue that is normally sterile, they multiply and cause an infection. Once the infection becomes established, characteristic signs appear. The signs and symptoms provide clues to the location of the infection and the possible or probable organisms that are involved.

Many microbiologic laboratory tests are used to identify the presence of a current or past infection. Serologic tests identify the activated immunologic response, the presence of the antigen, and the presence of antibodies that indicate a past or present infection of a specific type. Microscopy may be used to count the number of organisms and to identify the organism on slide preparations. A third method is to culture the specimen. Cultures are used to incubate and grow the infectious agent under controlled conditions. Once the source of infection is established in the culture medium, the organism can be examined by microscope and identified. Susceptibility or sensitivity tests are performed to determine the antibiotics or antimicrobial drugs that are effective in killing the organism.

Specimen collection is a vital part of the microbiologic testing process. Measures are taken to obtain an adequate specimen, avoid external sources of contamination, and deliver the sample to the laboratory without delay. Improper technique or failure to apply quality control measures can result in false-positive or false-negative findings.

Specimen collection and specimen handling is of particular importance for all health care workers because of the risk of transmission of infection. Hand washing and the use of latex or plastic gloves is essential. Care is taken to avoid needlestick injury. Specimen containers or tubes are closed tightly and secured before they are transported. To protect health care workers, universal precaution guidelines must be followed in handling blood and body fluids.

LABORATORY TESTS

EPSTEIN-BARR VIRUS SEROLOGY

(SERUM)

Synonym:

Epstein-Barr titer

NORMAL VALUES

Viral Capsid Antigen (VCA)–IgM:	<1:10
VCA–IgG:	<1:10
Epstein-Barr Nuclear Antigen (EBNA):	<1:5
Early Antigen (EA):	<1:10

Background Information

As presented in Table 7–1, the Epstein-Barr virus is a herpesvirus that is responsible for most cases of infectious mononucleosis. The virus infects the B

TABLE 7-1
HERPES GROUP OF VIRUSES

Virus Type	Infection
Herpes simplex	
Type 1	"Cold sores," infection of the mouth, lips, eye, skin, encephalitis (adult)
Type 2	Genital herpes, neonatal infection, encephalitis (newborn)
Epstein-Barr	Infectious mononucleosis, chronic Epstein-Barr virus infection, Burkitt lymphoma, nasopharyngeal carcinoma
Cytomegalovirus	Cytomegalovirus infectious mononucleosis, congenital infection
	In immunocompromised patients: interstitial pneumonia, gastroenteritis, retinitis
Varicella zoster	Chickenpox (varicella), shingles (herpes zoster)

---

lymphocytes and causes fever, swollen lymph glands, and an inflamed oropharynx. In the blood, there is an increase in the number of B lymphocytes and a transient rise in the heterophil antibodies. In most cases of childhood illness, the infection produces a mild upper respiratory tract illness. Infectious mononucleosis can develop in adolescents and young adults with the Epstein-Barr virus. The virus is transmitted via infected saliva.

As the body develops its immunologic response to combat the infection, antibodies are formed against several Epstein-Barr virus–specific antigens, including VCA, EBNA, and EA.

ANTIBODY FORMATION. The antibody VCA-IgM appears in the blood at an early stage of illness and remains in the blood for 1 to 2 months. The antibody VCA-IgG also appears early in the illness, but it remains in the blood for life. This antibody is the most often used test and is reported as the standard Epstein-Barr virus titer. It is the marker for current or prior infection.

There are three other Epstein-Barr–specific antibodies that form in response to viral antigen early antigen-D (EA-D), early antigen-R (EA-R), and EBNA. Epstein-Barr antibody titer may be measured in cases of acute or chronically progressive infection. In the usual pattern, acute primary infection causes an initial rise in the EA and VCA-IgM titers. With convalescence, these titers are reduced or absent, with a rise in VCA-IgG. Months later, VCA-IgG and EBNA titers rise and persist for many years or remain elevated throughout life. With chronic, progressive disease, all antibody titers remain elevated.

Several of the Epstein-Barr antibody titers also are elevated in certain malignant disorders, but a tissue biopsy must confirm the presence of malignancy. Previously, an elevated Epstein-Barr antibody titer was used to help diagnose chronic fatigue syndrome, but it is now known that there is poor correlation of these tests with the chronic fatigue syndrome because of poor specificity and sensitivity of the tests (Jacobs, 1990).

Purpose of the Tests

These serologic tests are used to diagnose Epstein-Barr viral infection in patients with infectious mononucleosis in whom heterophil antibody titers are negative.

Procedure

A red-topped tube is used to collect 10 ml of venous blood.

Findings

ELEVATED VALUES

Infectious mononucleosis
Nasopharyngeal cancer

Burkitt lymphoma
Hodgkin disease

Interfering Factors

* None

Nursing Implementation

Pretest

Schedule this test to be performed at the onset of illness and again after 2 to 3 weeks. This provides data during the periods of acute and convalescent phases of illness.

Posttest

On the requisition slip, write the date of the onset of illness.
Arrange for prompt transport of the specimen to the laboratory.

QUALITY CONTROL

In the laboratory, the serum must be frozen if the specimen is not tested promptly.

HERPESVIRUS ANTIGEN, DIRECT FLUORESCENT ANTIBODY

(CELL SCRAPINGS)

Synonyms:

─────────────── **NORMAL VALUES** ───────────────

Negative

Background Information

In the herpes family of viruses, there are several types that cause different infections. As seen in Table 7–1, the virus types include herpes simplex, types 1 and 2, Epstein-Barr virus, cytomegalovirus, and varicella zoster.

The herpes simplex virus (HSV) infection is caused by one of two viral types. In general, type 1 causes characteristic lesions in and around the mouth, and type 2 causes lesions of the genitalia. Type 1 virus can also cause HSV encephalitis in adults, and type 2 HSV infection can cause disseminated HSV neonatal disease. Once there has been a primary infection, the individual is a carrier of the virus, and antibodies are present throughout life.

Using immunofluorescence methodology, the antigen of HSV can be detected in cell preparations and inflammatory exudate. Using specific antibodies, the two serotypes of HSV can be differentiated. Possible tissue sources include scrapings of a lesion or vesicle from the conjunctiva, throat, bronchus, or genitalia. Tissue biopsy or spinal fluid can also be used.

Although this test is not as sensitive as a viral culture, it is faster. It takes 24 hours to obtain this test result and several days to obtain culture results. Because of the rapid results, this test is used in urgent situations such as when there is brain involvement or when chemotherapy must be started and a herpes infection could erupt as the patient becomes immunocompromised.

Purpose of the Test

The herpesvirus antigen direct fluorescent antibody test identifies herpes simplex virus type 1 or type 2.

Procedure

A sterile swab is used to collect cells and secretions from the base of a fresh ulcerated eruption. The specimen is then placed in a sterile culture tube. Universal precautions are used in the presence of an open, weeping lesion.

Findings

POSITIVE VALUES
Herpes simplex virus type 1 (HSV-1)
Herpes simplex virus type 2 (HSV-2)

Interfering Factors

- Delay in the analysis of the specimen
- Use of a fixative in the culture tube

Nursing Implementation

Pretest

If an operative biopsy specimen or spinal fluid specimen is obtained, it must be processed immediately. Notify the laboratory beforehand when the specimen is to be analyzed for immunofluorescence.

During the Test

Do not mix a fixative with the specimen in the tube.
Label the culture tube and requisition slip with the patient's identification data and the tissue source of the specimen.

Posttest

Arrange for prompt transport of the specimen to the laboratory.

QUALITY CONTROL
The analysis must be performed on a fresh or frozen specimen.

HISTOPLASMOSIS SEROLOGY

(SERUM)

Synonyms:

--- **NORMAL VALUES** ---

Complement Fixation titer:	<1:4
Immunodiffusion Test:	negative

Background Information

Histoplasmosis is a fungal disease caused by the *Histoplasma capsulatum* organism. The histoplasmosis infection results from the inhalation of spore-laden dust that is in the infected excreta of birds, bats, chickens, or turkeys. In the acute form, the spores usually cause pulmonary infection. The infection can also become chronic in the lungs and chest or disseminated in the reticuloendothelial system or any organ of the body.

The *complement fixation test* is used to diagnose all forms of the disease. A complement fixation titer of greater than or equal to 1:8 to 1:16 is highly suspicious of infection. A higher titer (>1:32) is even more indicative of infection in an active state. In follow-up testing, a rising titer indicates the progression of infection, and a decreasing titer indicates a regression of the infection.

The *immunodiffusion test* demonstrates M and H bands as an indication of infection. The M band alone indicates early or chronic infection. The presence of an H band also indicates active infection. The immunodiffusion test may be used as a screening tool or as a supplement to the complement fixation test.

Purpose of the Test

These serologic tests are used to help diagnose histoplasmosis and to monitor the response to therapy.

Procedure

A red-topped tube is used to collect 7 ml of venous blood.

Findings

ELEVATED VALUES
Histoplasmosis

Interfering Factors

- A recent skin test for histoplasmosis

Nursing Implementation

Pretest

Plan to obtain the first blood tests early in the infectious process and before the histoplasmosis skin test is performed. A recent skin test can cause a positive serologic result in 20% of patients (Teitz, 1990).

Posttest

Schedule repeat blood tests in 2 to 3 weeks to elevate the convalescent phase of the infection.

HUMAN IMMUNODEFICIENCY VIRUS SEROLOGY

(SERUM)

Synonyms:

human immunodeficiency virus (HIV) serology tests, acquired immune deficiency syndrome serology, AIDS serology, AIDS screen

────────────── **NORMAL VALUES** ──────────────

No human immunodeficiency virus (HIV)-antigens or antibodies are demonstrated

Background Information

HIV is from the retrovirus family of RNA viruses. Retrovirus behavior involves viral invasion of the RNA material into the nucleus of the host's cells, with a resultant reversal of the flow of genetic information. The retrovirus stores its instructions in the host's RNA and manufactures new, defective DNA material. The damaged DNA becomes incorporated into the host's DNA, and new cells that contain the virus are slowly but continuously manufactured.

The HIV retrovirus invades and infects the helper T (T4) lymphocytes, B lymphocytes, monocytes, and macrophage cells. This results in lysis of the infected cells and loss of the body's immune defenses. Once the immune system collapses or is compromised by the HIV infection, the person is susceptible to opportunistic infection, cancer, and neurologic disorders. There is growing evidence that the number of infected cells is much greater in the lymphatic system, central nervous system, and lungs than in the peripheral blood (Lebeck and Lewis, 1992).

HIV has a characteristic, identifiable structure (Fig. 7–1). The proteins (p) and glycoproteins (gp) that make up the structure of the virus are the target antigens

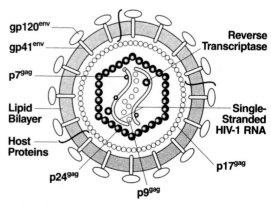

FIGURE 7–1. Basic structure of the human immunodeficiency virus. (With permission from Sande, M.A., & Volberding, P.A. [1995]. *The medical management of AIDS* [4th ed., p. 24]. Philadelphia: W.B. Saunders.)

used in the HIV antigen and antibody tests. Within 7 to 10 days after infection is initiated, the HIV antigen can be identified in the blood. This initial response disappears within 2 weeks, as p24 (core) antibody and gp41 (envelope) antibody emerge. The p24 antibody disappears within several weeks, and the gp41 antibody persists at an elevated level. Months to years later, HIV antigen may reappear in the blood before the development of the acquired immunodeficiency syndrome (AIDS).

The diagnosis of HIV infection is carried out by testing for viral markers. Some tests detect specific antibodies that are present in response to the antigen. The newer tests detect either the antigen or the virus itself, thus identifying the presence of the virus in the asymptomatic person.

HUMAN IMMUNODEFICIENCY VIRUS ANTIBODY TESTS. There are a number of tests that use the enzyme immunoassay (EIA) method to detect antibodies to HIV antigen in the patient's serum. HIV antibody tests are used to screen blood donors, applicants for life insurance, and individuals entering the armed forces. Antibody testing is also used to test other individuals, but they must give consent for the blood test (Henry and Campbell, 1992).

EIA or enzyme-linked immunosorbent assay (ELISA)-methodology is widely used to detect HIV antibodies, and test results are available in 2 to 4 days (Farzadegan, 1994). When the results are positive, the patient's antibodies bind to the HIV antigen that is in the test reagent, and there is a subsequent development of color in the solution. Positive results are verified with repeat testing by the EIA method or by additional testing with an alternate method such as Western blot, indirect immunofluorescence, or radioimmune precipitation.

The Western blot test demonstrates antibodies to specific viral proteins (Fig. 7–2). In this procedure, the different viral proteins and glycoproteins of the test reagent are separated electrophoretically. The patient's serum is placed over each of the antigens. If antibodies are present in the serum, they will bind to the test antigens. When radiolabeled proteins are used, the antigen-antibody complexes can be visualized radiographically. The formation of various bands of the viral proteins is considered a positive result because the bands confirm the presence of specific HIV antibodies in the patient's blood. When only one band is present, the test is repeated in 6 months. Because the Western blot test is technically difficult and expensive, it is used to confirm a positive ELISA test. Western blot test results are available in 1 to 2 weeks.

HUMAN IMMUNODEFICIENCY VIRUS ANTIGEN TESTS. There are new EIA tests that directly detect the presence of viral proteins in the serum. The HIV antigen tests detect p24 core antigen in the early stage of acute infection, before there is an antibody response. These tests are used as a screening tool in patients who are at high risk and are asymptomatic at the time of testing (Lebeck and Lewis, 1992).

POLYMERASE CHAIN REACTION VIRAL GENOME TEST. The polymerase chain reaction (PCR) is a new technique used to diagnose a very early stage of HIV infection. It detects the viral HIV-DNA molecules in the nuclei of monocytes from the peripheral blood (Ferre, 1994). The PCR is used to identify the infected DNA in the patient in whom antibodies have not yet developed. It also helps

Critical Thinking: The patient has a positive HIV antibody test. After he has been told of the result, he acts bewildered and cannot believe that it is true. How would you respond to him at this time?

Critical Thinking: It takes weeks to months after exposure before an HIV infection can be detected by antibody or antigen test. The PCR test can identify the HIV-DNA molecules at an earlier time. Should the more costly PCR test be used to screen the high-risk patients and the blood supply?

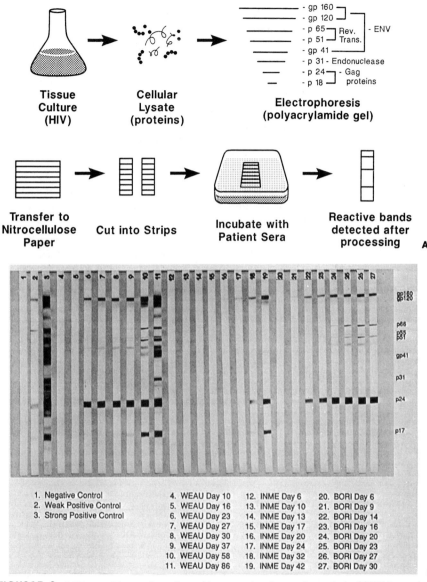

FIGURE 7–2. *A,* Western blot test is performed by separating tissue culture–derived HIV-1 proteins (p) and glycoproteins (gp) via polyacrylamide gel electrophoresis, transferring (blotting) the separated proteins onto nitrocellulose paper, incubating the cut strips of nitrocellulose paper with patient serum, and detecting anti-HIV antibodies that have bound to the HIV-1–associated proteins at the precise point at which they migrated in the gel. Through this procedure, the antibody reactivity against specific antigens can be determined (e.g., anti-Gag, anti-Env, or antiendonuclease antibodies). *B,* Examples of Western blot tests from three patients (*WEAU, BORI,* and *INME*) identified at the time of acute HIV-1 infection (seroconversion). Each lane represents a time point (in days) from the time of presentation with symptomatic acute HIV-1 disease or a positive or negative control (lanes 1 to 3). (With permission from Sande, M.A., & Volberding, P.A. [1995]. *The medical management of AIDS* [4th ed., p. 71]. Philadelphia: W.B. Saunders.)

quantify or measure the amount of virus or viral load that the patient has (Lebeck and Lewis, 1992).

T4:T8 RATIO. Once AIDS develops, the T4:T8 ratio is used to help measure the severity of the disease. T4 cells (helper T lymphocytes) and T8 cells (suppressor T lymphocytes) are part of the immune system defense against infection. In AIDS infection, the T4:T8 ratio is less than 1, indicating that the T4 cell count is severely reduced. When the T4 count is less than 300 cells/mm^3, azathioprine (AZT) therapy may be started. This test does not diagnose AIDS but is used to measure the severity of the illness.

Purpose of the Tests

The HIV serologic tests are used to diagnose current or latent infection, to screen the blood donated for transfusion purposes, and to monitor progression of the disease.

Procedure

For each test, a red-topped tube is used to collect 7 ml of venous blood.

QUALITY CONTROL

With venipuncture, the tourniquet should be tied lightly for a brief time to prevent pooling of cells in the vein at the site of blood collection. Venipuncture technique must be smooth, with a blood flow that fills the vacuum tube readily. If the blood has excessive turbulence because of flawed venipuncture technique, the hemolysis of the erythrocytes will alter the test results.

Findings

POSITIVE VALUES
Antigen tests: HIV infection
Antibody tests: HIV infection

DECREASED VALUES
T4:T8 ratio: AIDS

Interfering Factors

• Hemolysis

Nursing Implementation

Pretest

Many states have requirements to preserve confidentiality of results. An informed consent is often required before the test can be performed.

Posttest

A positive EIA (ELISA) antibody screen requires repeat testing or confirmation (or both) by a Western blot or alternate antibody test. A positive Western blot antibody test result or a positive antigen test result means that the patient is infected with, and is a carrier of, HIV. AIDS is likely to develop sometime in the future.

For the patient with positive blood tests:

1. Inform the patient that he or she cannot donate blood.

2. Explain that safe sex practices or abstaining from sexual intercourse will help prevent transmission of the infection.

3. Instruct that intravenous needles must not be shared.

4. Instruct the patient to continue with regular periodic examinations and follow-up laboratory testing. In addition, the obstetrician of the pregnant female patient should be informed of the positive test results. The virus can be transmitted from the infected mother to the fetus.

5. Teach the patient to seek health care assistance for symptoms of AIDS, including recurrent respiratory or skin infections, fatigue, diarrhea, weight loss, fever, or lymphadenopathy, or a combination of these conditions.

INFECTIOUS MONONUCLEOSIS TESTS

(SERUM)

Synonyms:

monotest, monoscreen, slide test, spot test, heterophil antibody test

---

NORMAL VALUES

Monotest: negative, nonreactive
Heterophil Titer: <1:56

Background Information

The Epstein-Barr virus is a herpesvirus that is responsible for most cases of infectious mononucleosis. This viral infection involves the reticuloendothelial system, including B lymphocytes, lymphoid tissues, and epithelial tissues of the oropharynx. Once there is infection by the virus, the immune response produces a rise in heterophil antibodies of the IgM class and a rise in Epstein-Barr antibodies. In most patients, the heterophil antibodies begin to rise in the prodromal period, 1 to 2 days before symptoms appear. There is a measurable presence of the heterophil antibodies 6 to 10 days after the symptoms appear. The level peaks in 2 to 3 weeks and persists 4 to 8 weeks to 1 year later.

The monotest detects the presence of heterophil antibodies. The sample of the patient's serum is mixed with horse erythrocytes. When the heterophil antibodies of infectious mononucleosis are present, the antibodies bind to the antigen of the horse cells. With the visible agglutination or clumping that results from the antigen-antibody reaction, the test result is positive (Smalley, 1990). The monotest is a rapid, simple, and effective test that identifies the source of infection. If the titer is to be measured, the heterophil titer test is used. If the heterophil titer is greater than or equal to 1:128, the test result is positive.

About 10% of patients who have infectious mononucleosis have a false-negative result on the Monospot and heterophil agglutination tests. These patients may be tested for the Epstein-Barr virus, cytomegalovirus, and toxoplasmosis antibodies to determine the specific diagnosis. Additionally, there are a small number of cases that produce a false-positive result on the monotest. The causes of a false-positive test result include Hodgkin disease, lymphoma, acute lymphocytic leukemia, infectious hepatitis, pancreatic cancer, rheumatoid arthritis, measles, cytomegalovirus, and malaria.

Purpose of the Test

These serologic tests help to diagnose infectious mononucleosis.

Procedure

A clotted red-topped tube is used to collect 7 ml of venous blood.

QUALITY CONTROL

With venipuncture, the tourniquet should be tied lightly for a brief time to prevent pooling of cells in the vein at the site of blood collection. Venipuncture technique must be smooth, with a blood flow that fills the vacuum tube readily. If the blood has excessive turbulence because of flawed venipuncture technique, the hemolysis of the erythrocytes will alter the test results.

Findings

POSITIVE VALUES
Infectious mononucleosis

Interfering Factors

• Hemolysis

Nursing Implementation

Pretest

Schedule this test a few days after the onset of illness.

A very early test result can remain negative until antibodies have time to develop.

Posttest

On the requisition slip, include the date of the onset of illness.
Arrange for prompt transport of the blood to the laboratory.

METHYLENE BLUE STAIN

(FECES)

Synonyms:

fecal leukocyte stain; Gram stain, stool; stool for white cells; white cells, stool; Wright stain, stool

---

NORMAL VALUES

No presence of polymorphonuclear leukocytes in the fecal matter

---

Background Information

Intestinal bacterial infection can cause the abrupt onset of severe diarrhea, sometimes accompanied by the passage of blood and mucus in the feces. When the bacteria are invasive, they cause the release of polymorphonuclear leukocytes from the injured intestinal tissue. These white cells are released into the lumen of the intestine and are present in the feces. A fecal smear, stained with methylene blue, Gram stain, or Wright stain, reveals the presence and quantity of leukocytes in the stool.

Leukocytes are usually present in diarrheal infection that is caused by invasive bacteria including *Salmonella*, *Shigella*, *Campylobacter*, and *Yersinia*. Leukocytes usually are absent in diarrheal infection caused by the toxigenic bacteria *Escherichia coli*, *Vibrio cholerae*, and *Clostridium difficile*.

Purpose of the Test

Methylene blue staining of a fecal smear is a rapid but nonspecific screening test that helps differentiate among the many causes of acute diarrhea and helps determine the need for a follow-up stool culture.

Procedure

About 2 gm of fresh stool and mucus is placed in a clean, plastic container with a lid. Although it is a less preferable alternative, a rectal swab may be used to obtain some fecal matter from the rectum (see also Chapter 2, Collection Measures).

Findings

ELEVATED VALUES
Infection with
Campylobacter
Yersinia
Shigella
Salmonella
Antibiotic-associated colitis
Ulcerative colitis
Amebiasis

Interfering Factors

- Barium in the fecal specimen
- Insufficient volume of fecal matter
- Delay or cooling of the specimen

Nursing Implementation

Pretest

Obtain the stool specimen before any barium studies are performed.
Wear gloves to obtain a fresh random stool sample.

Posttest

Place the lid securely on the collection container, discard gloves, and wash hands.
Send the specimen to the laboratory without delay. Do not refrigerate the specimen.

| QUALITY CONTROL |
Prolonged storage and cooling cause deterioration of the leukocytes and invalidate the test.

OVA AND PARASITES

(FECES)

Synonyms:

parasites, stool; parasitology examination; stool for ova and parasites; stool for O and P

━━━━━━━━━━━━━━━━━━━━━ **NORMAL VALUES** ━━━━━━━━━━━━━━━━━━━━━

No parasites or ova are found in the feces

Background Information

Numerous parasites can infect individuals and then live in the human intestinal tract during part of the parasitic life cycle. Many ova, cysts, larvae, or spores from fecal-contaminated soil enter the person via a fecal-oral route. As these forms of the parasite reach the intestine, they mature to the adult stage of development and deposit new ova into the patient's intestinal tract.

Common methods of transmission are from unwashed hands, eating contaminated raw fruits and vegetables, and drinking from a fecal-contaminated water supply. Some intestinal parasites, such as *Schistosoma* and hookworm, invade the body through the skin and then migrate through body tissue to the intestinal lumen. Others, including tapeworm and flukes, are transmitted by eating undercooked meat, raw fish, or plants that are contaminated by the parasite.

As seen in Table 7–2, protozoa, nematodes, trematodes, and cestodes reside in different parts of the intestinal tract and have different methods of attachment or degree of tissue invasion. Some lodge primarily in the intestinal tract; others are in the intestinal tract for part of the time but also migrate to other body cavities or organs.

The schedule and procedure for stool collection is based on the type of parasite infection that is suspected. Because of the distinct life cycle of each species, the ova may or may not be present in the intestine at a particular time. Additionally, some species deposit many ova each day and others deposit only a few at a time. Traditionally, the method of collection of fecal samples is to obtain three specimens on different days (Henry, 1991). This maximizes the chance of identification of the ova in at least one of the samples. Newer trends suggest obtaining one sample and awaiting the results before ordering additional tests. At times, multiple samples are indicated, but there is some question as to the number of specimens and the time interval for their collection (Proctor, 1991; Issac-Renton, 1991).

Using microscopic examination of the feces, the specific parasite is identified by the presence of its ova, larvae, trophozoites, cysts, or oocysts. In some cases, the egg count per gram of feces helps to determine the intensity of infection. Additionally, a patient may be infected with more than one parasite.

Purpose of the Test

The microscopic examination of the feces is used to identify the presence of specific parasites in the intestinal tract.

TABLE 7–2
GASTROINTESTINAL LOCATION OF PARASITES

Name	Anatomic Sites	Characteristics of Residence
Protozoa (Unicellular Parasites)		
Giardia lamblia	Small bowel	Mucosal attachment
Entamoeba histolytica	Colon, rectum	Lumen dweller, mucosal invasion
Balantidium coli	Colon, rectum	Lumen dweller, mucosal invasion
Isospora belli	Small bowel	Epithelial cell invasion
Dientamoeba fragilis	Small bowel, colon	Lumen dweller, mucosal invasion
Sarcocystis spp.	Small bowel	Epithelial cell invasion
Trypanosoma cruzi*	Esophagus, colon	Smooth muscle cells and autonomic nerve plexuses
Cryptosporidium parvum	Small bowel	Epithelial cell invasion
Nematodes (Roundworms)		
Trichuris trichiura	Colon	Mucosal attachment
Ascaris lumbricoides	Small bowel	Lumen dweller
Ancylostoma (hookworm)	Small bowel	Mucosal attachment
Strongyloides stercoralis	Small bowel	Mucosal invasion
Trichostrongylus	Small bowel	Mucosal invasion
Enterobius vermicularis (threadworm)	Colon, rectum	Lumen dweller
Oesophagostomium*	Cecum	Mucosal invasion
Anisakis*	Stomach, small bowel	Mucosal invasion
Ternidens	Ileocecal region	Mucosal attachment and invasion
Capillaria philippinensis	Small bowel	Mucosal invasion
Trematodes (Flukes)		
Opisthorchis (clonorchis)	Duodenum	Lumen dweller, epithelial attachment
Schistosoma spp.	Ileum, colon	Mesenteric veins, gut wall, mucosa, lumen
Fasciola hepatica	Small bowel	Mucosal attachment
Gastrocoides hominis	Colon	Mucosal attachment
Paragonimus westermani*	Small bowel, abdominal cavity, peritoneum	Peritoneal lesions
Echinostoma spp.	Small bowel	Mucosal attachment
Cestodes (Tapeworms)		
Hymenolepsis nana	Small bowel	Mucosal attachment
Taenia spp.	Small bowel	Mucosal attachment
Diphyllobothrium latum	Small bowel	Mucosal attachment
Dipylidium caninum	Small bowel	Mucosal attachment

*These parasites are not diagnosed by fecal examination.

Procedure

Critical Thinking: The nurse is assigned to obtain one stool sample from each of the 30 children in the kindergarten class and to send the samples to the laboratory. How can the nurse organize the project and obtain the cooperation of the parents?

Stool Collection: Collect a small sample of feces directly into a clean, wide-mouthed container and close the lid. A common requirement is to collect one specimen each day for 3 days.

Perianal Swab: Transparent tape is placed on a tongue depressor, sticky side out. Press the tape firmly on the perianal skin. Remove the tape and place it on a glass slide, sticky side down.

Findings

POSITIVE VALUES

Amebiasis

Giardiasis

Cryptosporidiosis

Tapeworm

Ascariasis

Hookworm

Pinworm

Others (see Table 7–2)

Interfering Factors

- Antibiotic therapy in the 3- to 4-week pretest period
- Soil, water, or urine contamination of the sample
- Barium sulfate administration in the 2- to 3-week pretest period
- Mineral oil, castor oil, antacids, or antidiarrheal medication in the week before the test

Nursing Implementation

Pretest

Schedule this test prior to any barium studies because the barium obscures the microscopic visualization of the ova.

Instruct the patient regarding correct collection procedure (see also Chapter 2). The feces should not be removed from the toilet bowl.

QUALITY CONTROL

The specimen must be free of contact with water or urine because these liquids will kill any trophozoites that are present. The specimen must also be free of soil contamination because amebae and other parasites of the soil will contaminate the specimen (Proctor, 1991).

Posttest

Place the lid on the specimen container. Remove gloves and wash your hands thoroughly.

QUALITY CONTROL

Intestinal parasites are a highly transmissible source of infection via the fecal-oral route or via contact with the skin. Precautions are taken to prevent self-inoculation from poor hygiene practices.

Include the time and date of the collection on the laboratory slip and the container. Send the specimen to the laboratory immediately because the examination of the specimen must begin within 30 to 60 minutes.

QUALITY CONTROL

Time delay and exposure to heat or cold temperatures will result in the death of trophozoites and cysts.

OVA AND PARASITES

(URINE)

Synonyms:

parasites, urine; urine for parasites; urine for *Schistosoma haematobium*

NORMAL VALUES

No ova or parasites are identified.

Background Information

Schistosoma haematobium, a parasitic fluke, dwells in fecal-contaminated water. It penetrates the skin of the person who comes into contact with the infective stage of the parasite during bathing or swimming in the polluted water. There are four species of *Schistosoma*, but the migration in the body and final destination of *S. haematobium* is somewhat different from that of the others. This difference is the basis for a different method of specimen collection for diagnostic testing.

After penetration of the skin and migration to the lungs, all species of developing *Schistosoma* migrate to the portal vein and mesenteric veins. Three species of *Schistosoma* penetrate the intestinal wall and deposit ova in the lumen of the gastrointestinal tract. *S. haematobium* continues the vascular migration downward into the inferior mesenteric veins that surround the bladder and urethra. The female flukes deposit ova that penetrate the bladder wall and pass into the urine.

Trichomonas vaginalis and *Enterobius vermicularis* are other parasites that may be present in the urine. In the infected human female, the ova of *T. vaginalis* are located in the vagina and endocervix but may pass into the bladder and urine by localized contamination. In the human male, the *T. vaginalis* ova are located primarily in the urethra and exit from the body in the urine. The ova of the intestinal parasite *E. vermicularis* are deposited in the perianal area by the adult female. The ova enter the urinary tract through fecal contamination of the urinary meatus or by local migration of the gravid female parasite into the urinary tract.

Purpose of the Test

The urine is examined to detect the presence of the ova of *S. haematobium* and *T. vaginalis.*

Procedure

Daily urine specimens are obtained for 2 to 3 consecutive days.

Findings

POSITIVE VALUES
Schistosomiasis
Trichomoniasis
Enterobiasis

Interfering Factors

- Refrigeration of the specimen
- Delay in transport of the specimen to the laboratory

Nursing Implementation

Pretest

Instruct the patient to use clean, dry containers to collect a specimen of urine each day for 2 to 3 days. When *S. haematobium* is suspected, instruct the patient to collect the urine at about noon each day. Additionally, the desired sample of the urine is collected toward the end of micturition. For unknown reasons, the ova deposits are heaviest at midday and are released in the greatest quantity in the terminal portion of the urinary stream.

Posttest

Wash the hands thoroughly after removing gloves or handling the urinary container.

┌───┐
│ **QUALITY CONTROL**   │
└───┘
Parasites are highly infectious. The ova of *Schistosoma* burrow through the skin, and *Enterobius* is transmitted via a fecal-oral route.

Arrange for transport of each specimen to the laboratory within 3 to 4 hours after collection. Do not refrigerate the specimen.

┌───┐
│ **QUALITY CONTROL**   │
└───┘
When urine is cold or old, the yield of *Schistosoma* is reduced.

PARASITE CULTURE

(FECES)

Synonym:

stool culture for parasites

─────────────────────────── **NORMAL VALUES** ───────────────────────────

┌───┐
│ No parasites or their ova are present in the fecal culture.   │
└───┘

Background Information

Many protozoa and helminths can live in the intestinal tract for part of the parasitic life cycle. Normally, the microscopic examination of the feces for ova and parasites is the best and easiest method for detection and identification of parasitic infection. Sometimes, however, the parasitic infection is light. The ova remain elusive and undetected by routine microscopic analysis.

The stool sample can be cultured until the parasites and ova mature and multiply. Then there are sufficient numbers that the ova can be located and identified. Only some of the parasites can yield positive results by stool culture method.

Purpose of the Test

This test detects light intestinal parasitic infections caused by amebae, nematodes, and schistosomes.

Procedure

A clean container with a tightly covered lid is used to collect about 2 gm of fresh feces from a random stool. In most instances, three stool samples are required—one each day or one every other day (Proctor, 1991).

Findings

POSITIVE VALUES

Amebiasis
Entamoeba histolytica
Giardia lamblia
Schistosoma spp.

Ancylostoma (hookworm)
Strongyloides stercoralis
Trichostrongylus

Interfering Factors

- Barium administration
- Antibiotic or antiamebic medication
- Intestinal medications: bismuth, Metamucil, castor oil
- Refrigeration or delay in transport of the specimen

Nursing Implementation

Pretest

The stool culture must be obtained before the patient has any barium studies performed.

Instruct the patient to discontinue antibiotics, antihelminthics, and intestinal medications for 1 week before the fecal specimens are collected. These medications reduce the yield of ova or interfere with the microscopic view of the culture medium.

Teach the patient to evacuate a small sample of the feces into a clean, dry container and then secure the container lid. If the patient requires assistance, use gloves to collect the specimen and wash your hands immediately after removal of gloves.

QUALITY CONTROL

Intestinal parasites are highly infectious. Some are transmitted by fecal-oral spread and others by contact with the skin. Self-inoculation can be prevented by effective hygiene measures.

The fecal samples must not be contaminated by water, urine, or soil. The trophozoites of amebae are destroyed by water and urine. The soil introduces a new source of contaminants to the culture specimens.

Posttest

Place the date and time of the specimen collection on each laboratory slip and container. Do not refrigerate the specimen. Arrange for prompt transport of the specimen to the laboratory (within 2 hours).

> **QUALITY CONTROL**
>
> The yield of trophozoites and other ova will be reduced by cooling or a time delay before the laboratory culture is started.

ROTAVIRUS, DIRECT EXAMINATION BY ENZYME IMMUNOASSAY

(FECES)

Synonyms:

rotavirus EIA; rotavirus, direct examination; EIA

━━━━━━━━━━━━━━━━ **NORMAL VALUES** ━━━━━━━━━━━━━━━━

No virus detected

Background Information

The rotavirus causes acute gastroenteritis with vomiting, dehydration, and moderate to severe diarrhea. This viral infection tends to affect infant and toddler age groups, particularly in the winter months.

The virus is maximally present in the feces during the first 3 days of illness. The shedding of the virus then gradually decreases until only minimal amounts are present in the feces by the eighth day of illness.

The virus cannot be cultured in vitro. The best method of identification of the rotavirus is by examination of the feces by EIA or radioimmunoassay. It is also possible to examine this virus by electron microscopy, but most laboratories do not have the equipment. If electron microscopic examination for enteroviruses is requested, the procedure and nursing implementation are the same as described for this test.

Purpose of the Test

This test identifies the rotavirus in feces of patients in whom a viral cause of gastroenteritis is suspected.

Procedure

A sterile container is used to collect a random sample of diarrheal fecal matter. The timing of the collection is early in the course of illness or within 3 to 5 days after the onset of diarrhea. More than one specimen may be required to reduce the possibility of a false-negative result.

Findings

POSITIVE VALUES
Rotavirus infection
Viral gastroenteritis

Interfering Factors

• Delay in transport of the specimen
• Warming of the specimen

Nursing Implementation

Pretest

Since this virus is easily transmitted, use gloves when collecting the specimen.

Collect a small amount (4 to 8 gm) of diarrheal stool in a sterile collection container or tube. A sterile tongue blade may be used to help in the collection.

Posttest

Close the container with the appropriate lid or stopper. After removing the gloves, wash your hands immediately.

Appropriately label the laboratory requisition slip and specimen container, including the time and date of the collection.

Arrange for immediate transport of the specimen to the laboratory.

QUALITY CONTROL

Excessive delay contributes to warming and drying of the specimen, with a resultant loss of virion particles. If there is delay in the laboratory, the specimen must be cooled to −70° C to preserve the virion.

STOOL CULTURE

(FECES)

Synonym:
stool culture for enteric pathogens

NORMAL VALUES

Negative for *Campylobacter, Salmonella,* and *Shigella*

Background Information

Stool culture may be used when the patient experiences severe, persistent or recurrent bloody diarrhea, with fever and tenesmus. There may be a history of travel to a developing country, a recent dietary intake of seafood, or exposure to a known bacterial agent.

The diarrhea is usually associated with one of three syndromes and indicates infection in a specific anatomic location. *Gastroenteritis* affects the stomach and causes vomiting. *Enteritis* affects the small bowel and causes fewer episodes of diarrhea. The fecal matter is profuse and very watery. *Dysentery* or *colitis* affects the colon and causes many episodes of diarrhea. The volume of fecal matter is small and it is mixed with blood, mucus, and leukocytes.

Once the fecal specimen is brought to the laboratory, samples of the feces are inoculated into several types of culture media. Under incubation, enteric pathogens grow and multiply while routine enteric pathogens are inhibited from growth. Routine microscopic examination is performed in 18 to 24 hours. When culture growth is negative, a final report is completed within 48 hours. When culture growth is positive, it will take several days to continue testing and identification of the microorganism.

In standard methodology, stool culture identifies *Salmonella* spp., *Shigella* spp., and *Campylobacter* spp. If specified on the requisition slip, other bacterial pathogens also can be identified by stool culture, including *Staphylococcus aureus*, *Clostridium difficile*, *Yersinia* spp., and *Vibrio* spp.

Stool culture is expensive, particularly when several days of testing are required to yield positive test results (Jacobs et al., 1990). As a preliminary test, methylene blue staining of stool may be used to identify bacterial diarrhea and indicate the need for stool culture.

Purpose of the Test

Critical Thinking: The patient has profound diarrhea, and a stool culture has been ordered. What other assessments of the stool are indicated?

The stool culture is used to identify the bacterial organism that causes intestinal infection.

Procedure

Random Stool Method: A small amount of freshly passed feces is placed directly into a clean, dry container.

Rectal Swab Method: The swab is inserted past the anal sphincter and into the rectum. The swab is gently rotated around the canal. To attain maximum absorption, the swab is kept in place for 15 to 20 seconds before it is withdrawn. Once the swab is placed in the culturette tube, the media compartment is crushed to moisten the specimen.

Findings

POSITIVE VALUES

Shigellosis

Enteric fever

Salmonella infection

Acute gastroenteritis

Cholera

Typhoid fever

Bacillary dysentery

Food poisoning

Infant botulism

Interfering Factors

- Contamination of the specimen with urine, detergent, or soap
- Improper technique of specimen collection
- Refrigeration or delay in transport of the specimen
- Antibiotic therapy

Nursing Implementation

Pretest

Obtain the specimen before any antibiotic therapy is started.

Instruct the patient to evacuate a small amount of feces directly into the container. If a bedpan is used, it must be rinsed with water and dried thoroughly before use. No urine can be mixed with the feces.

QUALITY CONTROL

Urine, soap, detergent, and drying of the specimen act to destroy the bacteria before they can be cultured.

Posttest

Use gloves to handle the open container or culturette until it is sealed. Remove gloves and wash hands thoroughly.

QUALITY CONTROL

The bacteria are highly transmissible via a fecal-oral route.

Arrange for direct transport of the specimen to the laboratory without delay. If a delay of more than 2 to 3 hours is anticipated, the specimen should be placed in a laboratory-determined type of transport medium to maintain a moist environment.

┌───┐
│ **QUALITY CONTROL**   │
└───┘

Refrigeration of the specimen may be necessary when there is a delay in transport for more than 2 to 3 hours. Cooling, however, will make the feces more acidic and destroy the *Shigella* spp.

SYPHILIS SEROLOGY

(SERUM)

Synonyms:

Venereal Disease Research Laboratory Test (VDRL), rapid plasma reagin (RPR), fluorescent treponemal antibody absorption test (FTA-ABS), micro-hemagglutination–*Treponema pallidum* (MHA-TP)

──────────────── **NORMAL VALUES** ────────────────

┌───┐
│ Negative; nonreactive   │
└───┘

Background Information

Treponema pallidum is the spirochete that causes syphilis. The spirochete is usually transmitted as the result of sexual contact with an infected partner. In addition, a pregnant woman with primary or secondary stage syphilis can also transmit the spirochete to her fetus.

Syphilis in the primary stage causes a chancre or ulcerated lesion on the external genitals or cervix or in the vagina. It can also appear on the anus or any other mucosal or nonmucosal surface. In the secondary stage, the spirochete has become systemic. There is a skin rash, and the central nervous system, bones, eyes, and liver may be involved. In the latent phase, there are no clinical complaints. If the infection proceeds to the tertiary stage, the patient develops granulomatous inflammation, called gummas, in the organs and tissues of the body. There is also spirochete damage to the cardiovascular system and brain.

There are several laboratory tests that can be used to detect antibodies produced in response to the infection. Each blood test has distinct advantages and disadvantages at the various phases of the disease. The Venereal Disease Research Laboratory (VDRL), rapid plasma reagin (RPR), and automated reagin test (ART) are reagin tests that are used to screen for the disease and monitor the response to treatment. The fluorescent treponemal antibody absorption test (FTA-ABS) and microhemagglutination assay–*Treponema pallidum* (MHA-TP) are specific antibody tests that are used to confirm the diagnosis. The results are reported as reactive, weakly reactive, or nonreactive.

VENEREAL DISEASE RESEARCH LABORATORY TEST. The VDRL is an effective screening test for syphilis. In most cases, the blood becomes reactive 1 to 3 weeks after the chancre appears. It is 100% reactive in the secondary phase and remains reactive in most cases of latent syphilis. The VDRL may convert back to a nonreactive state in tertiary or late stage syphilis. VDRL results are negative or nonreactive after effective treatment has eradicated the spirochete.

This test may also be performed on a sample of cerebrospinal fluid to assess for neurosyphilis. The VDRL testing of the spinal fluid is very specific but not very sensitive. It will identify only 25 to 40% of patients who have central nervous system syphilis (Edelstein, 1994).

There are a number of nontreponemal diseases that can cause a false-positive VDRL blood test. These are infectious mononucleosis, infectious hepatitis, malaria, brucellosis, systemic lupus erythematosus, rheumatoid arthritis, typhus, atypical pneumonia, Hansen disease, pregnancy, and drug addiction. Because of the possibility of a false-positive result, a reactive VDRL test should be followed up by one of the specific treponemal tests to confirm the diagnosis.

RAPID PLASMA REAGIN. The RPR assay is an effective screening test for primary and secondary phase syphilis. Like the VDRL, it produces serum agglutinin (reagin) in the presence of the syphilis antigen. The agglutinin indicates a positive or reactive serum. When a positive result occurs, the test is often followed up with one of the specific treponemal laboratory tests to confirm the diagnosis. Like the VDRL, this test also produces false-positive results in patients with collagen disease, infection, pregnancy, and drug addiction.

AUTOMATED REAGIN TEST. The ART is similar to the RPR plasma reagin test. Because the analysis is performed by automated equipment, the test is used to screen large numbers of serum samples. A positive test result should be followed up with one of the specific treponemal tests to confirm the diagnosis.

FLUORESCENT TREPONEMAL ANTIBODY ABSORPTION TEST. The FTA-ABS identifies the specific antibodies to *T. pallidum* that are present in the serum. This test is the most sensitive test for all stages of syphilis. It is used to confirm positive test results with the VDRL, ART, or RPR reagin screening tests, but it cannot itself be used as a screening test. This test also cannot be used to monitor treatment because once the results are reactive, they remain reactive for life (Jacobs et al., 1990). Because this test is highly sensitive and specific, even in detecting the third phase of syphilis, it is particularly useful for patients who have symptoms that suggest neurosyphilis. There are some false-positive results among the general population and in patients with collagen vascular disorders, pregnancy, and drug addiction.

MICROHEMAGGLUTINATION–*TREPONEMA PALLIDUM*. The MHA-TP also identifies specific antibodies to *T. pallidum* in the serum. The antibodies in the serum agglutinate when exposed to the antigen of this spirochete. The test is specific and sensitive in identification of all phases of syphilis except the primary stage. It is somewhat less sensitive than the FTA-ABS in the detection of early stage disease. The test is used to confirm a positive result on a reagin screening test. It is not used as a screening test itself and cannot monitor the results of treatment. This is because once it is reactive, the results remain reactive throughout life. False-positive results can occur in systemic lupus erythematosus, infections, mononucleosis, and Hansen disease.

Purpose of the Tests

These blood tests are used to screen for or confirm the diagnosis of syphilis. The VDRL test is used to monitor the response to therapy.

Procedure

A red-topped tube is used to collect 7 ml of venous blood.

QUALITY CONTROL

With venipuncture, the tourniquet should be tied lightly for a brief time to prevent pooling of cells in the vein at the site of blood collection. Venipuncture technique must be smooth, with a blood flow that fills the vacuum tube readily. If the blood has excessive turbulence because of flawed venipuncture technique, the hemolysis of the erythrocytes will alter the test results.

Findings

POSITIVE VALUES
Syphilis

Interfering Factors

- Lipemia
- Alcohol
- Hemolysis

Nursing Implementation

Pretest

Instruct the patient to avoid alcohol intake for 24 hours before the test. Fasting for 8 hours is also recommended to reduce the serum lipid content.

Posttest

Arrange for prompt transport of the specimen to the laboratory. The MHA-TP specimen requires refrigeration when there is a delay before analysis can be performed.

Instruct the patient to abstain from sexual contact until the results are known.

When the test results are positive for this sexually transmitted disease, instruct the patient to inform all sexual partners of the test results. Sexual contacts are advised to undergo testing.

Positive test results are reported to the state health department.
Instruct the patient to refrain from sexual contact until the infection is treated and cured.

TOXOPLASMOSIS SEROLOGY

(SERUM)

Synonym:

toxoplasmosis titer

NORMAL VALUES

IgM antibody titer: <1:8

Background Information

Toxoplasma gondii is a sporozoan parasite that infects feline animals, including household cats. The oocysts are excreted in feces and mature to the infective stage as sporocytes in the environment (soil, cat litter). In addition, the sporozoites may be present in raw or uncooked meat. When the sporocytes are ingested by a person, they produce infection of any nucleated cell.

Most infections are asymptomatic or produce mild lymphadenopathy and may resemble infectious mononucleosis. When the primary infection is acquired by a pregnant woman, the sporozoites are transmitted to the fetus via an infected placenta or infected maternal blood. Congenital toxoplasmosis can have devastating consequences for the fetus. This damage can include intrauterine death, brain damage, central nervous system disturbance, or chorioretinitis. The disease is also devastating to the immunocompromised patient. This parasitic infection can cause central nervous system involvement or infection of many different organs.

ANTIBODY TITER. In acute toxoplasmosis, antibodies of the IgM class appear in 1 to 2 weeks, and the titer peaks at 6 to 8 weeks. Many individuals already have antibodies from a previous asymptomatic infection, and the low or insignificant elevations persist for years. Titers that are less than or equal to 1:64 by the immunofluorescent method or less than or equal to 1:256 by the indirect hemagglutination method are considered insignificant or questionable. These results may be indicators for follow-up testing.

Titers that are greater than or equal to 1:64 by the immunofluorescent method or greater than or equal to 1:1024 by the indirect hemagglutination method are considered positive for acute infection within the past 3 months (Henry, 1991). In neonatal infection or in infection in the immunocompromised patient, the titer may be lower. This is because the infection increases faster that antibodies are produced. The various antibody titer tests are useful, but they also can produce false-positive or false-negative results.

POLYMERASE CHAIN REACTION. PCR assay testing is a new laboratory test developed to assess the fetal amniotic fluid or blood when the mother has toxoplasmosis. The research shows promise because of its greater accuracy, reliability, and validity in determining the health of the fetus who has been exposed to infection. The assay test method is not yet widely available, but in the future it will provide a greater amount of information about possible toxoplasmosis infection of the fetus (Campos, 1992).

Purpose of the Test

The antibody tests help in the diagnosis of toxoplasmosis, and it identifies antibody formation that results from exposure to the sporozoan parasite.

Procedure

A red-topped tube is used to collect 7 ml of venous blood.

Findings

ELEVATED VALUES
Toxoplasmosis

Interfering Factors

• None

Nursing Implementation

Pretest

Schedule the test to be performed at the onset of illness and 2 to 3 weeks later during the convalescent phase.

DIAGNOSTIC PROCEDURES

BLOOD CULTURE

(BLOOD)   *Synonyms:*

—————————— **NORMAL VALUES** ——————————

Negative; no growth of organisms

Background Information

Critical Thinking: On the same day, four different physicians order blood cultures for an acutely infected patient. How does the nurse respond to these multiple requests?

Septicemia, an infection of the blood, can be caused by almost any bacterial organism. To detect and identify the organism and to perform susceptibility tests to determine effective antibiotic treatment, the blood must be cultured. The indications of sepsis and the need for a blood culture include fever, a change in pulse rate, and hypotension or prostration. Shaking chills may or may not be present. The patient may also have a history of intermittent or persistent fever and a heart murmur, creating suspicions of bacterial endocarditis.

In sepsis, the bacteria are often present in the blood on an intermittent basis only. Specimen collection is timed to try to obtain the blood when the bacteria are present. The best time to collect the specimen is just before a chill or temperature spike, with two additional specimens taken at hourly intervals thereafter. Generally, after the bacteria enter the blood there is an onset of chills or fever about 1 hour later. By the time the fever begins, the bacteria may have moved out of the blood. It can take several blood culture attempts before the bacteria are identified.

There are variations in the timing of specimen collection in an effort to isolate the elusive organism. Sometimes, instead of three hourly specimens on 1 day, two consecutive blood culture specimens are obtained on 1 day and two more are obtained 24 hours later. The maximum total number of specimens, however, is four. Each blood culture specimen must be collected at a different vascular site with a separate venipuncture. There must be at least a 5-minute interval between collections of specimens. These guidelines help one obtain at least one successful culture, and they prevent blood loss that results from excessive specimen collection (Adams, 1991).

False-positive results will occur when the normal flora of the skin contaminate the specimen. The microorganisms can be introduced into the specimen during the venipuncture procedure. The skin bacteria then grow in the culture medium and appear to be the cause of the sepsis. To prevent this confusion, there must be careful antiseptic skin preparation before the venipuncture is performed. False-negative results can also occur. This means that there are pathogens in the blood, but they did not grow in the culture medium. The causes include an inadequate sample of blood and the administration of antibiotics before the specimen was drawn.

A preliminary culture report is available in 48 hours or more. To avoid any further delay in treatment, the report is usually delivered verbally, by phone, or by computer. The written confirmation follows by mail. A final report is available in 7 to 10 days.

Purpose of the Test

The blood culture confirms the presence of an infection in the blood stream and identifies the causative organism. Susceptibility testing measures the sensitivity of the pathogen to various antibiotics.

Procedure

For each blood culture specimen, there is preliminary careful skin antisepsis. Sterile technique is used to cleanse the skin and collect the blood.

For the adult, a needle and syringe, a transfer set, or a special set of blood tubes with culture media is used to collect 20 ml of venous blood.

For infants and small children, the procedure is the same, but 0.1 to 1 ml of venous blood is sufficient for each blood culture specimen. From 1 to 5 ml of blood may be obtained from older children, based on the larger body size and blood volume.

For the neonate, 0.5 to 1 ml of blood is sufficient for each specimen. The heelstick method and capillary tube blood sample are used only as a last resort because of the problem of contamination (Paisley and Lauer, 1994).

QUALITY CONTROL

With venipuncture, the tourniquet should be tied lightly for a brief time to prevent pooling of cells in the vein at the site of blood collection. Venipuncture technique must be smooth, with a blood flow that fills the syringe or tube readily. If there is excessive turbulence because of flawed venipuncture technique, the hemolysis of the erythrocytes will alter the test results.

Findings

POSITIVE VALUES

Bacterial endocarditis
Bacterial meningitis
Septic arthritis
Typhoid fever
Toxic shock syndrome

Sepsis or septicemia
Osteomyelitis
Bacterial pneumonia
Brucellosis

Interfering Factors

- Contamination of the specimen
- Hemolysis
- Antibiotic therapy

Nursing Implementation

Pretest

Inform the patient about the procedure, including the series of blood specimens and the skin asepsis. Ask the patient about any history of skin sensitivity to iodine.

Schedule the tests before antibiotic therapy is administered.

To assist with the timing of the blood sampling, monitor the patient's temperature, pulse, respirations, and blood pressure at frequent and regular intervals. Record the results in the patient's chart.

During the Test

Once the venipuncture site is identified, the skin is cleansed. The typical procedure is to first scrub the site in concentric circles and in an outward direction with 70% alcohol and then let it dry. Follow with a second scrub in the same pattern using povidone-iodine solution. This solution remains on the skin for at least 1 minute. By using this method to cleanse the skin, most of the normal flora are killed, and dirt and debris are removed from the pores. If there is a sensitivity to iodine, green soap may be substituted, or the alcohol preparation alone can be used.

The tops of the culture bottles or tubes are cleansed with alcohol or povidone-iodine before the blood is injected into them. If a blood collection system is used, only alcohol may be applied to clean the stoppers.

Using gloves and aseptic technique, the blood is drawn from the vein. The blood is then divided among the different bottles or tubes.

QUALITY CONTROL

If there is an *intravenous* catheter in place, the specimen is obtained from a venous site *below* the catheter or from the opposite extremity. This prevents hemodilution with intravenous fluids. Blood is never drawn from the intravenous line or the heparin-lock device because of the risk of external contamination. Additionally, heparin can inhibit bacterial growth. The blood is not usually drawn from a *central line,* although this guideline is controversial, and not all researchers agree (Washington, 1994). Central line catheters may harbor bacteria that are not necessarily present in the blood stream. The central venous line may be used to obtain the specimens from children or neonates. With careful aseptic preparation of the port or hub of the catheter, contamination of the specimen is infrequent (Paisley and Lauer, 1994).

Posttest

Ensure that each requisition slip and all collection containers or tubes are correctly identified. The time, date, and venous site are included.

Record each blood culture specimen collection, the time, date, and venous site in the patient's chart. These data help by keeping track of the number and timing of the blood cultures specimens and ensuring that alternative venous sites are used.

Arrange for prompt transport of the specimens to the laboratory.

DARKFIELD EXAMINATION, SYPHILIS

(CELL SCRAPINGS)

Synonyms:

Treponema pallidum darkfield examination, darkfield microscopy

──────────────────── **NORMAL VALUES** ────────────────────

Negative

Background Information

Treponema pallidum is the spirochete that causes syphilis, which is a sexually transmitted disease. During the primary stage of infection, an ulcerated lesion called a chancre appears on a mucosal or nonmucosal surface. The spirochete is present in the cell scrapings and in the moist exudate at the base of the lesion. In the secondary stage of disease, it is also present in the rash and the enlarged lymph nodes.

The best specimen of cell scrapings is obtained from a young, moist lesion. If present, dried serum must be removed before the scrapings are obtained. Oral and rectal lesions are not used because of the inevitable contamination from the normal flora and other organisms present.

Using darkfield microscopy, the slides of the cells and secretions reveal the absence or presence and characteristic movements of the syphilis spirochete. *Treponema pallidum* is a corkscrew-shaped organism that has rapid bending, flexing, and rotational movements.

A positive darkfield examination reveals syphilis at an early stage. Syphilis serologic tests are used to confirm the diagnosis, but these blood tests do not produce positive results for several weeks after the spirochete has caused infection.

Purpose of the Test

The microscopic examination of infected cells and exudate is used to diagnose the syphilis infection.

Procedure

Pipette method: After the surface of the chancre is cleansed with a saline-moistened swab, a sterile pipette is used to aspirate cells and exudate from the base of the ulcer. The secretions are placed on a sterile glass slide.

Slide method: After cleansing the surface of the chancre with a saline-moistened swab, a sterile glass slide is pressed directly on the ulcerated lesion.

QUALITY CONTROL

Once the specimen is obtained, a coverslip is placed over the slide to prevent drying of the secretions and cells.

Findings

POSITIVE VALUES

T. pallidum infection

Interfering Factors

- Contamination of the specimen
- Drying of the specimen
- Antibiotic therapy
- Healed lesion

Nursing Implementation

Pretest

Schedule this test before antibiotic therapy is started.

Instruct the patient to avoid placing lotions or creams on the lesion before the test is performed.

During the Test

Wear gloves during the test and when handling the specimen slide. If the test result is positive, the lesion and secretions are contaminated.

Posttest

Ensure immediate transport of the specimen to the laboratory. The darkfield examination must be performed within 15 minutes of collection. The secretions cannot become dry before the examination is completed.

Instruct the patient to abstain from sexual contact until the results are known.

When the test result is positive for this sexually transmitted disease, instruct the patient to inform all sexual partners of the test results. Sexual contacts are advised to undergo testing.

Positive test results are reported to the state health department.

Instruct the patient to refrain from sexual contact until the infection is treated and cured.

GENITAL CULTURE

(SECRETIONS)

Synonyms:

genitourinary culture, cervical culture, endocervical culture, prostatic fluid culture, vaginal culture, *Candida* culture, gonorrhea culture

——————————————— **NORMAL VALUES** ———————————————

Negative; normal flora present

Background Information

Critical Thinking: The 13-year-old patient is diagnosed with a sexually transmitted disease. Which communication techniques can help the adolescent and provide a complete history and nursing assessment?

A genital infection in the female is indicated by vaginitis, vulvovaginitis, or vaginal secretions. In the male, it is indicated by urethritis and urethral discharge. The infection may be caused by a sexually transmitted disease or it may be the result of other causes that are not related to sexual contact. There are numerous pathogens that can be responsible for a sexually transmitted disease, as presented in Table 7–3. The culture of the secretions or tissue scrapings is used to identify the causative organism.

NONSPECIFIC VAGINITIS. This is a common infection in women. The cause is often a yeast infection called candidiasis. The organism is *Candida albicans*, which is normally present in the flora of the vagina. The infection may be sexually transmitted, but it is often caused by a change in the host's resistance or by changes in the combination of bacteria in the normal flora of the vagina. Bacterial vaginosis can also produce the vaginal discharge. When the balance of bacterial flora changes because of antibiotic therapy or hormonal therapy, some of the normal flora increase. These normal flora include *Gardnerella vaginalis*, *Bacteroides*, and *Mycoplasma hominis*.

GONORRHEA. This is caused by the organism *Neisseria gonorrhoeae*, and remains the most frequently reported sexually transmitted disease (Kwa and Pentella, 1993). It has a high incidence in young adults of both sexes. There are two drug-resistant strains of gonococcus that are increasing in incidence: penicillinase-producing and tetracycline-resistant strains.

The initial infection involves the urethra of the male or the vagina and endocervix of the female. The gonococcus is capable of ascension to the upper

TABLE 7–3

DISEASES THAT MAY BE TRANSMITTED SEXUALLY AND THE ORGANISMS RESPONSIBLE

Disease	Organism(s)
Acquired immunodeficiency syndrome (AIDS)*	Human immunodeficiency virus
Bacterial vaginosis	Gardnerella vaginalis
	Bacteroides
	Mycoplasma hominis
Chancroid	Haemophilus ducreyi
Chlamydial infection†	Chlamydia trachomatis
Cytomegalovirus infections	Cytomegalovirus
Enteric infections	
Hepatitis A	Hepatitis A virus
Amebiasis	Entamoeba histolytica (protozoan)
Giardiasis	Giardia lamblia (protozoan)
Shigellosis	Shigellae (bacteria)
Genital herpes†	Herpes simplex virus
Genital Mycoplasma infections	Mycoplasma hominis
	Ureaplasma urealyticum
Genital (venereal) warts†	Human papillomavirus
Gonorrhea†	Neisseria gonorrhoeae
Granuloma inguinale (donovanosis)	Calymmatobacterium granulomatis
Group B streptococcal infections	Group B-hemolytic streptococcus
Molluscum contagiosum	Molluscum contagiosum virus
Pubic lice	Phthirus pubis
Scabies	Sarcoptes scabiei
Syphilis†	Treponema pallidum
Trichomoniasis	Trichomonas vaginalis

*U.S. Public Health Service fact sheet "Facts About AIDS" is available from NIAID.
†Discussed in individual fact sheets available from NIAID.
From National Institute of Allergy and Infectious Disease (1987). *Miscellaneous STDs.* Washington, D.C.: U.S. Department of Health and Human Services, National Institutes of Health, NIH Publication No. 87-909H.

pelvic organs, causing pelvic inflammatory disease. Because the infection can exist in other zones of sexual activity, cultures of the anus and throat may be needed in addition to a genital culture.

GENITAL HERPES. This condition is caused by the herpes simplex virus. It is transmitted by contact with the infected secretions or during asymptomatic shedding of the virus. Of the two different types of HSV, type 1 is transmitted by oral secretions, and type 2 is transmitted by genital secretions. The neonate may experience HSV, type 2 infection during delivery when he or she is in contact with the virus of the infected mother. The infection causes vesicle formation as sores on or near the mouth, in or around the vagina, on the penis, and around the anus, thighs, or buttocks.

The viral culture is used to confirm the diagnosis of genital herpes, but current test methods are not fully effective. To obtain the best chance for an accurate diagnosis, more than one urogenital or anorectal site should be cultured (Koutsky et al., 1992).

CHLAMYDIA. This is the leading cause of sexually transmitted disease in the United States, but the exact number of cases is unknown because it is not a reportable disease in most states (Body, 1993). Caused by *Chlamydia trachomatis,* the infection is transmitted by vaginal or anal sexual contact with an infected partner. Transmission can also occur during delivery, with transmission from the infected mother to the neonate. The infected male experiences a discharge of mucus or pus from the penis. There may also be some pain on urination or swelling of the scrotal area. The infected female experiences pain on urination, vaginal discharge, or abdominal pain. In an early stage of disease, the patient may be asymptomatic. Culture of genital secretions is one way to diagnose this infection, but the bacteria do not always grow under laboratory conditions. Alternative methods include screening the first voided urine by various laboratory methods.

CHANCROID. This is a soft chancre or genital ulcer that is caused by *Haemophilus ducreyi* and is spread by sexual contact with an infected partner.

TRICHOMONIASIS. This is the most common cause of sexually transmitted parasitic infection. The disorder usually involves the vagina, vulva, and urethra and is caused by the protozoan parasite *Trichomonas vaginalis* (Fig. 7–3). In the female, it causes vaginal secretions and an abnormal discharge. In the male, the urethral infection is often asymptomatic. In addition to culture of the genital area, the protozoan can be identified by microscopic examination of the urine sediment (Brunzel, 1994).

TOXIC SHOCK SYNDROME. This condition is caused by *Staphylococcus aureus.* Commonly, the bacteria are present on the skin and may also be present in other locations, including the vagina. Certain strains of the organism can produce toxins that enter the blood stream. When this occurs, the septic infection is severe.

Preliminary reports of a genital culture are usually available in 24 hours. When the culture is negative, the report is final in 48 hours. For a culture positive, there is a minimal wait of 48 hours before the report is completed.

Purpose of the Test

The genital culture is used to identify the pathogenic organism that causes abnormal discharge and inflammation of the vagina or urethra.

Procedure

Female: With the assistance of a speculum, a sterile swab or wire loop is inserted into the cervical canal to obtain secretions or endocervical cell scrapings.

Male: A sterile cotton swab is used to collect secretions from the penile discharge. The physician may insert a wire loop into the urethra to obtain cell scrapings.

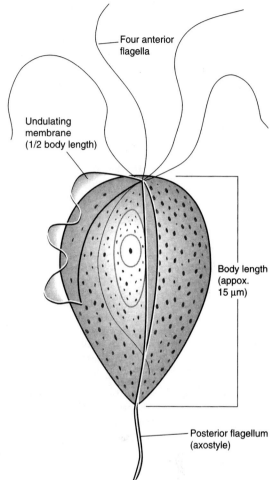

Four anterior
flagella

Undulating
membrane
(1/2 body length)

Body length
(appox.
15 μm)

Posterior flagellum
(axostyle)

FIGURE 7–3. Schematic diagram of *Trichomonas vaginalis*. (With permission from Brunzel, N.A. [1994]. *Fundamentals of urine and body fluid analysis* [p. 258]. Philadelphia: W.B. Saunders.)

Chancroid: The base of the genital ulcer is irrigated with saline. The fluid is aspirated with a sterile pipette or a moist, sterile cotton swab.

Herpes simplex: A sterile cotton swab is used to remove epithelial cells from the base of fresh lesions. Fluid from vesicles may also be obtained by aspiration with a sterile pipette.

For any of these procedures, a sterile culture tube is used to receive the specimen or specimens of cell scrapings or fluid aspirate.

Findings

POSITIVE VALUES

Neisseria gonorrhoeae
Candida albicans

HSV
Trichomonas vaginalis

Staphylococcus aureus	*Chlamydia trachomatis*
Group B streptococcus	Human papillomavirus
Gardnerella vaginalis	*Haemophilus ducreyi*
Enterobius vermicularis	*Giardia lamblia*

Interfering Factors

- Recent urination
- Recent douching
- Improper collection technique
- Contamination of the specimen
- Antibiotic administration

Nursing Implementation

Pretest

Instruct the patient regarding pretest conditions:

Male: Do not urinate within 1 hour of the test because there would be fewer organisms available for culture.

Female: Do not douche for 24 hours before the test because douching results in fewer organisms available for culture.

Inquire about any current use of antibiotics. The culture should be performed before any antibiotic therapy is started.

During the Test

Place the male in the supine position. The female is placed in the lithotomy position, as for gynecologic examination.

Provide emotional support to the patient during the collection of the specimen. For the female, the procedure may produce mild apprehension or discomfort, but it is not painful. The male may experience nausea, sweating, fainting, or weakness as the wire loop or swab is inserted into the urethra. These discomforts are temporary.

To avoid contamination, place the swab or tissue specimen into the culture tube carefully.

Posttest

The requisition slip should include information regarding the source of the specimen, the patient's name and age, the clinical diagnosis, the time and date of the specimen collection, and any current antibiotic therapy.

Arrange for transport of the specimen to the laboratory within 2 hours.

> **QUALITY CONTROL**
>
> The specimen must not be refrigerated because cooling would reduce the microbial count.

Instruct the patient to abstain from sexual contact until the results are known.

When the culture is positive for a sexually transmitted disease, instruct the patient to inform all sexual partners of the test results. Sexual contacts are advised to undergo testing.

Positive test results for gonorrhea are reported to the state health department.

Instruct the patient to refrain from sexual contact until the infection is treated and cured.

With gonorrheal infection, instruct the patient to have the culture repeated 1 week after the completion of antibiotic therapy.

MANTOUX SKIN TEST

(INTRADERMAL SKIN TEST)

Synonyms:

PPD skin test, tuberculosis skin test

NORMAL VALUES

Negative: Induration <5 mm

Background Information

Purified protein derivative (PPD) is a protein substance extracted from dead tuberculosis bacilli. The extract is injected intradermally to observe for a delayed hypersensitivity reaction. A positive reaction may indicate past or present infection with *Mycobacterium tuberculosis.*

Forty-eight to 72 hours after the intradermal injection, the injection site is examined for a reaction. The test result is considered negative when there is no change in the appearance of the skin or there is only redness, which is called erythema. When there is a hard, raised, and reddened area, the diameter of the induration is measured. A measurement of 5 to 10 mm of induration is considered a borderline result, and a repeat test with a stronger concentration of PPD is indicated. Induration greater than 10 mm is considered a positive result.

If the first strength of PPD produces a negative reaction, sometimes a repeat test is done, using an intermediate or second strength dose of PPD. This helps identify false-negative results from a minimal strength dose PPD test result. The Mantoux test does not provide a definitive diagnosis of tuberculosis, and it does not differentiate between active and dormant infection. A positive result is to be followed up with a chest x-ray study to provide a specific diagnosis and the status of the tubercular disease.

Patients who should not have the Mantoux test are those who already have had a positive Mantoux test result, those who have had tuberculosis in the past, and those who received the bacille Calmette-Guérin (BCG) vaccine. Once the Mantoux test result is positive, it remains positive for life. These patients are monitored by chest x-ray to provide data regarding the status of possible infection.

Patients with AIDS or other sources of immunosuppressive disorder may have a false-negative skin test result. Their immunocompromised condition sometimes prevents an adequate PPD skin response even though the tuberculosis bacilli are present.

Purpose of the Test

The Mantoux test screens for tuberculosis exposure, a previously healed tubercular infection, or active tuberculosis disease.

Procedure

An injection of 0.1 ml of PPD solution is injected intradermally, with an assessment of the skin site 48 to 72 hours later.

Findings

POSITIVE VALUES
Tuberculosis infection

Interfering Factors

- Corticosteroid medication
- Immunosuppressive disorder
- Previous tuberculosis infection
- Previous vaccination with BCG vaccine
- Other recent vaccinations

Nursing Implementation

Pretest

Ask the patient if there is a known history of a positive skin test result, a history of tuberculosis, or immunization with BCG vaccine. If the answer is yes, do not administer the Mantoux test.

Explain that the test is mildly uncomfortable while the needle is inserted and the solution injected, but the sensation is temporary.

Ensure that epinephrine hydrochloride, 1:1000, is at hand. There is a small risk of an anaphylactic reaction to the PPD solution.

During the Test

Inspect the inner aspect of the forearm. The site of the skin test should be free of skin eruption, infection, and excess hair.

Draw up 0.1 ml of the PPD solution in a tuberculin syringe.

Cleanse the skin at the test site with alcohol.

Hold the skin taut and introduce the needle between the layers of skin until the bevel of the needle is fully enclosed.

Inject the PPD solution. When the needle is positioned correctly, an intradermal blister-like formation occurs.

QUALITY CONTROL

The test is invalid if the solution is placed in the subcutaneous tissue beneath the layers of skin.

Posttest

Record the Mantoux test administration in the patient's record, including the site of the injection, the dose and strength of the solution, the time, and the date.

Instruct the patient that normal activities including bathing can be resumed. If the test site itches, it must not be scratched or rubbed.

Instruct the patient to return for a reading of the test result in 48 to 72 hours.

To read the test result, inspect and palpate the test site for a red, raised area of tissue reaction. If induration exists, use a millimeter tape to measure the diameter of the induration from the edge of one side to the edge of the other.

Record the measurement result in the patient's record.

Inspect the skin for integrity at the site of the injection. Some indurations are quite large and may develop an erosion or necrotic area in the center.

NASOPHARYNGEAL CULTURE

(SECRETIONS)

Synonym:

nose culture

NORMAL VALUES
Normal nasopharyngeal flora

Background Information

There is a variety of normal flora in the nose and nasopharynx, including *Staphylococcus aureus*, *Streptococcus pneumoniae*, *S. pyogenes*, *Branhamella catarrhalis*, *Neisseria* sp., and *Haemophilus influenzae*. These normal organisms may multiply and cause illness, particularly in children, the elderly, the immunocompromised individual, or the individual in a weakened condition. A nose culture positive for one of these organisms may indicate infection in the nasopharynx, sinuses, oropharynx, or tonsils. Infection can also occur elsewhere in the body, with the source of the infection being in the nose or throat. Additionally, some individuals are asymptomatic carriers of *S. aureus* or *N. meningitides*.

STAPHYLOCOCCUS AUREUS. The anterior nasal cavity is a major reservoir of *S. aureus*. In drug addicts with bacterial endocarditis, or in renal dialysis patients with septicemia, the nasal passageway may be the source of infection. This bacteria is also implicated in postoperative wound infection and in bacterial infection of the skin (furunculosis).

A large number of normal individuals harbor this organism, and the incidence is higher in hospital personnel and hospitalized patients. When there is an outbreak of this infection, the nasopharyngeal culture may be performed as a screening test to identify asymptomatic carriers.

BORDETELLA PERTUSSIS AND BORDETELLA PARAPERTUSSIS. These organisms cause pertussis or whooping cough. This respiratory tract infection usually infects infants and school-aged children who are not vaccinated or who are incompletely vaccinated and are in close contact with an infected individual.

The nasopharyngeal culture is performed early in the course of the illness to verify the diagnosis. Once the specimen is obtained, the pathogens are placed in a culture medium. After there is growth of the organism in the culture, microscopic examination can identify the cause of infection. Preliminary reports are usually available in 24 hours, and reports of no growth are complete in 48 hours. In a positive culture, the bacterial and fungal causes can be identified in 48 hours, but viral cultures require 1 to 2 weeks to complete.

Purpose of the Test

The nasopharyngeal culture is performed to identify the bacteria that cause upper respiratory tract infection and to detect carriers of the organism.

Procedure

A sterile, flexible, wire swab is used to collect a specimen from the posterior nasopharynx. Once collected, the specimen is placed in a culture tube.

S. aureus *testing:* In the culture for this pathogen, a sterile, cotton-tipped applicator stick is used instead of a wire for the collection of a specimen from the anterior nasopharynx.

Findings

POSITIVE VALUES

Pharyngitis   Pertussis
Thrush   Diphtheria
Scarlet fever   S. *aureus* carrier

Interfering Factors

• Antibiotic therapy
• Improper technique in specimen collection

Nursing Implementation

Pretest

If possible, obtain the specimen before antibiotics are started.
Inform the patient that the sterile wire swab will be put into the back of the nose and throat. Any mild discomfort disappears after the swab is removed.
Instruct the patient to cough before the swab is inserted.

During the Test

Help the patient sit up and tilt the head back.
Use a light or sterile nasal speculum, or both, to visualize the posterior nasal passage and nasopharynx.
Nasopharyngeal culture: Insert the sterile wire through the nasal passage into the nasopharynx. Allow the wire to remain for about 5 seconds. The patient may gag.
S. aureus *culture:* Insert the sterile wire 1 in. into the nares and rotate it against the nasal mucosa.
Fungal culture: Take scrapings of the plaque or lesion. Once the specimen is obtained, gently remove the swab or wire, without touching the mucosal walls.

Posttest

Place the swab or wire in the sterile culture tube, with or without culture medium.
On the requisition slip, write the time, date, specific site used to obtain the culture specimen, and the patient's name and age. Include the suspected clinical diagnosis and any current antibiotic therapy.
Arrange for prompt transport of the specimen to the laboratory.

SPUTUM CULTURE AND SENSITIVITY

(SPUTUM)

Synonym:

sputum C and S

―――――――――――――――――――― **NORMAL VALUES** ――――――――――――

> No growth

Background Information

Sputum is a product of the lower respiratory tract, not a product of the oropharynx, such as saliva. Sputum cultures are obtained to identify pathogenic organisms in patients with suspected pulmonary infections. If bacteria are present, a sputum *Gram stain* is performed to classify the bacteria as gram-positive or gram-negative. This knowledge may be used to initiate appropriate antibiotic therapy until the bacterial sensitivity portion of the test is completed. The sensitivity results identify which antibiotics are effective against the organism that is present in the sputum and which antibiotics are not effective because the organism is resistant.

Sputum culture results, like other culture results, are usually reported after 24 to 48 hours. The report of the Gram stain and the sensitivity study will follow the culture report. Some studies, however, including those of fungus and tuberculosis, may take weeks before the final report is obtained.

Purpose of the Test

Sputum culture and sensitivity testing are performed to diagnose respiratory infections, identify the pathogenic organism responsible for the infection, and determine the appropriate antibiotic therapy. It is also performed to evaluate the effectiveness of the antibiotic or antibiotics.

Procedure

Expectoration method: A sputum specimen may be obtained by the patient coughing up the sputum into a wide-mouthed sterile container with a cap.

Aspiration method: A bronchial sputum specimen may be obtained by aspiration. If a bronchial specimen is needed, suctioning equipment and a sterile sputum trap are used.

Bronchoscopy or transtracheal methods: A sputum specimen may also be obtained during a bronchoscopy or via transtracheal aspiration. The nurse may assist with these procedures but does not perform them.

Findings

POSITIVE VALUES

Pneumonia	Tuberculosis
Diphtheria	Gonorrhea
Influenza	Parasitic infection of the lungs

Interfering Factors

- Contamination of the specimen
- Antibiotic therapy

Nursing Implementation

Pretest

Perform this test before antibiotic therapy is started. This timing helps prevent a false-negative result.

Assess the patient's ability to follow instructions in coughing up the sputum as well as his or her ability to expectorate.

Provide a sterile container with a cap.

Instruct the patient to:

1. Collect the specimen on arising in the morning before eating or drinking.
2. Take several deep breaths.
3. Cough up the sputum from deep within the lungs.
4. Expectorate into the sterile container.

QUALITY CONTROL

Demonstrate the procedure and have the patient perform a return demonstration to ensure that the container and lid are not contaminated during the collection procedure. A major problem with the expectoration method is contamination of the specimen by the "normal flora"—the microorganisms normally found in the mouth and throat.

During the Test

Support and encourage the patient's attempts to produce sputum. If it is not contraindicated, postural drainage, clapping, and vibration may assist in raising the sputum. If the sputum is very tenacious, aerosol therapy may be necessary.

Approximately 1 tsp. of sputum is necessary for a sputum culture and sensitivity test. When the patient is unable to produce this amount in one attempt, the container should be capped between attempts to expectorate.

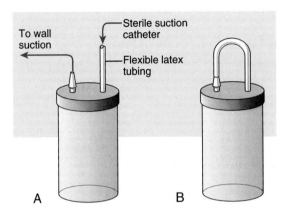

FIGURE 7–4. Sputum aspiration. *A,* Sputum trap. *B,* Closed sputum trap.

If the patient is extubated, a sputum trap is used to obtain the specimen (Fig. 7–4). In this case, the patient is suctioned as usual except that the sputum trap is inserted between the sterile suction catheter and the suction tubing attached to the wall suction regulator.

To use the sputum trap:

1. Tighten the cap to obtain an airtight seal.
2. Attach the wall suction tubing to the plastic "chimney" on the cap.
3. Connect the distal end of the sterile container to the latex tubing.
4. Suction as usual, but do not flush the catheter while the trap is in place.
5. After suctioning, disconnect the suction tubing and catheter.
6. Connect the latex tubing to the "chimney" of the cap.

Posttest

Ensure that the lid is tightly sealed and that the container is labeled correctly.
Send the specimen to the laboratory as soon as possible.
Do not refrigerate the specimen.

Complications

There are no specific complications in obtaining a sputum culture and sensitivity test. The nurse should, be cognizant of the complications of endotracheal suctioning, however, if that method is used to obtain the specimen.

THROAT CULTURE

(SECRETIONS)   ***Synonyms:***

NORMAL VALUES

Negative; normal organisms in the oropharynx

Background Information

There is a variety of flora found in the normal oropharynx. These flora do not cause respiratory illness unless there is some change in the patient's health. When acute pharyngitis occurs or there is a clinical illness that indicates an oropharyngeal source of infection, a throat culture may be indicated. The routine throat culture is used to screen for group A beta-hemolytic streptococcus. Another reason to perform a throat culture is to identify specific bacteria or fungi that cause infection of the oropharynx. When a specific organism is suspected because of the clinical condition of the patient, the laboratory is notified so that an appropriate and specific culture medium can be prepared. A routine throat culture may be ordered simultaneously with the specific throat culture.

ROUTINE THROAT CULTURE. This is used to screen for group A beta-hemolytic streptococcus—*Streptococcus pyogenes*. This bacterial cause of acute pharyngitis can result in the sequelae of rheumatic fever, scarlet fever, glomerulonephritis, wound infection, and sepsis. With early identification of the bacteria and effective antibiotic therapy, the potential development of a serious complication is diminished or eliminated. The colonization of the bacteria is in the pharynx and tonsils.

THROAT CULTURE FOR *CORYNEBACTERIUM DIPHTHERIAE*. This test is used to screen for the bacterium that causes diphtheria. In diphtheria, there is a gray pseudomembrane that appears on the tonsils and oropharynx. It spreads upward to the palate and nasopharynx and downward toward the larynx and trachea. Under the membrane, there are ulcers in the tissue. Culture results of no growth of this bacteria require 72 hours to report. A culture positive for *C. diphtheriae* requires at least 4 days for a complete report. Generally, a routine throat culture and a nasopharyngeal culture are performed simultaneously to identify or eliminate other possible organisms that may be the cause of respiratory disease.

Critical Thinking: The throat culture report for a 5-year-old male patient is positive for *Neisseria gonorrheae*. What nursing response is indicated?

THROAT CULTURE FOR *NEISSERIA GONORRHOEAE*. This gonorrheal throat culture is used to identify the gonococcal organism that has infected the oropharynx. The infection may be asymptomatic or may cause tonsillitis and acute pharyngitis. The throat is a primary site of sexually transmitted infection in homosexual males. Often, cultures of the genitalia and anal canal are performed at the same time. In children, a throat culture positive for this pathogen is indicative of child abuse–sexual abuse. The throat culture requires a minimum of 48 hours to identify this organism.

Purpose of the Test

The throat culture identifies the bacteria that cause infection of the oropharynx, pharynx, and tonsils. It is also used to screen for an asymptomatic carrier of the infection.

Procedure

A sterile, cotton-tipped swab is used to obtain a specimen of exudate from the throat. The swab is then placed in a culture tube and capped tightly.

Findings

POSITIVE VALUES

Pharyngitis	Scarlet fever
Thrush	Pertussis
Diphtheria	Gonococcal infection

Interfering Factors

- Antibiotic therapy
- Contamination of the specimen

Nursing Implementation

Pretest

Obtain the culture specimen before antibiotic therapy is started.

Inform the patient that the test involves swabbing the throat. The swabbing may cause a brief gagging sensation. The discomfort disappears as soon as the procedure is finished.

In cases of acute epiglottitis or suspected diphtheria, do not perform this test unless prepared to establish an alternate airway if needed.

If diphtheria is suspected, notify the laboratory in advance so that a special isolation medium can be prepared.

During the Test

Instruct the patient to tip the head back.

Use a tongue blade to depress the tongue.

The sterile swab is used to rub the inflamed sites and areas of exudate in the oropharynx and on the tonsils.

The swabs from a routine culture are placed in a regular culture tube. Throat culture for suspected diphtheria or gonococcal infection requires a special swab and culture-transport medium.

QUALITY CONTROL

During the swabbing of the throat, ensure that the tongue, cheeks, and uvula are not touched. Many organisms are commonly present in the oropharynx. Poor technique will cause a false-positive result.

Posttest

Ensure that the specimen is placed in the sterile culture tube or transport medium as appropriate for the specific test.

On the requisition slip, identify the source of the specimen, the name and age of the patient, the clinical diagnosis, and any antibiotic therapy that the patient is currently undergoing.

Arrange for prompt transport of the specimen to the laboratory.

Complications

There are no complications from a routine throat culture. In cases of acute epiglottitis or suspected diphtheria, however, assess the patient for a possible laryngospasm immediately after the specimen is obtained. In such cases, prepare to support oxygenation and assist with the establishment of an airway as needed. Record the results of the respiratory assessment in the patient's chart.

URINE CULTURE

(URINE)

Synonyms:

midstream urine culture; urine culture, midvoid specimen; urine culture, clean catch; urine culture, indwelling catheter

--- **NORMAL VALUES** ---

No growth

Background Information

The normal urinary tract and urine are sterile except for the normal flora that reside in the distal urethra and at the urinary meatus. Bacteriuria is the presence of bacteria in the urine. A lower urinary tract infection consists of an infection in the bladder or urethra, or both. An upper urinary tract infection involves the renal pelvis or renal interstitial tissues, or both. Any bacterial or fungal organism can cause a urinary tract infection, but the most common pathogens are those that are present in normal feces (Brunzel, 1994). An infection in the urinary tract produces bacteria in the urine.

In urine culture, the detection of significant bacteria is diagnostic of a urinary tract infection. A bacterial count of less than or equal to 10^5 colony-forming units per ml (CFU/ml) is considered positive and indicates significant bacteriuria. In the female, the test may be repeated once or twice to ensure the accuracy of the diagnosis because contamination of the specimen could

Critical Thinking: The urine culture report shows that the specimen was contaminated. For the repeat test, how should the nurse intervene to correct the technique of mid-stream urine collection?

cause a false-positive result. In the male, only one specimen is needed for a correct diagnosis.

The automated culture system is rapid and requires only 5 to 13 hours to detect bacteriuria accurately (Pappas, 1991). Routine culture methodology identifies the organism or organisms and the sensitivity study identifies the antimicrobial medications that are effective or ineffective against the pathogen. Culture results with no growth are available after 24 hours. Positive cultures require 24 to 48 hours to complete (Nachamkin, 1993).

Purpose of the Test

Culture of the urine is used to diagnose a urinary tract infection and to monitor the number of microorganisms in the urine.

Procedure

Midstream catch: A clean-voided midstream technique is used to obtain 15 ml or more of urine in a sterile container. A first voided specimen of the day is used because it has the highest colony count after an overnight incubation period.

Indwelling catheter: A sterile needle and syringe are used to obtain 4 ml or more of urine from the urine sample port of the catheter. The urine is then placed in a sterile container.

Mycobacterium culture: For a tuberculosis culture of the urine, first voided morning specimens are collected on three separate days.

Findings

POSITIVE VALUES

Urinary Tract Infection

Escherichia coli   *Streptococcus faecalis*
Proteus spp.   *Staphylococcus aureus*
Enterobacter spp.   *Candida albicans*
Pseudomonas   *Mycobacterium* spp.
Klebsiella spp.

Interfering Factors

- Contamination of the specimen
- Antimicrobial therapy

Nursing Implementation

Pretest

Instruct the patient regarding the proper procedure for collection of a clean-catch midstream urine sample. Hands must be washed with soap before the specimen is collected. As described further on, the perineum and urinary meatus must be cleansed carefully.

| **QUALITY CONTROL** |
Contamination of the specimen from the external genitalia, hair, vagina, or rectum would introduce microbes into the urine sample and cause a false-positive result.

During the Test

Midstream or Clean-Catch Method

Female: Instruct the female that after spreading the labia, the perineum, vulva, and urinary meatus are cleansed with three soapy sponges, using one downward stroke for each sponge. Each sponge is used only once and is discarded and then a sponge with water is used to remove the soap. The same single downward stroke is used, and the sponge is discarded. After the cleansing is completed, the labia must be maintained in that separated position until after the urine is collected.

Male: Instruct the male to cleanse the urethral meatus with the three soapy sponges and then rinse with the water sponge. Each sponge is used once and discarded. If uncircumcised, the prepuce must be retracted and the glans cleansed.

Collecting the urine: Instruct the patient to begin the urinary stream and void about 1 oz. and then as the urine flow continues, collect the urine by catching it midstream into the container. The first and last parts of the urinary stream are not used for the collection of the specimen. During the collection process, the container must not touch the perineal skin or hair. Once the specimen is obtained, the patient places the lid on the container without touching the inner surfaces.

Indwelling Catheter Method

When the catheter is already in place, the urine is removed from the catheter port.

Clamp the tubing below the urine collection port for 10 minutes. Cleanse the port with an alcohol sponge. Use a sterile needle and syringe to collect the urine sample through this port. Place the urine in a sterile container. Unclamp the tubing.

| **QUALITY CONTROL** |
Urine must not be collected from the drainage bag because bacteria can be on the outside of the bag. Additionally, the urine is not fresh and has had an opportunity to colonize bacteria while it remained at room temperature.

WOUND CULTURE

(SECRETIONS)

Synonym:

pus culture

─────────────────────── **NORMAL VALUES** ───────────────────────

> No growth

Background Information

Under normal conditions, microorganisms reside on surface tissues or in body cavities, or both, and do not invade or harm the person. These normal flora, however, produce infection when they are transmitted to other parts of the body or to sterile areas of tissue. In addition, there may be foreign debris in a wound that promotes the infection. Soft tissue infections affect various depths of tissue layers, including the epidermis, dermis, subdermis, fascial planes, and muscle tissue. The infectious organism may be enclosed or contained, such as in an undiagnosed abscess. The pathogens may also be in an open, ulcerated, or necrotic wound or fistulous tract that is exposed to the external environment.

Surgical microbes may include *Streptococcus pyogenes*, *Staphylococcus aureus*, or numerous other possible bacteria. The organisms may be aerobic or anaerobic. A routine wound culture screens the purulent material for aerobic organisms. If there is purulence but the culture result is negative, the culture is repeated and a screen for anaerobic organisms is performed.

One of the problems in culturing the infected wound is that there are many normal flora that grow in an open, draining wound, fistula, or opened abscess. The culture report identifies predominant organisms, but the information is of doubtful use in identifying the cause of infection.

In the case of an ulcerated or necrotic infection, the wound must be cleansed and debrided first to remove many of the bacterial flora. Sometimes, a biopsy of the ulcer or a curettage of the sinus tract is helpful. The tissue specimen contains the causative bacteria, and they can be identified by histopathology examination. This measure can be performed in addition to the wound culture. A closed wound, such as an unopened abscess, usually yields the causative organism in the wound culture of the purulent material.

The preliminary report from a wound culture is usually available in 24 hours. The isolation of the pathogen requires 48 hours or more, and a final negative result takes 72 hours to complete.

Purpose of the Test

The wound culture is used to determine the presence of infection and to identify the causative organism.

Procedure

A syringe and needle can be used to aspirate purulent material from a wound. Sterile swabs may also be used to absorb purulent matter from within a draining wound or fistula. For transport to the laboratory, the swabs are placed in a culture tube that contains culture medium.

Findings

POSITIVE VALUES

Staphylococcus aureus
Streptococcus pyogenes
Staphylococcus epidermidis
Escherichia coli
Proteus spp.

Pseudomonas spp.
Bacteroides spp.
Clostridium spp.
Group D streptococci
Klebsiella spp.

Interfering Factors

- Antibiotic therapy
- Contamination of the specimen

Nursing Implementation

Pretest

If possible, schedule this procedure before antibiotic therapy is started.
Explain that there is only minor discomfort as an open wound is swabbed. If an abscessed area must be opened surgically or a tissue biopsy, debridement, or tissue scraping are required, a local anesthetic may be used.
A written consent is needed for these surgical procedures.

During the Test

To express the purulent material, the tissue surrounding the wound is pressed. The cotton swab absorbs the fluid that appears.
The swab may also be inserted into the open lesion or drainage tract. Once the swab is in place, it is rotated against the side walls of the tissue.
A needle and syringe may be used to aspirate fluid from the purulent area or the drainage tract.

QUALITY CONTROL

Ensure that the syringe or swab does not touch the surface of the skin, vagina, rectum, or other body tissues. The contamination of the specimen with surface organisms produces invalid results.

Posttest

Ensure that the requisition slip indicates the patient's name and age, specific culture site, time, date, clinical diagnosis, and any current antibiotic therapy.

Arrange for prompt transport of the specimen to the laboratory.

QUALITY CONTROL

A delay in starting the culture growth can produce a reduced yield of microorganisms. If there is delay in the processing of the specimen in the laboratory, the specimen must be refrigerated.

REFERENCES

Adams, S. (1991). Critical issues in blood culture collection. *Clinical Laboratory Science, 4*, 276–278.

Avalos-Bock, S. (1994). Getting a rise out of tuberculosis with the PPD skin test. *Nursing 94, 24*, 51–53.

Bishop, W.P, & Ulshen, M.H. (1988). Bacterial gastroenteritis. *Pediatric Clinics of North America, 35*, 69–87.

Body, B.A. (1993). Screening of males for *Chlamydia trachomatis. Clinical Microbiology Reports, 2*, 46–47.

Brunzel, N.A. (1994). *Fundamentals of urine and body fluid analysis.* Philadelphia: W.B. Saunders.

Campos, J. (1992). Rejection criteria for stool ova and parasite examinations. *Clinical Microbiology Reports, 1*, 27–28.

Current, W.L., & Garcia, L.S. (1991). Cryptosporidiosis. *Clinics in Laboratory Medicine, 11*, 873–895.

Edelstein, P.H. (1994). Specific diagnosis of central nervous system syphilis. *Clinical Microbiology Reports 3*, 13.

Farzadegan, H. (1994). HIV-1 antibodies and serology. *Clinics in Laboratory Medicine, 14*, 257–269.

Ferre, F. (1994). Polymerase chain reaction and HIV. *Clinics in Laboratory Medicine, 14*, 313–333.

Garcia, L.S., & Brucker, D.A. (1988). *Diagnostic medical parasitology.* New York, N.Y.: Elsevier.

Gutierrez, Y., & Little, M.D. (Eds.). (1991). Diagnosis of important parasitic diseases. *Clinics in Laboratory Medicine, 11*, 811–1050.

Henry, J.B. (1991). *Clinical diagnosis and management by laboratory methods* (18th ed.). Philadelphia: W.B. Saunders.

Henry, J.K., & Campbell, S. (1992). Routine HIV antibody testing of hospitalized patients. *Public Health Reports, 107*, 138–141.

Hospital Infection Control. (1991) Improper disinfection causes diarrhea outbreak. *18*, 116–117.

Issac-Renton, J. (1991). Laboratory diagnosis of giardiasis. *Clinics in Laboratory Medicine, 11*, 811–827.

Jacobs, D.S., et al. (Eds.). (1990). *Laboratory test handbook* (2nd ed.). Baltimore: Williams & Wilkins.

Koutsky, L.A., et al. (1992). Underdiagnosis of genital herpes by current clinical and viral-isolation procedures. *New England Journal of Medicine, 326*, 1533–1539.

Kwa, B., & Pentella, M. (1993). Sexually transmitted diseases: Risks, transmission, and laboratory diagnostic update. *Clinical Laboratory Science, 6*, 85–89.

Lebeck, L.K., & Lewis, J. (1992). HIV infection: Immunobiology and laboratory diagnosis. *Clinical Laboratory Science, 5*, 28–30.

Little, M.D. (1991). Laboratory diagnosis of worms and miscellaneous specimens. *Clinics in Laboratory Medicine, 11*, 1041–1050.

Morris, A.J., et al. (1992). Application of rejection criteria for stool ovum and parasite examinations. *Journal of Clinical Microbiology 30*, 3213–3216.

Nachamkin, I. (1993). Incubation time for urine cultures. *Clinical Microbiology Reports, 2*, 24.

Paisley, J.W., & Lauer, B.A. (1994). Pediatric blood cultures. *Clinics in Laboratory Medicine, 14*, 17–30.

Pappas, P.G. (1991). Laboratory in the diagnosis and management of urinary tract infections. *The Medical Clinics of North America, 75*, 313–327.

Perry, J.L. (1993). New culture and identification procedures in mycobacteriology. *Clinical Laboratory Science, 6,* 163–164.

Pritchard, V., et al. (1991). Multistix versus laboratory urinalysis in the detection of urinary tract infection. *Journal of Gerontology Nursing, 17,* 39–42.

Proctor, E.M. (1991). Laboratory diagnosis of amebiasis. *Clinics in Laboratory Medicine, 11,* 829–859.

Seigel, D., et al. (1987). Predictive value of stool examination in acute diarrhea. *Archives Pathology Laboratory Medicine, 111,* 715–718.

Senay, H., & MacPherson, D. (1989). Parasitology: Diagnostic yield of stool examination. *Canadian Medical Association Journal, 140,* 1329.

Smalley, D.L., et al. (1990). Enzyme immunoassay for antibodies to Epstein-Barr virus nuclear antigen. *Clinical Laboratory Science, 3,* 397–398.

Swenson, P.D. (1994). Detection of HSV DNA in pregnant women by PCR. *Clinical Microbiology Reports, 3,* 39–40.

Teitz, N.W. (Ed.). (1990). *Clinical guide to laboratory tests* (2nd ed.). Philadelphia: W.B. Saunders.

Washington, J.A. (1994). Collection, transport and processing of blood cultures. *Clinics in Laboratory Medicine, 14,* 59–68.

Yannelli, B., et al. (1988). Yield of stool cultures, ova and parasite tests and *Clostridium difficile* determinations in nosocomial diarrheas. *American Journal of Infection Control, 16,* 246–249.

PART III

MULTISYSTEM DIAGNOSTIC PROCEDURES

CHAPTER 8

Ultrasonography

Ultrasonography, or ultrasound, sends pulsed, high-energy sound waves into the body and records the pattern of the echo as the sound waves bounce back from the tissues and organ structures. The echoes are converted to images that are seen on a monitor and photographed for later analysis.

Ultrasound has many advantages as a diagnostic procedure. Because it is noninvasive and does not use ionizing radiation, it is very safe for the patient. The scanning can be performed on the coronal, sagittal, or transverse planes, or in a combination of planes, to give a complete visualization of the targeted tissue (Fig. 8–1). When compared with the cost of computed tomography or magnetic resonance imaging, ultrasonography is inexpensive (Tempkin, 1993).

General information about ultrasound is presented in this chapter. Specific applications of ultrasound in different body systems are presented in the appropriate chapters in Part IV of this text.

ULTRASOUND

(SOUNDWAVE IMAGING)

Synonyms:

sonogram, diagnostic sonography

NORMAL VALUES

> There are no anatomic or functional abnormalities. The organs are normal in size, shape, contour, and position. The internal structures of the organs and nearby tissues are within normal limits.

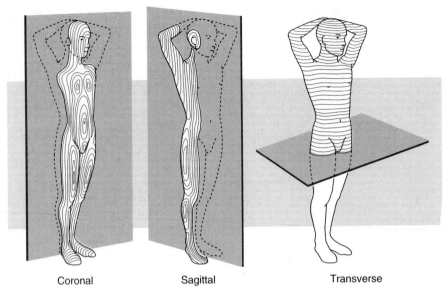

| Coronal | Sagittal | Transverse |

FIGURE 8–1. Scanning planes for ultrasound examination. (Redrawn with permission from Tempkin, B.B. [1993]. *Ultrasound scanning: Principles and protocols.* Philadelphia: W.B. Saunders.)

Background Information

Sound waves are transmitted through fluid and they bounce back or "echo" off more solid substances. In ultrasound, the sound waves are transmitted from the tissue surface through the body tissues in a directed path. Parts of the beam are reflected back quickly when they encounter a structure or substance of different acoustic character (Fig. 8–2). The remaining parts of the beam continue to a greater depth and are also reflected back as they ultimately encounter tissues of differing densities. The sound waves transmit through fluid but do not transmit through air, bone, or barium (Squire and Novelline, 1990).

There are many ultrasound scans used to examine organs, tissues, lymph nodes, and the vascular circulation. The more common scans are listed in Table 8–1.

TRANSDUCERS. The transducer, sometimes called the probe or the scan head, converts electric energy to high-frequency ultrasound energy. The ultrasound waves are sent by the transducer and also are received as they are reflected back. Once the transducer receives the echoes, they are converted back to electric impulses and are then converted to audio signals or visual images.

In the ultrasound procedures that are performed externally, the hand-held transducer moves over the skin in defined directions. The patterns of movement are determined by the anatomic location of the target organ (Fig. 8–3). Before the procedure begins, acoustic gel is applied to the skin. This creates an air-free surface for the transducer and eliminates the interference caused by air (Kremkau, 1993).

Critical Thinking: Just before the thyroid ultrasound examination begins, the 5-year-old sees the transducer and becomes visibly apprehensive. Which nursing approaches can be effective in helping the child cope with the experience?

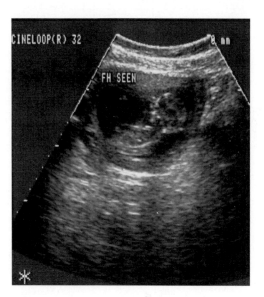

FIGURE 8–2. Pregnancy ultrasound. The varying density and composition of tissues allow visualization of the uterine contents. A normal 4-month fetus is seen in this ultrasound image.

Some transducers are designed as specialized probes that enter the body. These probes are used in the esophagus, vagina, rectum, or lumen of a blood vessel. The internal application is useful because the sound waves are placed nearer the particular organ or tissue. The procedure reduces or eliminates the interference of other tissues and the air of the lungs or bowel.

TECHNOLOGIC VARIATIONS. In ultrasound technology, there are several modes of examination available. The selection is based on the qualities and physiologic functions of the target tissues. *Diagnostic ultrasound* produces cross-sectional anatomic images of tissues or organs. *Doppler ultrasound* is used to detect and measure the movement of body fluids as it applies to blood flow. *Duplex Doppler ultrasound* combines the cross-sectional view of the blood vessel with the Doppler measurement of the movement of the blood (Foldes, 1993).

TABLE 8–1
ULTRASOUND PROCEDURES

Popliteal artery scan	Pelvic scan
Inferior vena cava scan	Female pelvic scan
Abdominal aorta scan	Obstetric scan
Carotid artery scan	Endovaginal scan
Abdominal scan	Male pelvic scan
Liver scan	Thyroid scan
Gallbladder–biliary tract scan	Scrotum scan
Pancreas scan	Breast scan
Renal scan	Neonatal brain scan
Spleen scan	Transesophageal echocardiography

Diagnostic ultrasound produces the wedge-shaped cross-sectional image of tissues or organs. The ultrasound pulsations pass through all tissues in their path until they reflect off solid structures. Some of the pulses echo quickly and others pass through fluid-filled structures until they encounter firm structure or high-density tissue at a more distant point. In diagnostic ultrasound, there are three variations or characteristics of the displayed images.

One way of displaying the ultrasound image is called a *B-scan* because of the

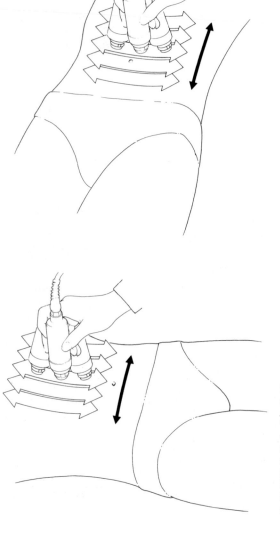

FIGURE 8–3. Technique of ultrasound examination of the abdomen. *A*, The transducer moves in a "rock-and-slide" motion in transverse planes. *B*, Using the same motion, the transducer scans the abdominal organs in sagittal planes. (With permission from Tempkin, B.B. [1993]. *Ultrasound scanning: Principles and protocols* [p. 11]. Philadelphia: W.B. Saunders.)

intensity of *brightness* of the image. The image is made of white dots on a black background, and the human eye sees tones of white, gray, and black. The strength of the echo produces varying intensities of brightness. The image of a strong echo is white and bright, as produced by sound impulses passing through fatty tissue. The absence of an echo is black, as produced by sound impulses passing through fluid. A second characteristic is that homogeneous tissues appear in shades of gray. This variation is called the *gray scale*. The third variation in the image display is called *real-time* scanning. Real-time refers to the ability to display two-dimensional images of tissues that are in motion. For example, in echocardiography, the heart valves can be seen as they open and close (Kremkau, 1993).

Doppler ultrasound detects the presence, direction, speed, and character of arterial or venous blood flow within the vascular lumen. The Doppler pulses echo off the moving erythrocytes in the blood in patterns that correlate with the flow of the blood. The echoes are converted to an audio signal or a linear graphic reading on a paper strip, similar to an electrocardiogram strip.

The audio signal changes according to the character of the blood flow. The blood flow may be characterized as *normal*; *disturbed*, as at the bifurcation of a blood vessel; or *turbulent*, as encountered beyond the point of a partial obstruction (Fig. 8–4). Severely obstructed circulation produces a weak signal or silence. In the graphic printout, the changes in circulation produce characteristic patterns in the linear tracings. A complete discussion of Doppler ultrasound in peripheral vascular disease is presented in Chapter 15.

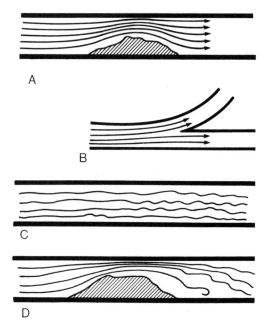

A

B

C

D

FIGURE 8–4. Patterns of blood flow detected by ultrasound. *A*, Disturbed blood flow at a stenosis. *B*, Disturbed flow at a bifurcation. *C*, Turbulent flow caused by too rapid a speed of flow. *D*, Turbulent blood flow resulting from partial obstruction. (With permission from Kremkau, F.W. [1993]. *Diagnostic ultrasound: Principles and instruments* [4th ed., p. 193]. Philadelphia: W.B. Saunders.)

Critical Thinking: A pregnant woman wants to stay with her confused, elderly mother during the ultrasound examination but explains that she is afraid of "exposure to radiation." How do you respond, and what arrangements can be made?

Duplex Doppler ultrasound combines the measurement of blood flow with the imaging of the lumen of the blood vessel or a cross-sectional, anatomic view of a particular structure or organ. The disturbance and turbulence of blood flow is located and visualized. It may be used to assess the circulation within an artery or vein or to detect the vascular or avascular characteristics of a tumor. It may also be used to evaluate the blood flow before or after a kidney or liver transplant.

When a color flow instrument is used with the duplex Doppler ultrasound, the images provide a color map or two-dimensional view of the blood flow and its characteristics. The colors primarily indicate the direction of the flow and sometimes indicate the speed and turbulence of the flow. In the image, the red indicates blood flow that moves toward the transducer and the blue indicates blood flow that moves away from the transducer. Green indicates a wide range of velocities that are present in the blood flow. Yellow, white, or mosaic patterns indicate high-velocity or complex blood flow patterns.

Purpose of the Test

Ultrasound examines organs, blood vessels, and structures of the body to identify malposition, malformation, or malfunction.

Procedure

High-frequency sound waves are directed into an area of the body in a specific pattern. The echoes of the ultrasound are converted to visual images, linear tracings, or audible sounds.

Findings

ABNORMAL VALUES

Cyst	Vascular occlusion
Tumor	Venous thrombosis
Hypertrophy	Atherosclerotic plaque
Obstruction or stricture	Abscess
Calculus	Congenital anomaly
Aneurysm	Hematoma, bleeding
Foreign body	Pregnancy, fetal development

Interfering Factors

- Air
- Overlying bones
- Bowel gas
- Barium
- Obesity

Nursing Implementation

Pretest

Obtain a written consent for any ultrasound procedure that involves insertion of a transducer into a body cavity or blood vessel. No consent is needed for the routine ultrasound examination that uses an external transducer and a noninvasive method of examination.

Schedule the ultrasound examination before or several days after any barium studies.

QUALITY CONTROL

Barium is an opaque substance that would block the transmission of ultrasound impulses. Residual barium causes an ultrasound problem for about 24 hours after a barium x-ray examination.

Instruct the patient about any dietary restrictions or modifications. Any abdominal ultrasound examination requires fasting from food for 12 hours. If the patient has a tendency toward bowel gas, a low-residue diet is implemented for 24 to 36 hours, followed by a 12-hour fast from all foods. Some abdominal ultrasound protocols require an enema before the examination. Schedule the abdominal tests for the early morning, before breakfast. Gynecologic ultrasound procedures often require drinking 40 oz. of water without voiding before the test. This fills the urinary bladder and moves it upward and away from the uterus.

QUALITY CONTROL

Intestinal gas must be removed from the colon because ultrasound impulses cannot pass through air. In addition, visualization of the abdominal organs and vasculature would be impaired by the overlying colon and its contents.

Inform the patient that the examination is safe and painless. Provide reassurance to alleviate anxiety.

A small child or agitated, anxious patient may be accompanied by a calming parent or other adult. Sedation may be needed, particularly for the small child (Torres, 1993).

Assist the patient in removing all clothes, jewelry, and metallic objects. A hospital gown is worn.

During the Test

Position the patient on the examining table.

Instruct the patient to remain still during the examination.

Apply the acoustic gel to the skin surface in the area to be examined. The gel serves as a conducting agent and eliminates the thin layer of air that causes a barrier to the transmission of impulses.

Posttest

Remove the acoustic gel to prevent the soiling of the patient's clothes.

If the patient received sedation, monitor vital signs until the patient is responsive. This patient cannot drive and must be accompanied by a responsible adult on the return home or return to the hospital room.

REFERENCES

Apple, S., & Thurkauf, G.E. (1992). Preparing for and understanding transesophageal echocardiography. *Critical Care Nurse, 12,* 29–34.

Blickman, J.G. (1992). The inroads of ultrasound, CT, and MR in pediatric imaging. *Applied Radiology, 21,* 38–47.

Foldes, M.S. (1993). The role of duplex and color Doppler imaging in the operating room. *Journal of Vascular Nursing, 11,* 108–110.

Keachie, J. (1992). Making sense of . . . Doppler ultrasound. *Nursing Times, 88,* 54–56.

Kremkau, F.W. (1993). *Diagnostic ultrasound: Principles and instruments* (4th ed.). Philadelphia: W.B. Saunders.

Snopek, A.M. (1992). *Fundamentals of special radiographic procedures* (3rd ed.). Philadelphia: W.B. Saunders.

Squire, L.F., & Novelline, R.A. (1990). *Fundamentals of radiology* (4th ed.). Cambridge, MA: Harvard University Press.

Sturman, M.F. (1993). *Effective medical imaging: Signs and symptoms approach.* Baltimore: Williams & Wilkins.

Tempkin, B.B. (1993). *Ultrasound scanning: Principles and protocols.* Philadelphia: W.B. Saunders.

Torres, L.S. (1993). *Basic medical techniques and patient care for radiologic technologists* (4th ed.). Philadelphia: J.B. Lippincott.

Radiography

There are many different radiographic methods that use a source of radiation for the imaging of the patient's tissues. These include x-ray studies, computed tomography (CT), radioisotope scans, and contrast studies. Although these methods vary in complexity of technique and equipment, all are based on the same principle. Electromagnetic energy passes partially through opaque tissues of varying radiodensities. The radio waves that pass through the patient's body are captured by the photographic film and produce a corresponding image of the tissues. The radio waves that are absorbed by body tissues do not affect the photographic film.

Discussions of radioisotope scans, contrast studies, and CT scans are presented in different chapters in Part III. This chapter concentrates on conventional x-ray studies, as they are used to image many tissues and organs of the body.

X-RAY STUDIES

(RADIOGRAPHY)

Synonyms:

plain film, conventional x-ray, simple radiography

NORMAL VALUES

The size, shape, appearance, thickness, and position of the organs and tissues are within normal limits for the patient's age. No anatomic or functional abnormalities are noted.

Background Information

The source of the x-ray emissions comes from high-voltage electric current that passes through a special vacuum tube in the x-ray machine. Within the vacuum tube, the electric current is converted to x-ray waves. As the x-rays are emitted from the machine, they pass through the patient and onto a photographic plate called the x-ray film (Fig. 9–1).

In the imaging process, the x-ray beam passes freely through air and almost as freely through fatty tissue. As all or most of the x-ray beam strikes the radiographic film, the resultant film image is black or very dark. As an example, the air cavities of lung tissue appear very dark to black on the chest x-ray film.

In soft tissues that are somewhat dense, some of the x-ray beam is absorbed by the tissues, and the remainder passes through the tissues and strikes the photographic plate. The resultant images are of soft gray tones that vary in intensity of shading. Thus, muscles, blood, organs, and other soft tissues are seen in shades of gray and are lightly visible on the x-ray film.

Most x-rays are absorbed or blocked by bone because of the calcium content of osseous tissues. Thus, the film image of bone is white, particularly in dense, healthy bone tissue that has a high concentration of calcium. In bones that are fractured, the crack, break, or displacement of bone is quite visible. In the patient

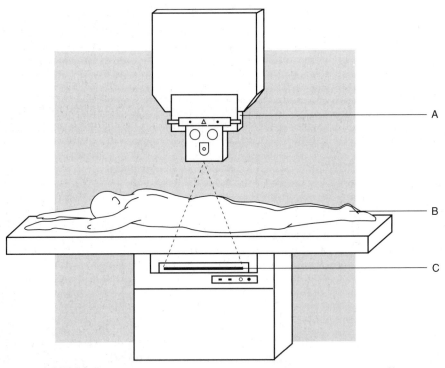

FIGURE 9–1. Simple radiograph. *A,* X-ray machine; *B,* patient; and *C,* x-ray film.

with osteoporosis, there is less calcium content in the bones, and the film image of the bone is more gray and porous.

The imaging of body tissues is affected by several variables. As already discussed, the composition of the various tissues creates differences in shading. The thickness of the tissues is also a variable. Some tissues are thicker and more dense or radiopaque. Others are thinner and therefore more radiolucent. The size, shape, and position of the organs or tissues are accurately reproduced because of the differences in the densities of the tissues.

All metals absorb x-rays. Because the x-ray beam is absorbed or blocked, the metal object appears totally white on the film, and any tissue behind the metallic object cannot be seen. For this reason, the patient must remove all jewelry and metallic objects from the body area that is to be imaged.

The radiopacity of metals also works to benefit the patient and personnel. X-ray beams cannot pass through lead of a particular thickness. Thus, a lead shield or apron is worn to protect reproductive organs and other radiosensitive tissues from undesired exposure to radiation (Fig. 9–2). Radiography rooms have lead-lined walls to prevent the passage of radiation into offices and corridors. This protects workers and others from inadvertent exposure.

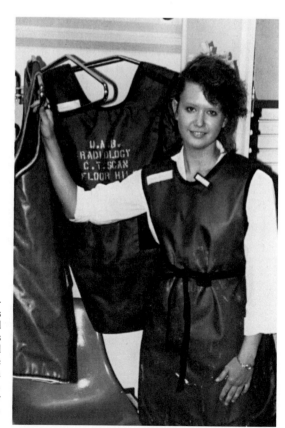

FIGURE 9–2. Protection from radiation exposure. Lead aprons should be handled carefully and stored on special holding racks when not in use. Film badges should be worn at the collar level, outside the lead apron. (With permission from Thompson, M.A., et al. [1994]. *Principles of imaging science and protection* [vol. 2, Slide 371]. Philadelphia: W.B. Saunders.)

Three-dimensional views of the tissue are obtained by filming from the front to back of the body as well as from the side. In radiology, these views are called *anteroposterior and lateral* (AP and lateral) (Fig. 9–3). If the patient is radiographed from the back-to-front and side views, the positions are called *posteroanterior and lateral* (PA and lateral). Other positions, such as oblique views, may be requested to image a particular section of anatomy that is less visible from a traditional position.

All anteroposterior x-ray films are viewed as if the patient was facing you. This means that the patient's left side is on your right side. Conversely, the posteroanterior x-ray film is viewed as if you are behind the patient and face his or her back. To prevent confusion and possible error in the interpretation of the film, the technician places the letters R and L on the film to indicate the *patient's* right and left sides.

CHEST X-RAY. This film is obtained routinely for hospitalized and preoperative patients to screen for tuberculosis and other serious pulmonary or cardiac disease. It also provides a preoperative comparison film for the postoperative patient in whom a pulmonary or cardiac complication develops, and it is a basic radiologic procedure for the patient with a suspected pulmonary disorder.

The film produces images of the lungs, trachea, bronchi, diaphragm, mediastinum, part of the heart, the bony thorax, and the pulmonary vasculature. It reveals characteristic patterns of opacity that help differentiate pneumonia from other conditions of similar symptomatology, such as atelectasis, pulmonary embolism, heart failure, or pneumothorax (Curtis et al., 1992). The opacities may also reveal the presence and location of a pulmonary tumor, lesion of the rib, enlarged mediastinal lymph nodes, cavitation, or abscess of the lung. The chest x-ray film does not always produce a definitive diagnosis, but it can identify abnormal findings that are suggestive of or compatible with a particular pulmonary disorder.

This same imaging process provides data about the heart, including its size and shape. In congenital and acquired cardiac disease, the enlargement of the heart and its atria or ventricles provides information about the improper function of the cardiac valves, pulmonary or aortic arterial hypertension, and venous pulmonary conditions that affect heart size.

ABDOMINAL X-RAY. There are various abnormal findings on the abdominal film useful in obtaining a diagnosis. The patterns of air and gas appear light and bright on the abdominal film. In normal findings, the air remains contained within the intestinal tract. With a perforation of either the stomach or intestines, the gas escapes into the abdominal cavity. When the patient is seated or in an erect position, the air rises and gathers under the diaphragm, where it is visible on the abdominal x-ray film. In intestinal obstruction, air and fluid collect above the area of obstruction, distending the lumen of the intestine. The abnormal width of the intestinal tissue and the air within the lumen are visible and diagnostically significant.

In the biliary tract, opaque stones or calculi produce a white, bright image on the abdominal film. The location of the stone is identified in the gallbladder or the cystic or common duct. Cholesterol stones are nonopaque, however, and

Critical Thinking: The x-ray finding of a 68-year-old female describes moderate osteoporosis of the hips. What health care teaching measures can help control this problem in the patient's future?

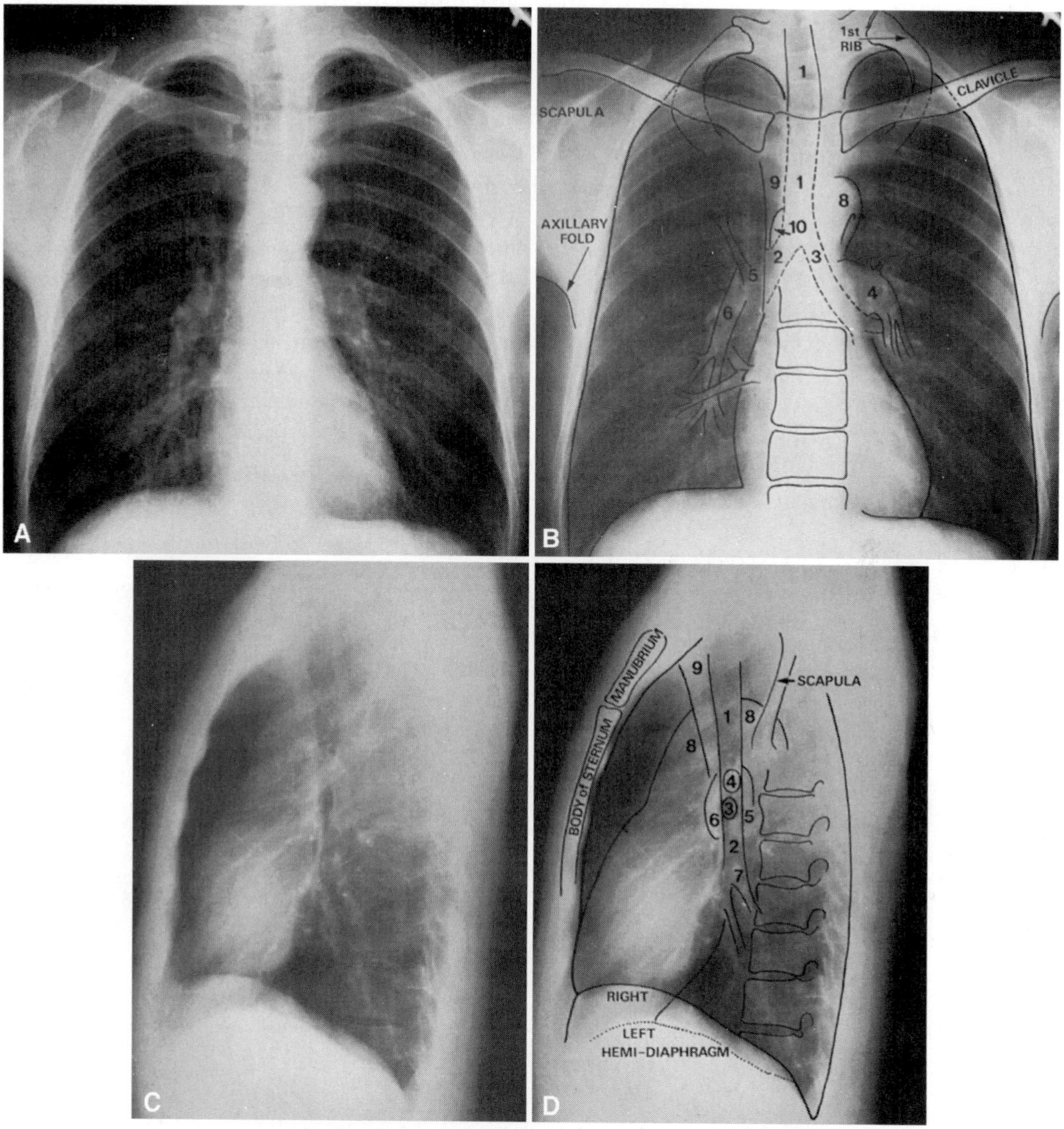

FIGURE 9–3. Normal chest roentgenograms—posteroanterior and lateral projections. *A*, A chest roentgenogram in an asymptomatic 26-year-old man taken in the erect position. *B*, A diagrammatic overlay shows the normal anatomic structures numbered or labeled: (*1*) trachea; (*2*) right main bronchus; (*3*) left main bronchus; (*4*) left pulmonary artery; (*5*) right upper lobe pulmonary vein; (*6*) right interlobar artery; (*7*) right lower and middle lobe vein; (*8*) aortic knob; and (*9*) superior vena cava. *C*, A chest roentgenogram in an asymptomatic 26-year-old man taken in the erect position. *D*, A diagrammatic overlay shows the normal anatomic structures numbered or labeled: (*1*) tracheal air column; (*2*) right intermediate bronchus; (*3*) left upper lobe bronchus; (*4*) right upper lobe bronchus; (*5*) left interlobar artery; (*6*) right interlobar artery; (*7*) confluence of pulmonary veins; (*8*) aortic arch; and (*9*) brachiocephalic vessels. (With permission from Fraser, R.G., et al. [1988]. *Diagnosis of diseases of the chest* [3rd ed., vol. 1, pp. 287–290]. Philadelphia: W.B. Saunders.)

cannot be seen on the abdominal film. This type of stone is visualized only on x-ray examination using contrast medium.

KIDNEY-URETER-BLADDER X-RAY. This x-ray film is also known as a flat plate of the abdomen. It images the structure, size, and position of the kidneys, ureters, and bladder, screening for abnormality in these organs and nearby tissues. Calcification of the renal calyces or renal pelvis is visible, as are any radiopaque calculi that are present in the upper urinary tract.

BONE AND JOINT X-RAY. X-ray studies are a vital tool in the assessment of bones and joints. In cases of trauma, the x-ray film is used to identify the presence, location, and type of fracture; the potential for injury to the surrounding soft tissues; and the healing activity after the fracture has been treated. The dislocation of a joint, bone tumor, bone infection, or loss of bone mass is also visible radiographically. In arthritic disorders or metabolic diseases such as gout, x-ray studies are used to visualize the size and structure of the joints and soft tissues and the alignment of the bones that articulate at the joints (Fig. 9–4).

SKULL-VERTEBRAL X-RAY. The x-ray films of the skull can detect abnormality of shape, size, and contour, including detection of a skull fracture. The skull series

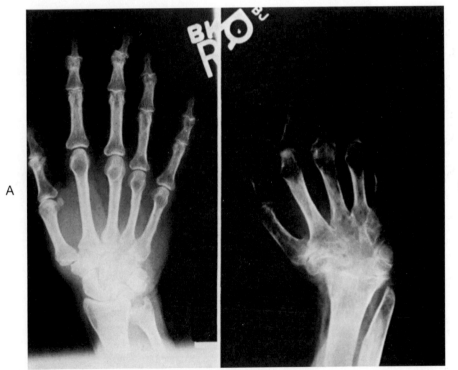

A

B

FIGURE 9–4. Effects of calcium on bone density. *A*, A 28-year-old patient with good calcium deposits in bone. *B*, A 72-year-old patient whose bones appear transparent as the result of calcium loss. This radiographic appearance is also attributed to pathologic changes caused by rheumatoid arthritis. (With permission from Thompson, M.A., et al. [1994]. *Principles of imaging science and protection* [vol. 2, Slide 290]. Philadelphia: W.B. Saunders.)

can be used to help identify changes in the skull that cause increased intracranial pressure, bleeding into the brain, bleeding within the skull cavity, or infection of the bone. Usually, a CT scan or magnetic resonance imaging is used instead of skull radiographs because tomography is more accurate and detailed in the imaging of both skull and brain tissues.

The vertebral x-ray films provide visualization of a fracture, dislocation, or deformity of the spine. They demonstrate degeneration or faulty alignment of the spinal vertebrae, causing a disorder in the intervertebral discs.

Findings

ABNORMAL RESULTS

Chest and Heart

Pneumothorax	Pneumonia
Atelectasis	Tuberculosis
Pleural effusion	Pulmonary abscess
Pleurisy	Fracture
Cystic fibrosis	Scoliosis
Pulmonary fibrosis	Chronic obstructive
Tumor or cyst	pulmonary disease
Mediastinal nodes	Silicosis
Aortic aneurysm	Atherosclerosis
Congestive heart failure	Cor pulmonale
Adult respiratory distress syndrome	Cardiac hypertrophy

Intestinal Tract

Intestinal tract perforation	Subphrenic abscess
Intestinal tract obstruction	Swallowed foreign body
Paralytic ileus	Foreign body in the
Volvulus	abdomen
Intussusception	Gastroenteritis
	Biliary tract calculus

Urinary System

Renal abscess	Congenital malformation
Renal tuberculosis	Tumor or cyst
Pyelonephritis	Renal or ureteral calculus
Glomerulonephritis	Polycystic renal disease
Hydronephrosis	Hematoma
Amyloidosis	

Bones and Joints

Fracture	Osteoarthritis
Dislocation	Rheumatoid arthritis
Subluxation	Gout
Bone cyst or tumor	Osteomyelitis
Congenital malformation	Osteoporosis

Vitamin D deficiency, rickets	Osteomalacia
Paget disease	

Skull

Congenital anomaly	Fracture
Neoplasm, skull	Paget disease
Osteomyelitis	Acromegaly

Spinal Vertebrae

Ankylosing spondylitis	Fracture
Lordosis	Subluxation
Scoliosis	Ruptured disc
Kyphosis	Osteoarthritis
Tuberculosis	Osteoporosis
Pott disease	Paget disease

Interfering Factors

- Excessive movement
- Failure to remove metal or jewelry from the x-ray field
- Improper positioning
- For abdominal and kidney-ureter-bladder films: retained barium or contrast medium, feces, ascites, gas, obesity

Nursing Implementation

Pretest

For the patient who requires an abdominal or kidney-ureter-bladder film, schedule the x-ray study before any radiologic study that uses barium or contrast medium. The contrast medium is radiopaque, and the residual contrast interferes with the visualization of the underlying tissues.

For most imaging procedures, instruct the patient to remove all clothes and put on a hospital gown. The exceptions are the skull radiograph and x-ray films of the distal extremities.

Instruct the patient to remove all jewelry and metallic objects from the area that is to be imaged.

Provide reassurance to the patient. Young children often fear the equipment, strange room, isolation, and separation from the parents. Adults may also feel somewhat apprehensive.

Critical Thinking: In the waiting room, the elderly patient complains to you that every time that she has an x-ray, she becomes stiff and cold. What nursing measures can help relieve or prevent the discomfort?

During the Test

Ensure the patient's safety at all times, particularly when there is a risk of the patient falling. There are no side rails on the radiography table, and restraints may interfere with positioning or imaging (Torres, 1993).

Position the patient for the specific views needed.

Instruct the patient to remain motionless during the imaging. Sometimes the patient is instructed to inhale deeply and hold the breath until the image is taken.

The patient must often wait in the imaging area as the decision is made whether to take additional x-ray films. Provide a blanket or extra gown for the patient who is chilled in the cool room.

Posttest

Assist the patient in dismounting from the radiography table and getting dressed, as needed.

REFERENCES

Curtis, A.M., et al. (1992). Pneumonia: Reading chest films right. *Patient Care, 26,* 40–46, 53–55, 58–60, 65, 69, 70–72.

Hoffman, E.B., et al. (1993). Radiologic imaging of children with spinal tuberculosis. A comparison of radiography, computed tomography, and magnetic resonance imaging. *Journal of Bone and Joint Surgery, 75,* 233–239.

Koehler, C. (1991). Why a radiology nurse? *Images, 10,* 1–3.

Pinner, J. (1991). Patient teaching for x-ray and other diagnostics. *RN, 54,* 32–36.

Snopek, A.M. (1992). *Fundamentals of special radiographic procedures* (3rd ed.). Philadelphia: W.B. Saunders.

Squire, L.F., & Novelline, R.A. (1990). *Fundamentals of radiology* (4th ed.). Cambridge, MA: Harvard University Press.

Sturman, M.F. (1993). *Effective medical imaging: Signs and symptoms approach.* Baltimore: Williams & Wilkins.

Torres, L.S. (1993). *Basic medical techniques for patient care for radiologic technologists.* Philadelphia: J.B. Lippincott.

CHAPTER 10

Nuclear Imaging

Nuclear imaging consists of several radiologic methods that are used to visualize the functions of particular organs or tissues. In comparison with other radiologic procedures, nuclear imaging is less precise in providing anatomic information, but it is helpful in demonstrating physiologic activity.

With a few exceptions, nuclear scans provide full-thickness images of organs. The two nuclear scans that are exceptions are positron emission tomography (PET) and single-photon emission computed tomography (SPECT). These nuclear scans also produce tomographic views that locate the abnormal function more precisely.

Nuclear scanning can locate the site of abnormal physiologic function. It often detects the abnormality at an earlier stage than is possible with other radiologic techniques. It has a high degree of accuracy and sensitivity, with few false-negative results (Mettler and Guiberteau, 1991). Because the nuclear scan cannot identify the cause of the pathologic change, its function is to provide supportive data in conjunction with other diagnostic procedures.

NUCLEAR IMAGING

(RADIONUCLIDE STUDY)

Synonyms:

nuclear scan, nuclear medicine scan, isotope scan

NORMAL VALUES

There is a normal uptake, distribution, and excretion of the radionuclide by the targeted organ or tissue.

Background Information

In most radiologic procedures, the source of the radiation is in a machine that emits radio waves that are aimed to pass through the patient from the external source. In the nuclear scan, the radionuclide is within the patient and provides a small source of radiation. Once it is within the patient's body, the radionuclide is taken up, concentrated, and distributed in the targeted organ or tissue. For a short time, it emits gamma rays in the pattern and concentration that corresponds to the physiologic uptake by the target organ or tissue.

A gamma camera or scintillation scanner detects and records the emission of the gamma rays as the equipment rotates around the patient. The data are converted into a visual image by the computer and its special software. The image appears on a monitor and is reproduced by paper tracing or photograph. This allows additional study of the images after the procedure is completed (Fig. 10–1).

RADIONUCLIDES. These are artificially produced, unstable, radioactive isotopes that emit small amounts of gamma rays. The radionuclides in nuclear medicine have a short half-life, which is the time needed for the nuclear material to decay and the radioactivity to become reduced to half of the original strength. By the end of the half-life period, the radioactive emissions of the radionuclide are considerably reduced or negligible.

Technetium-99m is one of the most common radionuclides used in nuclear scans. It emits a low level of gamma rays and has a half-life of 6 hours. After it is released from the target organ or tissues of the body, most of it is filtered out of the blood by the kidneys and excreted in the urine. Some of the ion is secreted directly into the colon and excreted in the feces.

Other common radionuclides include the isotopes of iodine, xenon, gallium, indium, and thallium. They all vary in their characteristics, including radioactive strength and half-life. Each radionuclide has a binding capacity that allows it to work as a radiopharmaceutical.

RADIOPHARMACEUTICALS. A radionuclide is the radiation source needed for imaging, but it cannot enter the target tissue by itself. A radiopharmaceutical is a combination of a radionuclide that is bound to a specific element, compound, or cellular component. The bound substance is taken up by specific target tissues and the radionuclide is absorbed with it.

In one example of how a radiopharmaceutical works, technetium-99m is bound to phosphorus or calcium to form the radiopharmaceutical that is used in a bone scan. Active bone cells absorb the calcium or phosphorus as part of bone metabolism, and the radioactive isotope is absorbed at the same time. Concentrations of active bone cells are identified because they emit the gamma rays that are recorded in the scan. Nonactive bone cells, such as those in a bone cyst or a nonhealing fracture, do not absorb the mineral element or radiopharmaceutical, and the deficit is seen on the scan.

In other examples, the radiopharmaceutical that contains heat-damaged erythrocytes is used in the spleen scan because the spleen collects and destroys damaged red blood cells. The radiopharmaceutical that contains leukocytes is

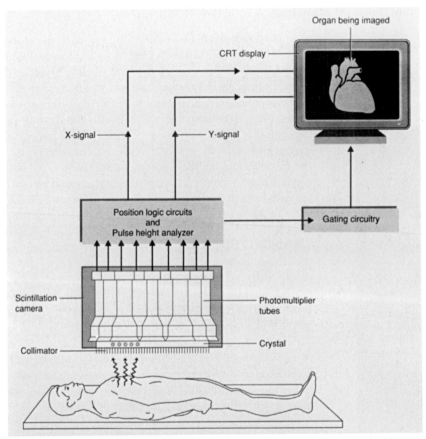

FIGURE 10–1. Diagram of the nuclear medicine scanning process. After administration of the radionuclide, the nuclear imaging is performed with a scintillation scanner and sensitive radiation detector. The nuclear emissions are computer-converted to produce an image of the targeted organ on the monitor. (With permission from Thompson, M.A., et al. [1994]. *Principles of imaging science and protection* [vol. 2, Slide 391]. Philadelphia: W.B. Saunders.)

Critical Thinking: The college student with a suspected nonhealing fracture arrives for his bone scan. He wants to know how the bone scan provides better information about healing than an x-ray. What explanation can you give him?

used in the gallium scan because white blood cells will sequester in areas of infection. When human cells are used, the cells are obtained from the patient's own blood to prevent problems of incompatibility.

Most radiopharmaceuticals are injected intravenously. Exceptions are those used in the lung ventilation scan, which requires a radiopharmaceutical that is inhaled as a gas, and those used in upper gastrointestinal scans, which require orally ingested radiopharmaceuticals.

IMAGING PROCESS. The gamma camera or scintillation scanner moves in an orbit around the patient, detecting the concentrations of gamma rays from all angles. The scanner never touches the patient, and the equipment is relatively quiet. The patient is positioned appropriately so that the scanner can detect the emissions from the targeted organ clearly. When a whole body scan is performed,

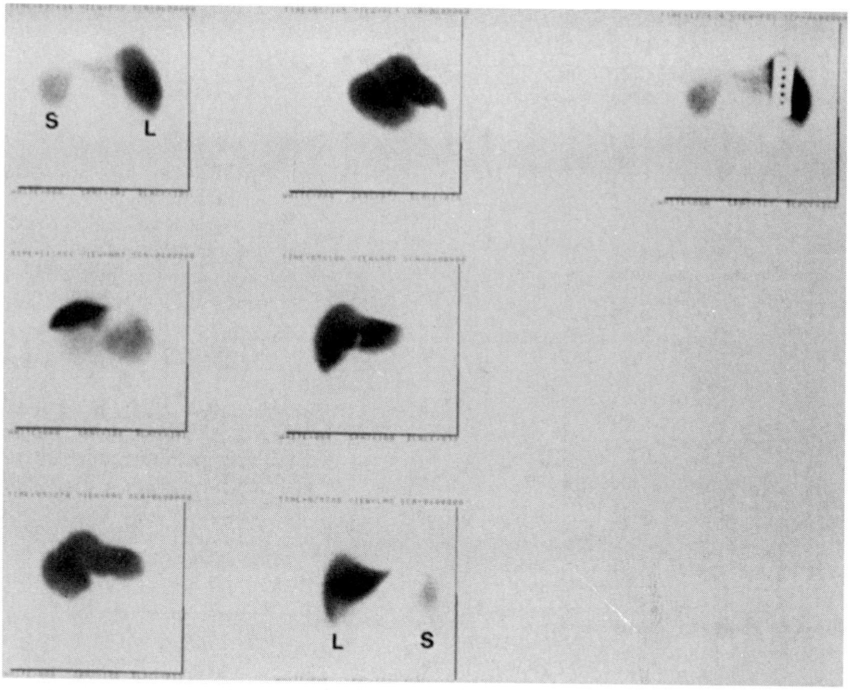

FIGURE 10–2. Normal liver-spleen scan. L = liver; S = spleen. (With permission from Gore, R.M., et al. [1994]. *Textbook of gastrointestinal radiology* [p. 1537]. Philadelphia: W.B. Saunders.)

such as a bone scan or gallium scan, the patient is placed on a moving table that gradually passes through the arcs of the scanner.

Imaging begins as soon as the radiopharmaceutical is absorbed by the targeted tissue. The images become more clearly defined as a greater amount of radioisotope is concentrated in the targeted tissue (Fig. 10–2). In some scans, the imaging is rapid and begins as soon as the radiopharmaceutical is injected. In other scans, it takes hours for the radiopharmaceutical to be absorbed, so the imaging is performed after a specific time interval.

EMISSIONS COMPUTED TOMOGRAPHY. The process of emissions computed tomography (ECT) combines the use of special radionuclides with a gamma camera or a scintillation camera, and a computer to produce three-dimensional tomographic images of specific tissues or body organs. As with traditional nuclear scans, the radiopharmaceutical is injected intravenously and localizes in the target tissue or organ. The gamma camera or scintillation scanner rotates around the patient, detecting the concentration and pattern of the radioactive material (Fig. 10–3). The emissions data are collected and converted to numeric (digital) data and then into visual images by the computer.

The difference with the ECT process is that the computer and software can produce many thin slices or tomographic views of the targeted area. The three-dimensional views can be produced from any angle and provide clear

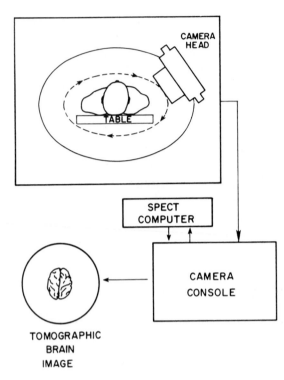

FIGURE 10-3. Single photon emission computed tomography (SPECT) nuclear scan. A schematic representation of a SPECT system. The camera detector rotates around the patient in an orbital path while acquiring data to be fed into the computer. Reconstructed tomographic images are created by the SPECT computer and are then displayed on the monitor. (With permission from Mettler, F.A., & Guiberteau, M.J. [1991]. *Essentials of nuclear medicine imaging* [3rd ed., p. 38]. Philadelphia: W.B. Saunders.)

localization and visualization of an abnormality. Nearby tissues that overlie or underlie the targeted area are less likely to obscure the view.

The ECT process is differentiated by the type of radioactive isotope used. The two types of ECT are PET and SPECT. Each of these processes has benefits and limitations.

PET uses cyclotron-produced isotopes such as fluoride-18, carbon-11, or oxygen-15 as the source of radioactivity. These radioisotopes all produce excellent contrast of the tissues and measure glucose metabolism. Oxygen-15 has been used for oxygen metabolism and to visualize regional cerebral blood flow.

The major limitations are the limited access to a cyclotron for the production of the radioisotopes, the short half-life of the radioactive material, and the costs involved. The cyclotron is a sophisticated machine that splits atoms to make the isotopes. It is expensive and not readily available for many institutions. Additional costs are incurred from the numerous personnel, including physicists and technicians, who are involved in the production of the nuclear material. The newly produced materials must then be delivered rapidly to the nuclear medicine laboratory and administered without delay because the radioisotope decays within a few hours. Because of the limitations, this procedure has been used primarily for research purposes.

SPECT uses radioisotopes such as technetium-99 or iodine-123, with a SPECT camera for the imaging process. The major advantages are the use of standard radiopharmaceuticals and scanning equipment to perform the procedure. Thus, it is more available and has lower costs. There are some limitations because the radiopharmaceuticals vary in their depth of activity and have a more scattered distribution that can interfere with the imaging.

ABNORMAL FINDINGS. There is abnormal uptake and distribution of the radionuclide when the pathologic condition affects the target organ or tissue. The abnormality may be a space-occupying lesion or tumor, nonfunctioning tissue such as scar tissue, a loss of structural integrity such as a fracture, or other abnormality. The types of abnormalities include deficiency of uptake, excessive uptake, localization of activity in focal areas of tissue, disseminated activity throughout the organ, and asymmetry when the results should be bilateral and symmetric.

When there is little to no uptake, the image appears faint gray or clear. With the diminished uptake of radioactive material in the tissue, there is a limited emission of gamma rays or photons to transmit the image. With normal or excessive uptake, the image appears dark or black because of the concentration of the radionuclide and the strength of the emissions.

NONVISUALIZATION. When the targeted organ or tissue is not visualized, there is no uptake of the radionuclide. One possible cause is that there is vascular or ductal obstruction that blocks the radionuclide from reaching the target site. Another possible cause is that the organ is nonfunctional. For example, nonvisualization can occur in the spleen scan of a patient with advanced sickle cell anemia. The lack of uptake of the radionuclide can be caused by organ atrophy from repeated infarct or mechanical obstruction of the splenic blood flow by sickled, clumped erythrocytes.

DECREASED ACTIVITY. When there is decreased activity in the target organ, it is called a *defect* or a *cold spot*. One or more focal areas of tissue are nonfunctional because of the pathologic change in the tissue. For instance, an abnormal liver scan can demonstrate a defect because of a cyst or abscess that has formed a space-occupying lesion. Multiple focal defects are often due to metastatic disease.

INCREASED ACTIVITY. When there is increased activity in the target organ, it is called a *focal abnormality* or *hot lesion* in otherwise normally functional tissue. The excess activity may also involve the entire organ. For instance, the thyroid scan of the patient with Graves disease demonstrates increased activity throughout the gland. All the thyroid tissue is hyperactive and absorbs a maximum amount of radionuclide. In bone fracture, a bone scan reveals normal excess activity at the fracture site 24 to 48 hours after the fracture occurs. The increased focal activity correlates with the osteogenic changes that are needed for normal bone repair and healing.

LOSS OF TISSUE OR VASCULAR INTEGRITY. This is demonstrated by a pooling or compartmentalization of the radionuclide in the area where blood has collected as a result of trauma or tissue damage. In trauma, the scan can demonstrate a linear defect, peripheral indentation, or displacement of the injured organ or tissue. The pooled blood has a high concentration of the radionuclide, with the emission of many gamma rays or photons in an abnormal pattern. A frank rupture, subcapsular hematoma, and a bleeding episode are all examples of losses of tissue integrity that produce excessive radioactivity at the site of the tissue injury. Lower gastrointestinal bleeding is detected when the injected radionuclide leaves the circulation and enters the lumen of the intestine. Over time, the pooled radionuclide demonstrates movement by peristalsis.

VERSATILITY OF NUCLEAR SCANS. There are many nuclear scans that can be used to visualize the function of different organs or tissues. There are also a variety of radionuclides that can be used to identify the area of abnormality. Some of these scans, the purposes, and the pertinent patient care information are presented in Table 10–1. Scans that are used more frequently are presented in greater detail throughout Part IV of this text.

Critical Thinking: In the pretest period for a bone marrow scan, the 2-year-old child is sedated with phenobarbital. What nursing assessments are performed during and after the test?

Purpose of the Test

A nuclear scan is used to assess the physiologic function and assist in the localization and diagnosis of abnormality in a designated organ or tissue.

Procedure

A radiopharmaceutical is administered to the patient, and a gamma camera or scintillation scanner records the radioactive emissions. These emissions are then converted to images that correspond to the location, distribution, and concentration of the radionuclide in the targeted organ or tissue.

Findings

ABNORMAL RESULTS

Organ atrophy or fibrosis
Congenital defect
Tumor or cyst
Metastatic lesions
Inflammation or abscess
Hyperactivity of organ function

Hematoma
Traumatic disruption of tissue
Vascular obstruction
Obstruction of a duct
Ischemia or necrosis of tissue

Interfering Factors

• Failure to follow specific pretest dietary or medication restrictions
• Recent intake of iodine

Nursing Implementation

Pretest

Obtain an informed consent from the patient or person responsible for the patient's health care decisions.
Provide the pretest patient instructions, which vary for each scan. Some scans have dietary restrictions to prevent an increase in the circulation to

Text continued on page 240

TABLE 10-1
NUCLEAR SCANS

Name of Scan	Purpose	Patient Position During Scan	Special Measures
Brain scan and cerebral flow scan	To evaluate brain tissue, internal carotid arteries and their intracranial branches, for the detection of cerebrovascular abnormality such as stroke or atherosclerosis To identify brain tissue abnormality such as tumor, hematoma, cyst, atrophy, or edema	Seated and supine	Initial views are obtained immediately after the injection of the radiopharmaceutical to document the circulation in the arteries and brain Additional images, taken 1–4 hours later, provide views of the brain tissue
Brain imaging (SPECT)	To visualize the function of brain tissue, particularly in the evaluation of dementia, cerebrovascular disease, and the location of foci of seizure activity	Supine	In the pretest and test periods, the patient must remain in an unstimulated state The room is kept dark, quiet, and without traffic
Cerebrospinal fluid imaging (cisternogram)	To investigate the passageway and flow of cerebrospinal fluid in the ventricular system of the brain To help diagnose hydrocephalus To investigate brain trauma, with leakage of cerebrospinal fluid	Supine and possibly Trendelenburg	If there is suspected leakage of cerebrospinal fluid from the ears or nose, packing is placed in these orifices A lumbar puncture is performed to instill the radiopharmaceutical intrathecally For adults, images are taken at 2, 6, 24, and 48 hours For children, images are taken at 1, 2, 4, 6, 8, and 24 hours

Table continued on following page **235**

TABLE 10–1
NUCLEAR SCANS *Continued*

Name of Scan	Purpose	Patient Position During Scan	Special Measures
Thyroid scan with technetium-99m	A rapid method of assessing thyroid function and structure To help diagnose hypothyroidism, thyroid nodule, cancer, and Graves disease	Supine, with neck in hyperextension	This test is preferred for patients who receive propylthiouracil because there is no iodine in the radiopharmaceutical The radiopharmaceutical is injected intravenously The patient should not swallow during the imaging stage
Thyroid scan with iodine-123	To assess thyroid function and structure To help diagnose hypothyroidism, thyroid tumor or nodule, and Graves disease	Supine with neck in hyperextension	Thyroid medications and iodine interference with iodine uptake in the test; these are discontinued in the pretest period per physician's orders and test protocol Pretest, no solid foods are permitted for 4–6 hours The radiopharmaceutical is given orally, 4–24 hours before imaging begins This test provides excellent images, but it is expensive; the iodine isotope is produced by the cyclotron process
Liver-spleen scan	To assess the physiologic functions of the liver and spleen To identify focal or diffuse areas of deficit, caused by tumor, fibrosis, circulatory abnormality, or trauma	Supine	The radiopharmaceutical is injected intravenously

Hepatobiliary scan	To assess for patency of the hepatic ducts, biliary ducts, and gallbladder To identify defects, abnormal function, and blockage	Supine	Nothing by mouth for 6–8 hours pretest (some protocols require nothing by mouth for a minimum of 2 hours)
Thallium scan with thallium-201 resting or exercise	To determine the blood flow to the myocardium, at rest or after maximal stress-exercise	Upright before and during administration of the radiopharmaceutical Supine and lateral for imaging	Nothing by mouth for 4–6 hours pretest to reduce radiopharmaceutical uptake in nearby organs Blood pressure and electrocardiogram are monitored during treadmill exercise and imaging phases Exercise is performed to the maximum heart rate, using the treadmill After injection of the radiopharmaceutical, imaging is performed immediately and after 3–4 hours
Myocardial infarction scan	To assess the cardiac tissue for damage caused by acute myocardial infarction, particularly when other tests are inconclusive	Supine	Scan is performed 10–72 hours after a possible myocardial infarction or cardiac insult Imaging is performed 2–3 hours after the radiopharmaceutical is injected

Table continued on following page

TABLE 10–1
NUCLEAR SCANS *Continued*

Name of Scan	Purpose	Patient Position During Scan	Special Measures
Gated blood pool ventriculography (ventriculogram)	To measure cardiac ventricular performance at rest and during stress or exercise To evaluate coronary artery disease, acute cardiomyopathy, valvular disease, and intracardiac shunting	Supine	The patient's erythrocytes are tagged to form the *blood pool*; the image sequence is *gated* (timed or triggered by the R wave of the electrocardiogram) Stress or exercise studies may be performed The patient has nothing by mouth for 4–8 hours before the test The imaging is performed immediately after the injection of the radiopharmaceutical
Pulmonary perfusion scan	To assess the integrity of the pulmonary circulation and to identify obstruction as from pulmonary embolus	Seated or supine	The radiopharmaceutical is given intravenously and the imaging is performed immediately thereafter
Pulmonary ventilation scan	To assess the ventilatory ability of the lungs, particularly in chronic obstructive pulmonary disease and inflammatory lung disease	Seated or upright	After the rapid imaging begins, the patient exhales deeply and inhales xenon-133 gas delivered by mask for 15 seconds; the patient then rebreathes oxygen for 2–3 minutes followed by normal air for 2–3 minutes, to clear the lungs

Meckel diverticulum scan	To assess for bleeding in the ilium, the distal part of the small intestine	Supine	After administration of the intravenous radiopharmaceutical, scanning of the lower abdomen is carried out every 5 minutes for 30 minutes and then scanning of the right lateral midabdomen is performed for 30 minutes
Gastrointestinal scan	To identify and locate the source of lower gastrointestinal bleeding; the causes include diverticulitis, vascular abnormality, neoplasm, or inflammatory bowel disease	Supine	After intravenous injection of the radionuclide, images are obtained at intervals for up to 24 hours
Testicular scan	To differentiate among the causes of a painful, swollen testicle; To assess for the vascular integrity of the testicle	Supine	After intravenous administration of the radiopharmaceutical, the imaging is performed immediately and again in 15 minutes
Bone marrow scan	To identify malignant tumor or abnormal distribution of bone marrow; To locate active sites for biopsy	Supine, prone, or sitting	Twenty minutes after intravenous administration of the radiopharmaceutical, imaging begins and lasts for 1 hour; Shield the liver and spleen during imaging

the liver or intestines. Many medications interfere with the absorption of the radiopharmaceutical. Often, after consultation with the patient's physician, medications are withheld and the patient remains under medical supervision during the period of the test.

If the scan involves the uptake of radioactive iodine (iodine-123, iodine-125, or iodine-131), instruct the patient to avoid the intake of iodine from food (shellfish, kelp preparations, and some vitamins) and medication sources (some cough medicines, Lugol solution) for 3 to 5 days before the test.

On the day of the test, assist the patient in removing all clothing, jewelry, and metal objects. A hospital gown is worn.

Provide reassurance regarding the scanning process. Other than the venipuncture, the procedure is painless. Some patients confuse this procedure with the computed tomography or magnetic resonance imaging and fear a claustrophobic sensation. Because there is no chamber for the patient to enter, this reaction is not a problem (McDonagh, 1991).

If the patient is anxious, a family member or friend can plan to be in the room during the scanning procedure. Unlike x-ray imaging, there is no external source of radiation exposure and therefore no risk.

Sedatives are usually used for the infant or child less than 3 years old, particularly when the scan requires an extended period of immobility. Administer the prescribed sedative. The medication is usually chloral hydrate, 25 mg/kg (by mouth or per rectum), or phenobarbital, 5 mg/kg (intramuscularly) (Cook et al., 1992).

During the Test

If sedatives are administered, monitor vital signs on a regular basis. This ensures early detection of any untoward response to the medication.

Instruct the patient to remain in the preestablished position while a bolus dose of radionuclide is administered intravenously and during the scanning process, which may begin immediately after the injection.

Posttest

As with the handling of all body fluids or waste products, wear gloves to dispose of any urine or feces and then wash your hands. The radionuclide is excreted in urine and feces for several days, although the radioactivity level is minimal after a few hours. The body wastes can be disposed of in the toilet.

Instruct the patient to wash his or her hands after voiding or a bowel movement. Parents and others should wash their hands after changing the diapers of the infant who had a nuclear scan. Reassure the patient that the amount of radioactivity is negligible, but it can remain on the hands unless they are washed.

REFERENCES

Bernier, D.R., Christian, P.E., & Langan, J.K. (1994). *Nuclear medicine technology and techniques* (3rd ed.). St Louis: C.V. Mosby.

Cimini, D.M. (1992). Indium-111 antimyosin antibody imaging: A promising new technique in the diagnosis of M.I. *Critical Care Nurse, 12,* 44–48, 50–51.

Cook, B.A., et al. (1992). Sedation of children for technical procedures: Current standard practice. *Clinical Pediatrics, 31,* 137–142.

McDonagh, A. (1991). Getting your patient ready for a nuclear scan. *Nursing 91, 21,* 53–57.

Mettler, F.A., & Guiberteau, M.J. (1991). *Essentials of nuclear medicine imaging* (3rd ed.). Philadelphia: W.B. Saunders.

Sharp, P.F., Gammell, H.G., & Smith, F.W. (1989). *Practical nuclear medicine.* Oxford: IRL Press.

Snopek, A.M. (1992). *Fundamentals of special radiographic procedures* (3rd ed.). Philadelphia: W.B. Saunders.

Squire, L.F., & Novelline, R.A. (1990). *Fundamentals of radiology* (4th ed.). Cambridge, MA: Harvard University Press.

Sturman, M.F. (1993). *Effective medical imaging: Signs and symptoms approach.* Baltimore: Williams & Wilkins.

Torres, L.S. (1993). *Basic medical techniques and patient care for radiologic technologists* (4th ed.). Philadelphia: J.B. Lippincott.

Yudd, A.P., et al. (1992). Bone scintigraphy: Lumbar spine SPECT imaging. . . Single photon emission computed tomography. *Applied Radiology, 21,* 46–51.

CHAPTER 11

Angiography

This chapter addresses the various radiologic techniques used to visualize the lumen of arteries and the arterial blood flow. In each technique, an iodinated contrast medium is injected into an arterial or a venous site, and rapid, multiple radiographs provide visualization of the contrast material as it moves through the vascular area of concern.

The focus of this chapter is an angiography as it is used to image the arterial circulation in many areas throughout the body. Additional discussions, such as coronary and cerebral angiography and angiography in the assessment of peripheral vascular disease, are presented in detail in subsequent chapters in Part IV of this text.

ANGIOGRAPHY

(RADIOLOGY)

Synonyms:

arteriography, digital subtraction angiography (DSA), digital vascular imaging (DVI), intravenous digital subtraction angiography (IVDSA)

Background Information

Angiography is an invasive test that uses an arterial injection of contrast medium to visualize the lumina of arteries. Radiographic images are taken with fluoroscopy and x-rays to illustrate the arterial abnormality.

DIGITAL SUBTRACTION ANGIOGRAPHY. This consists of angiography combined with a digital subtraction system to enhance the radiographic image. The system compares the images taken before and after the arrival of the contrast medium and subtracts the images of bone, soft tissue, and surrounding structures (Fig. 11–1). Additionally, the computer application can focus and sharpen the

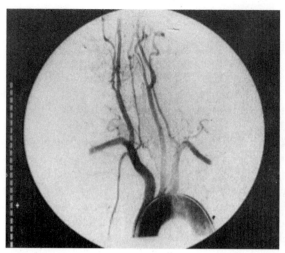

FIGURE 11–1. Digital angiogram of the thoracic aorta and the main arteries it supplies. Vessels appear dark because of the computer manipulation that is used in digital subtraction angiography. (With permission from Adler, A.M., & Carlton, R.R. [1994]. Introduction to radiography and patient care [vol. 1, Slide 208C]. Philadelphia: W.B. Saunders.)

NORMAL VALUES

No anatomic or functional abnormalities of the arteries are noted. There is no visualization of stenosis, occlusion, aneurysm, bleeding, tumor, or cyst.

image, alter the shades of gray, and provide diagnostic information that the human eye is unable to see without computer system assistance (Kim and Orron, 1992). Digital subtraction angiography has an additional advantage over conventional angiography because it uses a smaller, safer dosage of the contrast medium.

INTRAVENOUS DIGITAL SUBTRACTION ANGIOGRAPHY. This procedure uses an intravenous route for administering the contrast medium. Once the contrast material is in the venous circulation, it flows through the heart and enters the arterial circulation. Despite the advantage of easier and safer venipuncture technique with a reduced risk of hemorrhage, this method is used infrequently. It has a higher rate of nondiagnosis and requires a larger bolus of contrast material to obtain the images. It is occasionally used in selected circumstances, such as when aortic occlusion is suspected (Kim and Orron, 1992).

PATHOPHYSIOLOGY OF ARTERIAL DISEASE. *Atherosclerosis* is a common cause of arterial disease. The atheromas, or deposits of fibrofatty plaque, grow on the tissue surfaces of the lumen of arteries, impeding the blood flow. Thrombus formation can also develop at the site of the atherosclerotic deposit, increasing the size of the blockage and causing further restriction of the circulation.

In severe atherosclerotic disease, the atheromas are greater in number and also larger. In atherosclerosis, many arteries of the body contain the atheromatous deposits, although some arteries may be more occluded than others. The arteries affected most commonly are the aorta, renal arteries, coronary arteries, femoropopliteal arteries, internal carotid arteries, and the arteries of the circle of Willis.

Arteriography provides visualization of the atherosclerotic deposits and the stenosis or occlusion of the artery. It also demonstrates the diminished circulation to the distal tissue beyond the site of the obstruction and the presence of any collateral circulation that helps to provide blood flow to the distal tissue.

EMBOLI. These may also cause stenosis or obstruction in the arterial circulation. Commonly, the original cause of the clot is atrial fibrillation with the formation of a mural thrombus. As particles of the clot break off, they move into the arterial circulation and lodge in a distal part of the arterial tree (Fig. 11–2). Emboli also may originate from the thrombus that develops on atheromatous plaque. Particles of thrombus or the fibrofatty plaque break off and travel to a more distal arterial site. Angiography demonstrates the location of the embolus or emboli and the extent of the circulatory impairment caused by embolic activity.

ANEURYSMS. These are often caused by atherosclerosis, although in some instances, they result from infection or trauma. An aneurysm is a dilation of the artery that results from the degeneration and weakening of the muscular layer in the wall of the artery. Once the aneurysm develops, it interferes with the arterial blood flow. It tends to enlarge over time and a thrombus may develop on the luminal surface. The abdominal aorta is a common site for the development of an aneurysm; it can extend in size and involve the iliac arteries as well (Fig. 11–3). Other sites of aneurysmal disease are the femoral, popliteal, and cerebral arteries.

DISSECTION OF AN ARTERY OR ANEURYSM. On the luminal surface, blood penetrates and separates the tissue layers of the artery. As a result, there is hematoma formation, expansion of the tear, and creation of a blood-filled channel in the arterial wall. The dissection can occlude arteries (Fig. 11–4), and a dissecting aneurysm is prone to rupture. The aorta, particularly the ascending aorta just above the aortic valve, is a common site of dissection.

Angiography provides visualization of the size, type, and location of the aneurysm or dissection. It also defines the location of other arterial vessels that originate in or near the aneurysm or dissection. These arteries can be occluded or stenosed because of the aneurysmal defect. In the angiographic procedure, there is always a risk of rupture of the aneurysm during the injection of the contrast material under high pressure. Therefore, computed tomography or magnetic resonance imaging may be the preferred diagnostic procedure to identify these defects. These noninvasive techniques provide a clear diagnosis of an aneurysm or dissection with less risk to the patient.

ARTERIOVENOUS FISTULA AND ARTERIOVENOUS MALFORMATION. These are false or abnormal communications between an artery and vein. The fistula usually develops as a result of trauma, and the malformation is of congenital origin. Angiography is used to identify the condition and its precise location. When embolization or surgery is planned for correction of the condition, angiography provides specific location and landmarks. These conditions and their vascular sources can be hard to locate visually.

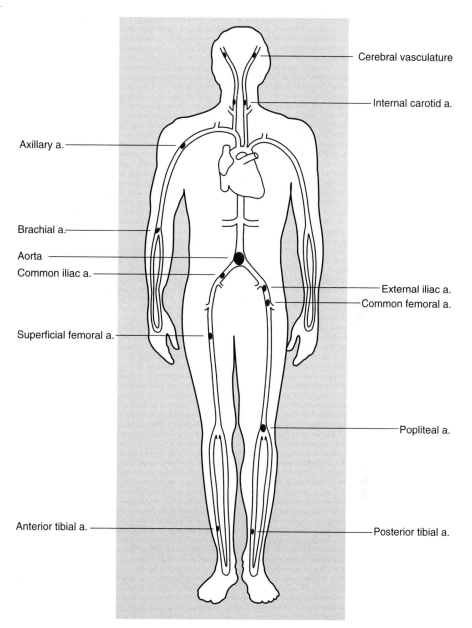

FIGURE 11–2. Common locations of arterial emboli. Eighty per cent of all emboli lodge in the lower extremities.

TUMORS AND CYSTS. These conditions produce characteristic changes in the circulation that supplies the tumor or in the tissue surrounding the tumor. Arteriography is no longer used as the primary diagnostic test to identify tumor or malignancy because the alternative noninvasive tests such as computed tomography, magnetic resonance imaging, and ultrasound are effective and safe.

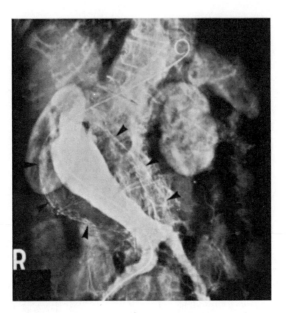

FIGURE 11–3. X-ray film of an abdominal aortic aneurysm. In addition to visualization of the aneurysm, the concerns include the size of the aneurysm and possible involvement of the renal or femoral arteries. Calcification in the wall of an abdominal aortic aneurysm gives a good indication of the aortic size *(arrows)*. (With permission from Fahey, V.A. [1994]. *Vascular nursing* [2nd ed., p. 260]. Philadelphia: W.B. Saunders.)

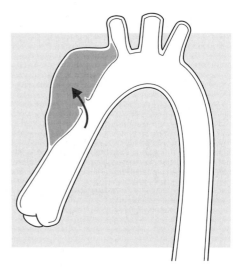

FIGURE 11–4. Dissection of the ascending aorta. In addition to visualization of the dissection, the concerns include the size of the dissection and any occlusion of the main arteries that arise from the aortic arch.

Angiography is still used, however, to assess certain tumors for vascularity and malignancy. It is also used to guide certain interventions in the treatment of tumors.

TECHNIQUE OF ANGIOGRAPHY. Angiography is performed using a 2% lidocaine solution for local anesthesia. The patient may also receive sedative-analgesia to promote relaxation. The procedure is performed under sterile conditions to minimize the risk of septicemia.

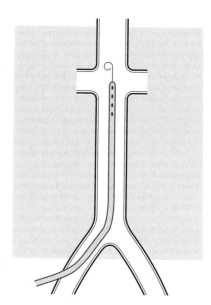

FIGURE 11-5. Transfemoral catheterization of the abdominal aorta. Once the catheter is inserted into the femoral artery, it is advanced in a retrograde direction through the aorta until it reaches the desired level.

Arterial access is achieved by the use of a special needle or catheter that passes through the skin and is inserted directly into an artery. When a needle is used, the access is by puncture technique. Once the needle has been properly placed in the lumen of the artery, the contrast medium is instilled by an automatic injection through the hollow core of the needle.

When a catheter is used, a small incision in the skin is made, and a needle is then used to enter the artery. Once the needle is in place, a specifically shaped guidewire is inserted through the core of the needle and is advanced into the artery. The needle is then removed and an arterial catheter inserted, gliding over the guidewire. The combined guidewire and catheter, called a guided catheter, is carefully manipulated and advanced through the arterial structure until the tip reaches the area to be examined (Fig. 11-5). The guidewire is removed, leaving the catheter in place. The contrast medium is injected by automated technique.

When the catheter is used to enter a specific branch of the aorta, the procedure is called a *selective arteriogram*. For example, *arch arteriography* means that the catheter is advanced to the aortic arch for arteriographic study.

Angiography using the digital subtraction system can be performed to visualize the whole arterial tree, the arteries of the upper extremities, or those of the lower extremities. Selective arteriography provides a view of the arterial circulation to specific sites or organs, including the heart, brain, lung, kidney, liver, spleen, and pancreas.

ARTERIAL PUNCTURE SITE. The selection of the puncture site is based on several variables, including the goal or purpose of the study, the arterial problem that exists, and the condition of the arteries. The common femoral artery is often used because of its wide diameter and superficial location. In the transfemoral approach, the needle puncture site is in the groin, usually on the side with the best pulses.

When the femoral approach cannot be used because of pulselessness or occlusion of the aorta or iliofemoral arteries, an alternative route is selected. The transaxillary and translumbar approaches may be used as alternatives.

In the transaxillary approach, the catheter is placed in the proximal brachial artery of the left arm in the section that overlies the head of the humerus. Once it is in the artery, it is advanced into the descending aorta. In the translumbar approach, the needle or catheter is inserted through the back, past the anterolateral edge of the vertebra, and into the aorta. Translumbar aortography is performed at the level of T12–L1 (high) for examination of the abdominal aorta. The level of L2–L3 (low) is used for examination of the peripheral or pelvic arterial circulation.

Critical Thinking: After angiography with a trans-axillary approach, how would you assess the patient for a possible brachial nerve plexus injury?

The location of the puncture site is important because in the postoperative period, the nurse must assess for bleeding, neurologic deficit, and the presence of distal pulses. The assessments vary based on the location of the possible arterial obstruction or bleeding source. The three sites generally used for arterial puncture are presented in Figure 11–6.

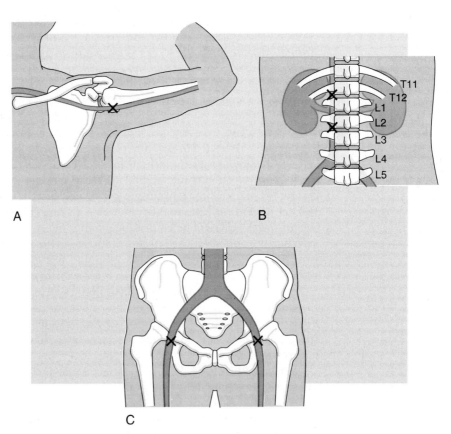

FIGURE 11–6. Arterial access sites for angiography. *A,* Transaxillary arterial puncture. *B,* Translumbar aortography arterial puncture, dorsal view. *C,* Femoral arterial puncture.

CONTRAST MEDIUM. There are numerous intravascular agents available and all of them contain iodine. The iodinated contrast material provides the radiopacity and enhances the imaging of arteriography procedures. The different contrast preparations vary in their osmolarity to the blood. Those that are hyperosmolar provide the best contrasted image, but there is also a higher degree of toxicity.

The sensation of pain, heat, a warm feeling, or burning on injection is related to the hyperosmolarity of the contrast medium. Contrast material with high osmolarity will cause greater discomfort, and low-osmolarity preparations cause markedly decreased sensations of pain. Problems of nausea and vomiting are also related to the hyperosmolarity of the contrast medium, but the relationship is not clear.

All contrast media have the potential to affect the heart, including the myocardial cells, the coronary arteries, and the conduction system. As contrast material is injected into the heart or its coronary arteries, or as it passes through the heart in the circulatory route, there is potential for sudden hypotension, bradycardia, or altered conductivity. The changes are generally small or insignificant, but on rare occasion, they can lead to cardiorespiratory arrest (Kim and Orron, 1992).

All iodinated contrast material is eliminated from the body by glomerular filtration with no tubular reabsorption. The contrast medium is somewhat nephrotoxic, however, and does alter the renal blood flow and filtration rate temporarily. In almost all cases, the contrast material is easily eliminated without damage, but occasionally there is renal failure. The cause is not clearly understood, but it is important to maintain hydration before, during, and after angiography to promote complete excretion of the contrast medium.

Allergic reactions to the iodine can also occur. The mild form is a temporary urticaria and flushing that responds to the administration of an H_1 antagonist such as diphenhydramine (Benadryl). The more severe but uncommon reactions include bronchoconstriction, laryngeal edema, and cardiopulmonary arrest. Patients who are most vulnerable are those with a history of allergy to iodine, a history of previous reaction to a contrast medium, a history of asthma, or current hemodynamic instability.

Patient Characteristics

Patients with chronic arterial occlusive disease often have coexisting conditions of hypertension, diabetes, atherosclerosis, and a history of cigarette smoking (Massey, 1986). Many patients experience anxiety regarding the diagnosis, the degree of damage to the arteries, and the possibility of surgical intervention based on the results of the test (Fahey and Riegel, 1989).

Purpose of the Test

Angiography is used to investigate arterial vascular disease, to provide visualization of the arteries during treatment procedures, and to evaluate the effectiveness of vascular surgery in the postoperative period.

Procedure

Iodinated contrast medium is injected into an artery using a percutaneous approach with a needle or an arterial catheter. Fluoroscopic images and serial x-ray films are taken to demonstrate the vasculature and any arterial abnormalities that are present. The procedure requires 30 to 90 minutes to complete.

Findings

ABNORMAL VALUES

Peripheral vascular disease   Arterial spasm
Arterial occlusion   Tumor
Aneurysm   Pseudoaneurysm
Vascular fistula   Arteriovenous malformation
Traumatic arterial injury   Inflammatory vasculitis
Thromboangiitis obliterans   Giant cell arteritis
Fibromuscular dysplasia   Raynaud disease or phenomenon
Collagen vascular disease   Cystic medial necrosis

Interfering Factors

- Severe allergy to contrast medium (iodine)
- Recent myocardial infarction
- Coagulation disorder
- Renal failure
- Sickle cell disease
- Homocystinuria

Nursing Implementation

Pretest

To help reduce distress and anxiety, instruct the patient regarding the procedure. Most patients do not know much about the test and will benefit from information about what they will experience, feel, see, or hear. The discussion can help with accurate expectations and reduction of the anxiety associated with the unknown (Rice et al., 1988; Fahey and Riegel, 1989).

The discussion should include the following information:

1. The patient should drink extra fluids on the day before the test and after the test. No oral fluids or food can be taken for a specific period just before the test, but intravenous fluids will be administered during the test. An intravenous line is established before the test begins.
2. Analgesic and sedative medication is usually given in the pretest period to help with relaxation.

3. A local anesthetic is injected to numb the tissue surrounding the arterial puncture site.
4. The patient will lie on the radiography table and will not be able to move during the test. There is a lot of equipment in the room, used for the imaging, computer calculations, and radiographs. The patient will hear clicking and whirring sounds during the procedure.
5. As the contrast medium is injected, the patient may feel a burning sensation or feelings of heat, pain, or nausea. Although there is momentary discomfort, the sensations are normal and brief.

Critical Thinking: During the pretest assessment interview, what type of information makes you suspect that the patient has an allergy to iodine?

Identify and report any patient history of allergy to iodine or seafood or a previous reaction to a radiologic procedure that used a contrast medium or dye.

Obtain written consent from the patient or the person legally responsible for the patient's health care decisions.

Ensure that recent laboratory tests results are posted in the patient's chart. Blood urea nitrogen and creatinine determinations are needed to verify adequate renal function. Activated partial thromboplastin time, prothrombin time, and platelet determinations are needed to verify adequate clotting ability (Vogelzang, 1988).

Begin the nothing-by-mouth status 2 to 6 hours before the test, as prescribed. The time variable is based on the protocol of the physician or institution and the type of angiographic study planned.

Monitor the vital signs and record the results in the chart. Hypertension should be under control before this test is performed.

On the morning of the test, assess the peripheral pulses and record the findings. A small ink mark should be placed on the skin to record the distal sites of pulsation. When a cerebral angiogram is planned, an assessment of mental status is carried out.

Have the patient void to empty the bladder before going to the radiology department. The contrast medium acts like a diuretic and can cause the discomfort of a full bladder.

Assist the patient in removing all clothing and putting on a hospital gown. All metallic objects such as jewelry must be removed from the area of the x-ray field.

Administer the on-call, pretest sedation. This usually consists of an intramuscular injection of the narcotic-analgesic meperidine (Demerol) and a sedative-relaxant such as midazolam (Versed) or diazepam (Valium).

Posttest

Place the patient on bedrest for 6 to 8 hours. The punctured extremity is to be kept straight. When the aorta has been used as the puncture site, the patient must remain in the supine position for the same amount of time.

Monitor vital signs and peripheral pulses every 15 minutes for 1 hour, every 30 minutes for 2 hours, and every hour for 2 hours (Vogelsang, 1988). With a femoral puncture site, the pertinent pulses are those of the popliteal, dorsalis pedis, and posterior tibialis arteries. With an aortic puncture site, the bilateral pulses include the femoral sites as well as those of the lower extremities. With an axillary puncture site, the brachial, radial, and ulnar pulses are significant.

Assess and compare the extremities bilaterally for signs of occlusion of the circulation and neurologic deficit. The data include color, warmth, movement, and the absence of neurologic signs such as pain or paresthesias.

Frequently observe the pressure dressing and the tissue surrounding the puncture site for signs of swelling or hematoma. Gentle palpation of the tissue near the puncture site also may be performed.

Extra fluid intake is essential to prevent nephrotoxicity from the contrast medium. The patient should drink extra fluids to achieve a 2000- to 3000-ml intake in the 24-hour posttest period. Because of the high volume of fluids and the diuretic effect of the contrast material, there will be a frequent need to urinate. Remind the patient that a urinal or bedpan must be used during the period of bedrest (Fahey and Riegel, 1989). Keep intake and output measurements.

Complications

The overall complication rate for the angiography procedure is 1 to 3%. The axillary approach has the most complications and the femoral approach has the fewest (Kim and Orron, 1992). Complications at the puncture site are the largest group of problems. Hemorrhage and hematoma are the most frequent complications, particularly when the axillary approach is used. During a translumbar puncture, a poorly placed needle can puncture the pleural lining or lung, causing a hemothorax. Hypertension, atherosclerotic disease, and coagulation problems are factors that contribute to the risk of bleeding.

Dissection, pseudoaneurysm, and perforation of the artery are usually caused by incorrect insertion of the needle, passage of the guidewire, or the high pressure of the contrast medium as it is injected.

Thromboembolic complications can develop because thrombi tend to form at the puncture site, on the catheter or guidewire, or at the area of arterial wall abnormality.

Neurologic complications are varied, depending on the underlying cause or location. In the axillary approach, the brachial nerve plexus is near the puncture site. If hemorrhage or hematoma occurs and the brachial nerve plexus is compressed, the compression can result in paralysis of the arm and hand. When cerebral angiography is performed, the patient can experience cerebral ischemia from a thrombus or embolus.

Complications from the contrast medium can range from mild to severe. They consist of an allergic response, cardiorespiratory complications, and renal failure.

TABLE 11–1
COMPLICATIONS OF ANGIOGRAPHY

Complication	Nursing Assessment
Hematoma or hemorrhage	**Femoral Puncture Site** Ecchymosis and swelling in the thigh or inguinal or abdominal area Inability to void Hypotension Tachycardia **Axillary Puncture Site** Ecchymosis and swelling in the axilla and inner aspect of the arm Paresthesias (numbness, tingling, "pins and needles" sensations) Severe pain **Translumbar Site** Dorsal ecchymosis Dyspnea-hemoptysis Hypotension Tachycardia
Dissection or pseudoaneurysm	Pain Obstruction of distal circulation Diminished or absent pulses Cyanosis of distal tissue Palpable mass at puncture site
Thrombus or embolus	Diminished or absent pulses Pain Cool, dusky, cyanotic extremity Loss of sensation in distal part of extremity
Neurologic deficits	**Peripheral** Pain Paresthesias (numbness, pins and needles sensation) Loss of motor function distally **Cerebral** Hemiplegia Confusion Aphasia Loss of consciousness Pupillary changes
Contrast reaction	Urticaria (hives, itching) Flushed skin Wheezing, stridor, dyspnea Hypotension Cardiac arrhythmias Cardiac arrest
Renal failure	Oliguria or anuria Elevated blood urea nitrogen–creatinine levels

The complications of angiography and the nursing assessments are presented in Table 11–1.

REFERENCES

Appleton, D.L., & La Quaglia, J.D. (1988). Vascular disease and postoperative management. *Critical Care Nurse, 5,* 34–42.

Bright, L.D., & Georgi, S. (1992). Peripheral vascular disease: Is it arterial or venous? *American Journal of Nursing, 92,* 34–43, 45–47.

Fahey, V.A. (Ed.). (1994). *Vascular nursing* (2nd ed.). Philadelphia: W.B. Saunders.

Fahey, V.A., & Riegel, B.J. (1989). Advances in diagnostic testing for vascular disease. *Cardiovascular Nursing, 25,* 13–18.

Griffith, H.W. (1989). *Instructions for patients: Medical tests and diagnostic procedures.* Philadelphia: Lea & Febiger.

Kim, D., & Orron, D.E. (1992). *Peripheral vascular imaging and intervention.* St Louis: Mosby-Year Book.

Massey, J.A. (1986). Diagnostic testing for peripheral vascular disease. *Nursing Clinics of North America, 21,* 207–218.

Mills, P. (1991). High tech, human touch: Care study . . . arteriography. *Nursing Times, 87,* 36–38,40.

Prevost, D.B. (1990). Diagnostic arteriography and percutaneous transluminal angioplasty of the lower extremities. *Journal of Vascular Nursing, 8,* 6–12.

Rice, V.H., et al. (1988). Development and testing of an arteriography information intervention for stress reduction. *Heart Lung, 17,* 23–27.

Vogelzang, R.L. (1988). Vascular imaging techniques and percutaneous vascular intervention. In V.A. Fahey (Ed.). *Vascular nursing,* Philadelphia: W.B. Saunders.

CHAPTER 12

Tomography

Computed tomography (CT) and magnetic resonance imaging (MRI) are diagnostic scanning procedures that provide multidimensional images of an organ or body section. Each test provides many cross-sectional images that are called tomographic slices or axial slices. These slices give two-dimensional detailed views of the anatomy and internal structure of the target area. Since axial slices can be obtained every few millimeters, the dimension of depth can also be achieved. The transverse, sagittal, coronal, and other planes can be selected to obtain the best view of the target tissue and its relationship to the surrounding tissues (Fig. 12–1). The different planes are selected by computer operations rather than by moving the patient into awkward positions.

CT uses ionizing radiation to produce the images, which are seen in black, white, and gray, depending on the density of the tissue. MRI uses a large magnet and radio waves to measure the rapidly changing magnetic fields of specific tissues. This procedure is based on the biochemical and physical properties of different tissues, including measurement of the movements of hydrogen ions. The distinct movements of the electrons are converted to images in shades of gray (Shankar and Montanera, 1991).

Both procedures use the computer and specialized software to integrate the images, provide clear definition or focus, and assist in the selection of axial slices. The image quality is precise and accurate so that even the smallest abnormalities can be visualized. These modalities have the ability to image the target tissue without the need for invasive procedures such as arterial catheterization or surgery. CT and MRI are used for similar purposes, but each has distinct advantages that determine the selection of one of them as the diagnostic tool of choice (Table 12–1).

Initially, both of these procedures were used to provide imaging of the brain. The results were so impressive that CT and MRI revolutionized the diagnostic methods of neurology and neurosurgery. Today the diagnostic uses have been

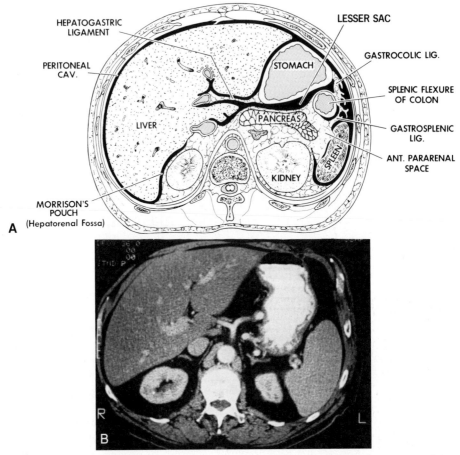

FIGURE 12–1. Cross-sectional views of the abdomen. *A,* Diagram of a transverse section of the upper abdomen showing the relationship of the organs and structures. *B,* A transverse computed tomography (CT) image of the abdomen. (*A,* Reproduced with permission from Moss, A.A., Gansu, G., & Genant, H.K. [Eds.]. [1992]. *Computed tomography of the body with magnetic resonance imaging* [2nd ed., vol. 3, Abdomen and pelvis, p. 1140]. Philadelphia: W.B. Saunders. *B,* Reproduced with permission from Thompson, M.A., et al. [1994]. *Principles of imaging science and protection* [vol. 2, Slide 390]. Philadelphia: W.B. Saunders.)

expanded to include the torso and all the organs and structures within it. As new computers and software evolve, there will be ongoing improvements in the areas of scanning speed, time, cost, enhanced capabilities, and new applications for both these diagnostic modalities (Moss et al., 1992).

DIAGNOSTIC PROCEDURES

TABLE 12–1
COMPARISON OF COMPUTED TOMOGRAPHY AND MAGNETIC RESONANCE IMAGING

Advantages of Computed Tomography	Advantages of Magnetic Resonance Imaging
Detailed view of bones and intra-osseous pathologic conditions	Visualization of any anatomic plane
Shorter time for procedure	Visualization of the vascular structures
Lower cost	Sharper contrast between soft tissues and the pathologic mass
More comfortable for the patient	

The basic procedures of tomography are presented in this chapter. The uses of the procedures in specific body systems are summarized in subsequent chapters.

COMPUTED TOMOGRAPHY

(RADIOLOGIC SCAN)

Synonyms:

CT scan, computerized axial tomography, CAT scan

NORMAL VALUES

No structural or anatomic abnormalities are noted.

Background Information

Computed tomography uses a fan of x-ray beams in a multidimensional scanning process to produce cross-sectional images of the body. As the x-rays pass through the body tissues, they fall on a circle of detectors located in the scanner ring. In some models, the x-ray source remains stationary while the detectors rotate around the patient. In other models, the detectors remain stationary while the x-ray sources rotate (Fig. 12–2). Regardless of the model, the scanning process uses the images taken from many angles to form a 360-degree composite scan for each axial slice.

As the radiation passes through the body, some of the energy is absorbed, based on the density of the tissue that is examined. The detectors register the photons that are able to pass through the tissue. The impulses are converted to numeric data by computer operations. The computer then translates the numbers to specific images that reflect the cross-sectional views of the targeted tissue. The images appear on the monitor and are photographed for further study.

Depending on the type of scanner and its speed, it takes from 1 to 10 seconds to obtain a single, two-dimensional axial slice. The patient lies on a movable

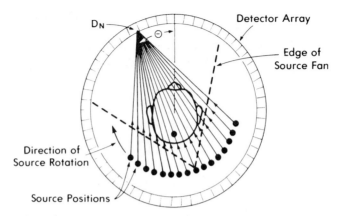

FIGURE 12–2. Computed tomography that uses a stationary ring system. In this system, the detectors (D_N) are aligned in a stationary ring. The radiation sources are in a fan-like array that moves clockwise around the patient. Each source of radiation transmits photons through the patient so that they fall on a particular detector on the opposite side of the body. As the sources move circularly, new detectors receive the radiation signals and record the data until the entire circle and a single axial slice are completed. (Modified with permission from Moss, A.A., Gansu, G., & Genant, H.K. [Eds.]. [1992]. *Computed tomography of the body with magnetic resonance imaging* [2nd ed., vol. 3, Abdomen and pelvis, p. 1365]. Philadelphia: W.B. Saunders.)

Critical Thinking: After a car accident, a 14-year-old boy is scheduled for a CT scan of the abdomen, STAT. He is frightened and in moderate pain, but his vital signs are stable. What nursing interventions can help him follow instructions and complete the scan without delay?

table that gradually advances through the scanner ring. Every few seconds the table advances a small but precise distance, and another axial slice is imaged. Using the sum of many axial slices and the computer resolution of the views, the entire target organ or area of the body can be viewed. The computer rapidly integrates hundreds to thousands of images to provide the final views desired.

The differences in tissue density and composition are reflected clearly in the final images. As the x-ray photons pass through dense tissue such as bone, calcium, metallic implants, or thrombi, many of the photons are absorbed. Thus, few photons reach the detectors in the scanner ring, and the image of this dense tissue appears whiter or brighter on the monitor or film. Conversely, less dense, more radiolucent tissue allows more photons to pass through the tissue to the detectors. These tissues appear in various shades of gray, according to their density and structure. Air and fat are very radiolucent and produce dark or black tones.

The CT scan can image the head or torso with or without contrast medium. When it is used, the contrast medium provides a sharper, more enhanced view of the tissue. In the head, the CT scan clearly identifies the intracranial or extracerebral abnormalities that are present. In the torso, it is effective in its imaging of the liver, pancreas, kidneys, adrenal glands, lungs, heart, great vessels, abdominal lymph glands, retroperitoneal area, abdominal cavity, vertebrae, and spinal cord. It can differentiate between a cyst and a malignant tumor.

The research of Peteet and associates (1992) investigated the psychologic needs of patients who undergo CT scanning. The data revealed that patients who had this diagnostic test for the first time appreciated the explanation of the procedure and information about what to expect. Patients who repeated the test demonstrated less need for explanations because they were already experienced and knowledgeable. Both the "first-time" patients and the "repeaters" reported anxiety, discomfort, and fear of the test results, fear of the machine, and some feelings of claustrophobia. Relaxation techniques were helpful in controlling the anxiety or discomfort.

Purpose of the Test

CT provides precise visualization of the structure, size, shape, and density of soft tissue, bone, major blood vessels, and organs of the head and torso. It distinguishes between benign and malignant tissue and is used in the staging of cancerous tumors. It can also be used to analyze the bone mineral content of the vertebrae in the assessment of osteoporosis (Moss et al., 1992).

Procedure

With or without the use of an iodinated contrast medium, the patient moves through a scanner ring, and multiple x-ray beams pass through the tissue. As the x-ray photons fall on the scanner, images of the tissue are produced. Depending on the speed of the scanner and the use or nonuse of contrast medium, the procedure requires 1 to 2 hours to complete.

Findings

ABNORMAL RESULTS

Tumor	Congenital malformation
Malignancy	Abscess
Cyst	Calculus
Stenosis	Inflammation
Thrombus	Fluid collection
Embolus	Bleeding or hemorrhage
Arteriosclerotic plaque	Organ atrophy
Calcification	

Interfering Factors

- Jewelry or metal in the x-ray field
- Uncooperative behavior
- Pregnancy
- Failure to maintain a nothing-by-mouth status (as indicated)
- Allergy to iodine (with the use of contrast material)
- Severe liver or kidney disease (with the use of contrast medium)

Nursing Implementation

Pretest

Ask the patient if there is any history of allergy to iodine or shellfish or an allergic reaction to dye or contrast material used in a previous x-ray study.

Explain the procedure to the patient and obtain written consent from the patient or person legally designated to make health care decisions for the patient.

If contrast medium is to be used, instruct the patient to discontinue all food and fluids for 4 to 8 hours before the test.

Instruct the patient to remove all clothes, jewelry, and other metal objects. A hospital gown is worn.

When no contrast material is used, reassure the patient that the procedure is painless. With the use of contrast medium, explain that the contrast agent is injected intravenously. The patient may feel warmth at the injection site, a salty taste, headache, or nausea as the agent is injected. These are temporary sensations that will disappear in a few minutes.

Provide appropriate orientation and reassurance so that fear of the unknown is diminished. Many patients feel some degree of apprehension as they enter the enclosed space of the machine.

Encourage the patient to relax during the scanning process by using techniques such as visual imagery, meditation, or prayer (Peteet et al., 1992).

Sedatives are usually used for the infant or child less than 3 years old, particularly when the scan requires an extended period of immobility. Administer the prescribed sedative. The medication is usually chloral hydrate, 25 mg/kg (by mouth or per rectum), or phenobarbital, 5 mg/kg (intramuscularly) (Cook et al., 1992).

During the Test

Instruct the patient to remain motionless while in the scanner and to hold his or her breath when instructed to do so.

Keep an emesis basin in the nearby area in case the patient vomits after receiving the contrast medium.

Posttest

If sedatives were administered, monitor the vital signs on a regular basis until the patient is responsive and awake.

No other special nursing measures are needed.

MAGNETIC RESONANCE IMAGING

(MAGNETIC FIELD SCAN)

Synonyms:

MRI, nuclear magnetic resonance, NMR

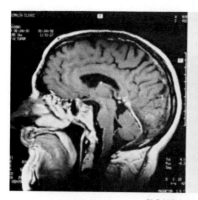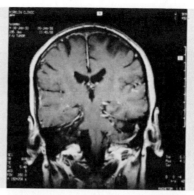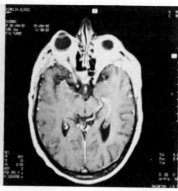

FIGURE 12–3. Magnetic resonance imaging (MRI) of the head. MRI can produce images in almost any body plane: *Left,* sagittal; *middle,* coronal; *right,* transverse. (Reproduced with permission from Thompson, M.A., et al. [1994]. *Principles of imaging science and protection* [vol. 2, Slide 393]. Philadelphia: W.B. Saunders.)

NORMAL VALUES

No structural or anatomic abnormalities are noted.

Background Information

MRI is a noninvasive imaging technique that uses a large, powerful magnet and a radiofrequency coil to obtain cross-sectional images of body tissues. The images of axial planes are similar to those produced by CT, but MRI has a greater ability to produce images of any plane (Fig. 12–3). This is particularly useful in imaging of the head, neck, brain, and spinal cord (Shankar and Montanera, 1991).

MRI is based on the biochemical differences among cells. The nuclei of cells contain many atoms that have electric fields. For example, each hydrogen atom has one proton with a positive charge. These protons are distributed randomly in tissue and behave like tiny magnets. When in the presence of the strong magnetic field produced by the MRI magnet, the body protons spin and move to realign in a new axis formation. The machine then emits pulses of radio waves to stimulate and detect the magnetized protons. The pulsed signal first displaces the aligned protons and then, on cessation of the radiowave stimulus, the machine detects the proton return to magnetized alignment (Fig. 12–4).

Different tissues have different densities, water content, proton concentrations, and patterns of movement. Once these differences are identified by the radiofrequency coil, the messages are transmitted to the computer for number coding and translation into images of the tissue. In shades of black, white, and gray, the images are seen on the monitor and are photographed or taped for further diagnostic study. Fat and marrow produce high signal intensities and brighter images. Bone and air produce low intensity, weak signals, and dark images.

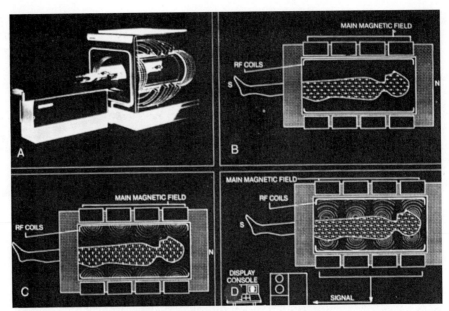

FIGURE 12–4. The process of MRI. *A*, Scanner consists of a cylinder (the magnet itself) into which the patient enters by a movable table top based on a large platform. *B*, The main magnetic field is oriented parallel to the long axis of the patient. The hydrogen nuclei of the patient's body water and fat point north in the direction of the main field. *C*, Radiofrequency (*RF*) coils acting like a radio transmitter send a radio signal of sufficient energy to tilt the nuclei 90 degrees, or at right angles to the main field. *D*, In the process of recovering alignment with the main field, the protons emit radio signals picked up by the RF coils, now acting like a radio receiver, and are transformed into an image. (Reproduced with permission from Nadolo, L.A., et al. [1991]. The neuroradiology of visual disturbances. *Neurologic Clinics*, 9, 5.)

Some of the pulse sequences are used to detect anatomic differences among tissues, including the difference between cystic and solid tissues or the difference among muscle, ligament, and tendon. Other pulse sequences are used to detect pathologic changes. Fluid-filled growths, edema, inflammation, hematoma, and neoplasm all produce weak signals, and the images are darker than those of the surrounding tissue.

ADVANTAGES AND LIMITATIONS. When compared with CT, MRI has several benefits. It does not expose the patient to ionizing radiation. It is also true, however, that the biologic effect and potential health risk of exposure to magnetic fields have not been fully defined (Moss et al., 1992). MRI is considered safer because there is no need for iodinated contrast medium. The use of contrast agents is in the developmental stage, however, and they may be used in the future. MRI appears to be effective in the imaging of the blood flow within the lumen of major arteries and veins.

MRI has some limitations in its cost and capability. The test is expensive because of the sophisticated machinery and the requirements for special housing. Because MRI cannot image bone, it cannot be used to measure bone density or to detect calcification or calcium stone formation. In addition, there are definite risks to the patient with a ferromagnetic metal implant. The magnetic forces of MRI are so great that they will twist or move the metallic object. Because the implant would become a missile and cause severe injury, metallic implants are a contraindication for this test. Examples of metallic objects in the body include aneurysmal vascular clips, shrapnel located near the eyes or neurologic system, pacemakers, joint implants, and intrauterine devices.

PSYCHOLOGIC NEEDS. The patient experiences no pain during MRI, but it is perceived as an unpleasant experience for many individuals. The patient may feel distress because he or she must enter the tubular chamber and cannot move or see outside. Throughout the test, the patient hears loud, harsh noise that sounds like the crushing of metal. In addition to the worry about the possible diagnosis, the patient feels uncertainty and sensory deprivation. All these factors contribute to a rise in anxiety (Flaherty and Hoskinson, 1989).

A variety of anxiety reactions can occur among patients, including nervousness, fear, palpitations, or sensations of choking. Although most patients report minor to moderate anxiety, a few can exhibit more acute disturbance, including panic disorder, claustrophobia, or depression. If the anxiety is too severe, the patient may not be able to tolerate the procedure.

Critical Thinking: Because of trauma to the joint, a promising young athlete must have an MRI scan of the shoulder. He expresses anxiety and dismay about his future athletic ability and asks you how MRI can help him. How would you respond to his question and feelings?

Purpose of the Test

MRI is used to assess anatomic structures, organs, and soft tissue, including visualization of any pathologic condition that is present. It can differentiate between benign and malignant growth and may be used to stage the cancer or evaluate the response to treatment of the malignancy.

Procedure

The patient enters the tube of the MRI machine, which contains a circular magnet and a radiofrequency coil. In the presence of the magnetic field and radio wave stimulation, there are changes in and movement of tissue protons. These movements are converted by computer to precise images of the tissue in any plane selected. The total time for test completion is about 90 minutes.

Findings

ABNORMAL RESULTS

Tumor
Stricture
Stenosis
Thrombus
Embolus
Malformation

Abscess
Inflammation
Edema
Fluid collection
Bleeding or hemorrhage
Organ atrophy

Interfering Factors

- Jewelry or metal in the magnetic field
- Metallic implant in the body
- Uncooperative behavior

Nursing Implementation

Pretest

Ask the patient if there is a history of any metallic implant having been placed in the body.

Explain the procedure and sensations that the patient will experience. Obtain written consent from the patient or person legally designated to make the patient's health care decisions.

To help minimize anxiety, encourage the patient to have a friend or relative stay during the procedure (Quirk et al., 1989).

To help minimize the emotional discomfort, encourage the patient to use relaxation strategies such as mental imagery of landscapes or seascapes, closing the eyes, and breathing for relaxation (Quirk et al., 1989).

Instruct the patient how to obtain help while inside the machine (Flaherty and Hoskinson, 1989).

Sedatives are usually used for the infant or child less than 3 years old, particularly when the scan requires an extended period of immobility. Administer the prescribed sedative. The medication is usually chloral hydrate, 25 mg/kg (by mouth or per rectum), or phenobarbital, 5 mg/kg (intramuscularly) (Cook et al., 1992).

During the Test

Instruct the patient to remain motionless on the narrow table during the test.

Posttest

If sedatives were administered, monitor the vital signs on a regular basis until the patient is responsive and awake.

No other special nursing measures are needed.

REFERENCES

Cook, B.A., et al. (1992). Sedation of children for technical procedures: Current standard practice. *Clinical Pediatrics, 31,* 137–142.

Flaherty, J.A., & Hoskinson, K. (1989). Emotional distress during magnetic resonance imaging. *New England Journal Of Medicine, 320,* 467–468.

Friedman, W.N., et al. (1992). Computed tomography in obstetrics and gynecology. *Journal of Reproductive Medicine, 37,* 3–18.

Moss, A.A., Gansu, G., & Genant, H.K. (Eds.). (1992). *Computed tomography of the body with magnetic resonance imaging* (2nd ed., vol. 3, Abdomen and pelvis). Philadelphia: W.B. Saunders.

Nadalo, L.A. (1991). The neurology of visual disturbances. *Neurologic Clinics, 9,* 1–35.

Peteet, J.R., et al. (1992). Emotional support for patients with cancer who are undergoing CT: Semistructured interviews of patients at a cancer institute. *Radiology, 182,* 99–102.

Quirk, M.E., et al. (1989). Evaluation of three interventions to reduce anxiety during MR imaging. *Radiology, 173,* 759–762.

Shankar, L., & Montanera, W. (1991), Computed tomography versus magnetic resonance imaging and three-dimensional applications. *Medical Clinics of North America, 75,* 1355–1366.

PART IV

LABORATORY
AND
DIAGNOSTIC TESTS
OF
SPECIFIC
BODY SYSTEMS

CHAPTER 13

Pulmonary Function

In the hierarchy of human needs, oxygen (O_2) is the primary basic need. Humans evolved to take in O_2 (pulmonary system) and deliver that O_2 (circulatory system) to meet cellular requirements. This chapter presents the laboratory and diagnostic tests used *today* to evaluate an individual's ability to ventilate and oxygenate the blood. Older tests, which have been replaced by advanced technology such as computed tomography (CT) and magnetic resonance imaging (MRI), are not included.

Unfortunately, today multiple environmental and personal habits place individuals at risk for pulmonary disorders. The experience of dyspnea, shortness of breath, breathlessness, and cough frequently brings the individual to the primary caregiver. Since many pulmonary disorders produce the same clinical manifestations, pulmonary laboratory and diagnostic testing is required for accurate diagnosis. This chapter presents many of the tests required to evaluate the patient with a respiratory dysfunction. Chapter 7 discusses tests related to respiratory infection.

The goal of the majority of tests included in this chapter is to identify the cause of the individual's distress so that appropriate therapy and relief may be provided. These tests are also used to evaluate the effectiveness of the therapies prescribed.

LABORATORY TESTS

ANGIOTENSIN-CONVERTING ENZYME

(SERUM)

Synonyms:

ACE, serum angiotensin-converting enzyme, SACE

NORMAL VALUES

ADULT*	**Male:**	12–36 IU/L *or* SI same
	Female:	10–30 IU/L *or* SI same

*Norms for individuals younger than 20 years of age are slightly higher

---

Background Information

Critical Thinking: After SACE results have been found to be elevated, how do you explain to your patient with hypertension why an ACE inhibitor has been prescribed for him or her?

Angiotensin-converting enzyme (ACE) is found primarily in the pulmonary epithelial cells. ACE converts angiotensin I to angiotensin II. Angiotensin II stimulates the adrenal cortex to produce and secrete the hormone aldosterone and is also a powerful vasoconstrictor. Since angiotensin II is a vasopressor, ACE levels are determined as part of the diagnostic work-up for hypertension.

ACE levels increase with sarcoidosis, a disease that causes widespread granulomatous lesions that may affect any organ, including the lungs. When sarcoidosis is suspected, ACE levels are determined to diagnose the disorder, assess its severity, and evaluate its therapy.

Purpose of the Test

ACE levels are determined to evaluate hypertension and to diagnose and treat sarcoidosis.

Procedure

A venipuncture is performed to collect 5 ml of blood in a red-topped tube.

Findings

Increase	Decrease
Cirrhosis	Adult respiratory distress
Gaucher disease (familial	syndrome
disorder of fat metabolism)	Diabetes mellitus
Hansen disease	Hypothyroidism
Histoplasmosis	Tuberculosis
Hodgkin disease	
Hyperthyroidism	
Myeloma	

Pulmonary fibrosis
Sarcoidosis
Scleroderma

Interfering Factors

• Steroids

Nursing Implementation

The nursing actions are similar to those for other venipuncture procedures.

ANION GAP

(SERUM)

Synonyms:
none

─────────────────── **NORMAL VALUES** ───────────────────

10–15 mEq/L *or* SI 10–15 mmol/L

Background Information

The anion gap is the sum of unmeasured anions in the serum: phosphates, sulfates, ketones, proteins, and organic acids. It is used to distinguish among causes of metabolic acidosis. Patients with diabetic ketoacidosis usually have a large anion gap, whereas those with metabolic acidosis due to intestinal fluid loss have a nearly normal anion gap.

Besides disease states that cause an increase or decrease in anions and cations in the blood, or both, fluid volume also affects the anion gap, because it may cause hemoconcentration (higher sodium and potassium concentration) or hemodilution (dilutional hyponatremia).

Purpose of the Test

The anion gap is calculated to determine the cause of metabolic acidosis.

Procedure

The anion gap is determined by subtracting the sum of measured anions (bicarbonate [HCO_3] and chloride [Cl]) from the measured cations (sodium [Na] and potassium [K]).

Findings

Increase	Decrease
Hypernatremia	Hypercalcemia
Hyperosmolar coma	Hypermagnesemia
Hypocalcemia	Hypoalbuminemia
Hypomagnesemia	Hyponatremia
Ketoacidosis	Multiple myeloma
Lactic acidosis	
Starvation	

Interfering Factors

- Dehydration
- Ingestion of licorice
- Excessive ingestion of
  Antacids
  Ethylene glycol
  Methanol
  Paraldehyde
  Salicylates
- Medications (partial listing)
  Adrenocorticotropic hormone   Diuretics
  Antihypertensive agents   Lithium
  Bicarbonates   Steroids
  Chlorpropamide   Vasopressin

Nursing Implementation

Critical Thinking: Calculate your patient's anion gap, when the Na^+ is 140, K^+ is 5, HCO_3^- is 30, and Cl^- is 100. How would the nurse interpret this result?

After the results of blood electrolyte determinations are obtained, calculate the anion gap during the test with the following formula:

$$(Na + K) - (HCO_3 + Cl) = anion\ gap$$

ARTERIAL BLOOD GASES

(ARTERIAL BLOOD)   *Synonym:*
                        ABGs

─────────────── **NORMAL VALUES** ───────────────

pH		7.35–7.45 *or* SI 7.35–7.45
PCO_2		35–45 mm Hg *or* SI 4.7–5.3 kPa
HCO$_3$		21–28 mEq/L *or* SI 21–28 mmol/L
PO_2	**Adult:**	80–100 mm Hg *or* SI 10.6–13.3 kPa
	Newborn:	60–70 mm Hg *or* SI 8.0–10.33 kPa
SaO_2	**Adult:**	>95% *or* SI Fraction saturated >0.95
	Newborn:	40–90% *or* SI Fraction saturated 0.40–0.90
Base excess		± 2 mEq/L *or* SI ± 2 mmol/L

Background Information

Arterial blood gases (ABGs) provide valuable information about the acid-base balance, ventilatory ability, and oxygenation status of the individual. The data derived from blood gas determinations support clinical assessments and are invaluable in evaluating medical treatment and nursing interventions. ABG determinations provide the pH, partial pressure of carbon dioxide (PCO_2), partial pressure of oxygen (PO_2) and bicarbonate HCO$_3$ levels, O_2 saturation (SaO_2), and base excess.

The pH (the partial pressure of hydrogen [H$^+$] ions in the blood) reflects the acid-base balance of the blood. A narrow normal range of pH reflects the body's need to maintain a relatively constant internal environment. There is an inverse relationship on the pH scale between H$^+$ concentration and pH. As the H$^+$ ion concentration goes up, the pH goes down. As the H$^+$ ion concentration increases in solution, H$^+$ ions can be given up. This is acidosis. As the H$^+$ ion concentration decreases in solution, H$^+$ ions could be taken on (H$^+$ ion receiver). This is alkalosis.

The pH of human blood is normally 7.35 to 7.45, which on the pH scale of 1 to 14 is above the neutral point of 7 and is therefore slightly alkaline. In the clinical setting, however, a pH of 7.35 to 7.45 is used as the neutral state. A pH below 7.35 is acidotic, and a pH above 7.45 is alkalotic. One must remember that other body fluids have a different normal pH (Fig. 13–1).

To maintain a normal pH, the body has evolved several mechanisms, including its buffering system and its respiratory and renal systems. Within seconds, the body buffers respond to changes in pH. Within minutes, the respiratory system adapts to changes in H$^+$ ion concentration, and in days the kidneys respond to the acid-base needs of the body. These changes reflect the body's ability to compensate for deviations in the acid-base balance and the need to maintain that balance within a narrow range.

PCO_2 reflects the ventilatory ability of the body to maintain a normal pH. Carbon dioxide (CO_2) in blood travels as an acid (carbonic acid) until it dissociates in the lungs to be exhaled as CO_2. When the blood becomes acidotic, the respiratory system increases its rate and depth of ventilation to blow off CO_2 and thus reduce the acid load in the blood. If the blood is alkalotic, the respiratory

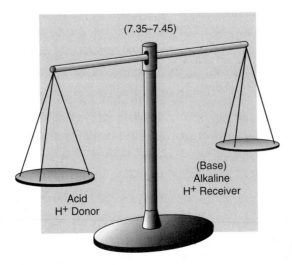

(7.35–7.45)

(Base)
Alkaline
H^+ Receiver

Acid
H^+ Donor

FIGURE 13–1. Acid-base balance.

system hypoventilates to retain CO_2 and thus move the pH toward normal. Pathologic conditions of the pulmonary system may interfere with this normal compensatory action. If an individual cannot adequately ventilate, CO_2 is retained and acidosis occurs. Since this acidosis is due to a pulmonary cause, it is called respiratory acidosis. If the lungs blow off too much CO_2, respiratory alkalosis occurs. Table 13–1 presents causes of respiratory acid-base imbalances and the nursing assessments for the imbalances.

The bicarbonate ion concentration in the blood (HCO_3) reflects the renal system's response to the acid-base balance. HCO_3 is made by the kidneys, and its production is increased whenever acidosis is present. However, it takes several days for the kidneys to respond fully to changes in pH. If the kidneys are unable to make HCO_3 to buffer the acid in the blood, the patient will be in a state of metabolic acidosis. If the patient has too much HCO_3 or has lost acid from the gastrointestinal or genitourinary tract, a state of metabolic alkalosis occurs (see Table 13–1 for causes of metabolic acid-base imbalances and the nursing assessments for the imbalances).

The pulmonary and renal systems are constantly balancing and adapting to maintain a normal pH. An abnormality in pH initiates a compensatory mechanism to restore the pH to normal or to achieve at least a partial compensation. For example, a patient with chronic obstructive pulmonary disease retains CO_2 and thus experiences respiratory acidosis. The kidneys respond to the decrease in pH and increase their production of HCO_3. This response results in a normal pH and high Pco_2 and HCO_3 levels. A serious clinical problem occurs with mixed acid-base imbalances, in which the patient has both respiratory and metabolic acidosis or respiratory and metabolic alkalosis, because compensation cannot take place.

The partial pressure of oxygen in the blood (Po_2) is the amount of O_2 dissolved in the plasma. Sao_2 is the percentage of hemoglobin saturated with O_2. Together, Po_2 and the Sao_2 form the O_2 *content*, the total amount of O_2 in the blood.

TABLE 13-1
CAUSES AND ASSESSMENTS OF ACID-BASE IMBALANCES

Cause	Clinical Assessment
Respiratory Acidosis	
Respiratory center dysfunction	Dyspnea
Opiates, anesthetics, sedatives	Tachycardia
Oxygen-induced hypoventilation	Headache
Central nervous system lesions	Confusion
Disorders of the respiratory muscles or	Pallor
chest wall	Diaphoresis
Myasthenia gravis, amyotrophic lateral	Apprehension
sclerosis	Restlessness
Kyphoscoliosis	Lethargy
Pickwickian syndrome	Drowsiness
Splinting caused by pain	Coma
Disorders of gas exchange	Hypertension
Chronic obstructive pulmonary disease	Papilledema
Acute pulmonary edema	
Asphyxia	
Hypoventilation while on a mechanical	
ventilator	
Respiratory Alkalosis	
Hyperventilation	Restlessness
Atelectasis	Dizziness
Severe anemia	Agitation
Pulmonary emboli	Tetany
Anxiety	Numbness
Central nervous system disorders	Tingling
Brain stem dysfunction	Muscle cramps
Subarachnoid hemorrhage	Seizures
Salicylate poisoning	Increased deep tendon reflexes
Hypermetabolic states	
Fever	
Thyrotoxicosis	
Sepsis	
Hyperventilation while on mechanical	
ventilation	

Table continued on following page

When interpreting the O_2 levels in the blood, barometric pressure must be considered. At sea level, barometric pressure is 760 mm Hg, at 5000 ft above sea level, barometric pressure is 630 mm Hg; thus, the norms for Po_2, Sao_2, and O_2 content must be adjusted. The normal arterial Po_2 at sea level is 95 mm Hg; at 5000 ft above sea level, it is 72 mm Hg (Hudak, 1994).

TABLE 13–1
CAUSES AND ASSESSMENTS OF ACID-BASE IMBALANCES *Continued*

Cause	Clinical Assessment
Metabolic Acidosis	
Diabetic ketoacidosis	Lethargy
Lactic acidosis	Nausea
Cardiac arrest	Vomiting
Anaerobic metabolism	Dysrhythmias
	Coma
Ingestion of acid	Hypotension
Salicylates	Hyperventilation
Ethylene	
Methanol	
Paraldehyde	
Loss of bicarbonate	
Diarrhea	
Fistulas	
Renal failure	
Metabolic Alkalosis	
Loss of acid	Dullness
Vomiting	Weakness
Excessive gastric suction	Dysrhythmias
Urine loss	Tetany
Diuretics	Hypokalemia
Excessive corticosteroids	Hyperactive reflexes
Exogenous	
Endogenous	
Hypokalemia	
HCO_3 overload	
Excessive ingestion of $NaHCO_3$	
Massive blood transfusions	
Excessive ingestion of licorice	
Nonparathyroid hypercalcemia	

$NaHCO_3$ = sodium bicarbonate.

When one assesses the patient's oxygenating ability, there may be a need to determine the ability of the O_2 to diffuse from the alveoli into the blood. This cannot be measured directly but can be estimated with the *alveolar-arterial* difference in partial pressure of O_2 ($P_{AO} - P_{aO_2}$), also known as the *alveolar-arterial (A-a) gradient*. The A-a gradient is the difference between the P_{O_2} in alveolar air and the P_{O_2} in the arterial blood. It is calculated by first estimating the alveolar P_{O_2}, which is done by subtracting the water vapor pressure from the barometric pressure, multiplying the resulting pressure by the

F_{IO_2} (percentage of oxygen the patient is breathing), and subtracting this from $1\frac{1}{4}$ times the arterial P_{CO_2}. To obtain the A-a gradient, the patient's arterial P_{O_2} is subtracted from the calculated alveolar P_{O_2}. Thus,

$$\text{A-a gradient} = \text{barometric pressure} - \text{water vapor}$$
$$\text{pressure} \times F_{IO_2} - 1\frac{1}{4} \times P_{ACO_2} - P_{aO_2}$$

The normal A-a gradient is less than 20.

An a:A ratio may also be calculated. The a:A ratio is the percentage of alveolar P_{O_2} that arterial P_{O_2} represents.

$$\text{a:A ratio} = \text{measured arterial } P_{O_2}\text{:calculated alveolar } P_{O_2}$$

The normal a:A ratio is greater than 0.75. The A-a gradient normally increases as the O_2 concentration the patient breathes increases, the a:A ratio does not. Therefore, for patients on mechanical ventilation with a changing F_{IO_2}, the a:A ratio is used to determine whether oxygen diffusion is improving.

Critical Thinking: A patient with chronic COPD presents with a pH of 7.34, a P_{O_2} of 64, and a P_{CO_2} of 68. How can the nurse plan to prevent O_2-induced hypoventilation in this patient?

The base excess or base deficit on the ABG determinations reflects the metabolic nonrespiratory contribution to the maintenance of normal pH. With a base excess, a positive balance greater than 2 correlates with metabolic alkalosis and with a base deficit, a negative balance less than −2 correlates with metabolic acidosis.

Purpose of the Test

ABG determinations are obtained for a variety of reasons, including the diagnosis of chronic and restrictive pulmonary disease, adult respiratory failure, acid-base disturbances, pulmonary emboli, sleep disorders, central nervous system dysfunctions, and cardiovascular disorders such as congestive heart failure, shunts, and intracardiac atrial or ventricular shunts, or both.

Arterial blood gases are used in the management of patients on mechanical ventilators and during the weaning process from the ventilators.

Procedure

An arterial blood sample of 5 ml is obtained via an arterial puncture or arterial line. The radial or femoral artery is usually used in adults, whereas the temporal artery is used in infants.

Findings

Acid-base imbalances (see Table 13–1)
Hypoxia

Interfering Factors

- Noncompliance with proper collection procedure, including air bubbles in syringe
- Low hemoglobin level

Nursing Implementation

Pretest

Critical Thinking: What
potential injury to a
patient may occur if
the Allen test is not performed before a radial
artery puncture?

Before a radial artery puncture is executed or a radial arterial line is inserted, perform an Allen test to ensure adequate collateral circulation to the hand. With the Allen test, occlude the radial and ulnar arteries with the fingertips while instructing the patient to tighten the fist (Fig. 13–2). Ask the patient to open the fist and remove pressure from the ulnar artery while maintaining pressure on the radial artery. If color returns to the palm and fingers within 5 seconds, there is adequate ulnar circulation. Prepare ice and heparinized syringe.

QUALITY CONTROL

Excessive amounts of heparin or an air bubble in the syringe will cause inaccurate results. Draw 1 ml of heparin up into a 5- to 10-ml glass syringe or plastic syringe with vented plunger. The plunger is

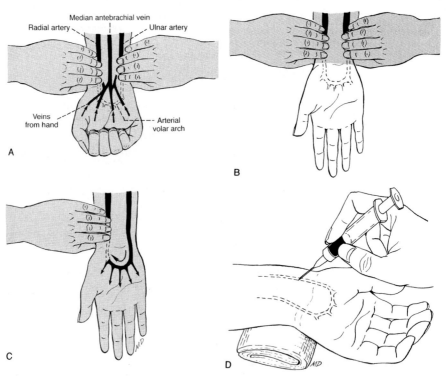

FIGURE 13–2. The Allen test. (Reprinted with permission from Black, J.M., & Matassarin-Jacobs, E. [1993]. *Luckmann and Sorensen's medical-surgical nursing* [4th ed., p. 927]. Philadelphia: W.B. Saunders.)

pulled back to coat the barrel of the syringe. Excess heparin is discarded, leaving the needle full of heparin. A 22- or 25-gauge needle is used.

QUALITY CONTROL

The patient's temperature affects results because the ABG machines are calibrated using gases at 37° C. Note on the requisition slip the patient's temperature at the time the blood is drawn.

Instruct the patient about the arterial puncture; it is painful. If the patient is anxious, hyperventilation may occur, giving false readings because CO_2 will be blown off.

Do not obtain an ABG reading for 20 to 30 minutes after a procedure or event that does not reflect the patient's current status (e.g., suctioning).

During the Test

Nurses in specialized units perform arterial punctures. The procedure is usually performed by a physician or a respiratory therapist.

If a radial artery is used, the wrist is hyperextended and the arm is externally rotated.

Palpate the artery for the point of maximal impulse. Cleanse the site with an alcohol swab.

The needle is inserted at a 45- to 90-degree angle at the point of maximal pulsation.

Observe the syringe; the plunger will move upward under arterial pressure.

Withdraw the needle and cork the syringe with the airtight rubber stopper.

Roll the syringe between your palms to mix the blood with the heparin.

Label the syringe and place it on ice.

Send the specimen to the laboratory immediately with a requisition slip marked with the patient's temperature, the F_{IO_2} value, and the time.

Posttest

Immediately after the needle is withdrawn, exert pressure on the arterial site for a minimum of 5 minutes. If the patient is taking anticoagulants, pressure on the site should be maintained for at least 10 minutes.

Complications

Complications from ABG determination result from the trauma of arterial puncture. They include arterial occlusion from hematoma formation or thrombosis, bleeding, and infection (Table 13–2).

TABLE 13–2
COMPLICATIONS OF ARTERIAL PUNCTURE

Complication	Nursing Assessment
Arterial occlusion	Loss of distal pulse Distal parts: pale, cool, cyanotic
Bleeding	Hematoma formation Restlessness Tachycardia Hypotension
Infection	Tachycardia Fever Elevated white blood cell count

LACTIC ACID

(VENOUS)

Synonym:

lactate

--- NORMAL VALUES ---

1–2 mEq/L *or* SI 1–2 mmol/L

Background Information

Lactic acid levels may be used to assess cellular oxygenation. If the cells do not receive adequate oxygen, anaerobic metabolism will occur. Lactic acid is the by-product of anaerobic metabolism. Rising lactate levels indicate a need to examine O_2 transport and consumption parameters.

Purpose of the Test

Lactate levels are used to support the diagnosis of cellular hypoxia. Lactate levels can also predict survival. High lactate levels (>4 mmol/L) indicate higher mortality rates.

Procedure

A venipuncture is performed to obtain 7 ml of blood which is placed in a gray-topped tube.

Findings

Increase	Decrease
Alcoholism	Hypothermia
Diabetic ketoacidosis	
Hyperthermia	
Liver failure	
Malignancies	
Peritonitis	
Shock states	

Interfering Factors

- Noncompliance with dietary and activity restrictions
- Medications
  - Acetaminophen (large doses)
  - Ethanol (large dose)
  - Epinephrine
  - Fructose
  - Sorbitol

Nursing Implementation

The nurse takes actions similar to those taken with other venipuncture procedures and:

Pretest

Instruct the patient not to eat or drink for 12 hours before the test and to ingest no alcohol for 24 hours before the blood is drawn.
Instruct the patient to lie quietly for 2 hours before the blood is drawn.

During the Test

Critical Thinking: When blood is drawn for a lactic acid level, why is the tourniquet omitted?

No tourniquet should be applied, and the patient should not clench the fist. Send the specimen to the laboratory immediately.

Posttest

Advise the patient to resume a normal diet and activity level.

MIXED VENOUS BLOOD GASES

(VENOUS)

Synonyms:

─────────── **NORMAL VALUES** ───────────

pH	7.33–7.43 *or* SI 7.33–7.43
Pco_2	41–51 mm Hg *or* SI 5.3–6.0 kPa
HCO$_3^-$	24–28 mm Hg *or* SI 24–28 mmol/L
Pvo_2	35–49 mm Hg
Svo_2	60–80%

Background Information

Mixed venous blood gases provide a method for evaluating the dynamic balance between O_2 supply and O_2 delivery to the body. Since the organs of the body use various amounts of O_2, mixed venous blood gases measure the blood in the pulmonary artery, which contains the venous return from all the body systems. Arterial blood gases reflect what is available for body use (supply), whereas venous blood gases tell how well the body delivered and used this supply.

Mixed venous blood gases may be obtained periodically, or the mixed venous oxygen saturation (Svo_2) may be monitored continuously.

Svo_2 monitoring has been made possible by the development of fiberoptic pulmonary catheters. It is measured by light emitted from the catheter and reflected onto red blood cells within the pulmonary artery. The wavelength of reflected light is interpreted by the Svo_2 computer and continuous readings of the Sao_2 in the blood *after* systemic circulation is provided. Since the hemoglobin normally unloads about 25% of its O_2 during systemic circulation, the normal Svo_2 is 75% with a range of 60 to 80%.

No specific value for Svo_2 is correlated with anaerobic metabolism. A Pvo_2 of 28 mm Hg does correlate with lactic acidosis, however, and this Pvo_2 corresponds to an Svo_2 of 53%, which seems to be a critical value.

The Svo_2 is used to evaluate the response to nursing care. For an unstable patient, changes in position, bathing, suctioning, and so forth can increase O_2 consumption, resulting in a corresponding lowering of the Svo_2. If the Svo_2 falls to less than 60% or varies by 10% from the patient's baseline for longer than 3 minutes (10 minutes after suctioning), a full assessment of the patient is needed, including a cardiac output determination.

Critical Thinking: As the nurse repositions the patient, it is noted that the Svo_2 decreases from 64 to 0%. What nursing assessments should be done and documented? What possible interventions should be taken?

Purpose of the Test

Mixed venous blood gases are obtained to assess the O_2 supply and tissue O_2 consumption. Changes in Svo_2 indicate a need to determine which factor in O_2 supply and delivery is abnormal: cardiac output, hemoglobin level, tissue O_2 consumption, or Sao_2.

Procedure

A mixed venous sample may be obtained in a heparinized syringe from the distal port of the pulmonary artery catheter, or continuous Svo_2 may be assessed from a fiberoptic pulmonary artery catheter attached to an oximeter.

Findings

Increase in Svo_2	**Decrease in Svo_2**
Anesthesia	Anemia
Cyanide toxicity	Anxiety
High Fio_2	Bleeding
Hypothermia	Cardiogenic shock
Left-to-right shunt	Congestive heart failure
Neuromuscular blockade	Fever
Relaxation	Hyperthermia
Sepsis	Hypovolemia
Sleep	Inadequate Fio_2
Vasodilation	Large burns
	Pulmonary disease
	Multiple trauma
	Position changes
	Seizures
	Severe pain
	Shivering
	Suctioning

Critical Thinking: The Svo_2 oximeter reads 40%. After assessing the patient, no clinical evidence of hypoxia or poor perfusion is present. What is an appropriate nursing intervention?

Interfering Factors

- Inadequate perfusion
- Poorly positioned pulmonary artery catheter

Nursing Implementation

Care is based on the technique used. With a random mixed venous blood gas determination, use the procedures that follow.

Pretest

Explain the procedure to the patient.
Assess the hemodynamic monitoring system.
Gather equipment: a 1- to 3-ml syringe, a 2- to 10-ml syringe, a syringe cap, heparin, and ice

During the Test

Wear gloves.

Draw up 1 ml of heparin into the 3-ml syringe and draw back to coat the barrel. Expel heparin, leaving heparin in the needle.

Attach an empty 10-ml syringe to the sampling stopcock at the distal port of the pulmonary artery catheter.

Turn the stopcock off to the infusion solution.

Aspirate 5 ml into the syringe to clear the distal line of solution. Close the stopcock to the infusion and syringe. Remove the syringe and discard. In special situations, such as in neonates, the blood is saved and returned to the patient after the sample is drawn.

Attach the 3-ml heparinized syringe to the stopcock.

Open the stopcock to the syringe and aspirate blood slowly.

Close the stopcock, remove the 3-ml syringe, and expel any air bubbles. Cap the syringe.

Gently roll the syringe in your hand to mix heparin and blood. Place on ice.

Attach a 10-ml syringe to the stopcock. Open the stopcock to the solution and flush to clear the stopcock of blood.

Turn solution off to the stopcock port used to obtain the sample and cap the sampling port.

Flush the line and ensure the patency of the distal port. Check the monitor for pulmonary artery waveform.

Send blood to the laboratory immediately; clearly indicate on the slip that the blood is a mixed venous sample.

Obtain and send an ABG sample, if ordered.

Posttest

Compare ABG and mixed venous blood gas samples.

With continuous Svo_2 monitoring, a special pulmonary artery catheter is inserted with Svo_2 sampling capability.

During the Test

Attach Svo_2 port to the oximeter.

Calibrate the oximeter when the catheter is inserted and once a day while it is in the patient.

Calibration or recalibration is needed if there is a 4% or greater difference between the mixed venous sample sent to the laboratory and the Svo_2 reading on the oximeter.

Set alarm parameter at plus and minus 10% of the displayed Svo_2. Adjust alarms as the patient's Svo_2 varies or the oximeter is recalibrated.

If intensity alarm signals, check catheter placement and patency. Check for air bubbles in the system or kinking of the catheter. Reposition the patient. Flush the catheter if needed.

Document hourly Svo_2 readings.

DIAGNOSTIC PROCEDURES

BRONCHOSCOPY

(ENDOSCOPY)

Synonyms:

NORMAL VALUES

No abnormalities visualized
No growth in culture specimen

Background Information

Bronchoscopy is an endoscopic diagnostic procedure involving the inspection and observation of the trachea, larynx, and bronchi. Bronchoscopy is ordered when patients have unexplained pulmonary signs and symptoms or when nonspecific radiologic abnormalities exist.

A bronchoscope permits direct visualization of the tracheobronchial tree down to the subsegmental bronchi. A biopsy of lung tissue may also be performed via the bronchoscope (*transbronchial lung biopsy*). It is usually done under fluoroscopy to permit proper positioning and opening of the forceps. A *transcatheter bronchial brushing* may also be carried out to obtain a biopsy. A small brush is inserted through the bronchoscope, which is moved back and forth until cells adhere to the brush. Once the brush is removed, the cells are brushed onto slides. Most bronchoscopy is performed with a fiberoptic bronchoscope, which is flexible. To remove foreign objects lodged in the larger airways, a rigid bronchoscope is usually used.

Purpose of the Test

Bronchoscopy may be performed for therapeutic or diagnostic purposes. Bronchoscopy is used diagnostically to visualize possible tumors, obstructions, secretions, bleeding sites, or foreign objects in the tracheobronchial system. It permits the collection of secretions for cytologic and bacteriologic study as well as for assessing tumors for potential resection. Tissue for lung biopsy may be obtained through the bronchoscope.

Bronchoscopy is used therapeutically to remove foreign objects from the tracheobronchial tree and to remove secretions that are obstructing the air passages. A bronchoscope may be used to fulgurate (electrodesiccate) and excise lesions.

Procedure

A rigid (metal) or flexible fiberoptic bronchoscope may be used. The rigid bronchoscope employs a hollow metallic tube with a light at its distal end. It is useful in removing secretions, in evaluating future surgical interventions, and in dilating endobronchial strictures. The rigid bronchoscope has almost been replaced by the flexible fiberoptic bronchoscope. However, the physician may prefer the metal scope under certain circumstances, such as endobronchial tumor resection, massive hemorrhage, foreign body removal, and in the treatment of small children.

The bronchoscope is inserted through the nose (most common) or through the mouth. The tube is inserted as the physician observes the condition of the upper airways through the eyepiece and guides the tube to the area of the lung to be evaluated (Fig. 13–3).

Findings

Atelectasis
Bleeding
Foreign objects
Infection
Lung cancer
Secretions
Tuberculosis
Tumors

Interfering Factors

• Patient distress (may require general anesthesia)

Nursing Implementation

Pretest

Ensure that a signed consent form has been obtained.
Obtain a medication history to determine whether the patient is receiving anticoagulant therapy or aspirin preparations.

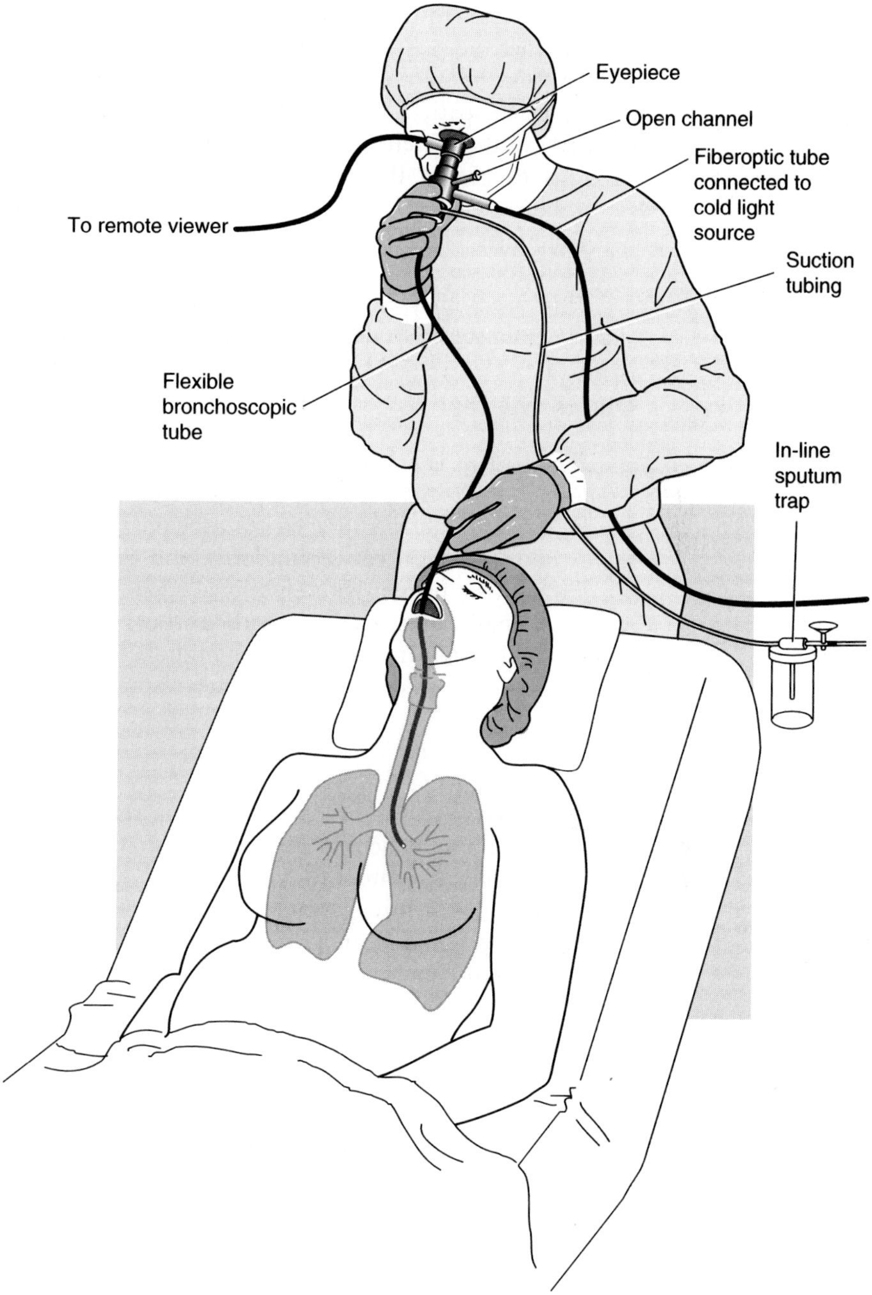

Eyepiece

Open channel

Fiberoptic tube
connected to
cold light
source

Suction
tubing

To remote viewer

In-line
sputum
trap

Flexible
bronchoscopic
tube

FIGURE 13–3. Flexible fiberoptic bronchoscopy.

If a prothrombin time (PT), a partial thromboplastin time (PTT), and a platelet count were ordered, check the results and report any clotting problems to the physician.

Instruct the patient not to eat or drink for 4 to 6 hours before the test.

Explain the purpose of and procedure for the test.

Warn the patient that the local anesthetic may taste bitter.

Inform the patient that as the tube is inserted it may feel like something is caught in the throat; provide reassurance that the airway is not blocked.

Administer atropine as prescribed to reduce tracheobronchial secretions and inhibit vagal stimulation. A sedative, such as midazolam hydrochloride (Versed), may also be ordered and given. Codeine may be ordered and administered to decrease the cough reflex.

Critical Thinking: A bronchoscopy is planned for a patient who expresses anxiety about gagging during the procedure. How can the nurse reassure the patient?

During the Test

The patient is positioned in the semi-Fowler or Fowler position.

Attach the patient to the pulse oximeter.

A local anesthetic is sprayed onto the pharynx, and the solution is dropped onto the vocal cords, epiglottis, and trachea to abolish the gag reflex.

Provide the patient with emotional support.

Encourage the patient to breathe through the nose or to pant.

Maintain supplemental O_2 for nonintubated patients.

Continuously monitor the patient's response, vital signs, and Sao_2.

Posttest

Critical Thinking: How can the nurse assess for the return of the gag reflex after bronchoscopy?

Withhold food and fluids until the gag reflex returns.

Reassure the patient that hoarseness, sore throat, and blood-streaked sputum are common.

Provide throat lozenges or throat sprays as comfort measures.

If a biopsy has been performed, send the specimen to the histology laboratory and the microbiology laboratory.

Complications

Complications are rare but include bleeding, drug reactions, hypotension, laryngospasm, bronchospasm, hypoxia, dysrhythmia, and cardiopulmonary arrest (Table 13–3).

CAPNOGRAM

Synonyms:

exhaled carbon dioxide, capnography, end-tidal carbon dioxide, $Petco_2$

TABLE 13–3
COMPLICATIONS OF BRONCHOSCOPY

Complication	Nursing Assessment
Bleeding	Hemoptysis Restlessness Hypotension Tachycardia Tension pneumothorax
Hypoxia	Low Sao_2 Restlessness Pallor, cyanosis Dyspnea Confusion Dysrhythmias
Bronchospasm	Wheeze Hypoxia
Laryngospasm	Stridor
Dysrhythmia	Abnormal electrocardiogram
Pneumothorax	(Dependent on size of the pneumothorax) Apprehension Feeling of tightness in chest Decreased or absent breath sounds over site Dyspnea Cough Depressed chest movement on affected side With a tension pneumothorax: mediastinal shift to unaffected side

Critical Thinking: Following a bronchoscopy, the nurse notes that the patient's larynx is shifting from the middle of the neck to the left side. Breath sounds are heard over the left lung fields, but sound is muted on the right side. What is the priority action of the nurse at this time?

─────── **NORMAL VALUES** ───────

35–45 mm Hg

Background Information

Capnography provides a CO_2 waveform, which produces a CO_2 elimination pattern during exhalation and a total percentage of CO_2 exhaled per breath.

Carbon dioxide is measured at the end of exhalation because at this point the exhaled CO_2 approximates arterial CO_2 levels. With normal perfusion of the lungs, arterial CO_2 will be a few millimeters higher (5 mm Hg) than end-tidal CO_2 (P_{ETCO_2}). When perfusion is not adequate, this assumption cannot be made. Figure 13–4 shows a typical tracing of a capnogram.

The P_{ETCO_2} increases in hypermetabolic states, which increases the production of CO_2, and in hypoventilation in which CO_2 is not blown off. The P_{ETCO_2}

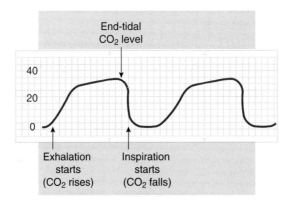

FIGURE 13–4. Capnograph tracing. On exhalation the capnograph tracing shows a rapid rise in carbon dioxide followed by a plateau. At the end of exhalation, the end-tidal carbon dioxide level is obtained. As inspiration begins, there is a dramatic decrease in carbon dioxide.

decreases when the metabolic rate decreases, as production of CO_2 decreases, and when there is decreased perfusion, causing a decrease in pulmonary blood flow.

Purpose of the Test

Monitoring exhaled CO_2 permits continuous evaluation of alveolar ventilation, reducing the number of ABG determinations needed. P_{ETCO_2} can be used to evaluate ventilator changes and weaning parameters from mechanical ventilation. It will confirm endotracheal intubation, since no capnographic waveform will occur if the tube is in the esophagus. P_{ETCO_2} is also used to assess the adequacy of cardiopulmonary resuscitation.

Procedure

Exhaled CO_2 is measured with exhaled gas analyzers. These analyzers measure the CO_2 by mass spectrometry or infrared analysis. Mass spectrometry requires aspiration of exhaled gas, whereas the infrared gas analyzer is usually attached to the exhalation tubing on a ventilator. The recorded value refers to the amount of infrared light absorbed by the exhaled breath. The higher the CO_2 level, the more infrared light absorbed, and the higher the reading.

Findings

Increase	Decrease
Burns	Acute cardiac failure
Hypermetabolic states	Anesthesia
Hypoventilation	Cardiac arrest
Malignant hyperthermia	Hypothermia
Multiple trauma	Hypothyroidism
	Hypovolemia
	Pulmonary edema
	Pulmonary embolism

Interfering Factors

- Cardiopulmonary abnormalities
- Metabolic disorders

Nursing Implementation

Critical Thinking: The capnographic waveform disappears. What immediate nursing assessments would be appropriate?

During the Test

Check the capnographic waveform. It should return to zero baseline on inspiration. If it does not, check the seal of the expiratory demand valve on the ventilator and the fresh gas flow in the tube.

If the waveform disappears or drops to zero, it may indicate accidental extubation, obstruction, esophageal intubation, or cardiac arrest.

COMPUTED TOMOGRAPHY OF THE CHEST

(TOMOGRAPHY)

Synonyms:

chest CT, CT scan of the chest

NORMAL VALUES

No abnormalities noted

Background Information

CT scans are used to diagnose pulmonary lesions (benign or cancerous). They can detect primary and metastatic processes. With some bronchogenic cancers, CT scanning can be used to determine the invasive extent of the cancerous process into the chest wall, diaphragm, or mediastinum as well as extrathoracic metastasis. CT scans are used to plan radiation therapy for the patient with cancer of the lung.

CT scans can be performed with or without contrast dyes. Vascular problems such as arteriovenous malformations, central pulmonary emboli, and septic emboli may be identified with CT scanning when a contrast agent is used. With orally ingested dyes, esophageal lesions can be evaluated.

CT scanning may be helpful in diagnosing silicosis, asbestosis, lung abscesses, and empyema. (See Chapter 12 for a complete discussion of CT scanning.)

LUNG BIOPSY

(PATHOLOGY)

Synonym:

open lung biopsy

━━━━━━━━━━━━━━━━ **NORMAL VALUES** ━━━━━━━━━━━━━━━━

Normal tissue

Background Information

Critical Thinking: Describe the psychologic implications of having an open lung biopsy, and the nurse's role in easing the patient's concerns.

A lung biopsy is performed to remove lung tissue so that the cells may be examined microscopically for pathologic features. A variety of methods are used to obtain these lung cells. Tissue samples may be obtained by bronchoscopy (see pp. 285–288), by fine needle biopsy (see pp. 298–300), or by open biopsy.

With an open biopsy, surgery is required, with its potential risks. It involves the resection of a small portion of tissue, which is sent to the laboratory for histologic examination.

Purpose of the Test

A lung biopsy is performed to diagnose pulmonary disorders such as cancer and sarcoidosis. Lung biopsy can confirm the diagnosis of fibrosis and degenerative or inflammatory diseases of the lung.

Procedure

For an open biopsy of the lung, a thoracotomy is required, which is a surgical procedure. After a small incision is made in the chest wall, the lung is exposed and tissue is excised. A chest tube or tubes are inserted to restore negative pleural pressure.

Findings

Carcinomas
Granulomas
Infections
Sarcoidosis

Interfering Factors

- Noncompliance with dietary restrictions
- Smoking
- Obesity

Nursing Implementation

Follow hospital protocol for the preoperative and postoperative care of a patient requiring a thoracotomy.

TABLE 13–4
COMPLICATIONS OF OPEN LUNG BIOPSY

Complication	Nursing Assessment
Bleeding	Tension pneumothorax Restlessness Tachycardia Hypotension
Pneumothorax	Dyspnea Tachypnea Decreased breath sounds Anxiety Restlessness
Empyema	Fever Tachycardia Malaise Elevated white blood cell count

Complications

Potential complications of an open lung biopsy are bleeding, pneumothorax, and empyema (Table 13–4).

LUNG SCANS

(RADIOGRAPHY)

Synonyms:

ventilation scan, perfusion scan, ventilation-perfusion scan, $\dot{V}/\dot{Q}$ scan, ventilation-perfusion scintiphotography

——————— **NORMAL VALUES** ———————

Normal ventilation and perfusion
Ventilation-perfusion ratio of 0.85 or greater

Background Information

For adequate oxygenation, the lungs must receive adequate alveolar ventilation and blood flow to the ventilated alveoli. Thus, there are two types of lung scans: a *ventilation scan* and a *perfusion scan.* Ventilation scans are performed to evaluate the distribution of gas within the lungs. The patient inhales a radioactive gas and a scanner records the distribution of the gas as it enters and leaves the lungs. Perfusion scans evaluate arterial pulmonary blood flow. A radioactive dye is given intravenously and a scintillation camera records the distribution of the dye as it passes through the right side of the heart to the pulmonary arterial bed.

Ventilation and perfusion scans (V/Q scans) may be performed together so that they can be compared to identify mismatching of ventilation and perfusion. V/Q scans are most often ordered to confirm the diagnosis of pulmonary emboli. The diagnosis of pulmonary emboli is difficult to confirm. Clinically, pulmonary emboli may be suspected because of chest pain, dyspnea, and hemoptysis, but pulmonary emboli are associated with other pulmonary and cardiac disorders, which makes the diagnosis difficult to confirm. Although pulmonary angiography is the most specific diagnostic tool for pulmonary emboli, it is invasive. A V/Q scan is less invasive and therefore less dangerous. It permits an evaluation of V/Q mismatching. Figure 13–5 demonstrates how alveolar-capillary blood flow must interface for adequate oxygenation.

When the radioactively tagged albumin is given intravenously, it circulates through the pulmonary vasculature. If a pulmonary artery is occluded, the part of the lung served by that vessel does not "take up" the radioisotope, and the scan is positive. The scan can verify a pulmonary occlusion. It cannot verify that the tissue is necrotic (pulmonary infarction). With the ventilation scan, decreased areas of ventilation are lighter, indicating poorly ventilated lung tissue.

Purpose of the Test

Ventilation studies may be performed to evaluate patients with decreased pulmonary function. V/Q scans are usually carried out to diagnose pulmonary emboli.

Procedure

For a perfusion scan, serum albumin is tagged with a radioisotope and given intravenously. As the tagged albumin passes through the right side of the heart into the pulmonary artery, a radiation detector scan of the lungs shows the diffusion of the radioactive albumin throughout the pulmonary vessels.

With a ventilation scan, xenon-133, xenon-127, or krypton-81m is given via inhalation. Multiple scans are taken during (1) washin, as the radioactive gas builds up in the lung; (2) equilibrium, as the gas reaches its plateau within the lung; and (3) washout, as the radioactive gas is exhaled.

Findings

Pulmonary vascular occlusion resulting from

Thrombus
Cysts
Abscesses
Carcinomas
Necrotizing pneumonia

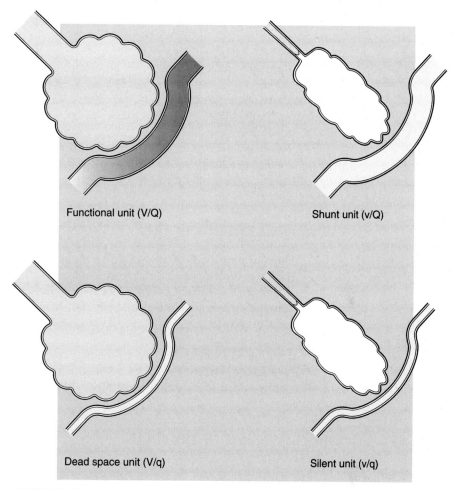

FIGURE 13–5. Alveolar-capillary interface. V = ventilated unit; Q = perfused unit; v = unventilated unit; q = unperfused unit.

Inadequate ventilation resulting from

Atelectasis
Chronic obstructive pulmonary disease
Adult respiratory distress syndrome
Retained secretions
Pleural effusion
Pneumonia
Pneumothorax

Interfering Factors

• Uncooperative patient

Nursing Implementation

Pretest

Critical Thinking: Develop a teaching plan for a patient with possible pulmonary emboli who is scheduled for a ventilation-perfusion scan.

Inform the patient about the procedure and ensure patient cooperation.

Explain to the patient that the ventilation scan must be performed in the nuclear medicine department. Some hospitals have portable perfusion scanners.

Advise the patient that with the ventilation scan the inhaled gas should be held in the lungs for 20 seconds when instructed to do so.

Schedule other radionuclide tests 24 to 48 hours after the perfusion scan.

During the Test

Maintain the patient in an upright position for the ventilation scan. This position is maintained for at least 15 minutes. If the patient is unable to maintain the upright position, a supine position may be used with the gamma camera underneath the patient.

After the radioactive gas is inhaled, encourage the patient to hold the breath for 20 seconds.

Radiolabeled albumin is given to the patient intravenously.

Six different views of the chest are obtained: anterior, posterior, right and left lateral, and right and left oblique.

MAGNETIC RESONANCE IMAGING OF THE CHEST

(TOMOGRAPHY)

Synonym:
MRI of the chest

Background Information

MRI of the chest is performed for cardiac, vascular, and neck imaging; however, its use for pulmonary evaluation at this time is limited, as CT scanning is more precise (Gamsu, 1992). It has proved useful in recurring tumors in the chest wall or pleural space after a pneumonectomy. MRI may also establish the diagnosis of arteriovenous malformation. (See Chapter 12 for a full discussion of MRI.)

Before chest MRI is performed, the patient is assessed for the presence of a permanent pacemaker. Cardiac pacemakers are considered a contraindication for MRI because they frequently contain ferromagnetic material and a magnetically activated relay switch. In addition, pacemaker leads may act as antennae, inducing electric current.

MEDIASTINOSCOPY

(ENDOSCOPY)

No pathologic cells

Background Information

Mediastinoscopy is a surgical invasive procedure in which the mediastinum is entered to determine whether cancer has invaded the mediastinum or its lymph nodes. The procedure involves the insertion of an endoscope into the mediastinum, permitting visualization of the lymph nodes and biopsy of mediastinal nodes and tissue.

Purpose of the Test

Mediastinoscopy is performed to determine invasion by lung cancer into the mediastinum, which can be used to "stage" lung cancer. This assists in determining appropriate treatment modalities. Mediastinoscopy may also be performed for suspected granulomatous infections and other intrathoracic diseases, including sarcoidosis.

Procedure

With the patient under general anesthesia, a small incision is made over the suprasternal fossa, and a mediastinoscope is gently inserted. The mediastinum, with its lymph nodes, is visualized; it may be photographed and tissue samples removed.

Findings

Bronchogenic carcinoma
Esophageal cancer
Granulomatous infections
Lymphomas
Sarcoidosis

Interfering Factors

- Noncompliance with dietary restrictions
- Phenytoin hypersensitivity (may cause false-positive cytologic findings)

Nursing Implementation

The nurse takes actions similar to those for thoracic surgery.

Pretest

Reassure the patient, who is usually fearful of the outcome.
Explain the procedure to the patient.
Ensure that an informed consent form has been obtained.
Instruct the patient not to eat or drink after midnight.
Perform preoperative care according to hospital protocol.

Posttest

Take vital signs every 15 minutes until they are stable and then every 4 hours for 24 hours.
Check the dressing to observe for bleeding or drainage.
Reassure the patient that chest discomfort is temporary.
Advise the patient to resume normal activities and diet when he or she has fully recovered from anesthesia.

Complications

Complications are rare but include accidental puncture of the esophagus, the trachea, or a blood vessel.

PERCUTANEOUS NEEDLE BIOPSY OF THE LUNG

(TOMOGRAPHY)

─────────────── **NORMAL VALUES** ───────────────

Normal tissue

Background Information

A fine needle biopsy of the lung has been made possible by the use of fluoroscopy and CT guidance. Intrathoracic lesions, especially of the lung parenchyma, can usually be visualized by biplane or C arm fluoroscopy technique. For small intrathoracic tumors or those located in the hilar or mediastinal area, a CT scan is used to guide the biopsy.

Purpose of the Test

A fine needle biopsy of the lung is performed to determine the pathology of a lung lesion such as cancer, granuloma, and sarcoidosis.

Procedure

Under the guidance of CT scanning or fluoroscopy, a biopsy needle is inserted into a lesion and a specimen is aspirated for histologic examination.

Findings

Carcinomas
Granulomas
Infections
Sarcoidosis

Nursing Implementation

Pretest

Assess the patient for bleeding disorders, as the needle path may be close to major vessels.
Instruct the patient about the procedure and the need to remain still and not cough when instructed not to move.
Assess the patient's history for contraindications to fine needle biopsy: pulmonary hypertension, severe chronic obstructive lung disease, or arteriovenous malformation.
Transport the patient to the CT laboratory; if fluoroscopy is planned, bring the patient to the radiology department.

Critical Thinking: If your patient has a pulmonary artery catheter in place, what measurements would indicate pulmonary hypertension and therefore be a contraindication to a fine needle biopsy of the lung?

During the Test

The patient is positioned according to the location of the lesion.
The skin is marked as a guide for needle insertion.
Skin preparation is carried out, and the area is draped.
A local anesthetic is given.
The biopsy needle is inserted, and samples are taken.
A pathologist may be present to prepare slides from the aspirated specimen. If a pathologist is not present, send the specimen in fixative to the laboratory.

Posttest

Observe the patient for a minimum of 2 hours.
A chest x-ray study is usually ordered 1 to 2 hours after the procedure to identify any pneumothoraces.

TABLE 13–5
COMPLICATIONS OF FINE NEEDLE BIOPSY OF THE LUNG

Complication	Nursing Assessment
Pneumothorax	Dyspnea, shortness of breath Anxiety, restlessness Tachycardia, tachypnea Diminished breath sounds Pallor
Hemorrhage	Restlessness Cool, pale skin Tachycardia Hypotension Oliguria
Bile leak	Abdominal pain Nausea and vomiting
Infection	Tachycardia Fever, malaise Elevated white blood cell count

Complications

The complications of percutaneous needle biopsy are pneumothorax, hemorrhage, bile leak, infection, and seeding of tumor cells (Table 13–5).

PULMONARY ANGIOGRAPHY

(RADIOLOGY)

Synonym:
pulmonary arteriography

━━━━━━━━━━━━━━━ **NORMAL VALUES** ━━━━━━━━━━━━━━━

Pulmonary vessels fill quickly and symmetrically, with no filling defects, narrowing, or obstruction

Background Information

Pulmonary angiography is an invasive diagnostic procedure in which radiocontrast medium is injected into the pulmonary artery or its branches to visualize the pulmonary vascular bed. It is usually performed when a pulmonary embolism is suspected and other less invasive procedures cannot exclude or confirm the diagnosis.

Risks are involved with pulmonary angiography; however, most of the problems are manageable, such as dysrhythmias, an allergic response to the contrast medium, and infection of the venous access site. Although there is no absolute contraindication for pulmonary angiography, certain conditions may require adaptations of the technique used. These conditions include systemic anticoagulation, pregnancy, an uncooperative patient, severe hypoxia, pulmonary hypertension, right-sided endocarditis (risk of dislodging vegetation), left bundle branch block (risk of complete heart block), and amiodarone pulmonary toxicity.

Purpose of the Test

Pulmonary angiography is used primarily to confirm the diagnosis of pulmonary embolism. It may be performed to diagnose congenital or acquired abnormalities of pulmonary vasculature.

Procedure

The procedure is performed in an angiography laboratory in which cardiac monitoring and emergency equipment is available. With the patient supine, a catheter is inserted via the antecubital or femoral vein into the right or left pulmonary artery, or both (decision is based on previous testing). Multiple films are taken after the dye is administered through the catheter.

Additional imaging techniques are available in some laboratories and may be part of the angiography. These techniques include *high-resolution cineangiography*, *balloon occlusion angiography*, and *digital subtraction angiography*. Cineangiography has the advantage of delineating flow and motion, helping distinguish questionable filling defects and overlapping structures. Balloon occlusion angiography involves occlusion of the pulmonary artery with a balloon catheter. A smaller amount of contrast dye is needed with balloon occlusion angiography, which permits excellent opacification. Digital subtraction angiography allows dye to be inserted into the superior vena cava or right atrium; thus, the procedure is less invasive.

Findings

Pulmonary embolism
Pulmonary artery stenosis
Pulmonary arteriovenous fistula

Interfering Factors

• Uncooperative patient
• Noncompliance with dietary restrictions

Nursing Implementation

Pretest

Perform and document baseline assessments.

Ensure that an informed consent has been obtained.

Instruct the patient about the procedure.

Check blood work for PT, PTT, and platelet determinations. If the patient is taking anticoagulants, the test is usually performed with the antecubital approach.

Check for a history of allergic reaction to contrast dyes or shellfish.

Maintain adequate hydration. A peripheral intravenous line is usually inserted.

Instruct the patient not to eat or drink, except for sips of water, for 4 to 6 hours before the procedure.

If a femoral vein is to be used as the access site, shave the area if necessary.

Ensure that a baseline electrocardiogram, electrolyte, blood urea nitrogen, creatinine, and ABG determinations are performed and that the results are in the patient's chart and abnormalities are reported.

Warn the patient that a warm, flushed, or nauseous feeling may ensue when the dye is injected but that this feeling passes quickly.

Critical Thinking: Before the nurse sent the patient for pulmonary angiography, the nurse evaluated the PT and PTT. The PT was 20 seconds, and the PTT was 54 seconds. What should the nurse do?

During the Test

The patient is awake and will need reassurance and explanations during the procedure.

Place the patient on a cardiac monitor and observe cardiac rhythm during the procedure.

Position the patient in the supine position. The site of venous entry is exposed, and the patient is draped.

After a local anesthetic is given, right heart catheterization is performed under electrocardiographic monitoring and intermittent fluoroscopy.

As the catheter is inserted, record pressure readings and cardiac output.

Warm contrast dye to body temperature.

Reassure the patient that any discomfort felt when the dye is administered is temporary.

Monitor the patient for complications related to the dye (allergic reaction, anaphylaxis, bronchospasms) or to catheterization (dysrhythmias, cardiac perforation).

Posttest

Maintain the patient on bedrest for 2 to 4 hours. Keep the patient warm.

Apply pressure to the site for a minimum of 5 minutes. Check the venous access site for hemostasis and assess distal pulses.

Observe the patient for complications.

Complications

Complications following pulmonary angiography are bleeding and arterial occlusion. In addition, observe for hypotension caused by osmotic diuresis and a delayed allergic reaction to the dye.

PULMONARY FUNCTION STUDIES

(SPIROMETRY)

Synonyms:

NORMAL VALUES

ADULT (70-KG MAN)	
(20–25% LOWER IN WOMEN)	
Tidal volume (V$_T$)	500 ml
Inspiratory reserve volume (IRV)	3100 ml
Expiratory reserve volume (ERV)	1200 ml
Residual volume (RV)	1200 ml
Vital capacity (VC)	4800 ml
Inspiratory capacity (IC)	3600 ml
Functional residual capacity (FRC)	2400 ml
Total lung capacity (TLC)	6000 ml
FEV$_1$	84%
FEV$_2$	94%
FEV$_3$	97%

Background Information

Spirometry is a method of measuring the volume of gas that moves into and out of the lungs. The patient breathes through a tube connected to the spirograph, which records on a moving sheet of paper the volume of gas displaced in the spirometer. Two or more volumes form a pulmonary capacity (Fig. 13–6).

The pulmonary volumes consist of the tidal volume (V$_T$), inspiratory reserve volume (IRV), expiratory reserve volume (ERV), and the residual volume (RV).

The V$_T$, the normal volume of air inhaled or exhaled during a single breath in a resting state, is normally 5 to 7 ml/kg body weight. *Minute volume (MV)* is obtained by multiplying the V$_T$ by the respiratory rate.

The IRV is the amount of air that can be inspired over and above the inspired V$_T$. The ERV is the air remaining in the lungs, which can be expelled after a normal exhalation. The RV is the amount of air remaining in the lungs that cannot be forcibly expelled.

Critical Thinking: The patient weighs 70 kg and has a tidal volume of 210 ml. What adaptations in nursing care will be required?

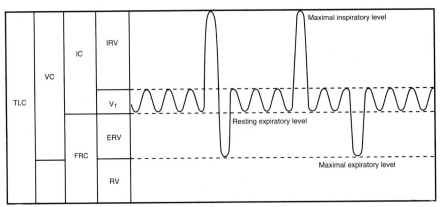

FIGURE 13–6. Pulmonary volumes and capacities. (From Black, J.M., & Matassarin-Jacobs, E. [1993.] *Luckmann and Sorensen's medical-surgical nursing* [4th ed., p. 930]. Philadelphia: W.B. Saunders.)

Pulmonary capacities consist of vital capacity (VC), inspiratory capacity (IC), functional residual capacity (FRC), and total lung capacity (TLC).

The VC is the amount of air that can be expelled from the lungs after a maximum inspiration: VC = V_T + IRV + ERV. A timed VC expresses the volume of air expelled forcibly over a certain amount of time. This *forced expiratory volume (FEV)* provides an index of pulmonary function. It is the amount of gas exhaled over a given period. It is reported with a subscript to indicate time in seconds. The FEV_1 is the amount of air expelled in the first second of forced exhalation after a maximal inspiration. FEV_2 refers to the amount of air expelled in the first 2 seconds, and FEV_3 is the amount of air expelled in 3 seconds. FEV is reported as a percentage of the *forced vital capacity (FVC)*.

In cases of obstructive and restrictive lung disease, FEV_1 decreases. With obstructive lung disease, this decrease in FEV_1 is due to increased resistance to outflow. With restrictive lung disease, the decrease in FEV_1 is due to a decreased ability to inhale an adequate volume of air. Therefore, with restrictive lung disease, an *FEV_1-to-FVC ratio* is a more accurate parameter for evaluating patient status and treatment.

In addition to FEV, the average rate of flow for a specific segment of the FVC may be measured while the FVC is being assessed. The segment measured is usually between 25 and 75% of the FVC. Previously called the *maximum midexpiratory flow rate (MMEF)*, it is now called *forced expiratory flow ($FEF_{25\%–75\%}$)*. The $FEF_{25\%–75\%}$ is the mean rate of expiratory air flow between 25 and 75% of the FVC.

The IC is the maximal amount of air that can be inspired: IC = V_T + IRV. The functional residual capacity, or FRC, is the amount of air left in the lungs after a normal resting exhalation: FRC = ERV + RV. The TLC is the amount of air in the lungs after a maximal inspiration: TLC = V_T + IRV + ERV + RV.

In addition to the volumes and capacities, a *maximum voluntary ventilation (MVV)* may or may not be determined. The MVV is the total amount of air that is moved into and out of the respiratory tract over 12 seconds with the patient's maximum effort to breathe quickly and deeply. The result is multiplied by 5 and expressed in liters per minute. It is sometimes called *maximum breathing capacity.*

An estimated volume of pulmonary function is called *dead space volume* (V_{DS}). The V_{DS} is that portion of inhaled air or gas that does not take part in gas exchange. It is made up of the anatomic dead space (V_D) (area from the nose and mouth to the terminal bronchioles) and alveolar V_D (areas of the lungs that are not perfused). Physiologic V_D consists of the anatomic and alveolar V_D. Normally, there is no measurable alveolar V_D. However, anatomic V_D usually is 1 ml V_D/lb of body weight or 2 ml V_D/kg of ideal body weight. The alveolar V_D increases with pathologic states that decrease blood flow to the lungs.

Pulmonary volumes may also be used to assess alveolar ventilation. *Alveolar ventilation* is estimated by taking the V_T and subtracting the V_{DS} ($V_T - V_{DS}$).

Varied measurements of the work of breathing can be obtained with pulmonary function studies, including the assessment of respiratory muscle strength. These measurements include the *P_{Imax} test, P_{Dimax} test, sniff test,* and *P_{Emax} test.* The P_{Imax} involves measuring the intrathoracic pressure while the patient attempts to inspire as forcibly as possible against an occluded airway after a maximal exhalation. The P_{Dimax} measures transdiaphragmatic pressure (P_{Di}) while the patient tries to inspire as forcibly as possible against an occluded airway after a maximal exhalation. The sniff test is similar to the P_{Imax} and the P_{Dimax}, only instead of attempting to inspire, the patient attempts a forceful maximal sniff. P_{Emax} is measured while the patient attempts to forcibly exhale against an occluded airway after a maximal inspiration (Cherniack, 1992).

A challenge or provocation test is included as part of the pulmonary function studies in patients with suspected hypersensitivities of the airways. *Bronchial provocation tests* or *bronchial challenge tests* are performed as part of the pulmonary function studies for patients who have symptoms suggestive of asthma but who do not show evidence of air flow limitations. They may also be used to assess airway function over time and to evaluate various therapeutic interventions. The provocation tests are contraindicated for anyone whose baseline FEV is less than 1.5 L, who has a history of severe responses to identifiable antigens, or who has had a viral infection of the upper airway within 8 weeks prior to the test.

Various substances can be used in the provocation test. Inhalation challenges are performed with methacholine or histamine. The *methacholine challenge test* and the *histamine challenge test* use nonspecific agents, which are usually administered with a nebulizer. Specific agents may also be given by inhalation. These specific antigens are given in varying concentrations. When indicated, the patient may be exposed to occupational inhalants through inhalation.

Instead of inhalational stimulants, oral challenges may be given, but these take several hours or days. Substances ingested are acetylsalicylic acid (aspirin), tartrazine, sodium salicylate, metabisulfite, and monosodium glutamate.

An *exercise challenge* may be used to induce bronchospasms, which are characteristic of hyperresponsive airways when they occur after short-term exercise. Before the test is performed, a baseline FEV_1 is obtained. The exercise challenge is accomplished with either a treadmill or an exercise bike under controlled environmental temperature and humidity. With 5 to 10 minutes of exercise, the heart rate usually reaches at least 80% of the predicted maximum heart rate. The exercise is stopped and the FEV_1 is measured.

The provocation tests are considered abnormal if there is a 20% or greater fall in FEV_1. At the end of the provocation test, a bronchodilator may be given by inhalation, and postbronchodilator pulmonary function evaluated.

Purpose of the Test

Pulmonary function studies are performed to evaluate the patient's respiratory status, especially in patients experiencing shortness of breath or other breathing difficulty. These studies may be used to evaluate the therapy for or progression of obstructive and restrictive lung disease. Portions of the test are used as parameters for weaning patients from mechanical ventilation and as part of preoperative evaluations.

Procedure

Pulmonary function studies are usually performed in the respiratory therapy department or in a physician's office. To establish a closed system with the spirometer, a nose clip is placed over the patient's nose and the spirometer's mouthpiece is held in the mouth with the patient's lips maintaining an airtight seal. The patient is then instructed when to breath normally, inhale maximally, and exhale maximally. This is repeated several times.

Findings

	Increase	Decrease
V_T		Atelectasis
		Fatigue
		Pneumothorax
		Pulmonary congestion
		Restrictive lung disease
		Tumors
IRV		Asthma
		Exercise
		Obstructive pulmonary disease
ERV		Ascites
		Kyphosis
		Obesity
		Pleural effusion
		Pneumothorax
		Pregnancy
		Scoliosis

RV		Elderly individuals
		Obstructive pulmonary disease
FRC	Chronic obstructive pulmonary disease	
FEV	Chronic obstructive pulmonary disease	Restrictive pulmonary disease
FRC	Chronic obstructive pulmonary disease	Adult respiratory distress syndrome
IC		Restrictive pulmonary disease
VC		Diaphragm restriction
		Drug overdose with hypoventilation
		Neuromuscular diseases
		Restrictive or depressed thoracic movement

Interfering Factors

- Fatigue
- Lack of patient cooperation
- Smoking
- Abdominal distention or pregnancy
- Poor seal around mouthpiece (or tube)
- Medications
     Analgesics, bronchodilators, sedatives

Nursing Implementation

Pretest

Assess the patient's cardiac status. Hold the test and notify the physician if the patient has a history of angina or recent myocardial infarction.

Maximize patient cooperation by explaining the procedure and the need for full participation. Demonstrate the nose clip and mouthpiece. The patient should wear dentures if necessary for a proper mouth seal.

Instruct the patient not to smoke for 6 hours before the test.

Check with prescriber about administering bronchodilator and intermittent positive-pressure breathing therapy before the test.

Ensure that no constricting clothes are worn.

Ensure that oral intake is light to prevent stomach distention.

Instruct the patient to void immediately before the test.

Schedule the test before any other tests or procedures that may fatigue the patient.

Critical Thinking: What would be the best time of day to schedule pulmonary function studies?

During the Test

QUALITY CONTROL

If an abnormal response to a specific substance occurs during a provocation test, a placebo substance should be given to ensure that the bronchospasms were not induced by the spirometry.

Posttest

Advise the patient to resume normal diet and activity.
Advise the patient to resume taking medications or receiving therapy if held.

PULSE OXIMETRY

Synonyms:

──────────── **NORMAL VALUES** ────────────

Sao_2 >95%

Background Information

Pulse oximetry provides a continuous, noninvasive measurement of an individual's Sao_2.

When the Sao_2 level is greater than 70%, pulse oximetry correlates accurately with Sao_2 measurements. When it is less than 70%, the reliability is questionable.

Purpose of the Test

Pulse oximetry is frequently used as part of the ongoing pulmonary assessment of patients at risk for hypoxia. This test permits the nurse to assess the patient's response to varied nursing procedures, guiding adaptations in patient care and activity. Continuous Sao_2 measurements can assist in weaning the patient from mechanical ventilation and decrease the number of ABG measurements required.

Procedure

The pulse oximeter is placed at the bedside and is attached to the patient by either a reusable or a disposable spectrophometric probe. The probe emits infrared and red light, which identifies arterial pulsation. It then measures the amount of infrared and red light absorbed. Oxyhemoglobin absorbs infrared light, and reduced hemoglobin absorbs red light. The microprocessor in the oximeter then calculates the percentage of hemoglobin that is saturated. A digital readout of the patient's pulse rate and Sao_2 is continuous.

Findings

Hypoxemia

Interfering Factors

- Inadequate pulsation
  Hypotension
  Hypothermia
  Vasoconstriction
- Carboxyhemoglobin
- Hyperbilirubinemia
- Radiopaque dyes
- Bright lights surrounding the probe

Nursing Implementation

Pretest

Assess potential sites (finger, earlobe, nose, toe) for arterial pulsation. The fingers are the most common site in an adult. Remove nail polish if present.

Apply warm packs if necessary to obtain adequate perfusion of the site.

QUALITY CONTROL

Evaluate the patient because the oximeter cannot distinguish between hemoglobin and carboxyhemoglobin. Was the patient at risk for smoke inhalation or carbon monoxide poisoning?

During the Test

QUALITY CONTROL

Ensure that light-emitting diodes, which transmit the dual wavelengths, are aligned. The plastic reusable probes are designed to align. The disposable probes require proper application.

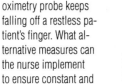

QUALITY CONTROL

If the earlobe is used, rub the lobe vigorously to arterialize the capillary blood in it. The earlobe can be used only for intermittent evaluation of the Sao_2.

Critical Thinking: The plastic reusable pulse oximetry probe keeps falling off a restless patient's finger. What alternative measures can the nurse implement to ensure constant and accurate measurement?

Set the alarm limits on the oximeter.
Shield the probe from bright light.

ROENTGENOGRAM, CHEST

(RADIOLOGY)

Synonyms:

chest x-ray, chest radiography

X-ray studies of the chest are an important diagnostic tool in assessing pulmonary and cardiac abnormalities as well as in evaluating therapies for these disorders. Chapter 9 discusses radiography in detail, including chest x-ray studies. Figure 13–7*A* presents a normal chest x-ray film. Compare this with a chest x-ray film showing emphysema (see Fig. 13–7*B*) and one showing pneumonia (see Fig. 13–7*C*).

THORACENTESIS

Synonyms:

pleural fluid analysis, pleural tap

───────────────── **NORMAL VALUES** ─────────────────

Normal pleural fluid
No pathogens or malignant cells

Background Information

Thoracentesis is an invasive procedure used to remove fluid (effusion) from the pleural space. It may be performed for diagnostic or therapeutic reasons, or both. In addition to removing fluid, a fine needle biopsy of the pleura may be performed to diagnose malignancy.

Pleural effusions (accumulation of fluid in the pleural space) may be due to neoplastic or infectious processes or leakage of fluid from the vascular system. If the effusion is due to neoplasms or infection, the fluid is usually called an exudate. If the fluid is due to leakage from the blood vessels, it is called transudate. To distinguish between exudates and transudates, pleural fluid is evaluated for protein, specific gravity, and glucose, and a blood cell count with differential is performed.

Pleural fluid is also obtained for cultures to identify tuberculosis and fungal and

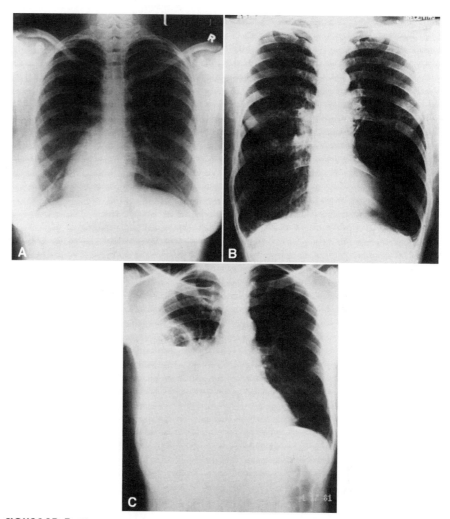

FIGURE 13–7. Chest roentgenogram. *A*, The normal chest x-ray film. *B*, Lung with emphysema. *C*, Lung with pneumonia. (Reprinted with permission from Thompson, M.A., et al. [1994]. *Principles of imaging science and protection* [vol. 2, Slides 207, 295, 296]. Philadelphia: W.B. Saunders.)

various bacterial infections. Cytologic examination of the pleural fluid is performed to rule out malignancy.

Purpose of the Test

Thoracentesis is performed to remove fluid from the pleural space for diagnostic or therapeutic reasons. An accumulation of fluid in the pleural space is abnormal. Examination of that fluid identifies or confirms diagnoses of cancer, infection, or severe fluid overload (congestive heart failure, liver failure, and systemic or pulmonary hypertension).

Procedure

After the patient is positioned in a seated, upright position, the lower posterior chest is exposed and prepared, and a local anesthetic is given. A needle is inserted into the pleural space. The fluid is aspirated. A pleural biopsy may be performed at this time.

If a *pleural biopsy* is planned, a special biopsy needle with a hooked biopsy trocar is used. Usually three specimens are obtained from three pleural sites. Specimens are placed in fixative and sent to the laboratory immediately.

Findings

Bacterial, viral, or fungal infection
Malignancy
Collagen disease
Lymphoma
Systemic lupus erythematosus
Liver failure
Nephrotic syndrome
Myxedema
Pancreatitis

Interfering Factors

• Uncooperative patient

Nursing Implementation

Pretest

Explain the procedure and the purpose of the test to the patient.
Ensure that a signed consent form has been obtained.
Perform and document a baseline assessment. A blood pressure cuff is left in place to permit easy monitoring of the blood pressure during the procedure.
Initiate supplemental O_2 if ordered.
Check the PT, PTT, and platelet count to identify potential bleeding problems.
Instruct the patient not to cough or move during the procedure.
Obtain a thoracentesis tray from supply room.

During the Test

Continuously monitor the patient's response to the procedure.
Observe the pulse oximeter, if in use, for changes in Sao_2.

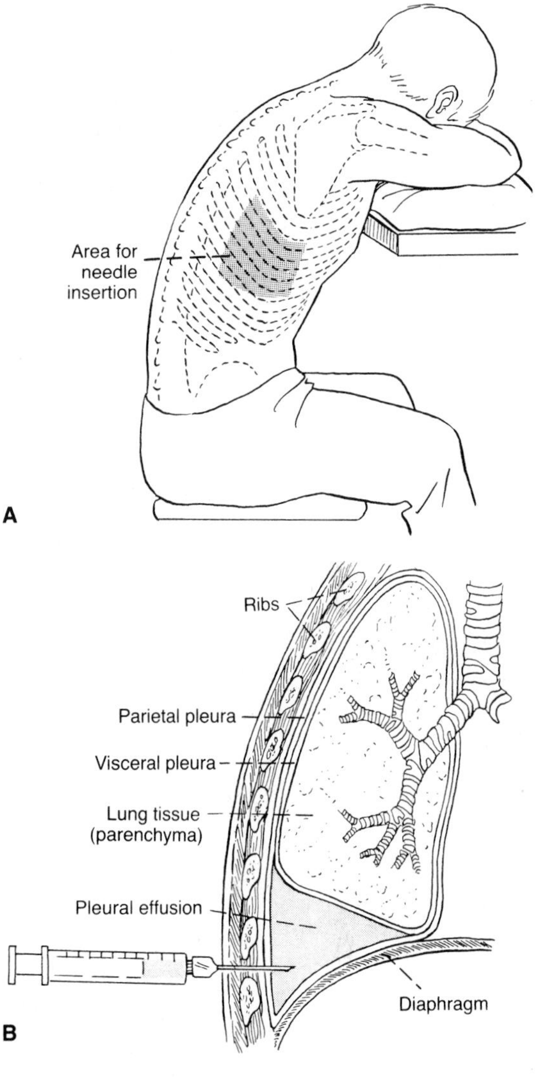

Area for needle insertion

FIGURE 13–8. Thoracentesis. *A,* Thoracentesis position. Arms are raised and crossed. Head rests on folded arms. This position allows the chest wall to be pulled outward in an expanded position. If an over-bed table is not available, the arms may be left down but positioned forward of the hips or crossed in front of the chest. *B* shows the usual site for the insertion of a thoracentesis needle for a right-sided effusion. The actual site varies with each client, depending on the location and volume of the effusion. The physician tries to keep the needle as far away from the diaphragm as possible while at the same time inserting the needle close to the base of the effusion so that gravity can help with drainage. (Reprinted with permission from Black, J.M., & Matassarin-Jacob, E. [1993]. *Luckmann and Sorensen's medical-surgical nursing* [4th ed., p. 938]. Philadelphia: W.B. Saunders.)

A

Ribs

Parietal pleura

Visceral pleura

Lung tissue (parenchyma)

Pleural effusion

Diaphragm

B

Position the patient in an upright position, seated on the side of the bed with the legs resting on a footstool. The patient's arms should be supported on a padded overbed table (Fig. 13–8). If the patient is unable to sit up, he or she may lie on the unaffected side with the back flush with the edge of the bed.

Provide emotional support to the patient, as pressure pain may be experienced even though local anesthesia is given.

After the needle is inserted with a stopcock attached, fluid is drawn off for analysis. A catheter may be inserted at this point if a large amount of fluid is to be drained.

TABLE 13-6
COMPLICATIONS OF THORACENTESIS

Complication	Nursing Assessment
Pneumothorax	Respiratory distress Diminished breath sounds Tracheal deviation to unaffected side (tension pneumothorax)
Pulmonary edema	Dyspnea, orthopnea Shortness of breath Crackles

Critical Thinking: Following a thoracentesis, a pneumothorax occurs. What emergency equipment should the nurse provide?

Critical Thinking: When a thoracentesis is done for a patient with a large pleural effusion, what changes in the patient's status are to be expected?

When a biopsy is performed, instruct the patient to exhale fully and perform the Valsalva maneuver to prevent air from entering the pleural space when the tissue sample is taken.

Posttest

Check vital signs every 15 minutes until they are stable.
Assess for bilateral breath sounds.
Document amount, color, and character of the fluid obtained.
Obtain a chest radiograph as ordered to check for pneumothorax.
Encourage the patient to lie on the uninvolved side for 1 hour to improve oxygenation.
Check small dressing over the site for bleeding or drainage. Palpate around the site for subcutaneous emphysema.

Complications

The major complication following thoracentesis is pneumothorax. Another complication is reexpansion pulmonary edema. It occurs if large amounts of pleural fluid are removed, which causes an increase in negative intrapleural pressure. If the lungs do not reexpand to fill the space, edema can result. Bleeding is a rare complication. Since thoracentesis is an invasive procedure, infection is possible but extremely rare because it is performed with sterile technique (Table 13–6).

REFERENCES

Capel, L.C., & Stolark, A. (1991). Continuous Svo₂ monitoring: A research review. *Dimensions in Critical Care Nursing, 10,* 202–209.
Cason, C.L., Desalvo, S.K., & Ray, W. T. (1994). Changes in oxygen saturation during weaning from short-term ventilator support after coronary artery bypass graft surgery. *Heart & Lung, 23,* 368–375.

Chernecky, C.C., Krech, R.L., & Berger, B.J. (1993). *Laboratory tests and diagnostic procedures.* Philadelphia: W.B. Saunders.

Cherniack, R.M. (1992). *Pulmonary function testing* (2nd ed.). Philadelphia: W.B. Saunders.

Clark, A.P., Winslow, E.H., Tyler, D.O., & White, K.M. (1990). Effects of endotracheal suctioning on mixed venous oxygen saturation and heart rate in critically ill adult. *Heart & Lung, 19,* 552–556.

Clark, J., Votteri, B., Ariago, R., Cheung, P., et al. (1992). Noninvasive assessment of blood gases. *American Review of Respiratory Disease, 145,* 220–232.

Clochesy, J.M., Breu, C., Cardin, S., Rudy, E.B., & Whittaker, A.A. (1993). *Critical care nursing.* Philadelphia: W.B. Saunders.

Dolan, J.T. (1991). *Critical care nursing: Clinical management through the nursing process.* Philadelphia: F.A. Davis.

Durren, M. (1992). Clinical notebook: Getting the most from pulse oximetry. *Journal of Emergency Nursing, 18,* 340–342.

Ehrhardt, B., & Graham, M. (1990). Pulse oximetry: An easy way to check oxygenation. *Nursing '90, 90,* 50–54.

Flynn, J.M., & Bruce, N.P. (1993). *Introduction to critical care skills.* St. Louis: C.V. Mosby.

Gamsu, G. (1992). The lungs. In A.A. Moss, G. Gamsu, & H.K. Genant (Eds.), *Computed tomography of the body with magnetic resonance imaging* (pp. 157–236). Philadelphia: W.B. Saunders.

Gilbert, R. (1991). Spirometry and blood gases. In J.B. Henry (Ed.), *Clinical diagnosis and management* (18th ed.). Philadelphia: W.B. Saunders.

Halfmann, S.J., & Noll, M.L. (1990). Can continuous monitoring of mixed venous oxygen saturation be substituted for thermodilution cardiac output measurements? *Focus on Critical Care, 17,* 157–162.

Hayden, R.A. (1993). Trend-spotting with an Svo_2 monitor. *American Journal of Nursing, 93*(1), 26–33.

Healy, C.J., Fedullo, A.J., Swinburne, A.J., & Wahl, G.W. (1987). Comparison of noninvasive measurements of carbon dioxide tension during withdrawal from mechanical ventilation. *Critical Care Medicine, 15,* 764–768.

Hudak, C.M., & Gallo, B.M. (1994). *Critical care nursing: A holistic approach* (6th ed.). Philadelphia: J.B. Lippincott.

Hudak, C.M., & Gallo, B.M. (1994). *Handbook of critical care nursing.* Philadelphia: J.B. Lippincott.

Hurray, J., & Saver, C. (1992). Arterial blood gas interpretation: Improving perioperative skills. *American Operating Room Nurses Journal, 55,* 180–185.

Jacobs, D.S., Kasten, B.D., DeMott, W.R., et al. (1990). *Laboratory test handbook* (2nd ed.). Baltimore: Williams & Wilkins.

Mettler, F.A., & Guiberteau, M.J. (1991). *Essentials of nuclear medicine imaging* (3rd ed.). Philadelphia: W.B. Saunders.

Qureshi, N., Momin, Z.A., & Brandstetter, R.D. (1994). Thoracentesis in clinical practice. *Heart and Lung, 23,* 376–383.

Scanlan, C.L. (Ed.). (1990). *Egan's fundamentals of respiratory care.* St. Louis: C.V. Mosby.

Sox, H.R. (Ed.). (1990). *Common diagnostic tests: Use and interpretation* (2nd ed.). Philadelphia: American College of Physicians.

Speicher, C.E. (1990). *The right test: A physician's guide to laboratory medicine,* Philadelphia: W.B. Saunders.

Stratton, M.B. (1990). Ventilation-perfusion scintigraphy in diagnosis of pulmonary thromboembolism. *Focus on Critical Care, 17,* 287–293.

Tietz, N.W. (Ed.). (1992). *Applied laboratory medicine.* Philadelphia: W.B. Saunders.

Wallach, J. (1992). *Interpretation of diagnostic tests: A synopsis of laboratory medicine* (5th ed.). Boston: Little, Brown.

White, K.M., Winslow, E.H., Clark A.P., & Tyler, D.O. (1990). The physiologic basis for continuous mixed venous oxygen saturation monitoring. *Heart & Lung, 19,* 548–551.

Winslow, E.H., Clark, A.P., White, K.M., & Tyler, D.O. (1990). Effects of a lateral turn on mixed venous oxygen saturation and heart rate in critically ill adults. *Heart & Lung, 19,* 557–561.

CHAPTER 14

Cardiac Function

The laboratory and diagnostic evaluation of cardiac function has evolved into many sophisticated techniques. The number of diagnostic procedures is proliferating. The number of tests and the various names and abbreviations for the same or similar tests can be confusing. This chapter emphasizes the knowledge the nurse must have for each of the studies presented and provides guidelines for assisting the patient in preparing for the procedure as well as for caring for the patient during and after the procedure.

The emotional needs of the patient and family during the diagnostic testing vary with the clinical condition of the patient, the purpose of the procedure, and the possible risk of the test. Patients undergoing cardiac testing may or may not have experienced cardiac symptoms. The test may be a preamble to surgery or, because of the high incidence of cardiac disease, may be part of a routine physical examination.

Other tests not specific to the heart play an important role in identifying coronary problems. These tests include arterial blood gas and mixed venous gas determinations, a complete blood count, an erythrocyte sedimentation rate, a blood chemistry panel, and an electrolyte value. In addition, the importance of the patient's history and the clinical presentation cannot be overemphasized.

LABORATORY TESTS

ENZYMES AND ISOENZYMES, CARDIAC

(SERUM)

Background Information

Enzymes are complex compounds that are found in all tissues and that speed up the biochemical reactions of the body. Damage to body tissue causes release of the enzymes from the injured cells into the serum. Enzymes may be common to more than one type of tissue. Elevated serum levels of the enzymes reflect tissue damage, but since the enzymes are not specific, patterns of enzyme elevations are used to determine myocardial tissue damage.

Creatine phosphokinase (CPK) is an enzyme found in the heart, brain, and skeletal muscle. The individual with larger muscle mass has a higher CPK level than does the average person. CPK may be separated into three isoenzymes. Isoenzymes refer to the various forms of an enzyme, which differ chemically, physically, or immunologically, or a combination, but catalyze the same reaction. The CPK isoenzymes include CPK-MM, CPK-MB, and CPK-BB. With myocardial damage, the elevated fraction is CPK-MB.

Aspartate aminotransferase (AST), previously called serum glutamic oxalo-acetic transaminase (SGOT), is an enzyme found in the heart, kidneys, brain, red blood cells, liver, lungs, pancreas, and skeletal muscle.

Lactate dehydrogenase (LDH) is present in almost all metabolizing cells but is especially high in the heart, kidneys, brain, red blood cells, liver, and skeletal muscles. Since LDH is present in so many tissues of the body, the origin of its release cannot be determined without the use of electrophoresis, which separates out its five isoenzymes. LDH_1 and LDH_2 are used to assess myocardial damage.

NORMAL VALUES

Creatine phosphokinase (CPK) or creatine kinase (CK)	**Adult Male:**
	5–35 µg/ml
	20–170 IU/L
	<90 U/L
	5–55 mU/ml
	Adult Female:
	5–25 µg/ml
	10–135 IU/L
	<80 U/L
	5–35 mU/ml
	Male Child:
	0–70 IU/L
	Female Child:
	0–50 IU/L
	Newborn:
	65–580 IU/L
	10–200 U/L

━━━━━━━━━━━━━━━ **NORMAL VALUES** ━━━━━━━━━━━━━━━

CPK isoenzymes
    CPK-MM (skeletal   90–97% of total CPK *or* SI 0.90–0.97
    muscles)   (fraction of total CPK)
    CPK-MB (heart)   0–6% of total CPK *or* SI 0.00–0.06%
                           (fraction of total CPK)
    CPK-BB (brain)   Trace or 0% of total CPK *or* SI trace or
                           0.00 (fraction of total CPK)

Aspartate amino-   **Adult:** 8–20 U/L
transferase (AST)   **Older Adult:**
or serum glutamic   Male: 11–26 U/L
oxaloacetic   Female: 10–20 U/L
transaminase   **Child (<5 years):**
                           19–28 U/L
                      Infant: 15–60 U/L
                      Newborn: 16–72 U/L

Lactic acid   60–120 U/ml (Wacker scale)
dehydrogenase (LDH)   150–450 U/ml (Wroblewski–La Due
                         scale)

LDH isoenzymes   70–200 IU/L
LDH_1 14–26% *or* SI 0.14–0.26 (fraction of total
    Heart, red blood cells   LDH)
LDH_2
    Reticuloendothelial   29–39% *or* SI 0.29–0.39 (fraction of total
    cells and kidney   LDH)
LDH_3
    Lungs, lymphatics,   20–26% *or* SI 0.20–0.26 (fraction of total
    spleen, and others   LDH)
LDH_4 8–16% *or* SI 0.08–0.16 (fraction of total
    Kidney, placenta,   LDH)
    and liver
LDH_5
    Kidney, liver, and   6–16% *or* SI 0.06–0.16 (fraction of total
    skeletal muscle   LDH)
Serum alphahydroxy-
butyrate dehydrogenase   50–250 U/L

Serum alpha-hydroxybutyrate dehydrogenase (SHBD) is found in the heart, liver, and red blood cells. It is nonspecific and is not usually part of the cardiac enzyme protocol.

The cardiac enzyme protocol usually consists of CPK and its isoenzymes being collected three times, every 8 hours, after the onset of cardiac symptoms. CPK, CPK isoenzymes, LDH, LDH isoenzymes, and AST determinations are usually ordered at the onset of symptoms and thereafter every 24 hours three times.

Purpose of the Test

Cardiac enzyme and isoenzyme studies are used with clinical evaluation and electrocardiographic studies to diagnose myocardial injury.

Procedure

Critical Thinking: What nursing actions would ensure that the cardiac enzyme protocols are followed?

A venipuncture is necessary to obtain 5 to 10 ml of blood in a red-topped tube.

QUALITY CONTROL

Q/A: Cardiac enzyme protocols require that isoenzymes be determined at certain frequencies and times. A study carried out at a large teaching hospital found that the guidelines established for CPK-MB and LDH isoenzymes were not followed either in regard to the number required or the required timing (Saxema et al., 1993).

Findings

Multiple diagnoses cause changes in enzyme levels, as they are found in many body tissues. Because of this lack of specificity, enzymes alone do not establish diagnoses.

In diagnosing myocardial infarction, a pattern of enzyme changes *supports* the diagnosis. The first enzyme to rise is CPK. CPK levels begin to rise 6 hours after the infarction, peak in 18 hours, and return to normal in 2 to 3 days. CPK-MB levels rise within 3 to 6 hours after an infarction, peak in 12 to 24 hours, and return to normal in 12 to 48 hours. An increase in CPK-MB, expressed in a percentage of the total CPK, supports the diagnosis of myocardial damage. The percentage accepted as diagnostic of an infarction varies from laboratory to laboratory. If the CPK-MB level rises quickly and then drops quickly, myocardial contusion is suspected.

AST levels will begin to rise 6 to 10 hours after an infarction, peak in 24 to 48 hours, and return to normal after 4 to 6 days.

LDH elevations do not occur until 24 to 48 hours, peak in 3 to 4 days, and do not return to normal levels for 10 to 14 days after an infarction. LDH_2 levels are normally greater than LDH_1 levels. If LDH_1 levels become greater than those of LDH_2, it is called a "flipped" LDH and is indicative of a myocardial infarction. The "flipped" LDH is especially helpful if the person delayed seeking help when chest pain occurred. However, the "flipped" LDH will revert within 1 week in approximately half of patients with an infarction, even though the serum LDH levels will remain elevated (Henry, 1991).

Following a myocardial infarction, there is an elevation of the serum alpha-hydroxybutyrate level within 12 hours; it peaks in 48 to 72 hours and remains elevated for 1 to 3 weeks.

Because of their nonspecificity, other clinical problems may create changes in the enzyme levels. Common causes of these changes follow:

CPK

Increase	Decrease
Amyotrophic lateral sclerosis	Addison disease
Biliary atresia	Anterior pituitary hyposecretion
Burns	Connective tissue disease
Cancers, some	Cirrhosis, alcoholic
Cardiomyopathy	Metastatic cancer
Central nervous system trauma, including cerebrovascular accident	Steroid administration
Hypokalemia, severe	
Hypothermia	
Hypothyroidism	
Infarction	
Cerebral	
Bowel	
Myocardial	
Intramuscular injections	
Muscular dystrophy	
Myocarditis	
Organ rejection	
Pulmonary edema	
Pulmonary embolism	
Renal insufficiency or failure	
Surgery	

AST

Increase	Decrease
Cirrhosis	Severe liver failure
Congestive heart failure	
Hepatitis	
Myocardial infarction	
Pericarditis	
Pulmonary infarction	
Reye syndrome	

LDH

Increase	**Decrease**
Alcoholism	Radiation therapy
Anemia	Oxalates
Burns	
Cancer	
Cardiomyopathy	
Cerebrovascular accident	
Cirrhosis	
Convulsions	
Delirium tremens	
Hepatitis	
Hypothyroidism	
Infectious mononucleosis	
Codeine	
Lithium carbonate	
Meperidine	
Morphine	
Niacin	
Pneumonia	
Pulmonary infarction	
Procainamide	
Propranolol	
Shock	
Thyroid hormones	
Ulcerative colitis	

SERUM ALPHA-HYDROXYBUTYRATE DEHYDROGENASE

Increase	**Decrease**
Anemia	Clinically insignificant
Leukemia	
Lymphoma	
Melanoma, malignant	
Muscular dystrophy	
Myocardial infarction	
Nephrotic syndrome	
Orthopedic hip surgery	

Interfering Factors

CPK
- Cardioversion
- Drugs
    Alcohol

                Aspirin
                Halothane
                Lithium
                Succinylcholine

- Muscle trauma
- Recent vigorous exercise or massage
- Surgery

     AST

- Drugs
        Acetaminophen
        Antituberculosis agents
        Aspirin
        Chlorpropamide
        Dicumarol
        Erythromycin
        Methyldopa
        Sulfonamides
        Vitamin A
- Muscle trauma
- Not fasting
- Strenuous fasting

     LDH

- Pregnancy
- Prosthetic heart valves
- Recent surgery

Nursing Implementation

Pretest

Reassure the patient, who is usually frightened and having chest pain and may also be in denial.

Do *not* give intramuscular injections or perform repeated venipunctures, if possible, until all the initial enzyme studies are completed.

Instruct the patient about the need to repeat blood sampling.

Determine if alcohol or drugs that affect results have been ingested.

During the Test

If the tourniquet is in place too long, inaccurate results may occur.

Posttest

Nursing actions are similar to those for any venipuncture.

LIPIDS, SERUM

(SERUM)

Synonym:

lipoprotein-cholesterol fractionation

━━━━━━━━━━━━━━━ **NORMAL VALUES** ━━━━━━━━━━━━━━━

Lipids, total	400–800 mg/dl *or* SI 4.0–8.0 g/L
Cholesterol, total	120–200 mg/dl *or* SI 3.11–5.18 mmol/L
Low-density lipoprotein (LDL)	<130 mg/dl *or* SI <3.37 mmol/L
High-density lipoprotein (HDL)	**Male:** 44–45 mg/dl *or* SI 1.24–1.27 mmol/L **Female:** 55 mg/dl *or* SI 1.425 mmol/L
LDL:HDL ratio	<3
Triglycerides	**Male:** <40 years 46–316 mg/dl *or* SI 0.52–3.57 mmol/L >50 years 75–313 mg/dl *or* SI 0.85–3.5 mmol/L **Female:** <40 years 37–174 mg/dl *or* SI 0.42–1.97 mmol/L >50 years 52–200 mg/dl *or* SI 0.59–2.26 mmol/L

Background Information

Most lipids are bound to protein in the blood and are called lipoproteins. Lipoproteins are usually measured to identify persons at risk for coronary artery disease (CAD). In the laboratory, lipoproteins are separated by electrophoresis. Fractionation of the lipoproteins is then performed according to their density. The following groups have been identified:

- Very low-density lipoproteins (VLDL), which are made up of 70% triglycerides
- Low-density lipoproteins (LDL), which are made up of 45% cholesterol
- High-density lipoproteins (HDL)

Critical Thinking: Does gender and/or age influence who would benefit by having serum lipids done?

There is a high correlation between elevated VLDL and LDL and CAD. Research has shown that HDL may protect from CAD, since it seems to inhibit the uptake of LDL.

Purpose of the Test

Lipid levels are used to identify individuals at risk for CAD and as an evaluation tool to determine the effectiveness of "heart-healthy" changes in lifestyle.

Procedure

A venipuncture is necessary for a lipid profile. Two red-topped tubes of 7-ml capacity are required. If a cholesterol level determination is performed as a screening test, a drop or two of blood is obtained from a fingerstick using a sterile lancet, and the blood is collected in a capillary pipette.

Findings

CHOLESTEROL

Increase	Decrease
Alcoholism	Hyperalimentation
Arteriosclerosis	Hyperthyroidism
CAD	Liver disease
Diabetes mellitus	Malabsorption
Hepatitis (early stage)	Malnutrition
High-fat diet	
Myxedema	
Obstructed bile duct	
Pancreatitis	

HDL

Increase	Decrease
Alcoholism	Arteriosclerosis
Diabetes mellitus	Hyperalimentation
Exercise	Hypothyroidism
Myxedema	Malabsorption
Nephrotic syndrome	Malnutrition
Pancreatitis	

LDL

Increase	Decrease
Alcoholism	Arteriosclerosis
CAD	Hyperalimentation
Diabetes mellitus	Malabsorption
Nephrotic syndrome	Malnutrition
Pancreatitis	

TRIGLYCERIDES

Increase	Decrease
Alcoholism	Hyperalimentation
Arteriosclerosis	Malabsorption
Diabetes mellitus	Malnutrition
Myxedema	
Nephrotic syndrome	
Pancreatitis	

Interfering Factors

Diet affects the results of a lipid profile. The patient's diet affects the fractionation outcome. Has the patient been dieting to lose weight?

If the patient has had a recent traumatic event or infarction, results will also be affected. Medications such as estrogen, steroids, birth control pills, and hypolipid agents cause an inaccurate lipid picture.

For cholesterol screening, eating a diet high in saturated fats will affect the results.

Nursing Implementation

The nursing actions are similar to those of other venipunctures. In addition, review the following.

Pretest

Critical Thinking: Develop a teaching plan including diet and exercise education for a person whose cholesterol level is over 270 mg/dl (SI 6.99 mmol/L).

Instruct the patient to fast for 12 hours before the blood sample is taken. If a cholesterol screening only is planned, instruct the patient to refrain from eating a high-fat diet for 12 hours before the blood is drawn.

Posttest

Review results with the patient. If the patient is at risk for CAD, diet and exercise education may be necessary.

MYOGLOBULIN

(SERUM)

Synonym:
Mb

--- NORMAL VALUES ---

40–180 mg/dl
<55 ng/ml

Background Information

Myoglobulin is an oxygen-binding protein found in striated muscle. It releases oxygen at very low tensions. Any injury to skeletal muscle will cause a release of myoglobulin into the blood.

Purpose of the Test

Myoglobulin levels may be used with cardiac enzymes to diagnose myocardial infarction, evaluate muscle injury, or assess polymyositis.

Procedure

A venipuncture is performed to obtain 5 ml of blood in a red-topped tube.

Findings

Increase
Myocardial infarction
Muscle injury or breakdown
Polymyositis

Interfering Factors

Myoglobulin is nonspecific. Any trauma to skeletal muscle can cause an increase, which limits its usefulness in diagnosing a myocardial infarction.

Nursing Implementation

The nurse performs actions similar to those in other venipuncture procedures. No fasting is necessary.

DIAGNOSTIC PROCEDURES

CATHETERIZATION, CARDIAC

(RADIOLOGY) **Synonyms:**

angiocardiography, coronary arteriography

Background Information

Cardiac catheterization is an invasive procedure that permits the assessment of anatomic abnormalities of the heart. Cardiac catheterization may assess (1) pressures, oxygen content, and oxygen saturation in the various heart chambers; (2) cardiac output and index; (3) patency of the coronary arteries; and (4) pressure gradients across the valves.

Cardiac catheterization may be a right-sided catheterization, a left-sided catheterization, or both. A right-sided catheterization is performed today in specialized units under the category of hemodynamic monitoring; therefore, this section will focus on left-sided catheterization.

The reader may wish to review the general principles of angiography in Chapter 11 before reading the specifics of cardiac angiography.

Purpose of the Test

A cardiac catheterization is performed to (1) evaluate coronary artery disease with unstable, progressive, or new-onset angina or angina that is not responding to medical therapy; (2) diagnose atypical chest pain; (3) diagnose complications of myocardial infarctions such as septal rupture and refractory dysrhythmias; (4) diagnose aortic dissection; (5) evaluate the need for coronary artery surgery or angioplasty; (6) assess valvular function; and (7) determine the efficacy of a heart transplant. Rarely, a cardiac catheterization may be carried out to obtain a biopsy specimen.

Procedure

A left-sided catheterization is performed in a cardiac catheterization labora-tory. This laboratory is designed with fluoroscopy, electrocardiographic equip-ment, and emergency equipment and drugs (code cart). For a left-sided cathe-terization, a catheter must be threaded through an artery into the left side of the heart; therefore, arterial access is necessary. Pressure measurements are obtained in the aorta and left atrium and ventricle. Samples of blood are obtained for oxygen analysis. Cardiac output, stroke volume, and ejection fractions are measured.

When a *coronary angiogram* is included in the test, dye is instilled into the heart to visualize the size of the ventricles, wall motion, and contractility and to identify valvular dysfunction.

A *coronary arteriogram* may also be obtained. The catheter is withdrawn from the left ventricle and positioned at the coronary ostia, where small boluses of dye are injected into the coronary arteries while a series of x-ray films are taken.

NORMAL VALUES

Pressures	Right atrium: 1–16 mm Hg
	Neonate: 0–3 mm Hg
	Children: 1–5 mm Hg
	Right ventricle: 15–25/0–6 mm Hg
	Neonate: 30–60/2–5 mm Hg
	Children: 15–30/2–5 mm Hg
	Pulmonary artery pressure: 15–25/5–15 mm Hg
	Neonate: 30–60/2–10 mm Hg
	Children: 15–30/5–10 mm Hg
	Pulmonary artery wedge pressure: 6–12 mm Hg
	Left atrium: 4–12 mm Hg
	Neonate: 1–4 mm Hg
	Children: 5–10 mm Hg
	Left ventricle: 90–140/4–12 mm Hg
	Neonate: 60–100/5–10 mm Hg
	Children: 80–130/10–20 mm Hg
Cardiac output	4–8 L/minute
Cardiac index	2.5–4 L/minute
	Neonate and Children: 3.5–4 L/minute
Stroke index	30–60 ml/beat/minute
Ejection fraction	55–75%
Oxygen saturation	75% (right side of heart)
	95% (left side of heart)
Oxygen content	14–15 vol % (right side of heart)
	19 vol % (left side of heart)
Oxygen consumption	250 ml/minute
Volume	Left ventricular end-diastolic: 50–90 ml
	Left ventricular end-systolic: 14–34 ml
	Right ventricular end-diastolic: 70–90 ml
	Left atrium: 57–79 ml
Mass	Left ventricular thickness
	Males: 12 mm
	Females: 9 mm
	Left ventricular wall mass
	Males: 99 g
	Females: 76 g
Wall motion	Normal
Valve gradient	None
Valve orifice areas	Aortic valve: 0.7 cm^2
	Mitral valve: 1 cm^2

Findings

Cardiac catheterization provides a significant amount of data for analysis, which may support the following diagnoses:

CAD
Coronary occlusions and degree of blockage
Congenital abnormalities
Septal defects
Shunting
Aneurysms
Valvular defects

Interfering Factors

- Allergic reactions to contrast medium
- Uncontrolled congestive heart failure
- Dysrhythmias
- Renal insufficiency
- Electrolyte imbalances
- Infection
- Drug toxicity

Nursing Implementation

Pretest

Critical Thinking: Develop a teaching plan for a patient and significant other when cardiac catheterization is anticipated. How would age and culture influence the plan?

Verify that an informed consent has been obtained.
Instruct the patient about the purpose and procedure for the study. Explain to the patient that the table rotates and that the physician may ask the patient to change positions or cough.
Assist with the precatheterization evaluation—blood work, including a prothrombin time and a partial thromboplastin time; an electrocardiogram (ECG); and chest x-ray film if the procedure will be performed on an outpatient basis.
If contrast dye is going to be used, check for allergies.
Assess the patient's fears. Correct any misperceptions and reassure the patient that there will be a continuous presence by the nurse, physician, and technicians to assist during the procedure.
Prepare catheter site according to laboratory protocols. The femoral artery is commonly used for the percutaneous insertion of the catheter.

Critical Thinking: How would a patient express fears of a cardiac catheterization and its potential results? What if the patient is unable to communicate verbally?

The patient is to have nothing by mouth after midnight, except if the catheterization is planned for late in the afternoon. In that case, a clear liquid breakfast may be taken.
Premedication is given as ordered to reduce the patient's anxiety. In some catheterization laboratories, the patient is premedicated to decrease the risk of allergic reaction to the contrast dye.

Encourage the patient to wear glasses, if required, to the catheterization laboratory.

During the Test

Critical Thinking: What can the nurse in the catheterization laboratory do to reassure the patient during the procedure?

The patient is awake. The nurse provides emotional support and reinforces explanations given about the procedure.

Continuous cardiac monitoring is maintained.

A local anesthetic is used after the insertion site is prepared and draped.

The physician inserts the cardiac catheter under fluoroscopy.

The patient may be asked to change position or cough during the procedure.

Observe constantly for complications especially dysrhythmia from catheter irritation or sensitivity to the contrast dye.

Posttest

Observe the insertion site for signs of bleeding. Palpate around the puncture site to detect bleeding into tissue. If bleeding is present, exert pressure just proximal to the puncture site with a gloved hand for a minimum of 15 minutes.

Critical Thinking: If a femoral arterial approach is used during a cardiac catheterization, which distal pulses would the nurse assess?

Monitor vital signs and cardiac monitor according to hospital protocol.

Check distal pulses for arterial patency.

Report any significant changes in vital signs, rhythm, and circulation or the occurrence of chest pain.

Evaluate the patient's psychologic response to the procedure and its findings.

Review Chapter 11 for a complete discussion.

Complications

Table 14–1 summarizes the multiple complications that may occur with cardiac catheterization. Although there are many complications, their incidence is small.

ECHOCARDIOGRAM

(SONOGRAM)

Synonyms:
ECHO, heart sonogram, transthoracic echocardiogram

────────────────────── **NORMAL VALUES** ──────────────────────

No anatomic or functional abnormalities

TABLE 14–1
COMPLICATIONS OF CARDIAC CATHETERIZATION

Complication	Nursing Assessment
Ventricular tachycardia, ventricular fibrillation	Observe monitor and patient
Supraventricular tachycardia	Observe monitor for paroxysmal supraventricular tachycardia, atrial fibrillation, and atrial flutter
Asystole	Observe monitor and patient, especially if patient had preexisting blocks
Vasovagal reaction	Observe monitor and pulse rate
Contrast medium reaction	See Chapter 11
Retroperitoneal bleeding	Hypotension
	Tachycardia
	Low abdominal or flank pain
	Drop in hematocrit
Air embolism	See Chapter 11
Thrombus at catheter insertion site	Check distal pulses
	Observe extremity for color and temperature change
Hematoma at catheter insertion site	As above
Cardiac tamponade	Decreased cardiac output
	Muffled heart sounds
	Increased right atrial pressure
	Pulsus paradoxus
Myocardial infarction	Chest pain
	Electrocardiographic changes
	Elevated cardiac enzyme levels
Acute congestive heart failure, pulmonary edema	Crackles
	Dyspnea
	Pink, frothy sputum
	Cyanosis
	Skin—cold and clammy
Cerebrovascular accident	Change in level of consciousness
	Change in behavior
	Hemiparesis
	Aphasia
Infection	Fever
	Tachycardia
	Elevated white blood cell count

Background Information

An echocardiogram is a noninvasive test that uses ultrasound techniques to detect enlargement of the cardiac chambers or variations in chamber size during the cardiac cycle. It also assesses valvular function, septal defects, and pericardial effusion.

Purpose of the Test

An echocardiogram is performed for a variety of diagnostic reasons such as to evaluate abnormal heart sounds; evaluate heart size, chamber size, and valvular function; and detect tumors, pericardial effusion, and wall motion abnormalities.

Procedure

An echocardiogram may be carried out at the bedside, in a special laboratory, in a clinic, or in a doctor's office. A transducer is placed over the third and fourth intercostal spaces to the left of the sternum. The transducer emits ultrasonic beams of high-frequency sound waves that are inaudible to the human ear. The transducer then picks up the echos created by the deflection of the beams off the various heart structures. This creates a picture on the oscilloscope. The picture is created because the echo varies in intensity based on the differing densities of the structures.

Findings

Abnormal heart valves
Aneurysm
Cardiomyopathy
Congenital heart disorders
Congestive heart failure
Idiopathic hypertrophic subaortic stenosis
Mural thrombi
Myocardial infarction
Pericardial effusion
Restrictive pericarditis
Tumor of the heart

Interfering Factors

- Chest wall abnormalities
- Excessive movement
- Improper placement of transducer

Nursing Implementation

Pretest

Instruct the patient that the test is noninvasive. The patient is awake during the test and usually in a recumbent position.

Inform the patient that an electromechanical transducer will be positioned on the chest. The patient will sense only the conduction jelly and the movement of the transducer. No pain or risk is involved.

During the Test

The patient may be asked to breathe slowly or hold the breath.

Posttest

Evaluate the patient's response to the procedure.
Cleanse the chest of conduction gel.

ELECTROCARDIOGRAM

Synonyms:
ECG, EKG, 12-lead ECG or EKG

──────────────── **NORMAL VALUES** ────────────────

Normal rate and rhythm. No abnormalities noted.

Background Information

The ECG is an invaluable tool in the assessment of the heart. It records the heart's electric activity. There are four common systems for the measurement of the electric activity of the heart: 12-lead ECG, cardiac monitoring, telemetry, and Holter monitoring. The electrochemical physiology characteristics are the same for each of these systems; that is, each uses electrodes on the body surface, amplifies changes in electric potentials, and provides a graphic recording. This is made possible by the body's fluid system, which acts as a conductor of electric forces. A 12-lead ECG presents a graphic recording of 12 electric planes of the heart. By manipulating the skin electrodes, 12 various views of the heart's electric activity are seen.

In a 12-lead ECG, leads I, II, and III are limb leads. In lead I, the negative electrode of the electrocardiograph is connected to the right arm, and the positive electrode is attached to the left arm. In lead II, the negative electrode is placed on the right arm, and the positive electrode is placed on the left leg. In lead III, the negative electrode is on the left arm, and the positive electrode is placed on the left leg. Leads I, II, and III form a triangle, which is called the Einthoven triangle (Fig. 14–1).

The second three leads (aVR, aVL, and aVF) recorded by the electrocardiograph machine are called augmented limb leads. In these leads, two limbs are attached to negative electrodes, and a third limb is attached to a positive electrode. If the positive electrode is placed on the right arm, the lead is called aVR (augmented voltage right arm). If the positive electrode is on the left arm,

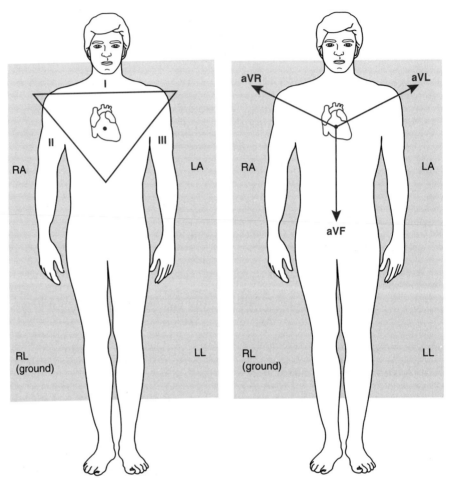

FIGURE 14–1. Einthoven's triangle.   **FIGURE 14–2.** Augmented limb leads.

it is called aVL (augmented voltage left arm). When the positive electrode is on the left foot, it is called aVF (augmented voltage foot) (Fig. 14–2).

If one takes the three sides of the Einthoven triangle and moves them to the center, they form three intersecting lines of reference (Fig. 14–3A). If one superimposes the augmented limb leads, the lines of reference and the six limb leads form six intersecting lines (one every 30 degrees). Each limb lead records a different angle and therefore a different view of the same electric activity (Fig. 14–3B).

For the precordial or chest leads, the positive electrodes are applied to the person's chest and the negative electrode is applied to the limbs. Usually, six chest leads are recorded. This is carried out by placing the positive electrode at six different positions across the chest. The chest leads are identified as V_1 through V_6. The chest leads give various views of the horizontal plane of the left ventricle.

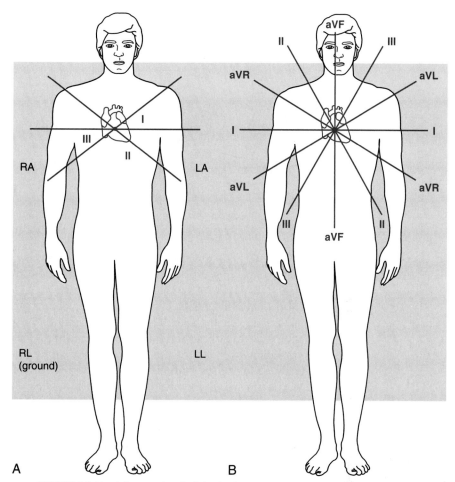

FIGURE 14–3. *A,* Intersecting limb leads. *B,* Intersecting limb and augmented leads.

The precordial leads can be visualized as spokes of a wheel, the center being the atrioventricular (AV)-node (Fig. 14–4).

There are other possible lead placements used to identify electric cardiac abnormalities, which are not recorded on the usual 12-lead ECG. Examples are a right-sided ECG when a right ventricle infarction is suspected, and posterior lead placement when a posterior infarction is suspected.

With increasing recognition of right ventricular infarction, right-sided ECGs are increasing in frequency. Right ventricular infarctions present with ST elevations of at least 1 mm in the right precordial leads V_{4r} and V_{5r}. Leads for right ventricular assessment are placed at the right fifth intercostal space at the midclavicular line (V_{4r}), at the right intercostal space at the anterior axillary line (V_{5r}), and at the right fifth intercostal space at the midaxillary line (V_{6r}).

Understanding the lead system of the ECG is important in its interpretation. The morphologic features or shape of the varied waveforms is dependent on the

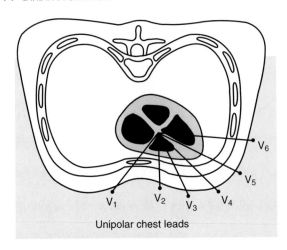

Unipolar chest leads

FIGURE 14–4. Precordial leads (V_1 to V_6).

lead. Whether the waveform is positive, negative, or biphasic depends on whether the mean electric axis is toward or away from the positive electrode of the lead.

CARDIAC MONITORING. This permits a continuous visualization of the electric activity of the heart. Usually, cardiac monitoring consists of a bedside oscilloscope, which has the capability of recording. The bedside monitor may have the ability to relay electric impulses to a central monitoring system, which is usually at the nurses' station. Most monitoring systems have both visual and auditory alarm systems, which trigger an alarm if preset deviations in rate occur.

Many central monitoring systems contain a memory tape loop, which will record and play back strips occurring immediately before and after the alarm has been discharged. Computerized electrocardiographic monitoring is also available. It provides continuous scanning for dysrhythmias and pattern changes, processes the information to determine trends, and has audio and visual alarms to alert the nurse to life-threatening situations.

The lead visualized on the oscilloscope is determined by the lead placement. Some nursing units use lead II for most of their patients, since lead II usually has a P wave, which is easily seen. Other units prefer MCL_1, a modified chest lead, since ventricular ectopy, QRS axis deviation, and conduction disturbances can be seen. MCL_1 is preferred when attempting to distinguish ventricular from supraventricular tachycardia or when assessing changes indicating myocardial ischemia. With MCL_1, the negative electrode is positioned under the left clavicle at the midclavicular line, the positive electrode is placed at the fourth intercostal space at the right sternal border, and the ground electrode is placed under the right clavicle at the right midclavicular line (Fig. 14–5).

Some newer monitor systems permit assessment of more than one lead simultaneously, and even continuous 12-lead electrocardiographic monitoring is available.

TELEMETRY. This is used for ambulatory cardiac patients. Telemetry permits the transmission of electrocardiographic readings without the patient being attached to a monitor. Telemetry requires that at least two electrodes be attached

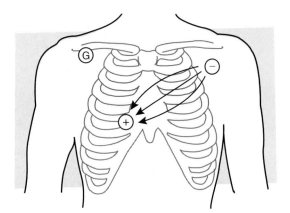

FIGURE 14-5. MCL$_1$ (modified lead).

to the patient (frequently MCL$_1$ without the ground electrode). The electrodes are plugged into a small pocket-sized transmitter, which is usually secured to the patient's robe pocket or carried. The transmitter emits a signal that is picked up and displayed on a central monitoring system.

HOLTER MONITORING. This type of monitoring is also called *ambulatory monitoring* and it permits the recording of cardiac electric activity over time (usually 24 hours) on a cassette tape recorder. It allows the patient to perform normal daily activities so that cardiac responses to these activities can be determined.

Purpose of the Test

Critical Thinking: As a community health educator, what are the priority instructions to be taught the public about what to do when an individual experiences chest pain?

The purpose of the 12-lead ECG is to diagnose myocardial infarction, injury, and ischemia. It also assists in identifying hypertrophy, axis deviations, and electrolyte abnormalities and distinguishes between ventricular and supraventricular tachycardias. Left versus right hypertrophy can be distinguished by comparing the morphologic characteristics of the QRS complex in leads V$_5$ and V$_6$, by determining axis deviation, and by the P wave.

The primary purpose of cardiac monitoring, telemetry, and Holter monitoring is dysrhythmia detection. These procedures are helpful in identifying conduction defects and responses to therapeutic measures.

Procedure

For a 12-lead ECG, the technician, the physician, or the nurse places the patient in a supine position. Conduction jelly is placed on the electrodes, and the electrodes are applied. The electrocardiograph's electrode wires are marked and color-coded. It is essential that the chest leads be positioned correctly for accurate interpretation.

The chest leads are applied as follows:

V$_1$: Fourth intercostal space at the right sternal border
V$_2$: Fourth intercostal space at the left sternal border

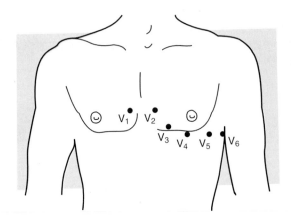

FIGURE 14–6. Chest lead placement.

V_3: Midway between V_2 and V_4
V_4: Fifth intercostal space at the left midclavicular line
V_5: Fifth intercostal space at the anterior axillary line
V_6: Fifth intercostal space at the midaxillary line (Fig. 14–6)

Electrocardiographs vary. Older machines record one lead at a time. Newer machines simultaneously record the 12 leads and automatically mark the leads.

With Holter monitoring, electrodes are applied to the patient's chest (placement varies with desired leads) and attached to a battery-operated tape recorder. Most recorders permit simultaneous recording of two channels (frequently lead II and V_5 are chosen). Recorders are equipped with an event marker, which alerts the scanning technician that the patient experienced some symptom. A diary is kept by the patient, who records daily activities and the times they were performed, when and what medications were taken, and the presence and time symptoms occurred. The recordings are analyzed at 60 to 120 times real time by a microcomputer program. Any abnormalities are then recorded on the usual electrocardiograph paper.

Findings

Axis deviations (right or left)
Conduction disturbances
Dysrhythmias
Hypertrophy of the ventricles
Electrolyte imbalances
Pericarditis
Pulmonary infarctions
Therapeutic drug effects or toxicity, or both

Critical Thinking: On admission to the hospital, a patient with substernal chest pain has ST elevations in leads II, III, and aVF. What should the nurse's response be?

As a myocardial infarction evolves, a sequence of electrocardiographic changes occurs. First, the ST segment changes. Elevation of an ST segment indicates myocardial injury. ST depression occurs as a reciprocal change in the ventricular

TABLE 14–2
ELECTROCARDIOGRAPHIC CHANGES WITH ACUTE MYOCARDIAL INFARCTION

	Lead Changes	Reciprocal Changes
Inferior wall	II, III, aVF	I, aVL
Lateral wall	I, aVL, V_5, V_6	V_1, V_2, V_3
Anterior wall	V_2, V_3, V_4	II, III, aVF
Anteroseptal	V_1, V_2, V_3, V_4	II, III, aVF
Posterior wall		V_1, V_2, V_3, V_4

wall opposite the infarction. The ST segment will return to normal within days or weeks after the infarction.

Within hours or days of the infarction, the T-wave inverts. It reflects ischemic changes in the heart. The T-wave will revert back to normal within weeks or months of the infarction.

Lastly, an abnormal Q-wave appears in the leads directly over the transmural myocardial infarction. An abnormal Q-wave is the presence of a Q-wave in a lead in which a Q wave is not normally seen or one that is wider than 0.04 seconds or a third of the height of the QRS complex. A non–Q-wave infarction occurs when there is a subendocardial infarction. A Q-wave indicates myocardial necrosis and may remain for years after the infarction.

Table 14–2 summarizes which leads reflect which walls of the left ventricle. Note that since no leads are usually placed over the posterior wall of the heart, posterior infarctions are diagnosed by reciprocal changes. Right ventricular infarctions are assessed by performing a right-sided 12-lead ECG.

Interfering Factors

• Patient movement, poor grounding, and poor skin contact can interfere with a clear recording of the ECG.

Nursing Implementation for a Twelve-Lead Electrocardiogram

Pretest

Explain to the patient the purpose and procedure for the ECG. No risk is involved.

No pretest restrictions are required.

Since electrodes are applied to the four extremities and the chest, clothing should permit easy access. If the male patient's chest is excessively hairy, the sites may need to be shaved.

During the Test

Establish a relaxed environment.
Place the patient in a supine position.
Conduction jelly is placed on the electrodes and the electrodes are applied.
The recording is made.

Posttest

Remove the conduction jelly.
Help the patient to a comfortable position.

Nursing Implementation for Cardiac Monitoring

Pretest

Inform the patient as to the purpose of the monitoring.
Briefly explain the effects of movement on the scope's display. Include an explanation of the alarm system.
Clarify that the monitor is an assessment tool and not a therapy.
Apply the electrodes as indicated or according to the nursing unit protocol. Shave the site if the chest is hairy.
Set alarms.

During the Test

Continuously monitor for rhythm or rate changes.
Check that the conduction jelly on the electrodes is moist. Replace if necessary.
If artifacts (electrocardiographic recordings not related to a cardiac event) occur, determine the source and correct if possible.

Posttest

Remove electrodes and cleanse site of jelly.
Observe skin for signs of irritation.

Nursing Implementation for Holter Monitoring

The nursing actions are similar to those in cardiac monitoring, except that the Holter monitor's indicator light is checked to determine if the battery is functioning. The patient is instructed to keep a diary of activities and is taught how to trigger the event marker.

Complications

Electrocardiography is a noninvasive procedure without complications.

ELECTROPHYSIOLOGIC STUDIES

(RADIOLOGY)

Synonym:
EPS

--- NORMAL VALUES ---

Normal cardiac rhythm
Normal conduction, refractory, and interval times

Background Information

Electrophysiologic studies are invasive procedures performed in special laboratories or in cardiac catheterization laboratories. These studies require the insertion of catheters into the right and sometimes the left side of the heart. Several procedures are included: atrial stimulation, ventricular stimulation, bundle of His studies, and ventricular mapping.

Purpose of the Test

Electrophysiologic studies are performed to diagnose dysrhythmias, identify causes of ectopy, and determine a person's risk for lethal ventricular dysrhythmias. They are used to determine appropriate therapy in patients who have not obtained the desired effect from usual therapies and in whom noninvasive evaluation techniques have not provided the information necessary to determine which therapy or combination of therapies will be effective.

Procedure

Several procedures are included in the category of electrophysiologic studies. The patient may have one or all of the studies performed based on the clinical state. During the test, three or four multipolar pacing catheters are inserted percutaneously. One is positioned high in the atrium, one in the low-septal right atrium, one in the coronary sinus, and one in the right ventricle. Conduction intervals are measured to locate conduction delays. Atrial pacing is carried out to assess sinoatrial node response, AV node response, and bundle of His and Purkinje conduction. If indicated, *atrial extrastimulus testing (AEST)* is performed. With this test, a premature atrial stimulus is initiated to assess atrial and AV node response. Atrial flutter or atrial fibrillation may be initiated. The focus or reentry pathway may then be identified. In some patients, *His bundle electrographic studies* are performed to evaluate His bundle conduction.

Ventricular extrastimulus testing (VEST) is performed to assess ventricular dysrhythmias. Ventricular tachycardia (VT) may be induced. If a right ventricular stimulus does not induce VT, a left-sided stimulation may be carried out. This requires the insertion of a multipolar pacing catheter through an artery. When VT is induced, its response to overdrive pacing or drugs, or both, can be evaluated. If the patient has recurrent VT, *ventricular endocardial mapping* may be performed to localize the origin of the dysrhythmia. If ventricular mapping is performed, VT is induced and the ectopic focus is delineated by multiple intracardiac tracings.

If the electrophysiologic studies involve evaluation of drug responses, the test must be repeated because only one drug or combination of drugs can be assessed at a time. If this is necessary, subclavian catheters are left in place between testings.

Findings

Electrophysiologic studies may identify dysrhythmias, conduction abnormalities, and appropriate treatment for these disturbances.

Interfering Factors

See section on cardiac catheterization.

Nursing Implementation

The nursing actions are similar to those for cardiac catheterization with the following additions.

Pretest

Reassure the patient that if dysrhythmias or blocks occur, resources are available to control and treat them.

Warn the patient that a "fluttering" sensation in the chest or hiccups may occur.

Antiarrhythmic drugs are usually discontinued for four half-lives (or four doses) before the test. In patients with potentially lethal dysrhythmias, cardiac monitoring is required.

The patient receives nothing by mouth for 6 hours prior to the procedure.

Premedication usually consists of diazepam (Valium), since it has no significant electrophysiologic effect. Avoid any medications with possible cardiac effect.

During the Test

Critical Thinking: What medications should the nurse have on hand during an EPS?

Actions are similar to those in cardiac catheterization except that only small doses of lidocaine are used as a local anesthetic to prevent systemic effects.

Posttest

Assess site of catheter placement. If further studies are to be carried out, a catheter may have been left in place.

Check distal pulses if left-sided catheterization was performed.

Bed rest is maintained. For a right-sided study, bed rest is maintained for 2 hours; for a left-sided study, bed rest is maintained for 6 to 12 hours.

Encourage the patient to turn from side to side.

Avoid hip flexion if a femoral insertion was performed.

Evaluate the dressings for bleeding and infection. They should be kept dry and intact.

Anticoagulant therapy may be ordered if prolonged catheterization was required or if left ventricular stimulation or mapping was performed.

Patient and family teaching will depend on the findings of the studies and the indicated therapy.

Complications

See the section on cardiac catheterization. In addition, if a subclavian insertion site was used, observe for pneumothorax.

ENDOMYOCARDIAL BIOPSY

(PATHOLOGY)

──────────────── **NORMAL VALUES** ────────────────

> Normal cardiac tissue

Background Information

Endomyocardial biopsy is an invasive procedure requiring cardiac catheterization. It permits sampling of right or left ventricular tissue.

Purpose of the Test

An endomyocardial biopsy is usually performed to determine if a transplanted heart is being rejected. Other purposes for the biopsy are to diagnose myocarditis or doxorubicin (Adriamycin) cardiomyopathy and to determine the cause of restrictive heart disease.

Procedure

The procedure involves a cardiac catheterization (see pp. 327–330). A catheter with a jaw-like tip is inserted under fluoroscopy, and several small tissue samples are obtained. A right or left ventricular sample may be taken. For patients at high risk, such as those with a history of left ventricular thrombus or infarction, a right ventricular biopsy may be preferred.

Findings

Doxorubicin-induced cardiomyopathy
Cardiac amyloidosis
Cardiac fibrosis (especially radiation injury)
Chagas cardiomyopathy
Myocarditis
Rejection of transplanted heart
Scleroderma
Toxoplasmosis
Tumor infiltrates
Vasculitis

Interfering Factors

- Bleeding disorders
- Severe thrombocytopenia
- Systemic anticoagulation
- Uncooperative patient

Nursing Implementation

See discussion of cardiac catheterization.

Complications

Although complications of endomyocardial biopsy are rare, they include accidental biopsy of papillary muscle or chordae tendineae, cardiac perforation,

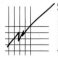

TABLE 14–3
COMPLICATIONS OF ENDOMYOCARDIAL BIOPSY*

Complication	Nursing Assessment
Accidental biopsy of papillary muscle or chordae tendineae	New onset of a mitral or tricuspid murmur
Hemopericardium	Decreased cardiac output
	Muffled heart sounds
	Increased right atrial pressure
	Pulsus paradoxus
Cardiac perforation	Same as hemopericardium
	Shock

*Complications other than those listed can occur, but they are related to cardiac catheterization.

and hemopericardium. Other complications can occur but are related to the catheterization rather then the biopsy itself. Table 14–3 provides assessments to be made by the nurse indicating a complication.

ERGONOVINE PROVOCATION TEST

(RADIOLOGY) ──────────────── **NORMAL VALUES** ────────────────

> No ST segment changes

Background Information

Ergonovine provocation testing is used to diagnose coronary artery spasm and vasospastic angina. Accurate diagnosis of coronary artery spasm is necessary, as treatment varies. Because of its risk, ergonovine provocation testing is limited to carefully selected patients.

Purpose of the Test

Ergonovine provocation testing is indicated in patients with atypical angina in whom coronary artery spasm is *suspected*.

Procedure

The ergonovine provocation test is usually performed as part of a cardiac catheterization. First, the cardiac catheterization must rule out severe coronary artery obstruction. A pacing wire is then inserted. Intravenous ergonovine maleate (Ergotrate maleate) is given, which usually will stimulate a spasm within 3 to 6 minutes. Its effect lasts 10 to 15 minutes. If a positive response occurs, the spasm is reversed by administering nitroglycerin intravenously.

Bedside ergonovine provocation testing can be performed in the coronary care unit in patients who have had a cardiac catheterization to verify that the coronary arteries are not severely obstructed. Ergonovine is given intravenously every 5 minutes up to seven times. The ergonovine is stopped when ST segment changes are seen on the monitor whether the patient has pain or not. Nitroglycerin is given to reverse the spasm.

Findings

A positive response to ergonovine includes chest pain with ST segment abnormalities (rarely, chest pain does not occur), spasms visible on the arteriogram, serious dysrhythmias, or a combination.

Interfering Factors

Ergonovine provocation testing should not be performed if there is severe obstruction of a coronary artery or multivessel obstructive cardiac disease or in the presence of severe congestive heart failure, uncontrolled hypertension, pregnancy, acute myocardial infarction, or possible cerebral hemorrhage. It is contraindicated in anyone with a history of hypersensitivity to ergonovine.

Nursing Implementation

Critical Thinking: What clinical assessments indicate severe congestive heart failure and possible postponement of the ergonovine provocation test? How would the nurse explain the test cancellation to the patient and/or significant other?

See the section on cardiac catheterization. In addition, review the following.

Pretest

Warn the patient that chest pain is expected but will be treated immediately.
Discontinue vasoactive medications—nitrates for 4 hours before the test, calcium blockers for 24 hours before the test, and beta-blockers for 48 hours before the test.

During the Test

Continuous cardiac and hemodynamic monitoring is performed.
If major adverse effects are noted, the ergonovine is stopped.

Posttest

Assess the patient for chest pain with or without ST segment changes, as spasms may recur after the nitroglycerin is stopped.
Maintain patient on the monitor and continue bed rest for 1 to 2 hours if the procedure is performed in the coronary care unit.

Complications

A variety of complications may occur with ergonovine provocation testing. Close observation of the patient as well as assessment of subjective data is essential. The complications range from nausea, vomiting, and headache to atypical chest pain, myocardial infarction, dysrhythmias, bronchospasms, and hyper- or hypotension. Table 14–4 summarizes the assessments with each of these complications.

GATED BLOOD POOL STUDIES

(RADIONUCLIDE
IMAGING)

Synonyms:

technetium-99 ventriculography, MUGA, multiple gated acquisition angiography

TABLE 14–4

COMPLICATIONS OF ERGONOVINE PROVOCATION TESTING

Complication	Nursing Assessment
Atypical chest pain	Patient report
Bronchospasms	Dyspnea
	Wheeze
Dysrhythmias	Monitor for ventricular tachycardia, ventricular fibrillation, complete heart block, sinus arrest
Nausea, vomiting	Patient report
	Emesis
Hypotension or hyper-tension	Monitor blood pressure
	Hemodynamic monitoring
Headaches	Patient report
Myocardial infarction	Chest pain
	Electrocardiographic changes
	Elevated cardiac enzyme levels

─────────── **NORMAL VALUES** ───────────

Normal wall motion
Ejection fraction = 55–75%
Response to exercise—increase in ejection fraction greater than 5%

Background Information

A gated blood pool scan is a noninvasive method of assessing myocardial function, particularly wall motion of the left ventricle. It also permits evaluation of left ventricular ejection without invasive catheterization.

Purpose of the Test

A gated pool study is performed to assess ventricular function by evaluating wall motion and determining ejection fractions.

Procedure

Critical Thinking: If the patient's ejection fraction is less than 20%, what adaptations in nursing care must be made?

The procedure for the gated pool study is similar to that for myocardial imaging. The red blood cells are tagged with technetium-99m pyrophosphate, a gamma-emitting radionuclide. Since the bound technetium cannot diffuse through cell membranes, it remains in the blood. Its emissions are more concentrated in body cavities with large blood volumes, including the heart chambers.

During the procedure, the patient is monitored with a cardiac monitor, and the ECG is synchronized with the imaging equipment. Multiple images can be obtained. Results usually report the "first pass," which analyzes the radiotracing during the initial flow through the heart. In addition, a "gated" analysis is performed, which reports cardiac chamber responses of 200 to 300 cardiac cycles. Since left ventricular size can be measured at the end of diastole and systole, the ventricular ejection fraction can be measured. After a gated analysis, the patient may or may not be reassessed with exercise stress testing.

Findings

Hypokinesis—slightly diminished wall motion
Akinesis—absence of wall motion
Dyskinesia—paradoxical wall motion or bulging
Decreased ejection fraction

Nursing Implementation

See section on cardiac imaging and stress testing.

Complications

See section on stress testing.

PERICARDIOCENTESIS

(PATHOLOGY)

Synonym:
pericardial fluid analysis

─────────────────── **NORMAL VALUES** ───────────────────

Fluid is sterile, clear, or straw-colored.

Background Information

Pericardiocentesis is a diagnostic and therapeutic procedure in which the pericardial space is accessed with a needle or cannula, and fluid is aspirated. For diagnostic purposes, the fluid is then analyzed. For therapeutic purposes, either fluid is drained on a one-time basis or a catheter is left in place for 1 to 48 hours (rarely, it may be kept in for 72 hours.)

Normally, the pericardial space between the visceral and parietal pericardium contains approximately 20 to 50 ml of clear serous fluid. If the pericardium becomes inflamed or diseased or is disrupted, pericardial effusion may occur. As fluid builds up in the pericardial space, cardiac tamponade may result. Cardiac tamponade will eventually lead to a decrease in cardiac output, with an increase in right atrial pressure, pulsus paradoxus, and hypotension. If progressive and untreated, cardiac tamponade will result in death.

Purpose of the Test

Analysis of pericardial fluid is performed to determine the cause of and appropriate therapy for acute pericarditis, subacute effusive-constrictive pericarditis, neoplastic pericardial disease, and pericardial effusion of unknown cause.

Procedure

A pericardiocentesis for diagnostic purposes is not an emergency situation and can be performed in the controlled environment of an operating room or special procedure room. The procedure begins after a skin preparation and infiltration of a local anesthetic, usually 1% lidocaine without epinephrine. A small incision is made in the skin, the site being determined by the desired approach.

The most common approach to the pericardial space is the left xiphocostal space. The needle is inserted through an incision made just under and to the left of the xiphoid process into the angle between the xiphoid process and the left costal margin. The physician points the needle toward the left shoulder and advances it until a "popping" or "giving" sensation is felt as the pericardium is entered. Traditionally, an electrocardiographic lead is attached to the pericardiocentesis needle. As the needle advances, a chest lead on the ECG is recorded. When the heart is punctured, a zone of injury pattern is noted, and the needle is withdrawn slightly. Some physicians do not recommend this technique because poor electrocardiographic tracings prevent the zone of injury from being seen, which may lead to cardiac lacerations. The sign of injury on the ECG also may not occur if the needle infiltrates an area of fibrosis, a tumor, or infiltrative cardiomyopathy tissue. There is a possibility of ventricular fibrillation if the electrocardiograph is not grounded properly, there is electric leakage or the individual performing the procedure accidentally touches the needle and electrocardiograph.

Other approaches for a pericardiocentesis include the following:

RIGHT XIPHOCOSTAL APPROACH. This is similar to the left xiphocostal approach except that the needle is directed toward the right shoulder. This approach carries the potential risk of puncturing the right atrium and inferior vena cava.

APICAL APPROACH. An incision is made just lateral to the cardiac apex (identified by fluoroscopy, radiography, or echocardiography). The needle is directed toward the right shoulder. This approach has the potential of lacerating the left pleural space and lung.

RIGHT-SIDED APPROACH. An incision is made between the right fourth and fifth intercostal spaces, and the needle is directed medially. The potential risk is a puncture of the right pleura or right atrium.

PARASTERNAL APPROACH. An incision is made between the right or left fifth and sixth intercostal spaces, and the needle is directed posteromedially. The potential risk if the right side is used is puncture of the right pleura and lung. If the left side is used, it is possible to puncture the left anterior descending artery or internal mammary artery.

Once the needle is in position, approximately 20 ml of fluid is removed for analysis. If cytologic studies are performed, a heparinized container is necessary. The fluid is usually analyzed for color; hemoglobin concentration; hematocrit value; red blood cell, white blood cell, and differential counts; and protein and glucose determinations. In addition, gram stains and culture, fungal stains and culture, and cytologic studies are performed. Additional fluid is removed if viral and parasite studies, immunologic and serologic screens, or lipoelectrophoresis is planned.

If therapeutic pericarditis is desired after the specimens are obtained, a catheter is inserted and positioned to allow drainage.

Findings

Bacterial, viral, or fungal infection
Malignancies

Interfering Factors

Pericardiocentesis requires a patient who is cooperative and who will lie still during the procedure. Uncooperative patients may require sedation. Those on anticoagulant therapy, with bleeding disorders or thrombocytopenia, are not appropriate candidates. If cultures of the fluid are planned, administration of antibiotics will affect the results.

Nursing Implementation

Pretest

Ensure that an informed consent form has been signed.
Explain the procedure to the patient.
Check laboratory work for bleeding problems.
Obtain a baseline ECG if ordered.
Document baseline vital signs and heart sounds.
Take medication history to check for anticoagulant use.
The patient maintains a nothing-by-mouth status for 4 to 6 hours before the test.
Administer sedation as prescribed.
Shave site as ordered.

Critical Thinking: Your patient with a pericardial effusion is scheduled for a pericardiocentesis. Which laboratory tests would you check?

TABLE 14–5
COMPLICATIONS OF PERICARDIOCENTESIS

Complication	Nursing Assessment
Puncture or laceration of cardiac chamber	Bloody pericardial fluid
	Acute cardiac tamponade
Laceration of coronary artery	Acute cardiac tamponade
	Ventricular fibrillation
Ventricular fibrillation	Observed on monitor
Pneumothorax	Dyspnea
	Absence of bilateral breath sounds
Peritoneal puncture	Straw-colored fluid if ascites is present

During the Test

Position the patient. Usually a recumbent position is used, with the torso and head elevated 30 to 45 degrees.

Ensure that an intravenous infusion is present and patent.

Maintain patient on telemetry or cardiac monitor.

Frequent vital signs are taken.

Have a defibrillator and emergency drugs on hand.

Continue to reassure and support the patient, who will feel the local anesthetic being infiltrated and may experience a sharp pain when the pericardium is infiltrated.

Critical Thinking: For a patient with a cardiac tamponade, as the fluid is drained during the pericardiocentesis, what clinical evaluations indicate that it is effective?

Posttest

The patient may return to pretest activities gradually if vital signs are stable. Assess for recurrence of symptoms.

Complications

Complications from pericardiocentesis include puncture or laceration of the cardiac chamber, laceration of a coronary artery, ventricular fibrillation, pneumothorax, and peritoneal puncture. See Table 14–5 for assessments of these complications.

PHONOCARDIOGRAM

(SONOGRAM)

──────────── NORMAL VALUES ────────────

No abnormalities

Background Information

A phonocardiogram is a graphic recording of cardiac sounds. It is a noninvasive test that amplifies cardiac sounds, which are recorded simultaneously with the electrocardiographic readings.

Purpose of the Test

The phonocardiogram is performed to determine the exact timing of heart sounds; differentiating the varied sounds such as murmurs, splits, and clicks; and evaluating valvular function.

Procedure

A phonocardiogram may be carried out at the bedside, in the physician's office, in the clinic, or in a cardiac laboratory. Electrocardiographic equipment is necessary, and electrodes are applied. Microphones are placed over the heart in various positions.

Findings

Valve disorders (stenosis or incompetence)
Estimate of ventricular function
Hypertrophic cardiomyopathies

Interfering Factors

Critical Thinking: What instructions can the nurse provide to prevent the Vaisalva maneuver from interfering with a phonocardiogram?

- Improper placement of microphone
- Muscle tremors
- Obesity
- Valsalva maneuver

Nursing Implementation

Pretest

Inform the patient as to the purpose and procedure of the study.
Explain to the patient that the test is painless and that no risk is involved.
Instruct the patient to remain quiet and still during the procedure.

During the Test

Electrocardiograph electrodes are applied and attached to the electrocardiograph recorder.
Conduction jelly is applied to the chest wall.

As the phonocardiogram microphone is positioned at various sites over the chest wall, the patient may be asked to change position, perform muscle tightening, or change breathing patterns.

Posttest

Remove conduction jelly from the chest and extremities.

ROENTGENOGRAM, CARDIAC

(RADIOLOGY)

Synonym:

cardiac x-ray

NORMAL VALUES

Normal size, shape, and positioning of the heart and great vessels

Background Information

A cardiac roentgenogram is a routine screening procedure in patients with suspected or known cardiac disorders. It provides information regarding the size of the heart, its shape, and the location of the cardiac structures and great vessels.

The x-ray study may also be used to evaluate pulmonary vasculature and determine the placement of evasive catheters and pacemaker wires.

See Chapter 9 for a full discussion of roentgenograms. The exception to the general preparation of the patient for a cardiac evaluation is that the electrodes used to monitor a patient are not usually removed when an x-ray film is taken.

Procedure

Various views of the chest are usually obtained in a cardiac x-ray series. The four views commonly obtained are anteroposterior; posteroanterior; lateral, right anterior oblique; and left anterior oblique. During acute cardiac states, only portable chest x-ray studies are available to evaluate the client's progress. Since the plate is positioned under the client, an anteroposterior view is obtained.

SIGNAL-AVERAGED ELECTROCARDIOGRAM

(ELECTROPHYSIOLOGY)

Synonym:

SAECG

──────────────── **NORMAL VALUES** ────────────────

Normal cardiac rhythm and conduction times

Background Information

Signal-averaged electrocardiography is a technique used to detect conduction defects that may precede VT. It is a noninvasive bedside test similar to a 12-lead ECG. With a signal-averaged ECG, the recording is obtained for 15 to 30 minutes, and the electric current from the heart is amplified 1000 times. The machine then integrates all these signals and removes extraneous electric signals.

Purpose of the Test

The cardiologist assesses the printout of the signal-averaged ECG for late potentials, which place the patient at risk for sustained VT. A late potential is seen as a QRS complex that extends 20 to 60 msec into the ST segment.

Procedure

The procedure is similar to the 12-lead ECG, except that no limb electrodes are necessary and the six chest electrodes and ground lead are positioned differently on the chest.

Interfering Factors

Since the signal-averaged ECG averages the cardiac cycle of the patient, a relatively regular rhythm is needed during the test. *Frequent* premature atrial contractures or premature ventricular contractures will interfere with the results. Signal-averaged electrocardiography is also unable to detect late potentials in patients with right or left bundle branch block.

Findings

Late potentials

Nursing Implementation

The nursing actions are similar to those for electrocardiography. In addition, review the following.

Pretest

Check with the prescriber regarding discontinuing or administering the patient's antiarrhythmic medication.

During the Test

Keep the environment quiet.
Instruct others to stay out of the patient's room.

STRESS TESTING, CARDIAC

(ELECTROPHYSIOLOGY)

Synonyms:

graded exercise testing (GEX), graded exercise stress testing (GEST), exercise stress testing, exercise electrocardiography

─────────── **NORMAL VALUES** ───────────

No unexpected changes in the ECG

Background Information

Critical Thinking: Who is at risk for coronary artery disease and would benefit from stress testing? How can the nurse reach this population?

Stress testing is an important noninvasive procedure for evaluating the cardiovascular status of patients who are known to have cardiac disease or who are at risk for cardiac disease. The test increases the demand placed on the heart by increasing physical activity. Through electrocardiographic tracings, it can be determined whether the heart is able to meet the increased oxygen demand.

Purpose of the Test

Stress testing is an invaluable technique in (1) assessing the at-risk population, (2) diagnosing chest pain syndromes and dysrhythmias associated with ischemia, (3) evaluating the effectiveness of therapy (surgical or pharmacologic), and (4) identifying the initial level of function in cardiac rehabilitation programs and evaluating the results.

Procedure

Critical Thinking: Develop a teaching plan to prepare an outpatient for cardiac stress testing. How should the plan be adapted, if the patient is an elderly female?

Stress testing requires the use of a bicycle ergometer or a treadmill with continuous electrocardiac recording. The test is performed in a series of stages in which the patient exercises for 3 minutes. At the end of each stage, a 12-lead ECG is recorded. After each stage, the workload or "graded load" is increased. This is accomplished by increasing the speed or resistance of the bicycle or treadmill. The stress testing continues until the patient reaches the maximum heart rate, becomes symptomatic, or displays electrocardiographic changes consistent with ischemia. The maximum heart rate is usually determined by normograms. A gross estimate of the maximum heart rate is 220 beats per minute minus the patient's age.

If a patient is physically unable to exercise to the point of maximum heart rate, a *dipyridamole (Persantine) scan* may be performed. It is estimated that 25 to 30% of patients who are candidates for stress testing are not able to perform the exercise required because of peripheral vascular disease or pulmonary, orthopedic, or neurologic dysfunction (Marchiondo, 1994). Dipyridamole may be given intravenously or by mouth. It causes coronary artery dilation similar to the response of the coronary arteries to exercise. After peak effect is reached (85% maximum heart rate), a thallium scan is performed (see pp. 357–359). A follow-up scan is performed 4 hours later.

Findings

A 1-mm depression of the ST segment is a positive stress test, indicating myocardial ischemia.

Interfering Factors

Severe anxiety may interfere with the patient's ability to participate fully in the stress testing. False-positive results may be due to bundle branch block, ventricular hypertrophy, or digitalization. False-negative results may be due to the use of beta-blockers.

Nursing Implementation

Pretest

Instruct the patient about the purpose and procedure of the test.
Inform the patient to wear comfortable clothes and rubber-soled walking shoes.
Instruct the patient not to eat, smoke, or drink alcohol for 3 to 4 hours before the test.
Assess for contraindications to stress testing:
  Chest pain
  Hypertension
  Thrombophlebitis
  Second- or third-degree heart block
  Serious dysrhythmias
  Severe congestive heart failure
  Neurologic, musculoskeletal, or vascular problems that would impede mobility on the bicycle or treadmill

During the Test

Have emergency equipment and drugs available (code cart).
The patient is attached to electrodes for recording a 12-lead ECG.

TABLE 14–6
COMPLICATIONS OF CARDIAC STRESS TESTING

Complication	Nursing Assessment
Dysrhythmias	Monitor patient
Myocardial ischemia	Chest pain
	ST elevations or depressions

A blood pressure cuff is put in place for quick access. A baseline blood pressure reading is obtained.

As the graded exercises begin, a multichanneled ECG is recorded. A 12-lead ECG is recorded and the blood pressure is checked as each workload ends (every 3-minute increment).

Observe for signs to stop the stress testing, for example, falling blood pressure, three consecutive premature ventricular contractures, chest pain, or exhaustion. The stressing may or may not be discontinued if ST depressions occur, blood pressure does not rise, or frequent or coupled premature ventricular contractions or bundle branch block occurs.

If dipyridamole was used, assess for side effects: myocardial infarction, dysrhythmias, bronchospasms, chest pain, nausea, headache, flushing hypotension, and dizziness.

Posttest

Cardiac monitoring is continued for 5 to 10 minutes after the testing to evaluate the patient's physiologic response.

Blood pressure is checked.

Remove conduction jelly and assist in robing the patient if necessary.

Evaluate the patient's physical and emotional response to the testing.

Instruct the patient to rest and not to take hot showers or baths for 2 to 4 hours.

Complications

Stress testing is performed in a controlled environment; however, dysrhythmias and myocardial ischemia may occur (Table 14–6).

THALLIUM TESTING

(RADIONUCLIDE
IMAGING)

Synonyms:

thallium scan, thallium exercise imaging, resting thallium scan

━━━━━━━━━━━━━━━━━━━━━ **NORMAL VALUES** ━━━━━━━━━━━━━━━━━━━━

> Normal myocardial perfusion; no "cold" spots

Background Information

Thallium is a radioactive analog of potassium, which is rapidly taken up by myocardial cells. After thallium-201 is given, almost 90% of it is extracted by the myocardium within seconds. For this to occur, two factors are essential: (1) adequate perfusion and (2) cellular extraction efficiency. Since cellular ischemia does not seem to affect thallium uptake in the myocardium, its lack of uptake is an indication of an infarction.

Purpose of the Test

Thallium imaging is used to assess coronary blood flow to determine areas of infarction and ischemia. It is used to diagnose CAD and assess revascularization following coronary artery bypass surgery.

Procedure

Critical Thinking: How do you explain to patients the need to repeat thallium scans 3 to 4 hours after the initial scan is done?

Thallium scanning is performed with an Anger gamma camera combined with a computer. Continuous counts of emitted photons are made during the cardiac cycle. The scan identifies "cold spots," areas of decreased thallium uptake. Cold spots identify areas of ischemia and infarction. Thallium can be given under a state of no physical demand, which is known as a *resting thallium study*, or it can be part of a stress test, in which case it is called *exercise thallium imaging*. Exercise thallium imaging distinguishes ischemic sites from infarcted areas. Thallium scans are repeated, once during stress testing and then 3 to 4 hours after the thallium was given and the stress test was completed. With the second imaging, if a "cold spot" remains, it is assumed to be an infarcted area. If the "cold spot" disappears, it is recognized as an ischemic area.

Findings

Cold spots indicate and distinguish areas of infarction and ischemia.

Interfering Factors

See discussion of stress testing.

Nursing Implementation

Nursing care is similar to that in stress testing, except that the patient has an infusion of normal saline started.

Pretest

Usually, long-acting nitrates are held for 8 to 12 hours before the test.

During the Test

The thallium is given intravenously about a minute before the completion of the stress test.

After the completion of the stress test, the patient is placed supine on the table, and multiple scintigraphic images are taken.

Posttest

Assess the patient's response.

Three to four hours later, the patient returns for repeat films.

TRANSESOPHAGEAL ECHOCARDIOGRAPHY

(SONOGRAM)

Synonym:
TEE

──────────────── **NORMAL VALUES** ────────────────

No anatomic or functional abnormalities

Background Information

A transesophageal echocardiogram is an invasive procedure that uses ultrasound technique to detect enlargement of cardiac chambers and variations in chamber size during the cardiac cycle. It also assesses valvular function, septal defects, and pericardial effusion. Although these functions can be accomplished with a transthoracic echocardiogram, transesophageal echocardiography permits a better view of the posterior atrium and aorta. Transesophageal echocardiography is also indicated when a transthoracic approach is inadequate such as when the patient is obese or has chest wall structure abnormalities.

Purpose of the Test

Indications for transesophageal echocardiography include diagnosis of (1) a thoracic aortic pathologic condition, including suspected aneurysms; (2) mitral valve disease or assessment of a prosthetic valve; (3) suspected endocarditis; (4) congenital heart disease, for example, atrial septal defect; (5) left atrial intra-cardiac thrombi; and (6) cardiac tumors.

Procedure

Transesophageal echocardiography is similar to transthoracic echocardiography except that the ultrasound probe is fitted into the end of a flexible gastroscopy tube and advanced down the esophagus behind the heart.

Findings

See the discussion of the echocardiogram.

Interfering Factors

Transesophageal echocardiography should not be performed if the patient has a history of irradiation of the mediastinum, esophageal dysphagia, or structural abnormalities.

Nursing Implementation

Pretest

Ensure that a signed informed consent form has been obtained.

Maintain the patient on a nothing-by-mouth status for 6 to 8 hours.

Describe the procedure to the patient, especially the need for a mouthguard, positioning, and the need to swallow when asked.

If the patient has prosthetic heart valves, prophylactic antibiotics may be prescribed.

Administer antianxiety medication as prescribed.

During the Test

Administer medication to decrease secretions as ordered.

A topical anesthetic is sprayed into the throat.

Instruct the patient to gargle with viscous lidocaine and then to swallow it. Warn the patient that it will make the tongue and throat feel "swollen."

A mouthguard is placed to prevent the patient from biting down on the endoscope.

The patient is positioned on the left side in the chin-chest position. The head may be supported with a small pillow.

The probe is lubricated with lidocaine jelly and slowly inserted as the patient swallows.

Monitor the patient for a vasovagal response from the medication given to dry up secretions.

Check the patient for gagging.

Observe the oximeter for oxygen saturation readings.

TABLE 14–7

COMPLICATIONS OF TRANSESOPHAGEAL ECHOCARDIOGRAPHY

Complication	Nursing Assessment
Esophageal perforation	Bleeding Pain
Transient dysrhythmias	Observe on monitor
Transient hypoxia	Observe pulse oximetry Observe skin color and respiratory pattern
Vasovagal response	Observe monitor for bradycardia Check pulse

Posttest

Assess the patient for return of the gag reflex before resuming oral intake. Give lozenges for relief of throat discomfort.

Complications

Transesophageal echocardiography has several complications that are related to the placement of the probe in the esophagus, including esophageal perforation, transient hypoxia, dysrhythmias, and a vasovagal response. See Table 14–7 for a summary of assessments of each of these complications.

VECTORCARDIOGRAM

(ELECTROPHYSIOLOGY)   *Synonym:*
VCG

─────────────────── **NORMAL VALUES** ───────────────────

Normal cardiac axis

Background Information

A vectorcardiogram is a graphic recording of electric forces of the heart. It is a noninvasive procedure that graphically records the direction and magnitude of the heart's electric forces by means of a continuous series of vector loops. Three planes of the heart are recorded (frontal, sagittal, and horizontal).

Purpose of the Test

A vectorcardiogram is used to assess ischemia, conduction defects, and chamber enlargement (hypertrophy or dilation).

Nursing Implementation

See section on electrocardiography for nursing care.

REFERENCES

Apple, S., & Thurkauf, G.E. (1992). Preparing for and understanding transesophageal echocardiography. *Critical Care Nurse, 12*, 29–34.

Beattie, S., & Meinhart, S.L. (1992). Transesophageal echocardiography: Advanced technology for the cardiac patient. *Critical Care Nurse, 12*, 42–44, 45–48.

Bentley, L.J. (1987). Radionuclide imaging techniques in the diagnosis and treatment of coronary heart disease. *Focus on Critical Care, 14*, 27–36.

Chen, J.T.T. (1992). Radiographic diagnosis of heart failure. *Heart Disease and Stroke, 1*, 58–63.

Chernecky, C.C., Krech, R.L., & Berger, B.J. (1993). *Laboratory tests and diagnostic procedures.* Philadelphia: W.B. Saunders.

Chyun, D. (1993). The cutting edge in cardiovascular medicine [Supplement]. *Critical Care Nurse, June*, 16–17.

Currie, P., & Chandrasekaran, K. (1990). TEE: Current application and future directions. *Cardiology, 7*, 57–69.

Dossey, B.M., Guzzetta, C.A., & Kenner, C.V. (1992). *Critical care nursing: body-mind-spirit.* New York: J.B. Lippincott.

Drew, B.J. (1991). Continuous bedside electrocardiographic monitoring: State of the art for the 1990s. *Heart Lung, 20*, 610–623.

Drew, B.J., & Sparacino, P.S.A. (1991). Accuracy of bedside electrocardiographic monitoring: A report on current practices of critical care nurses. *Heart Lung, 20*, 597–607.

Grauer, K. (1992). *A practical guide to ECG interpretation.* St. Louis: Mosby–Year Book.

Hebner, C.S., Moseley, M.J., & Shank, T.L. (1993). What is transesophageal echocardiography? *American Journal of Nursing, 93*, 74–80.

Henry, J.B. (1991). *Clinical diagnosis and management by laboratory methods.* Philadelphia: W.B. Saunders.

Holloway, N.M. (1993). *Nursing of the critically ill adult* (4th ed.). Redwood City, CA: Addison-Wesley.

Hudak, C.M., & Gall, B.M. (1994). *Critical care nursing: A holistic approach* (6th ed.). Philadelphia: J.B. Lippincott.

Jalal, S., Naccarelli, P., Shis, H., & Dougherty, A.H. (1994). Role of electrophysiologic testing after MI. *Journal of Myocardial Ischemia, 6*, 30–40.

Kotar, S.L., & Gessler, J.E. (1993). Full-disclosure monitoring: A concept that will change the way arrhythmias are detected and interpreted in the hospitalized patient. *Heart Lung, 22*, 482–489.

Lansdowne, L.M. (1990). Signal-averaged electrocardiograms. *Heart Lung, 19*, 329–335.

Marchiondo, K. (1994). Pharmacologic stress testing: An alternative to exercise. *Critical Care Nurse, 14*, 41–45.

Merva, J. (1993). SAECG: A closer look at the heart. *RN, 56*, 50–53.

Miracle, V.A., & Hovekamp, G. (1994). Needs of families of patients undergoing invasive cardiac monitoring. *American Journal of Critical Care, 3*, 155–157.

Mizuno, K. (1992). Angioscopic examination of the coronary arteries: What have we learned? *Heart Disease and Stroke, 1*, 320–324.

Prytowsky, E.N., & Noble, R.J. (1992). Electrophysiological studies: Who to refer. *Heart Disease and Stroke, 1*, 188–194.

Saxema, S., Anderson, D.W., Kaufman, R.L., et al. (1993). Quality assurance study of cardiac isoenzymes utilization in a large teaching hospital. *Archives of Pathology and Laboratory Medicine, 117*, 180–183.

Schell, M. (1990). Cholesterol, lipoproteins, lipid profiles: A challenge in patient education. *Focus on Critical Care, 17,* 203–211.

Thelan, L.A., Davie, J.K., Urden, L.D., & Lough, M.E. (1994). *Critical care nursing diagnosis and management.* St. Louis: Mosby–Year Book.

Tilkian, A.G., & Daily, E.K. (1986). *Cardiovascular procedures: diagnostic techniques and therapeutic procedures.* St. Louis: C.V. Mosby.

Wackers, F.J.T. (1994). Myocardial perfusion imaging to assess myocardial viability. *Journal of Myocardial Ischemia, 6,* 41–44.

Peripheral Vascular Function

This chapter discusses the diagnostic procedures that identify abnormalities in the anatomic structure and the lumina of arteries and veins. Additionally, most of the procedures evaluate the alterations in blood flow that result from the disease processes.

When the lumen of the artery is partially blocked, the descriptive term is *stenosis*. When the lumen of either the artery or the vein is completely blocked, the descriptive term is *occlusion*. In arterial peripheral vascular disease, the most common causes of stenosis and occlusion are atherosclerosis and thrombus, particularly affecting the aorta and the iliac and femoral arteries. In venous disease of the lower extremities, the most common cause of occlusion is thrombosis or thrombophlebitis, particularly affecting the deep femoral vein.

Many of the vascular diagnostic procedures are *invasive*, meaning that the blood vessel is penetrated by needle, catheter, or insertion of an instrument into the vascular lumen. Transluminal ultrasound and angioscopy involve the insertion of instruments directly into the artery or vein. Additionally, an iodine-based contrast agent is sometimes used to outline the lumen of the vessel and the abnormalities present. Arteriography, venography, and lymphangiography all use a contrast agent that is administered by needle or catheter insertion into the vascular lumen.

There are also *noninvasive* testing modalities that offer minimal risk to the patient and provide excellent viewing of the blood vessels in the extremities. Ultrasound, plethysmography, computed tomography (CT), and magnetic resonance imaging (MRI) are used to assess the quality of the vascular system, quantify the amount of blood that can circulate through a partially occluded vessel, or identify tumors or other pathologic conditions that externally compress the blood vessel and impede the circulation. Because they are safe and painless, these noninvasive procedures can be repeated in the ongoing or long-term evaluation of the patient, as needed.

In recent years, there have been many improvements, refinements, and modifications in the design of catheters and guides and in the composition of contrast agents. These changes have resulted in greater safety for the patient. Also, there have been major improvements in the quality of imaging because of the invention and use of x-ray image intensifiers, high-definition monitors, videotape or disc recorders, instant replay, and real-time subtraction techniques. These technologic developments have improved diagnostic accuracy because the images are much clearer.

In the past, vascular diagnostic procedures provided information regarding diagnosis. Today, some of these diagnostic procedures are used as adjuncts to vascular surgery to provide both diagnostic and evaluative data during surgical repair. The roles and uses of these diagnostic modalities are still emerging, and newer techniques continue to be developed and refined (Astleford, 1990; Cavaye et al., 1991; Fogarty, 1991).

The nurse can help the patient by preparing him or her for the procedure and what to expect during the test. The advanced technology of the vascular laboratory can be intimidating. The results of the tests are a significant source of data for developing the patient's plan of care. The location, extent, and severity of peripheral vascular disease will require nursing modifications in regard to the patient's mobility, exercise, attainment of rest or comfort, and independence.

DIAGNOSTIC PROCEDURES

ANGIOGRAPHY

(RADIOGRAPHY)

Synonyms:

arteriography, digital subtraction angiography

Angiography uses an iodinated contrast agent, fluoroscopy, and x-ray studies to obtain images of the opacified artery and its target organ or organs. In peripheral arterial vascular disorders, angiography is used to investigate the origin, extent, and severity of arterial vascular disease. In peripheral vascular disease or arterial occlusive disease, the most common causes of stenosis or occlusion are atherosclerosis and thrombus, affecting the aorta and the femoral or iliac artery. A complete discussion of angiography is presented in Chapter 11.

ANGIOSCOPY

(ENDOSCOPY)

Synonym:

vascular endoscopy

─────────────────── **NORMAL VALUES** ───────────────────

The lumen of the artery or bypass graft is free from obstruction. The suture line is intact, and the graft is patent.

Background Information

In severe arterial occlusive disease, the artery is narrowed by thrombus, embolus, or atherosclerotic plaque. Patients who have nonhealing ulcers, gangrene, chronic infection, severe claudication, or constant pain in the lower leg are at risk of losing the leg unless intervention is successful. In venous disease, the veins can be thrombosed or inflamed or can have incompetent valves.

Angioscopy is used to visualize the lumen and endothelial surfaces of the affected artery or vein directly so that the cause of the obstruction or impaired blood flow can be identified. The small diameter of this vascular endoscope allows it to be placed in the lumina of the aorta and the carotid, coronary, iliac, femoral, popliteal, and tibial arteries and also into the larger veins, including the vena cava and the carotid and common femoral veins. Angioscopy cannot, however, visualize the small runoff vessels, measure the degree of stenosis, or determine the composition of the atherosclerotic deposits (Eton and Ahn, 1991).

Angioscopes are small, flexible endoscopes of different diameters designed to fit into narrow arteries. The angioscope contains fiberoptics and a light source for visualization of the obstruction. A video camera is connected to the viewing eyepiece, and the images of the lumen are projected onto a video monitor. Within the angioscope, there is an irrigation-instrumentation channel. The irrigating saline is used to remove blood from the lens, and small instruments can incise, suture, or remove small sources of obstruction.

The angioscope is inserted through a small surgical opening in the artery or vein and is passed into the lumen in an antegrade or retrograde direction (Fig. 15–1). The topographic information provided by the angioscope is used to help in the diagnosis, intervention, and evaluation of the treatment.

Angioscopy is usually performed as an adjunctive procedure during vascular surgery. It provides direct visualization and monitors the vascular surgical

Critical Thinking: The patient had a popliteal artery bypass with angioscopy. In the early postoperative period, what cluster of assessment data would validate a nursing diagnosis of *altered tissue perfusion (peripheral)?*

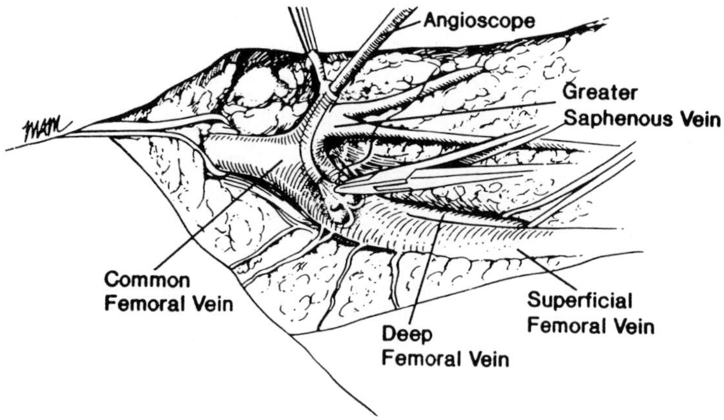

FIGURE 15–1. Angioscopy as an adjunct to surgical intervention. The angioscope has been placed in the common femoral vein to visualize the superficial femoral valve. (Reproduced with permission from Gloviczki, P., et al. [1991]. Femoral vein valve repair under direct vision without venotomy: A modified technique with the use of angioscopy. *Journal of Vascular Surgery*, 14, 645.)

interventions such as bypass grafting, endarterectomy, thrombectomy, embo- lectomy, angioplasty, or closed repair of a blood vessel (Fig. 15–2). On completion of a saphenous vein bypass graft, the angioscope is passed through the graft to inspect the lumen and distal anastomosis. After thrombectomy or atherectomy, the angioscope is used to inspect the lumen for residual fragments of plaque or clot. Residual particles are removed or the graft is revised, as necessary.

The use of angioscopy has now expanded to become a diagnostic procedure. Percutaneous angioscopy of pulmonary, peripheral, and coronary arteries is part of an experimental protocol in some medical centers. The percutaneous procedure is performed under local anesthesia, with a sedative analgesic used for relaxation. As the diagnostic techniques and procedures are further developed, angioscopy will likely become a routine part of vascular diagnosis and surgical procedures.

Intraoperative angioscopy is safe and reliable, with little reported damage to the arterial wall or vein graft. This procedure is safer than angiography because there is no risk of an allergic reaction or renal failure caused by iodinated contrast agents (Kim and Orron, 1992).

Purpose of the Test

Angioscopy provides three-dimensional visualization of the lumen and endo- thelial lining of an artery or saphenous vein bypass graft. This endoscopic pro- cedure is used to identify the cause of arterial obstruction and to evaluate the surgical vascular results during the intraoperative period. In the percutaneous approach, it can be used to diagnose the vascular cause of angina, graft failure, and chronic pulmonary embolus.

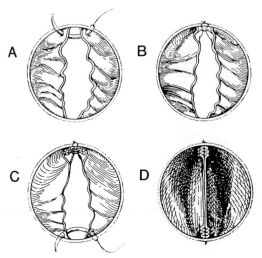

FIGURE 15–2. Angioscopic visualization of the surgical repair of an incompetent venous valve. *A,* Needle passage through the valve leaflets. *B,* Assessment of the valve after the placement of each suture. *C,* Sutures are usually required in both commissures to achieve complete valvular competence. *D,* Final angioscopic appearance of a competent valve after repair. (Reproduced with permission from Gloviczki, P., et al. [1991]. Femoral vein valve repair under direct vision without venotomy: A modified technique with use of angioscopy. *Journal of Vascular Surgery,* 14, 646.)

Procedure

The angioscope is inserted into a distal segment of an artery via an incision in the arterial wall. This may be performed through the skin (percutaneous approach) or through the open surgical incision. Once the area of concern is reached, the vascular lumen is inspected (Fogarty, 1991).

Findings

ABNORMAL RESULTS

Severe peripheral vascular disease
Residual valve leaflets in the venous bypass graft
Bypass graft torsion (twisting) or stenosis
Arterial thrombus or embolus
Platelet thrombus
Incompetent venous valve leaflets

Interfering Factors

• None

Nursing Implementation

Pretest

Provide preoperative instructions and obtain a written consent from the patient or person legally responsible for health care decisions.
Instruct the patient to ingest nothing by mouth for 8 hours before the test or surgery.

Collect baseline data and record the results in the patient's chart. These data include determinations of blood pressure, pulse, respirations, and appropriate peripheral pulses (those distal to the area of arterial surgery and angioscopy).

Administer the prescribed sedative analgesic for relaxation.

During the Test

Connect and test all equipment prior to the start of the procedure. The video camera is focused correctly.

Maintain and replace the supply of irrigation fluid, preventing air bubbles from entering the system or the patient's circulation.

Record the total volume of irrigation fluid used. Also include the irrigation total as part of the patient's fluid intake (Fogarty, 1991).

QUALITY CONTROL

The angioscope is cleaned, wrapped, and gas-sterilized after each use to prevent transmission of infection and the onset of sepsis.

Posttest

Observe the surgical or arteriotomy incision for signs of localized swelling, hematoma formation, or bleeding. When a percutaneous approach is used, the incision may be small, and it is often located in the groin.

Observe and assess the distal extremity for color, temperature, and the presence of pulses.

COLD STIMULATION TEST

(SKIN TEMPERATURE)

Synonym:

cold sensitivity test

NORMAL VALUES

The temperature in the fingers returns to normal within 15 minutes.

Background Information

In vasospastic disorders that affect the arterial circulation of the upper extremities, hypersensitivity to the cold is a common complaint. In normal circulation, exposure of the hands and fingers to cold causes temporary vasoconstriction and a lowering of the temperature in the fingers. Once the cold temperature source is eliminated, the circulation improves and the temperature of the fingers returns to normal within 15 minutes. Patients with upper extremity vasospastic disorders require a much longer time to recover normal skin temperature.

Purpose of the Test

The cold stimulation test assesses the symptom of upper extremity hypersensitivity to cold temperatures.

Procedure

The temperature of the fingers is recorded before and after the hands are immersed in ice water. The total time required for this test is 30 to 60 minutes.

Findings

ABNORMAL RESULTS
Raynaud syndrome
Rheumatoid arthritis
Scleroderma
Systemic lupus erythematosus

Interfering Factors

- Nicotine
- Caffeine
- Room temperature (excessively warm or cool)
- Gangrenous fingers
- Open wounds or infection in hands or fingers

Nursing Implementation

Pretest

Instruct the patient to refrain from smoking and ingesting caffeine (cola, cocoa, coffee, tea) for 24 hours before the test because they are vasoconstrictive substances.
Remove any jewelry from the patient's fingers and wrist.
Inform the patient that the ice water can cause some temporary discomfort in the fingers, but it will disappear after the fingers are warm.

During the Test

Apply the thermistors to the distal part of the fingers of both hands. The thermistors record the skin temperature.

Record the baseline thermistor temperature.

Immerse the hands in ice water for 20 seconds.

Record the temperature immediately after removal of the hands from the water.

Record the temperature every 5 minutes until the temperature returns to the pretest baseline value.

Posttest

Remove the thermistors.

COMPUTED TOMOGRAPHY, VASCULAR

(TOMOGRAPHY SCAN)

Synonyms:

CT scan, CAT scan, computed axial tomography

CT is a major diagnostic procedure in the assessment, diagnosis, and evaluation of vascular disease, particularly of the blood vessels of the torso. The procedure may use an intravenous iodinated contrast medium to sharpen the view of the lumina of the arteries and surrounding organs.

CT provides visualization of the arterial wall and identifies other abnormalities such as fluid or hematoma that exist in the perivascular tissue. The cross-sectional views provide definition of the normal vascular anatomy and any significant, measurable abnormality (Fig. 15–3).

Preoperatively, it is the diagnostic procedure of choice to assess an abdominal aortic aneurysm, including the size, location, and extent of involvement of other arteries or organs. It also is used to evaluate complications such as dissection and the presence of anomalies.

In arterial vascular disease, it is used to diagnose an aneurysm of the thoracic or abdominal aorta or the iliac, femoral, or popliteal artery. It can also detect

FIGURE 15–3. Diagram of a cross-section of a diseased arterial wall. Computer-generated analysis of the average thickness of the aneurysmal wall and periaortic fibrosis calculated from computed tomography (CT) scans of 12 patients with inflammatory abdominal aortic aneurysms. Note the increased thickness in the anterior wall. (Reproduced with permission from Fiorani, P., et al. [1991]. Extraperitoneal approach for the repair of inflammatory abdominal aortic aneurysm. *Journal of Vascular Surgery,* 13, 695.)

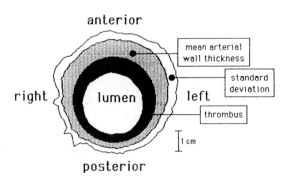

inflammation of the aneurysm and the postoperative complications of a vascular graft, including infection, abscess formation, hemorrhage, and fistula (Fahey and Riegal, 1989).

In venous abnormalities, CT will identify the inferior vena cava and the presence of a thrombus, anatomic abnormality, or complication related to the placement of a vena cava filter. The presence of a deep vein thrombus can also be identified in the iliac–vena cava segment (Kim and Orron, 1992).

A complete discussion of CT scanning is presented in Chapter 12.

DOPPLER ULTRASOUND

(ULTRASOUND)

Synonyms:

Doppler flow studies, Doppler testing

NORMAL VALUES

ARTERIAL OR VENOUS EXAMINATION
  Normal frequency and volume of audio signal
  Normal waveform pattern
  No evidence of vascular stenosis or obstruction
ANKLE BRACHIAL INDEX (ABI)
  0.9–1
SEGMENTAL PRESSURES
  >30 mm Hg difference in systolic pressure between
    the upper and lower segments of same extremity or
    the right and left extremity

Background Information

The Doppler ultrasound probe transmits low-intensity sound waves that are directed at a specific blood vessel. The transmitted sound waves strike moving red blood cells and bounce back to the transducer-receiver within the probe. The received impulses are translated into an audible signal or a waveform recording on graph paper. Additionally, the systolic pressure in upper and lower extremities can be measured.

AUDIBLE SIGNALS. These signals are heard as the blood cells circulate through the artery or vein and pass through the Doppler beam of sound waves. The instrument is sensitive and can detect even the most minimal blood flow. The *frequency* (pitch) of the sound is determined by the velocity of the blood flow. When erythrocytes circulate freely and rapidly in patent arteries or veins, the frequency is higher. Conversely, when blood flow is slowed because of stenosis, the pitch is lower.

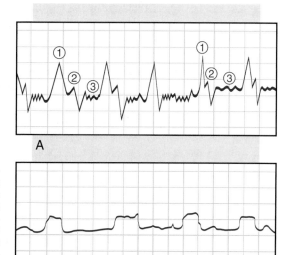

FIGURE 15–4. Normal versus abnormal Doppler arterial waveform patterns. *A,* Normal waveform with triphasic pattern of sharp upstroke and downstroke and good amplitude: *(1)* systolic component, *(2)* diastolic component, and *(3)* elastic wall rebound. *B,* Abnormal waveform with monophasic pattern of low amplitude and flat waves. This pattern indicates severe arterial obstruction.

The *loudness* of the sound is a measure of how many erythrocytes travel through the blood vessel and pass the Doppler beam. When the cells move rapidly and freely in a normal blood vessel, the sound is loud. Conversely, stenosis is indicated by softer, fainter sounds, and obstruction produces no sound at all.

Waveform recordings are Doppler signals that are transformed into a linear image. The waveforms are recorded on a graph paper strip in a manner similar to the recording of an electrocardiogram (ECG).

The normal venous waveform is spontaneous and in phase with respirations. When the extremity and vein are compressed manually, signal augmentation occurs as seen by the upward spike in the waveform pattern. In abnormal venous flow, as in partial or total venous occlusion, the augmentation signal is absent. Reflux flow is also evident on the waveform, such as that caused by incompetent venous valves.

The normal arterial waveform is characterized by three phases called the systolic, diastolic, and wall rebound phases (Fig. 15–4). When the artery is stenosed, the waveform pattern diminishes in height. In severe obstruction, the diastolic phase and wall rebound phase are absent.

The audio signal and waveform analysis are used to investigate peripheral vascular disease in the upper and lower extremities. In the diagnostic work-up for cerebrovascular disease, both components of the examination are used to assess the external carotid arteries in the neck.

ANKLE BRACHIAL INDEX AND SEGMENTED PRESSURES. These two measures assess systolic pressures within the arteries of the extremity. Both tests use blood pressure cuffs and the Doppler probe to obtain exact systolic readings at different levels of the extremities. They identify, locate, and quantify the drop of systolic blood pressure where it occurs. Stenosis or occlusion of the artery causes a drop in blood pressure distal to the site of the obstruction.

ANKLE BRACHIAL INDEX. The ABI compares the systolic pressure in the ankles with that of the arm. Normally, the systolic pressure in the ankle is almost equal to or equal to (90 to 100%) that of the arm. The ABI is a comparison of the ankle pressure to the arm pressure and is expressed by one of the following mathematical formulas:

$$\text{ABI} = \frac{\text{A (ankle pressure)}}{\text{B (brachial pressure)}} \qquad \text{ABI} = \text{A} \div \text{B}$$

An ABI value of less than 0.9 is abnormal. It means that somewhere between the heart and the ankle there is a low systolic pressure caused by stenosis or occlusion of an artery. The numeric value of the ABI is proportionate to the severity of the occlusion. An ABI of <0.5 indicates severe ischemia or gangrene.

SEGMENTED PRESSURES. These pressures are obtained when the ABI value is abnormal. The purpose is to locate the site of the diminished circulation in the extremity. Normal pressure differences should not exceed 30 mm Hg between the right and left limb or segmentally between the upper and lower segments of the extremity.

Critical Thinking: The patient is scheduled for bone surgery on his foot. How can you explain the Doppler ultrasound testing to this anxious patient?

QUALITY CONTROL

The accuracy of the examination and interpretation of results depend on the expertise of the examiner. Additionally, some of the findings are subjective interpretations rather than measurable data. Accuracy is increased when both technique and review of interpretations undergo periodic evaluation (Blackburn and Peterson, 1988).

Purpose of the Test

Doppler ultrasound detects stenosis or occlusion in an artery or vein, assists with the diagnosis of peripheral artery or cerebrovascular disease, evaluates the results of arterial reconstruction or vascular bypass surgery, and assesses for possible trauma to an artery.

Procedure

Venous and Arterial Doppler Tests: Acoustic gel and the Doppler probe are placed on the skin at the desired vascular sites. Audible signals are heard and interpreted. Three to five waveforms are recorded at each vascular site. The specific vascular sites and sides of the body (right or left) are identified to avoid confusion and error.

Venous sites of the lower extremities are the posterior tibial, greater saphenous, common femoral, superficial femoral, and popliteal veins. Venous sites of the upper extremities and neck are the brachial, axillary, subclavian, and jugular veins. Arterial pulse sites of the lower extremities are the common femoral, popliteal, dorsalis pedis, and posterior tibial pulses. Arterial pulses in the upper extremities and neck are the brachial, radial, ulnar, and carotid pulses.

Segmental Pressures: Blood pressure cuffs are applied bilaterally to the upper thighs, above and below the knees, and above the ankles. Gel is applied to the skin. The pressure cuffs are inflated one at a time. On deflation of each, the Doppler probe identifies the systolic pressure by audio signal, and the numeric value is recorded. The ABI is calculated from the ankle and brachial pressures.

Findings

ABNORMAL VALUES

Arterial stenosis or occlusion
Venous thrombosis
Venous valvular incompetency

Interfering Factors

- Nicotine, alcohol, and caffeine
- Anxiety
- Uncooperative behavior

Nursing Implementation

Pretest

Inform the patient about the test and obtain a written consent from the patient or the person legally designated to make health care decisions for the patient.

Instruct the patient to avoid nicotine, alcohol, caffeine, and other stimulants-depressants that will cause vasoconstriction.

Reduce the room lighting to promote relaxation.

Maintain a comfortable room temperature to prevent shivering and vaso-constriction.

Instruct the patient to remove all clothing and to wear a hospital gown.

For arterial tests, place the patient in the supine position. For venous tests of the lower extremities, position the patient in the supine position with two pillows under the legs to elevate them above the heart. The leg and hip are externally rotated and the knee is flexed.

During the Test

Venous Doppler Examination

Apply acoustic gel to the skin at the ankle, calf, thigh, and groin.

At each test point, use the probe and the audio mode to listen to the blowing sound that is in rhythm with the respirations.

Record three to five venous waveforms at each site, labeling each recording with the correct anatomic location.

Arterial Doppler Examination

Locate the pulse points on the upper or lower extremities and apply acoustic gel.

At each pulse point, apply the probe and the audio mode to listen to the blowing sounds.

Record three to five arterial waveforms at each site, labeling each recording with the correct anatomic location.

Ankle Brachial Index

Place blood pressure cuffs on each arm and above each ankle.

Apply acoustic gel at the sites of the brachial, dorsalis pedis, and posterior tibial pulses.

Inflate each cuff (one at a time). Use the probe to identify the initial systolic beat as the cuff is deflated slowly.

Record the systolic pressures on the chart.

Calculate the ABI, using the arm with the higher pressure reading.

If the ABI value is less than 0.9, continue the examination with the segmented pressure examination.

Segmented Pressure Examination

Place additional cuffs at the top of the thighs and above and below the knees.

At the femoral and popliteal pulse sites, obtain the pressure readings by repeating the technique described previously. Waveforms may also be recorded at these sites.

Record all results on the chart.

Posttest

Remove the blood pressure cuffs.
Remove the acoustic gel from the skin.

DUPLEX DOPPLER ULTRASOUND

Synonyms:

duplex scan, B-mode real-time imaging, duplex ultrasonography, vascular ultrasound

Duplex doppler ultrasound combines the techniques of Doppler ultrasound and radiographic imaging to detect and identify abnormalities of arteries and veins. B-mode imaging locates and provides images of the affected vessel, and the Doppler component identifies the disturbance of blood flow caused by atherosclerotic plaque or thrombus. The two methods are complementary; their combination provides information that is clearer than the data obtained from a single modality.

Duplex Doppler ultrasound has been widely used to assess cranial neck vessels and now is also used to assess the abdominal aorta and the peripheral vascular system. The technique can detect an embolus, stenosis, a thrombus, an aneurysm, and venous insufficiency.

It is now the diagnostic test of choice to verify the presence of a deep vein thrombus, particularly in the femoral or popliteal vein (White et al., 1989). It is as accurate as venography in the detection of venous thrombi. Additionally, it is advantageous because it is noninvasive, less painful, and uses no contrast medium.

Duplex Doppler ultrasound may also be used to assist with arteriography, angioplasty, placement of an inferior vena cava filter, thrombotic therapy, and the evaluation of bypass grafts and vascular access grafts.

A complete discussion of ultrasound is found in Chapter 8.

LYMPHANGIOGRAPHY

(RADIOGRAPHY)

Synonyms:

NORMAL VALUES

No evidence of obstruction, tumor, or enlarged nodes in the lymphatic system

---

Background Information

Critical Thinking: A Latino woman with endometrial cancer is scheduled for lymphangiography. Awaiting the test, she starts to cry and asks "Why am I so sick? I have not sinned and I am always faithful to my husband." How can you provide comfort and give consideration to her cultural belief?

The lymphatic system is an extensive network of capillaries, channels, and ducts that collect and transport lymphatic fluid. This system moves fluid from organs and tissues to the thoracic duct and then to the venous circulation. The lymph nodes are located at many sites within the system and serve as filters of the fluid. When there is obstruction of the lymphatic system, stasis and backflow of fluid will result. This causes lymphedema, which is the collection of lymphatic fluid in the interstitial spaces.

There are several possible causes for blockage in the lymphatic system, including congenital abnormality, irradiation or other causes of fibrosis, surgical excision of lymphatic tissue, filariasis, and advanced malignancy. In the case of malignancy, there is usually metastatic involvement of the lymph nodes, often located in the pelvis, groin, and abdomen.

Lymphangiography is used infrequently today because of the effectiveness of CT scans, MRI, and ultrasound in the imaging of enlarged lymph nodes and the staging of malignancy. Additionally, lymphangiography is painful and carries a greater risk of complications than do the noninvasive imaging alternatives.

Purpose of the Test

Lymphangiography is used to diagnose the cause of lymphedema of the lower or upper extremities. It may also be used to investigate metastatic disease, lymphoma, and other cancers, including the staging of the cancer and evaluation of cancer therapy.

Procedure

Under local anesthesia, methylene blue is injected subdurally in the webbing between the great toe and the second toe. The lymphatic system transports the dye upward along the dorsum of the foot, until a larger lymphatic vessel is identified.

A 1-in. incision is made over the dye-stained lymphatic vessel. After dissection, the vessel is cannulated with a fine needle that has tubing attached. Using a pump, iodized oil contrast material is instilled through the tubing and needle into the lymphatic vessel at a rate of 5 to 10 ml/hour. As the dye ascends through the lymphatic system, multiple x-ray films are taken to visualize the lymphatics and lymph glands of the lower extremities, groin, pelvis, and abdomen. The total time required for this test is 3 to 4 hours, with additional films taken after 24 hours.

Findings

ABNORMAL VALUES

Hodgkin lymphoma	Metastatic cancer
Retroperitoneal tumors	Trauma
Inflammation	Primary lymphedema
Filariasis	

Interfering Factors

- Allergy (iodine, shellfish, or contrast medium)
- Severe lung, heart, liver, or kidney disease

Nursing Implementation

Pretest

Identify any history of allergy to iodine or shellfish or any previous reaction to an x-ray study that used contrast material.

Provide instruction about the procedure and obtain informed consent from the patient or person who is legally responsible for making health care decisions for the patient.

Inform the patient of the following:

- The time required for the test and the need to return for additional films
- The need to arrange for transportation home when the test is performed on an outpatient basis
- The fact that the skin will have a blue streak and the stool will be blue for about 48 hours until the stain is cleared from the body
- The fact that there will be a 1-in. incision made on the back of the foot near the ankle

Take baseline vital signs.

During the Test

Instruct the patient to be still during the injections of the stain and the contrast medium and while x-ray films are taken.

Provide comfort and emotional support because the test is distressing and painful. Pain is to be expected in the foot, back of the leg, and groin as the contrast medium reaches each area.

Monitor vital signs and observe for cardiopulmonary complications.

Posttest

Monitor vital signs until they are stable.

To reduce swelling, apply an ice pack to the incision.

Maintain a sterile dressing on the incision site for 2 days. Inform the patient that the incision can feel sore, but it is to be kept clean and dry. The sutures are removed in 7 to 10 days.

Instruct the patient to rest in bed for 24 hours, with the foot elevated.

Complications

Lymphangiography can cause several complications. During the test, the patient can experience an allergic-type reaction to the contrast medium, including cardiopulmonary distress. After the test, lymphangitis, cellulitis, or wound infection can occur. Although the methylene blue stain should disappear, it sometimes remains for a long time. A summary of the complications of lymphangiography appears in Table 15–1.

MAGNETIC RESONANCE ANGIOGRAPHY

(TOMOGRAPHY)

Synonym:

MR angiography

TABLE 15-1
COMPLICATIONS OF LYMPHANGIOGRAPHY

Complication	Nursing Assessment
Lymphangiitis	Generalized edema
	Swelling of the extremity
	Fever and chills
	Enlarged nodes
Cellulitis and ascending infection	Redness
	Swelling
	Pain
	Tenderness
	Fever
Infection of suture line	Incisional redness, swelling
	Tenderness
	Purulence or serous drainage
	Fever
Allergic-type reaction	Urticaria or itching
	Erythema
	Tachycardia
	Respiratory distress or stridor
	Cyanosis
	Hypotension
	Chest pain
	Cardiac arrest

Magnetic resonance angiography is a noninvasive procedure used to study blood flow and the structure and location of the major blood vessels. The blood acts as a physiologic contrast medium, so no pharmacologic contrast medium is needed. The procedure can identify vascular stenosis, occlusion, thrombus, collateral vessels, tumor, aneurysm, and other abnormalities affecting an artery or vein. Additionally, the direction and rate of flow can be quantified (Kim and Orron, 1992).

In vascular diagnostic procedures, magnetic resonance angiography is used to identify aortic aneurysm, dissection, complications of vascular grafts, arteriovenous malformation, bleeding, and portal hypertension (Fahey and Riegal, 1989). In the study of the lower extremities, it provides a clear image of the circulation of the aorta, the iliac arteries and veins, and the femoral and popliteal veins. A complete discussion of MRI is presented in Chapter 12.

PLETHYSMOGRAPHY, ARTERIAL

(MANOMETRY)

Synonyms:

pulse cuff recording, PCR, pneumoplethysmography

—————————————————— **NORMAL VALUES** ——————————————————

> No evidence of arterial peripheral vascular disease; normal arterial waveform pattern

Background Information

Using blood pressure cuffs, plethysmography measures changes in the blood volume of the extremities. Normally, arterial flow is about equal to venous flow within an organ or extremity. If the venous blood flow of an extremity is interrupted by using low pressure in the air cuffs, there will be a subsequent increase in the arterial blood volume in the extremity. This change in arterial volume can be detected by the plethysmograph. The machine records the linear waveform pattern on a strip of graph paper, much like the recording of an ECG.

In normal arterial circulation, the waveform has a pulsatile pattern with a characteristic rise, sharp peak, dicrotic notch, and down slope in each pulsation (Fig. 15–5). When the artery is stenosed or obstructed, a smaller volume of blood can pass through the arterial lumen. The abnormal waveform pattern is of low amplitude and reduced slope, with the loss of the dicrotic notch.

Purpose of the Test

Plethysmography is a noninvasive test that evaluates the arterial blood flow in the extremities. It detects the presence of peripheral arterial vascular disease.

Procedure

Plethysmograph cuffs are inflated at different levels on the extremities, and arterial waveforms are recorded. The total test takes about 30 minutes to complete.

Findings

ABNORMAL VALUES
Peripheral vascular disease
Arterial occlusive disease
Arterial embolus
Arterial trauma

Interfering Factors

- Smoking
- Caffeine
- Alcohol

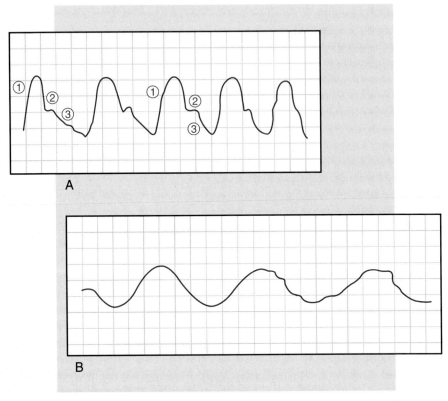

FIGURE 15–5. Normal versus abnormal arterial plethysmography waveforms. *A*, The normal waveforms have characteristic *(1)* sharp rise to peak, *(2)* dicrotic notch, and *(3)* downslope to baseline. *B*, Abnormal waveforms show a loss of the dicrotic notch, lower height, and rounding out of the peaks.

- Cold room temperature
- Anxiety

Nursing Implementation

Pretest

Explain the procedure to the patient and obtain written consent from the patient or person responsible for the patient's health care decisions.

Instruct the patient to refrain from smoking and alcohol and caffeine ingestion before the test because stimulants, depressants, and vasoconstrictive substances will alter the results.

Assist the patient in removing all clothing and putting on a hospital gown. Restrictive clothing can alter the circulatory flow to the extremities.

Place the patient in a supine position, with a pillow under the head.

Maintain a comfortable room temperature and dim the room lighting. Cool temperatures, anxiety, and muscle tension will alter the results.

Instruct the patient to refrain from talking and movement during the test.

During the Test

The pressure cuffs are applied to both legs at the level of the upper thighs, above and below the knees, and above the ankles.

At the first cuff site, inflate the cuff to 75 mm Hg for 2 to 3 seconds and then lower the pressure to 65 mm Hg. Record four to five waveforms. Label the recording with the correct identification of the cuff level and right or left side. Repeat this procedure at each cuff site.

Posttest

Deflate and remove the cuffs.

PLETHYSMOGRAPHY, VENOUS

(MANOMETRY)

Synonyms:

impedance plethysmography, venous cuff examination, maximal venous out-flow test, occlusive phlebography

━━━━━━━━━━━━━━━━━ **NORMAL VALUES** ━━━━━━━━━━━━━━━━━

Normal waveform patterns with adequate venous capacity and maximum venous outflow; no evidence of deep vein thrombosis

Background Information

Using blood pressure cuffs and electrodes, venous plethysmography measures the change in blood volume in the extremities. The electrodes and the recorder produce a linear waveform pattern that is recorded on a paper graphic strip, much like the recording of an ECG.

In normal venous circulation, the blood moves toward the heart from the distal extremities. If a vein is compressed temporarily by a blood pressure cuff, the venous flow is interrupted. Distal to that compression point, the veins become engorged. On deflation of the cuff and release of the compression, the vein quickly empties of its excess blood and resumes normal venous outflow.

When a deep vein is obstructed by a thrombus, there is also back-up of the venous blood and engorgement of the distal vessel. Once the vein is compressed temporarily by the blood pressure cuff, there is also further interruption of the blood flow. Increased engorgement of the distal vein cannot occur because the vein has already filled to capacity. On deflation of the cuff and release of the compression, there is resumption of only minimal venous blood flow because the thrombus continues to obstruct the lumen.

As the compression is applied to a normal vein, the venous plethysmography

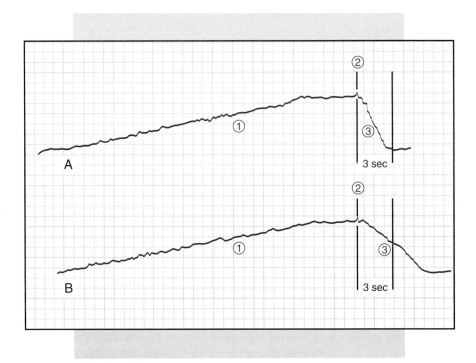

FIGURE 15–6. Normal versus abnormal venous plethysmographic waveforms. *A,* The normal waveform *(1)* demonstrates complete venous capacitance, *(2)* release of the thigh cuff, and *(3)* rapid venous outflow that completes in 3 seconds. *B,* The abnormal waveform demonstrates *(1)* venous capacitance, *(2)* the release of the thigh cuff, and *(3)* slow venous outflow. It takes longer than the normal 3 seconds for the waveform to return to the baseline level.

waveform pattern shows a gradual rise in height from the baseline. This phase is called venous capacitance and represents the filling of the distal vein to its fullest capacity. On release of the compression, the waveform drops rapidly and returns to baseline (Fig. 15–6). In an obstructed vein, the release of the pressure cuff relieves the venous compression, but there is limited venous outflow and slow emptying of the engorged vein. Correspondingly, the waveform demonstrates a limited, slow return to baseline.

Purpose of the Test

Venous plethysmography is used to detect deep vein thrombosis and to screen patients who are at high risk for the development of venous thrombosis.

Procedure

Plethysmograph cuffs and electrodes are applied to the thigh and calf to control and monitor venous blood flow. The cuffs are inflated, and the recorded waveforms demonstrate the filling of the vein to maximal capacity. On rapid release of the cuffs, the waveform demonstrates the venous outflow of the distal vein. The total time required to complete the test is 30 to 45 minutes.

Findings

ABNORMAL VALUES
Venous thrombosis
Thrombophlebitis
Venous obstruction (partial or complete)

Interfering Factors

- Nicotine, alcohol, and caffeine
- Anxiety and muscle tension
- Uncooperative behavior
- Compression of pelvic veins (tumor, tight bandages)
- Low cardiac output
- Shock
- Arterial occlusive disease

Nursing Implementation

Pretest

Inform the patient about the procedure and obtain written consent from the patient or person legally designated to make the patient's health care decisions.

Instruct the patient to refrain from smoking or injesting alcohol or caffeine before the test because stimulants and relaxants will alter the test results.

Help the patient to remove all clothing and to put on a hospital gown. Any compression from restrictive clothing alters the venous circulation from the extremities. Maintain a comfortable room temperature and dim the lights because anxiety or muscle tension alters the results.

Place the patient in the supine position, with the legs elevated above the heart and supported by pillows. The affected leg and hip are externally rotated, and the knee is flexed.

Instruct the patient to refrain from movement or talking during the test.

During the Test

Place blood pressure cuffs on the thigh and calf of the affected leg.

Apply the conductive gel and electrodes to the skin.

Inflate the cuff on the calf to 15 mm Hg of pressure. This cuff and electrode monitor the inflow of the venous system.

Inflate the cuff on the thigh to 55 mm Hg of pressure. This pressure level obstructs the venous outflow but allows the arterial flow to fill and engorge the distal vein segment.

Start the recorder to trace the waveform. Once the tracing has risen to its maximum and forms a plateau, the venous filling is completed.

Quickly release the pressure on the thigh cuff to open the venous outflow of the vein. The waveform pattern will continue and provide the linear recording of the return to the baseline reading.

Repeat the procedure until three to five waveforms are recorded. Label the paper, correctly identifying the extremity.

Repeat the entire procedure on the opposite extremity to provide comparison data.

Posttest

Remove the deflated cuffs and electrodes.
Wipe the conductive gel off the skin.

TRANSLUMINAL ULTRASOUND

(ULTRASOUND)

Synonyms:

TUS, endovascular ultrasonography, EUS, intravascular ultrasonography, IVUS

Transluminal ultrasound is a new, emerging procedure that uses catheter ultrasonography within the lumen of an artery. The technique provides high-quality images of the lumen and any atherosclerotic or arteriosclerotic deposits in the lumen or under the tissue surface layer. It provides visualization of the intima, media, and adventitia, the three tissue layers of the artery. It identifies the presence of lipid deposits, fibrous growth, surface irregularity, and stenosis of the lumen, and calcium deposits in the medial layer.

This specialized arterial catheter has one or more ultrasound transducers in its tip. This method of ultrasonography performs 360-degree scanning and cross-sectional imaging of the artery. As the ultrasound signals strike the tissue surfaces, they bounce back to the transducer for conversion to visual imagery. The images appear on the video monitor and are recorded on tape or film.

To perform the procedure, the flexible catheter is inserted percutaneously and advanced into the arterial lumen. A guidewire and fluoroscopic visualization are used to control the direction and depth of insertion. At present, the catheter is used to examine the arteries of the lower extremities through a small incision in the groin.

Transluminal ultrasound produces a much higher quality image than does noninvasive Doppler ultrasound. This is because the transluminal ultrasound operates at much higher frequencies, and the sound waves do not have to pass through skin, fat, muscle, and other tissues to produce the image.

Currently, this test is used as an adjunctive procedure to evaluate the lumina of stenosed arteries before and after percutaneous catheter therapy, such as atherectomy or balloon or laser angioplasty (Kim and Orron, 1992). In the future, as the technology and technique are developed, its use will expand to work in other vascular structures. It will be used more frequently in the removal of atheroma or the dilation of stenosed areas to prevent tissue damage to the medial and adventitial layers of the affected artery (Eton and Ahn, 1991).

A complete discussion of ultrasound is presented in Chapter 8.

VENOGRAPHY

(RADIOGRAPHY)

Synonyms:

phlebography, contrast venography

--- **NORMAL VALUES** ---

No evidence of intraluminal filling defects, obstruction, incompetent venous valves, calcifications, or dilations of collateral veins

Background Information

Venography is an invasive technique that provides radiographic visualization of the venous system, particularly in the lower extremities. In this location, the venous system consists of the superficial veins, the deep veins, and the perforating veins. The lower leg veins provide a passive conduit for the return of the blood to the heart and also serve as a reservoir for the large volume of circulating blood.

The valves within the veins are the most important functional feature. Each valve has a pair of fibrous leaflets that control the direction of the blood flow upward toward the heart and from the superficial to the deep veins. When valves are competent, there is no reflux or backflow. Incompetent valves cause a reflux of blood into the superficial vein system and the ultimate formation of varicosities. Incompetence of the perforating veins usually is caused by deep vein thrombosis or other source of obstruction.

Deep vein thrombosis and thromboembolism are caused by three general pathologic conditions, including damage to the blood vessel, venous stasis, and alterations in the ability of the blood to coagulate (Deutsche and Green, 1990). Thrombosis is the most common venous pathologic condition. As the thrombus enlarges, it occludes the lumen of the vein and ultimately destroys the venous valve or valves. In the early stage of formation, the thrombus is soft and friable. When located in the leg, a piece of the thrombus can break off, travel, and lodge in the lung as a pulmonary embolus. A thrombus that is 24 to 48 hours old becomes firm and adheres to the vein wall. Eventually, the thrombus will partially or completely resolve by fibrinolysis.

Examination of the veins by venography is carried out by several methods. *Ascending venography* is used to identify the presence and location of deep vein thrombosis and to assess the patency of the deep venous system. *Descending venography* is used to assess valve competency (Vogelzang, 1988). *Venography of the upper extremities* evaluates occlusion, lesions, or thrombosis in the subclavian or axillary veins. *Venacavography* evaluates the inferior vena cava for obstruction, malformation, traumatic injury, and placement of the inferior vena cava filter.

Today, noninvasive technologies such as ultrasound, plethysmography, and compression sonography are used to identify deep vein thrombosis of the lower extremities. CT and MRI are the preferred methods to image the vena cava. When these procedures are inconclusive, however, the venogram is used to clarify the data.

Purpose of the Test

Venography is used to investigate venous function, suspected obstruction, venous insufficiency, postphlebotic syndrome, and the source of pulmonary embolism. It also evaluates veins before and after bypass surgery, reconstructive surgery, or thrombolytic therapy to determine the effectiveness of treatment.

Procedure

Contrast medium is injected into the vein via a butterfly needle or an intravenous catheter. Using a tilt table, fluoroscopy, and x-ray studies, the contrast medium illustrates the flow patterns of the venous circulation and identifies the site of occlusion in the vein.

In venography of the lower extremities, either ascending or descending venography may be used. Ascending venography uses a butterfly needle placed in a small vein on the dorsum of the foot (Fig. 15–7). In descending venography, a catheter is placed in the common femoral vein via a percutaneous femoral approach.

Findings

ABNORMAL VALUES
Deep vein thrombosis
Tumor (extrinsic compression)
Vascular tumor (intrinsic blockage)
Venous compression syndrome
Venous insufficiency
Varicose veins
Congenital malformation
Traumatic injury to the vein

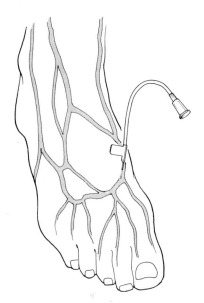

FIGURE 15–7. Technique of ascending venography. Diagrammatic representation of the ideal needle position to instill the contrast medium. (Reproduced with permission from Kim, D., & Orron, D.E. [1992]. *Peripheral vascular imaging and intervention.* St. Louis: Mosby–Year Book.)

Interfering Factors

- Allergy to iodine or contrast medium
- Renal failure
- Congestive heart failure
- Severe pulmonary hypertension

Nursing Implementation

Pretest

Identify any allergy to iodine or shellfish or an allergic reaction to a previous x-ray study that used contrast medium.

Instruct the patient regarding the procedure and pretest preparation. Obtain written consent from the patient or person legally designated to make health care decisions for the patient.

Ensure that the pretest blood urea nitrogen and creatinine determinations are performed and the results are posted in the patient's chart. This is carried out to ensure that renal function is adequate, since the kidneys must clear the contrast material from the body.

Solid foods are omitted for 4 hours before the test, but water is permitted.

Record baseline vital signs.

During the Test

Provide emotional support during the period of discomfort. The injection of contrast material is painful.

TABLE 15–2 COMPLICATIONS OF VENOGRAPHY	
Complication	**Nursing Assessment**
Cellulitis	Redness
	Swelling
	Pain or tenderness
Thrombophlebitis	Pain
	Redness
	Swelling
Allergic-type reaction	Urticaria or itching
	Erythema
	Respiratory distress or stridor
	Cyanosis
	Hypotension
	Tachycardia
	Chest pain
	Cardiac arrest

On completion of the test, an intravenous solution of 200 to 300 ml of heparinized saline is administered. This flushes the contrast medium from the veins.

Posttest

Obtain vital signs and record the results.
Assess the puncture site for signs of swelling, pain, redness, or hematoma.
Keep the patient on bed rest for 2 hours.
Resume the previous dietary status. Instruct the patient to drink extra fluids for 24 hours to help flush the remaining contrast medium from the veins and kidneys. Frequent urination is expected until the diuresis is complete.

Complications

Critical Thinking: After a venography, what does the professional nurse instruct the aide to report about the patient?

If more than 5 to 10 ml of contrast material infiltrates into the tissue, a chemical cellulitis will result. The contrast medium also can cause postvenographic thrombosis or phlebitis. The onset of these posttest complications can begin in 2 to 12 hours, peak in 12 to 24 hours, and gradually subside in a few days. During the test, an allergic-type reaction to the contrast medium can occur. A summary of the complications of venography is presented in Table 15–2.

REFERENCES

Appleton, D.L., & LaQuaglia, J.D. (1988). Vascular disease and postoperative management. *Critical Care Nurse, 5*, 34–42.

Astleford, P.M. (1990). The latest advances in vascular technology. *Journal for the Society of Peripheral Vascular Nursing, 8,* 9–13.

Blackburn, D.R., & Peterson, L.K. (1988). Noninvasive vascular testing. In V.A. Fahey (Ed.). *Vascular nursing.* Philadelphia: W.B. Saunders.

Blank, C.A., & Irwin, G.H. (1990). Peripheral vascular disorders: Assessment and intervention. *Nursing Clinics of North America, 25,* 777–794.

Bright, L.D., & Georgi, S. (1992). Peripheral vascular disease: Is it arterial or venous? *American Journal of Nursing, 92,* 34–43, 45–47.

Cavaye, D.M., et al. (1991). Intravascular ultrasound imaging of an acute dissecting aortic aneurysm: A case report. *Journal of Vascular Surgery, 13,* 510–512.

Deutsch, J., & Green, D. (1990). Deep vein thrombosis in the critically ill patient. *Critical Care Nursing Quarterly, 13,* 29–37.

Editorial. (1987). Radiographic contrast agents—a perspective. *New England Journal of Medicine, 317,* 891–893.

Eton, D., & Ahn, S.S. (1991). Trends in endovascular surgery. *Critical Care Nursing Clinics of North America, 3,* 535–549.

Fahey, V.A. (Ed.). (1994). *Vascular nursing* (2nd ed.). Philadelphia: W.B. Saunders.

Fahey, V.A., & Riegal, B.J. (1989). Advances in diagnostic testing for vascular disease. *Cardiovascular Nursing, 25,* 13–18.

Fiorani, P., et al. (1991). Extraperitoneal approach for the repair of inflammatory abdominal aortic aneurysm. *Journal of Vascular Surgery, 13,* 692–697.

Fogarty, A.M. (1991). Angioscopy: New developments in vascular surgery. *AORN Journal, 53,* 725–728.

Frost, F.S. (1991). High resolution real-time ultrasound for the diagnosis of venous thrombosis in the rehabilitation setting. *American Journal of Physical Medicine and Rehabilitation, 70,* 3–4.

Gloviczki, P., et al. (1991). Femoral vein valve repair under direct vision without venotomy: A modified technique with use of angioscopy. *Journal of Vascular Surgery, 14,* 645–649.

Griffith, H.W. (1989). *Instructions for patients: Medical tests and diagnostic procedures.* Philadelphia: Lea & Febiger.

Huether, S.E., & Jacobs, M.K. (1986). Determination of normal variation in skin blood flow velocity in healthy adults. *Nursing Research, 35,* 162–165.

Hyers, T.M. (1989). Deep vein thrombosis: Selecting the best diagnostic method. *Journal of Critical Illness, 4,* 37–48.

Kim, D., & Orron, D.E. (1992). *Peripheral vascular imaging and intervention.* St. Louis: Mosby–Year Book.

Looking at deep vein thrombosis. (1990). *Emergency Medicine, 22,* 43–44.

Massey, J.A. (1986). Diagnostic testing for peripheral vascular disease. *Nursing Clinics of North America, 21,* 207–218.

Mills, P. (1991). High tech, human touch: Care study...arteriography. *Nursing Times, 87,* 36–38, 40.

Peterson, L.K. (1985). Perioperative vascular monitoring. *Critical Care Quarterly, 8,* 1–9.

Prevost, D.B. (1990). Diagnostic arteriography and percutaneous transluminal angioplasty of the lower extremities. *Journal of Vascular Nursing, 8,* 6–12.

Rice, V.H., et al. (1988). Development and testing of arteriography information intervention for stress reduction. *Heart Lung 17,* 23–27.

Vogelzang, R.L. (1988). Vascular imaging techniques and percutaneous vascular intervention. In V.A. Fahey (Ed.). *Vascular nursing.* Philadelphia: W.B. Saunders.

White, R.H., et al. (1989). Diagnosis of deep vein thrombosis using duplex ultrasound. *Annals of Internal Medicine, 111,* 297–304.

CHAPTER 16

Hematologic Function

In hematologic testing, the laboratory tests provide information regarding the number, concentration, structure, and characteristics of the cells in the blood. The diagnostic procedures of bone marrow aspiration, biopsy, and nuclear scanning provide information about the marrow tissue that forms the blood cells.

There are many blood cell alterations that have their origin in abnormal bone marrow function. The marrow can be altered by malignancy, inadequate nutrition, infection, genetics, radiation, chemical toxins, or an adverse reaction to medication. The abnormal changes can include excess production of cells, diminished or lack of production of cells, errors in the maturation of cells, and the production of defective cells.

Some diseases, such as leukemia, directly affect the bone marrow and its ability to produce blood cells. Other diseases, such as renal failure, cause changes in hematopoietic function, even though the bone marrow cells are healthy. Additionally, there are diseases or conditions of the body that directly alter the blood cells. Examples include some parasitic infections and antigen-antibody reactions.

The cells of the blood consist of erythrocytes, leukocytes, and platelets (Table 16–1). The plasma also contains clotting factors, antibodies, and other plasma proteins, including albumin. In hematologic testing, the number and concentration of each type of cell provides important estimates about bone marrow function. The marrow responds to the signals of the microenvironment and to the presence of colony-stimulating factors for the regulation of its activity in formation, differentiation, and maturation of blood cells (Haeuber and DiJulio, 1989).

TABLE 16-1
FORMED ELEMENTS OF THE BLOOD

Erythrocytes	Agranular leukocytes
Reticulocytes	Lymphocytes
Leukocytes	Plasma cells
Granular leukocytes	T cells
Neutrophils	Monocytes
Eosinophils	Thrombocytes
Basophils	Platelets

The study of the structure and characteristics of the blood cells provides important data for accuracy in diagnosis of hematologic disorders. In the investigation of anemia, studies of blood cells and bone marrow help differentiate among the types of anemia, identify abnormal erythrocytes and cell membrane characteristics, and identify the source of the problem. Broadly defined, anemias are caused by acute or chronic blood loss, by abnormal formation of erythrocytes or their hemoglobin content, or by hemolysis or the early destruction of the erythrocytes.

Diseases of the phagocytic and immune systems are defined through the study of leukocytes. There may be excessive or diminished numbers of one or more types of leukocyte. There also may be immature or abnormal forms of these cells in the blood.

LABORATORY TESTS

The specific causes of problems of hemostasis and coagulation are identified by the estimate of the platelet count and the measurement of clotting factors and clotting times.

The quantitative measurement of the blood cells is presented in Chapter 4. The laboratory tests for clotting are presented in Chapter 6.

ANTIGLOBULIN TESTS

(BLOOD)

Synonyms:

antiglobulin test, direct; AGT; direct Coombs test; direct antiglobulin test; DAT

antiglobulin test, indirect; indirect Coombs test; indirect antiglobulin test; IAT

─────────── **NORMAL VALUES** ───────────

Negative

Background Information

The antiglobulin tests consist of direct and indirect tests. They are used to detect the presence of antibodies in the serum and antigens on erythrocytes (Fig. 16–1). When there is an antigen-antibody reaction in the blood, the erythrocytes become coated with antibody globins and the erythrocytes agglutinate. In severe conditions, there is phagocytosis of the cell membranes and lysis of the coated erythrocytes. The lysis of many erythrocytes results in hemolytic anemia.

DIRECT ANTIGLOBULIN TEST. The direct antiglobulin test, or direct Coombs test, looks for antibodies attached to red blood cells. In this antigen-antibody reaction, the immunoproteins, IgG, and complement cling to the erythrocytes and coat the red cells with globin. The coated cells are "sensitized" and then clump together in the process called agglutination. The severity of the reaction depends on the number of antibodies produced and the number of erythrocytes affected.

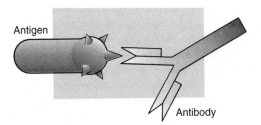

Antigen

Antibody

FIGURE 16–1. Antigen and antibody. A specific antibody matches the antigen based on the characteristic shape that protrudes from the antigen surface. Once the antibody locks onto the antigen, the antigen is destroyed by phagocytosis, an enzyme toxin from complement, or other biochemical response of the immune system.

In transfusion of incompatible blood, the recipient's anti-Rh_0 IgG antibodies detect the foreign antigens on the cells of the donor blood. The antibodies move to attack and destroy the foreign cells in a massive antigen-antibody response. During the pregnancy of an Rh_0-negative mother who carries an Rh_0-positive baby, the maternal Rh_0 antibodies and complement pass through the placenta and into the infant's circulation. Since the blood types of the mother and fetus are incompatible, the maternal antibodies attack the erythrocytes of the fetus. As the erythrocytes of the fetus become coated, agglutinate, and undergo hemolysis, erythroblastosis fetalis or hemolytic anemia of the newborn develops.

Some medications also cause elevation of the direct antiglobulin test. Methyldopa (Aldomet) and levodopa (Dopar) are the medications most often involved, but others are penicillin, cephalosporin, tetracycline, sulfonamides, quinidine, and insulin. Protein in the medication is the antigenic substance, and IgG or complement causes the erythrocytes to become coated. In most of these cases, the direct antiglobulin test result is elevated, but in a few cases, hemolytic anemia results (Jacobs, 1990).

The direct antiglobulin test examines the patient's erythrocytes for antibodies. The red blood cells of the specimen are immersed in laboratory antiglobulin serum. After the erythrocytes are washed to remove other serum proteins, the antibodies remain attached to the antigens on the cellular surfaces of erythrocytes.

INDIRECT ANTIGLOBULIN TEST. The indirect antiglobulin test, or indirect Coombs test, looks for the presence of antibodies in the patient's serum. In the laboratory analysis, the patient's serum is mixed with known reagents of red cells, and the result is observed for an antigen-antibody reaction. If there are circulating antibodies present in the patient's serum, they adhere to and coat the reagent red cells. Agglutination of the erythrocytes occurs when the level of antibodies is high.

In the first trimester of pregnancy, this test is used to screen Rh_0-positive and Rh_0-negative expectant mothers. When the test results are negative, the test is repeated in the 28th week of pregnancy and at delivery. Whenever the test becomes positive for the presence of antibodies, it is followed up with antibody identification, a titer reading, and possible amniocentesis. The development of maternal antibodies occurs in the Rh-negative mother who carries an Rh-positive fetus. The antibodies cross the placental barrier, enter the fetal circulation, and result in the coating and agglutination of fetal erythrocytes.

Purpose of the Test

The *direct antiglobulin test* detects antibodies on the erythrocytes. It is part of the posttransfusion work-up to detect red cell incompatibility between the donor and recipient blood. It is also used to help diagnose erythroblastosis fetalis, or hemolytic disease of the newborn, and helps confirm the diagnosis of hemolytic anemia.

The *indirect antiglobulin test* detects unknown antibodies in the serum. It is used as an antibody screen in type and crossmatch testing in preparation for blood transfusion. It detects maternal-fetal blood incompatibility and predicts the hematologic risk to the fetus. It is used to evaluate the need for Rh$_o$ (D) immune globulin administration and helps confirm the diagnosis of hemolytic anemia.

Procedure

Direct Antiglobulin: One red-topped and one lavender-topped tube are used to collect 7 ml of venous blood in each tube. In the newborn, venous cord blood may be collected.

Indirect Antiglobulin: A red-topped tube is used to collect 7 ml of venous blood.

QUALITY CONTROL

The tourniquet must not be applied tightly or for a prolonged time. Venipuncture technique must be smooth, with a blood flow that fills the tube readily. If the blood flow has excessive turbulence because of flawed venipuncture technique, hemolysis of the erythrocytes will alter the test results.

Findings

POSITIVE VALUES

DIRECT ANTIGLOBULIN TEST

Autoimmune hemolytic anemia
Hemolytic transfusion reaction
Hemolytic disease of the newborn
Lymphoma
Systemic lupus erythematosus
Mycoplasmal infection
Infectious mononucleosis
Sensitivity to particular medications

INDIRECT ANTIGLOBULIN TEST

Maternal-fetal blood incompatibility
Autoimmune hemolytic anemia
Sensitivity to particular medications

Interfering Factors

- Hemolysis
- Inadequate identification of the specimen

Nursing Implementation

Pretest

Include the following information on the requisition form:

- Recent history of blood transfusion or plasma expanders
- A list of the medications taken

Posttest

Ensure that the specimen and requisition slip include the patient's name, identification number, and the source of the blood (venous, cord). Arrange for prompt transport of the specimen to the laboratory

QUALITY CONTROL

The serum must be separated from the cells without delay.

COMPLEMENT, TOTAL

(SERUM)

Synonyms:

CH_{50}, total hemolytic complement, complement assay

--- **NORMAL VALUES** ---

75–160 U/ml *or* SI 75–160 kU/L

Background Information

Complement is a system of 25 plasma proteins and cell membrane–associated proteins that circulate as inactive precursors in the blood. When activated, they serve to mediate the defense system and protect against infection. In supporting the work of antibodies, the complement cells facilitate phagocytosis, eliminate antigen-antibody complexes, and puncture the cell membranes of bacteria. In an active form, complement induces an inflammatory response.

When complement is activated, it follows the "classical pathway" (Fig. 16–2) or an "alternative pathway." The activation of the classical pathway usually occurs when an antibody locks onto an antigen. In the alternative pathway, the process usually starts when complement C3 interacts with other factors. Ultimately, both pathways finalize with the formation of a membrane attack complex. This complex penetrates the wall of the molecule and causes lysis of the cell.

Complement proteins are increased in an acute response to inflammation or infection and are decreased or absent in hypercatabolism (autoimmune disease), hereditary deficiency, and overexpenditure of the complexes.

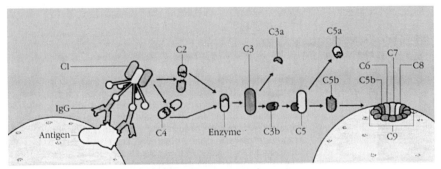

FIGURE 16-2. The complement cascade. The classic complement pathway becomes activated when the first complement molecule, C1, recognizes an antigen-antibody complex. Each of the remaining complement proteins, in turn, performs its specialized job, cleaving or binding the complement molecule next in line. The end product is the cylindrical membrane attack complex. (Reproduced with permission from Schlindler, L.W. [1988]. *Understanding the immune system.* [NIH publication No. 88-529, p. 10]. Washington, D.C.: U.S. Department of Health, Public Health Service, National Institutes of Health.)

Purpose of the Test

Total complement is used to evaluate or monitor systemic lupus erythematosus and its response to therapy. The test is also used to diagnose complement deficiency and to detect disease caused by the immune complex.

Procedure

A red-topped tube is used to collect 7 ml of venous blood.

Findings

ELEVATED VALUES

Chronic infection
Acute rheumatic fever
Diabetes mellitus
Obstructive jaundice

Rheumatoid arthritis
Ulcerative colitis
Thyroiditis

DECREASED VALUES

Systemic lupus erythematosus
Acute poststreptococcal glomerulo-
   nephritis
Advanced cirrhosis of the liver

Multiple myeloma
Hypogammaglobulinemia
Acute vasculitis

Interfering Factors

• None

Nursing Implementation

No specific patient instruction or intervention is needed.

FETAL HEMOGLOBIN

(WHOLE BLOOD)

Synonyms:
HbF, hemoglobin F

NORMAL VALUES	
Adult:	<2% HbF *or* SI <0.02 mass fraction HbF
Infant:	8-11 months: 1.6 ± 1% HbF *or* SI 0.16 ± 0.01 mass fraction HbF
	3 weeks: 70 ± 7.3% HbF *or* SI 0.7 ± 0.073 mass fraction HbF
	1 day: 77 ± 7.3% HbF *or* SI 0.77 ± 0.073 mass fraction HbF
Kleihauer Betke Method	
Adult:	<0.01% HbF *or* SI 0.0001 mass fraction HbF
Newborn, full term:	>90% HbF *or* SI >0.9 mass fraction HbF

Background Information

Hemoglobin F (HbF) is one of three distinct types of hemoglobin and the major hemoglobin in the fetus and newborn infant. During the first year of life, there is a gradual decrease in the production of HbF and a gradual increase in the production of hemoglobins A and A_2, (HbA and HbA_2), the predominant hemoglobins of childhood and adulthood. By the age of 1 year, there should be very little HbF in the erythrocyte pool. When HbF remains at an elevated level, it can be caused by a hereditary or acquired disorder.

HEREDITARY PERSISTENCE OF FETAL HEMOGLOBIN. This is a group of conditions that persist after infancy but cause little hematologic abnormality. The HbF content varies from 20 to 30% of total hemoglobin in those who have the heterozygous type of hereditary persistence of fetal hemoglobin. In those who have the homozygous type of condition, the hemoglobin is 100% HbF, with no HbA or HbA_2. These individuals demonstrate slight macrocytic, microchromic erythrocytes, but there is no anemia. The HbF is distributed uniformly throughout each erythrocyte.

HEMOGLOBINOPATHY. This is an alteration of the structure of hemoglobin that may or may not result in significant hematologic disease. Elevated levels of

HbF are found to coexist in some of these hemoglobin disorders. In beta-thalassemia disorders, there is an uneven distribution of HbF among the erythrocytes. This means that some of the erythrocytes have HbF present and others do not.

FETAL-MATERNAL HEMORRHAGE. The Kleihauer Betke method of analysis is used after fetal-maternal hemorrhage. It detects the amount of fetal cells and HbF in the maternal and newborn circulation. Based on the calculation of fetal blood contamination in the mother, she is given the proper dose of $RH_0(D)$ immune globulin to prevent the formation of anti-D antibodies and the development of erythroblastosis fetalis in a subsequent pregnancy. Maternal erythrocytes may have entered the blood of the newborn. The quantity of HbF is measured before blood transfusions are given.

Purpose of the Test

HbF is measured to help diagnose some forms of anemia in adults, assess the severity of fetal-maternal hemorrhage in the newborn and mother, and calculate the dosage of $RH_0(D)$ immune globulin to be given to the mother after a fetal-maternal hemorrhage.

Procedure

A purple-topped tube is used to collect 7 ml of venous blood. In cases of fetal-maternal hemorrhage, three separate purple-topped tubes are used to obtain 7 ml of blood from the mother, the newborn, and the cord blood. The cord blood serves as a control specimen.

Findings

ELEVATED VALUES

Hereditary Disorders	Acquired Disorders
Beta-thalassemia anemia	Pernicious anemia
Hereditary persistence of fetal hemoglobin	Refractory normoblastic anemia
Sickle cell anemia	Sideroblastic anemia
Trisomy 21 (Down syndrome)	Aplastic anemia
	Juvenile chronic myeloid leukemia
	Acute leukemia
	Erythroleukemia
	Benign monoclonal gammopathy
	Metastatic cancer of bone marrow
	Chronic renal disease
	Hyperthyroidism
	Pregnancy
	Molar pregnancy
	Fetal-maternal hemorrhage

Interfering Factors

- Hemolysis
- Improper labeling of specimens
- Delay in the preparation of specimens

Pretest

Ensure that all specimens and laboratory requisition slips are identified with the patients' names and sources of blood (i.e., mother, newborn, cord blood).

Posttest

Arrange for prompt transportation of the blood to the laboratory.

> **QUALITY CONTROL**
>
> The analysis is performed on fresh blood within 6 hours. Once slides are prepared, a fixative must be applied within the hour to prevent deterioration of the specimen.

GLUCOSE-6-PHOSPHATE DEHYDROGENASE SCREEN

(BLOOD)

Synonym:

G-6-PD screen, blood

―――――――――――――――――――――― **NORMAL VALUES** ――――――――――――――――

G-6-PD enzyme activity is present

Background Information

Critical Thinking: Could genetic screening tests become instruments of discrimination? How can the individual be protected from potential misuse of the information by others, resulting in unemployment or the inability to get health or life insurance?

Genetic defects in erythrocyte metabolism are responsible for many forms of hemolytic anemia. With deficient or diminished enzyme activity, the erythrocytes have a shorter life span. The deficiency of the glucose-6-phosphate dehydrogenase (G-6-PD) enzyme in the erythrocyte is the most frequent and important of this type of chronic hemolytic anemia. The deficiency of this enzyme is hereditary and linked to the X chromosome.

This type of hemolytic anemia is seen most frequently in black individuals, and it is usually a mild condition. There is a more severe, but rare, form of the disorder that affects Asian and Mediterranean individuals. It can cause hemolytic disease of the newborn.

A sudden, acute episode of severe hemolytic anemia is usually triggered by the administration of particular drugs, an infection, or illness. The medications include sulfonamides, antimalarial drugs, and a variety of other medications. The illnesses are usually acute bacterial or viral infections or metabolic disorders, including acidosis. In severe infection, the anemia can be life-threatening.

When the screening test result is positive, a quantitative blood test is performed to evaluate the severity of the defect. The screening test cannot detect the deficiency of the G-6-PD enzyme after the hemolytic episode is over because the defective erythrocytes are destroyed by hemolysis.

Purpose of the Test

This screening test is used to detect a G-6-PD enzyme defect in erythrocytes and determine that it is the cause of hemolytic anemia.

Procedure

A lavender-topped tube is used to collect 7 ml of venous blood.

Findings

DECREASED VALUES
G-6-PD anemia, mild to moderate
G-6-PD anemia, severe

Interfering Factors

• Sudden, severe hemolysis

Nursing Implementation

No specific patient instruction or intervention is needed.

HEINZ BODIES

(BLOOD)

Synonyms:
Heinz body stain, methyl violet stain for Heinz bodies

NORMAL VALUES

No Heinz bodies are identified.

Background Information

Heinz bodies are precipitates or particles present in abnormal hemoglobin and are visible in the presence of methyl violet stain. The Heinz bodies represent the end product of denatured hemoglobin and are associated with some form of hemolytic anemia.

The life span of the normal erythrocyte is 120 days. This time is shortened by intrinsic or extrinsic factors that alter the erythrocytes and result in their premature destruction and removal. There are five types of change that cause premature destruction of red cells and hemolytic anemia: (1) osmotic lysis, (2) phagocytosis of the erythrocytes, (3) complement-induced cytolysis, (4) fragmentation of the erythrocytes and denaturation, and (5) the alteration of the chemical or biologic properties of the erythrocytes. The premature destruction of red cells is observed in some hemolytic anemias, but the causes and importance of these five mechanisms are not fully understood.

In normal physiology, the iron in hemoglobin must remain in a reduced state so that oxygen molecules can be transported. The erythrocytes protect the hemoglobin from internal and external agents and prevent excess oxidation of iron. If these mechanisms fail, the hemoglobin becomes nonfunctional.

Abnormalities in the erythrocytes occur because of exposure to oxidant drugs or toxins, defects in the intrinsic protective mechanisms of the erythrocytes, and genetic abnormalities of hemoglobin. Once the hemoglobin is oxidized, the end product of the change produces precipitates called Heinz bodies.

The Heinz bodies exist within the damaged erythrocytes and may be attached to the cell membrane. With methyl violet staining of the erythrocytes, the microscopic examination of the slides reveals deep purple, small, irregular forms. Their presence reflects either metabolic derangement or altered hemoglobin. The formation of the Heinz bodies is usually followed by the destruction of the erythrocyte.

Purpose of the Test

The test is used to identify hemolytic disorders associated with Heinz body formation.

Procedure

A purple-topped tube is used to collect 7 ml of venous blood.

QUALITY CONTROL

The tourniquet must not be applied too tightly or for very long. Venipuncture technique must be smooth, with a blood flow that fills the vacuum tube readily. If the blood has excessive turbulence because of flawed venipuncture technique, the hemolysis of the erythrocytes alters the test results.

Findings

ABNORMAL VALUES
G-6-PD deficiency
Congenital Heinz body hemolytic anemia
Drug-sensitive hemolytic anemia

Interfering Factors

- Hemolysis
- Coagulation of the specimen

Nursing Implementation

Pretest

No specific patient instruction or intervention is needed.

Posttest

Arrange for prompt transport of the specimen to the laboratory.

| QUALITY CONTROL |
Clotting of the specimen renders it invalid for use. The specimen will require refrigeration until it can be examined.

HEMOGLOBIN ELECTROPHORESIS

(BLOOD)   *Synonyms:*
none

NORMAL VALUES	
HbA	95–98%
HbA$_2$	1.5–3.5%
HbF	0–2%
HbC	Absent
HbS	Absent

Background Information

In the normal adult, the three types of hemoglobin found in erythrocytes are HbA, HbA$_2$, and HbF. Abnormal hemoglobins are produced by a single amino acid substitution in one of the polypeptide chains in the globin part of the molecule.

There are more than 400 variants of hemoglobin now identified by letters other than A, A_2, and F. To further subclassify the variants, the name may include a geographic region, city, or place of discovery, such as HbM Boston. Of all the abnormal variants, HbS, sickle cell hemoglobin, is the most predominant. Others that are relatively common are HbC, HbD Punjab, and HbE.

Hemoglobinopathy is the general term used to describe altered hemoglobin and some forms of hemolytic anemia. There is a range of intensity of anemia that can exist in individuals with a hemoglobin defect. The differences include the type of general alteration of the globin molecule, a homozygous (pure) state that produces disease, and a heterozygous (mixed) state that produces the trait but not the disease.

HEMOGLOBIN A_2. Although this is a normal hemoglobin, there should be little of it. Hemoglobin electrophoresis evaluates the amount of HbA_2 in the investigation of beta-thalassemia trait and to differentiate beta-thalassemia diseases from iron deficiency anemia. The beta-thalassemia diseases are a group of disorders that produce a range of conditions that vary from no clinical change to severe hypochromic, microcytic anemia. The amount of HbA_2 is increased in beta-thalassemia trait. Abnormal elevations of HbA_2 may include up to 7% of the total hemoglobin content.

HEMOGLOBIN F. HbF is the hemoglobin present in fetal life; it is gradually replaced by HbA and HbA_2 during infancy. Adults can have abnormal quantities of HbF in hereditary persistence of fetal hemoglobin. The homozygous state produces mild microcytic, hypochromic erythrocytes without anemia. The hemoglobin electrophoresis test reveals 100% HbF. The heterozygous state produces no hematologic abnormality, but hemoglobin electrophoresis reveals 30 to 40% HbF.

HEMOGLOBIN S. In the homozygous state, HbS (HbSS) produces sickle cell anemia, a severe hemolytic anemia. Hemoglobin electrophoresis demonstrates no HbA, with a large percentage of HbS, and elevated amounts of HbF and HbA_2. In the heterozygous form, or sickle cell trait, hemoglobin electrophoresis demonstrates 30 to 35% HbS mixed in with HbA and HbA_2 and a normal percentage of HbF. Sickle cell trait (HbAS) produces no disease or hematologic abnormality unless the person experiences hypoxia, acidosis, or thrombotic phenomena. One of the thalassemia disorders may coexist with the sickle cell trait condition.

HEMOGLOBIN C. In the homozygous state of HbC disease (HCC), there is often a mild hemolytic anemia that is usually asymptomatic. On electrophoresis, there is no HbA present. Most of the hemoglobin is HbC, with smaller quantities of other forms of hemoglobin. In the heterozygous state (HbAC), 30 to 40% is HbC, with about 50 to 60% HbA present. One of the thalassemia disorders may coexist with the HbC trait.

Hemoglobin electrophoresis separates the normal from the abnormal hemoglobin in the blood sample. Hemoglobin molecules in alkaline solution have a net negative charge. The different types of hemoglobin molecules move

Critical Thinking: Develop a teaching plan for the mother of an infant with sickle cell anemia. The plan should focus on early recognition and intervention for a sickle cell crisis.

at different rates toward the anode of the electrophoresis test. For screening purposes, different media and buffers separate the distinct types of hemoglobin.

Purpose of the Test

Hemoglobin electrophoresis is used to detect hemoglobinopathy, help confirm the diagnosis of thalassemia, evaluate hemolytic anemia, identify the presence of HbC, identify sickle cell hemoglobin, and differentiate between sickle cell disease and sickle cell trait.

Procedure

A purple-topped tube is used to collect 7 ml of venous blood. A fingerstick or earlobe puncture is used to obtain two purple-topped capillary tubes of blood.

QUALITY CONTROL

The use of a tight tourniquet is to be avoided and it should not remain tied for a prolonged period. Venipuncture technique must be smooth, with a blood flow that fills the vacuum tube readily. If the blood has excessive turbulence because of flawed venipuncture technique, hemolysis of the erythrocytes will alter the results.

Findings

ELEVATED VALUES

Beta-thalassemia minor or major
Sickle cell disease
Sickle cell trait
HbH disease
Megaloblastic anemia

Hereditary persistence of fetal
   hemoglobin
HbC disease
HbC trait

DECREASED VALUES

DEFICIENCY OF HbA_2

Sideroblastic anemia
HbH disease
Erythroleukemia

Untreated iron deficiency anemia
Hereditary persistence of fetal
   hemoglobin

Interfering Factors

- Blood transfusion in the preceding 4 months
- Hemolysis
- Coagulation of the specimen

Nursing Implementation

Pretest

Ask the patient about any transfusion of blood within the preceding 3 to 4 months. A recent transfusion would make the findings of the test inconsistent.

Posttest

Gently rotate the tube several times to mix the anticoagulant with the blood. This prevents clotting of the specimen.

Arrange for prompt transport of the blood to the laboratory.

| QUALITY CONTROL |
The specimen must be fresh or refrigerated.

HEMOSIDERIN, URINARY

(URINE)

Synonyms:

──────── NORMAL VALUES ────────

Negative

Background Information

Hemosiderin granules are indicators of hemoglobin in the urine resulting from significant acute or chronic intravascular hemolysis. With the lysis of many erythrocytes, hemoglobin is released into the blood and is metabolized in the renal tubules to form ferritin and hemosiderin. The hemosiderin granules are present in the cells or casts in urinary sediment. They appear in the urine on the second or third day after the hemolytic episode. The source of the urinary hemosiderin may also be diseases that cause siderosis of the renal parenchyma, such as hematochromatosis.

The presence of hemoglobin in the urine may not be detected by a reagent strip. When the urinary sediment is stained with Prussian blue stain, however, the iron in hemosiderin appears as blue-stained granules. The results are seen by microscopic examination of the slides, which contain urinary cells and casts.

Purpose of the Test

Urinary hemosiderin is used to identify hemolytic anemia that is associated with intravascular hemolysis.

Procedure

A random sample of 30 to 60 ml of urine is collected in a clean glass container.

QUALITY CONTROL
To avoid the introduction of iron from extraneous sources, the container, slides, and covers must be free of iron.

Findings

ELEVATED VALUES

Blood transfusion reaction
Mechanical trauma to erythrocytes
G-6-PD deficiency
Thalassemia major
Sickle cell anemia
Paroxysmal cold hemoglobinuria
Severe infectious organisms (malaria, *Clostridium perfringens*)

Microangiopathic hemolytic anemia
Exposure to oxidant drugs or chemicals
Severe megaloblastic anemia
Hematochromatosis

Interfering Factors

• None

Nursing Implementation

No special patient instruction or intervention is needed.

HUMAN LEUKOCYTE ANTIGEN

(BLOOD)

Synonyms:

HLA typing; tissue typing, crossmatch; crossmatch lymphocyte; transplant tissue typing

———————— **NORMAL VALUES** ————————

No destruction of lymphocytes

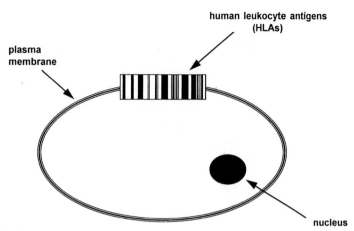

FIGURE 16–3. Human leukocyte antigens. Schematic representation of a cell with human leukocyte antigens on the cell surface. (With permission from Workman, M.L. The immune system: Your defensive partner and offensive foe. [1993]. *AACN Clinical Issues in Critical Care Nursing, 4,* 456.)

Background Information

The human leukocyte antigens (HLAs) are genetic products that are major determinants of histocompatibility. These antigens exist in an exact sequence or pattern that is specific and different for each individual. The only exception is in identical twins who have the same HLA antigens. The unique protein sequence is found on every cell of the body, including on leukocytes (Fig. 16–3).

HLA antigens are produced by chromosome 6. The chromosome loci are identified as HLA-A, HLA-B, HLA-C (class I) and HLA-DR, HLA-DQ, HLA-DP, and HLA-DW (class II). Class I antigens are derived from T lymphocytes and class II antigens are derived from B lymphocytes. The HLA-A, HLA-B, and HLA-C antigens are present on almost all nucleated cells. HLA-D antigens are present on B lymphocytes, monocytes, and possibly endothelial cells.

Circulating leukocytes are in contact with other cells. During that moment of contact, the leukocytes compare the HLA sequence on the cell surface with their own HLA sequence. When the HLA sequence is the same, the leukocyte perceives "self" in the other cell and does not react. When the HLA sequence is different, the leukocyte perceives "nonself" and initiates an inflammatory response. The nonself cell will be inactivated and destroyed (Workman, 1993).

In organ transplantation, HLA histocompatibility matching of the organ donor and transplant recipient is essential. Tissue matching improves the chance of acceptance of the tissue graft and increases the long-term survival of the transplanted tissue (Sanfillipo, 1991). When HLA matching is less than optimal, the recipient's immune system is activated with the recognition of a foreign HLA antigen. Mismatching results in graft-versus-host disease, graft failure, and possible increased sensitization of the recipient when retransplantation is needed.

Critical Thinking:
A 10-year-old child needs a renal transplant, and the 3-year-old sibling is the only family member who is HLA compatible. What are the ethical issues involved in a parental consent for one child to donate an organ to the sibling?

TABLE 16-2
HLA ANTIGEN-ASSOCIATED DISEASES

Specific HLA Antigens	Diseases
B27	Ankylosing spondylitis
	Reiter syndrome
	Anterior uveitis
B47	Congenital adrenal hyperplasia
B35	Subacute thyroiditis
B8	Chronic autoimmune hepatitis
Cw6	Psoriasis
D/DR3	Myasthenia gravis
	Systemic lupus erythematosus
	Celiac disease
	Graves disease
	Idiopathic Addison disease
D/DR4	Pemphigus
	Rheumatoid arthritis

HLA typing may also be used to exclude paternity or provide data regarding genetic counseling. A child inherits two sets of HLA antigens—one set from each parent. The HLA typing of the child and parent is used to confirm or exclude paternity. Exclusion of paternity occurs when there is no match between the father's and child's HLA type.

There are a number of disease syndromes associated with a single leukocyte antigen (Table 16–2), although the clinical significance of the tissue marker is not yet understood. The specific HLA antigens are statistically correlated with illnesses that are thought to have autoimmune characteristics. The discussion of HLA B27 is presented in Chapter 23.

Purpose of the Test

In organ transplantation, HLA tissue typing is used to determine tissue compatibility between the donor and the recipient. HLA leukocyte antigen testing may also be performed to exclude paternity when the identity of the father is questioned, and it may be used as a source of data in genetic counseling.

Procedure

Donor Specimen: Two green-topped tubes are each filled with 7 to 10 ml of venous blood.

Recipient's Blood: A red-topped tube is used to obtain 7 to 10 ml of venous blood.

HLA Typing: A green-topped, heparinized tube is filled with 7 to 10 ml of venous blood.

Findings

ABNORMAL VALUES

HLA-A, HLA-B, or HLA-DR mismatch
Incompatibility of donor and recipient tissues

Interfering Factors

• Recent blood transfusion
• Inadequate lymphocytes in the specimen

Nursing Implementation

Pretest

Schedule this test before or 72 hours after any blood transfusion.

Posttest

Arrange for prompt transport of the specimen to the laboratory. The analysis must be performed immediately on a fresh blood sample.

QUALITY CONTROL

A prolonged delay or refrigeration of the specimen will yield an insufficient number of lymphocytes for the test.

INTRINSIC FACTOR ANTIBODIES

(SERUM)

Synonyms:

antiintrinsic factor antibodies, anti-IF antibodies

━━━━━━━━━━━━━━━━ NORMAL VALUES ━━━━━━━━━━

Negative; no intrinsic factor antibodies are present

Background Information

Intrinsic factor is a glycoprotein manufactured by the parietal cells of the gastric mucosa. The function of intrinsic factor is to bond with ingested cobalamin (vitamin B_{12}) and then adhere to receptor sites in the distal ilium. At these receptor sites, the cobalamin is absorbed into the blood. Most of it is transported to the liver for storage and some goes to the bone marrow for hematopoiesis. Pernicious anemia is a megaloblastic anemia that results from inadequate manufacture of intrinsic factor, interference with the bonding of intrinsic factor–cobalamin, or interference with the bonding of the intrinsic factor–cobalamin complex at the ileal receptor sites.

The failure to produce intrinsic factor occurs with the surgical removal of the tissue source, as in total gastrectomy and some cases of partial gastrectomy. The production of intrinsic factor is also diminished in diseases that damage the gastric mucosa, including atrophic gastritis and gastric atrophy.

Interference with the function of intrinsic factor is caused by intrinsic factor antibodies. These antibodies are autoimmune complexes that are present in most cases of pernicious anemia. Adult pernicious anemia may be an autoimmune gastritis of genetic origin, but the relationship of the autoantibodies to the gastritis is unknown (Henry, 1991).

There are two types of intrinsic factor antibody. Type 1, the "blocking" antibody, interferes with the bonding of intrinsic factor to cobalamin. Type 2, the "binding" antibody, interferes with the attachment of the intrinsic factor–cobalamin complex to the ileal receptor sites.

It is unclear whether the antibodies cause the pernicious anemia or develop as a result of it. Intrinsic factor antibodies are also present in a small percentage of patients who have hyperthyroidism or insulin-dependent diabetes without pernicious anemia.

When pernicious anemia is diagnosed by the triad of megaloblastic anemia, decreased serum cobalamin, and the presence of intrinsic factor antibodies, there is no need to perform a Schilling test or gastric analysis.

Purpose of the Test

This test is performed to differentiate pernicious anemia from other causes of megaloblastic anemia.

Procedure

A red-topped tube is used to obtain 7 ml of venous blood.

Findings

POSITIVE VALUES
Pernicious anemia
Hyperthyroidism (Graves disease)
Diabetes mellitus (insulin-dependent)

Interfering Factors

• Recent radioisotope scan
• Recent vitamin B_{12} injection

Nursing Implementation

Pretest

Schedule this test before any radioisotope scan. The radioisotopes of the nuclear scan interfere with the radioimmunoassay method of analysis used in this test.

Instruct the patient to withhold any injection of vitamin B_{12} for 48 hours before the test. Recent injection of this vitamin could cause a false-positive result.

Posttest

Arrange for prompt transport of the specimen to the laboratory.

QUALITY CONTROL

The serum must be separated from the cells and then stored at $-20°$ C until it is analyzed.

IRON STUDIES

(SERUM)

Synonyms:

serum iron, Fe; transferrin, Tf; siderophilin; total iron-binding capacity, TIBC; transferrin saturation, iron saturation

Background Information

Iron is an inorganic ion that is essential to many vital body processes, including erythropoiesis, the transport of oxygen to tissues, and cellular oxidation mechanisms. In normal physiology, the total iron content remains relatively constant throughout life. The body has an efficient method to conserve the iron from senescent erythrocytes and reuse it in erythropoiesis and hemoglobin synthesis (Fig. 16–4).

ABSORPTION. Iron homeostasis is regulated by the function of intestinal absorption of the iron in foods. Because the body has a limited ability to excrete iron, the intestine absorbs only 5 to 10% of the daily iron intake. This prevents the retention of an excessive or toxic amount. Most of the iron is absorbed from the duodenum and jejunum, with enhanced absorption in the presence of gastric acids. In the time of greater demand, as in pregnancy or after blood loss, the intestinal tract absorbs a greater quantity of iron to meet the body's need.

TRANSPORT. Once absorbed, iron enters the blood and the unbound iron attaches to transferrin, a plasma protein. At the bone marrow, iron is passed into developing erythrocytes to become heme molecules and part of hemoglobin.

STORAGE. Some of the absorbed iron combines with apoferritin to form ferritin, and the remainder is deposited into tissues in the form of hemosiderin.

──────────────── **NORMAL VALUES** ────────────────

Serum Iron
Adult Male: 65–175 µg/dl *or* SI 11.6–31.3 µmol/L
Adult Female: 50–170 µg/dl *or* SI 9–30.4 µmol/L
Child: 50–120 µg/dl *or* SI 9–21.5 µmol/L
Infant: 40–100 µg/dl *or* SI 7.2–17.9 µmol/L
Newborn: 100–250 µg/dl *or* SI 17.9–44.8 µmol/L
Transferrin
Adult >60 Years: 180–380 mg/dl *or* SI 1.8–3.8 g/L
Adult 16–60 Years: 200–400 mg/dl *or* SI 2–4 g/L
Child 3 Months–16 Years: 203–360 mg/dl *or* SI 2.03–3.6 g/L
Newborn: 130–275 mg/dl *or* SI 1.3–2.75 g/L
Total Iron-Binding Capacity 218–385 µg/dl *or* SI 39–69 µmol/L
Transferrin Saturate 20–50%
Ferritin
Adult Male: 20–250 ng/ml *or* SI 20–250 µg/L
Adult Female: 10–120 ng/ml *or* SI 10–120 µg/L
Child 6 Months–15 Years: 7–140 ng/ml *or* SI 7–140 µg/L
Infant 2–5 Months: 50–200 ng/ml *or* SI 50–200 µg/L
Newborn: 25–200 ng/ml *or* SI 25–200 µg/L

Both ferritin and hemosiderin are used to store the iron reserves, and the stored iron can be released when there is a need. The stored iron reserves are located in the tissues of the liver (hepatic parenchymal cells) and in the reticuloendothelial cells of the bone marrow, spleen, and liver.

CIRCULATION. Iron is present in the hemoglobin content of erythrocytes. Each hemoglobin molecule has iron-containing pigment called heme. As the erythrocytes are damaged or become senescent, they are removed from the circulation by hemolysis. During this process, the reticuloendothelial tissues extract the iron. The iron is either bound to transferrin for transport or is stored as hemosiderin in the reticuloendothelial tissues and the liver.

IRON DEFICIENCY. A decrease in the level of iron occurs when the supply of iron is insufficient to meet the body's demand and the iron reserves are also depleted. The source of the problem can be insufficient intake, impaired absorption, blood loss, or increased demand because of pregnancy and lactation (Table 16–3).

IRON OVERLOAD. Excessive iron storage occurs in some anemias, in liver disease, in excessive iron replacement therapy, and after multiple transfusions.

LABORATORY TESTING. There is no one test that fully measures iron deficiency, iron overload, and iron storage. A battery of several tests is used to provide a complete assessment, including the complete blood count. The laboratory assessment of iron stores includes serum iron, transferrin, total iron-binding capacity, transferrin saturation, and ferritin.

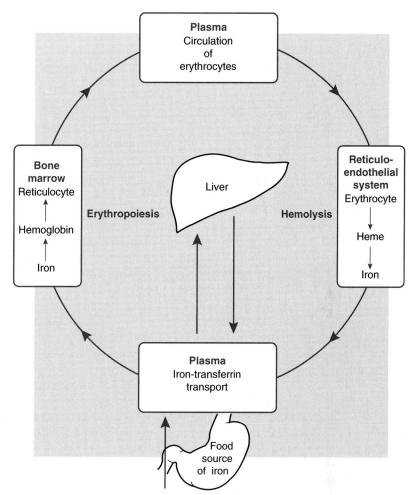

FIGURE 16–4. The use and conservation of iron. Some iron is readily available in the plasma and bone marrow for the synthesis of hemoglobin and erythropoiesis. After the hemolysis of old or damaged erythrocytes, the body is very efficient in the conservation and storage of iron in the liver and bone marrow. Whenever the immediate supply of iron is low, the liver releases the stored iron for erythropoiesis.

TABLE 16–3
FACTORS THAT CONTRIBUTE TO IRON DEFICIENCY

Insufficient Intake	Impaired Absorption	Blood Loss	Increased Demand
Fad diets	Gastric surgery	Gastrointestinal bleeding	Pregnancy
Pica	Celiac disease	Excessive menstruation	Lactation
Poverty	Achlorhydria		

Serum Iron. This is the amount of iron bound to transferrin. In the laboratory analysis, the iron must first be separated from the transferrin so that the measurement is accurate. As a single laboratory test, a serum iron determination is used to evaluate iron toxicity. The value is decreased in iron deficiency anemia and the anemia associated with chronic disease. The test is useful when measured with transferrin and transferrin saturation.

Transferrin. This is the major protein that binds serum iron and transports it in the blood. In normal physiology, about one third of the transferrin is bound with iron, and the remainder is available in reserve. Transferrin is elevated in iron deficiency anemia and is decreased with iron overload. It is a useful index of nutritional status because it is elevated in uncomplicated iron deficiency but is in the normal to low-normal range in other types of anemia.

Total Iron-Binding Capacity. This is the maximum iron-binding capacity of transferrin and other iron-binding globulins. The serum value also provides data regarding the nutritional status of the individual. The results of the total iron-binding capacity determination correlate with the transferrin value, meaning that the total iron-binding capacity rises in iron deficiency anemia and decreases in the presence of iron overload.

Transferrin Saturation. This is a calculation of the iron storage, expressed as the ratio of serum iron:total iron-binding capacity. The result is the percentage of transferrin that is saturated with iron. The value is decreased in iron deficiency, but a value of less than 15% indicates iron deficiency erythropoiesis.

Ferritin. This is a reliable indicator of total iron storage. The level is decreased in iron deficiency anemia and elevated in iron overload. When a ferritin determination is combined with other iron studies, the results distinguish among the different types of microcytic, hypochromic anemias. Iron deficiency anemia is indicated by a serum ferritin value of less than 10 ng/ml (SI, <10 µg/L).

Critical Thinking: The young adult patient has a serum iron level of 40 µg/dL (SI: 7.2 µmol/L) and a nursing diagnosis of *Nutrition alteration: Less than body requirements.* After you have obtained a nutritional history of this patient, what dietary practices would require nursing intervention?

Purpose of the Tests

These tests provide an estimate of total iron storage and information regarding the nutritional status of the individual. They help distinguish between iron deficiency anemia and the anemia of chronic disease. They also confirm the presence of iron overload and hematochromatosis.

Procedure

A red-topped tube is used to collect 7 ml of venous blood. This blood sample is drawn before other blood samples that require vacuum tubes with anticoagulant.

QUALITY CONTROL

The tourniquet is applied loosely and is not kept in place for long. The venipuncture must be smooth, with a blood flow that fills the vacuum tube readily. If the blood has excessive turbulence because of flawed venipuncture technique, the hemolysis of the erythrocytes will alter the results.

Findings

ELEVATED VALUES

Serum Iron

Anemias (pernicious, aplastic, hemolytic)
Hemochromatosis
Thalassemia
Excess iron replacement
Multiple transfusions
Iron poisoning
Lead poisoning
Vitamin B_6 deficiency
Acute leukemia
Acute hepatitis

Transferrin Saturation

Iron toxicity
Hemochromatosis
Viral hepatitis
Nephrosis
Thalassemia

Transferrin

Iron deficiency anemia
Elevated estrogen levels
Pregnancy

Total Iron-Binding Capacity

Hypochromic anemias
Iron deficiency anemia
Acute hepatitis
Pregnancy

Ferritin

Hemochromatosis
Liver disease
Iron overload
Acute leukemias
Inflammatory diseases
Infectious diseases

DECREASED VALUES

Serum Iron

Iron deficiency anemia
Pernicious anemia (in remission)
Nephrosis
Hypothyroidism
Acute or chronic infection
Malignancy
Starvation

Transferrin Saturation

Iron deficiency anemia
Anemia of chronic infection
Malignancy

Ferritin

Iron deficiency anemia

Transferrin

Inflammation or necrosis
Malignancy
Malnutrition
Multiple myeloma
Hepatocellular diseases
Nephrotic syndrome

Total Iron-Binding Capacity

Anemias (non–iron-deficient)
Hemochromatosis
Malignancy
Renal disease
Thalassemia

Interfering Factors

- Recent administration of radioisotopes (ferritin)
- Hemolysis (serum iron, iron saturation)

- Lipemia (transferrin)
- Recent blood transfusion (serum iron)

Nursing Implementation

Pretest

Schedule these laboratory tests before or a few days after a blood transfusion to obtain the most accurate results.

Schedule these laboratory tests before any nuclear scans, since the radioactive isotopes of the scan interfere with the radioimmunoassay method for testing of ferritin.

Schedule these tests to be performed in the morning. Serum iron has a diurnal rhythm, with the highest value in the early morning. The serum iron values fluctuate widely between day and night and also on different days.

Instruct the patient to fast from food and fluid for 8 hours before the tests for transferrin levels. Lipemia interferes with the transferrin values.

If the patient takes an iron supplement, include this information on the requisition slip.

Posttest

Arrange for prompt transport of the specimen to the laboratory.

QUALITY CONTROL

The cells must be separated from the serum without delay. This avoids false elevation due to hemolysis.

MALARIA SMEAR

(PERIPHERAL BLOOD)

Synonym:

blood smear for malarial parasites

─────────── **NORMAL VALUES** ───────────

No organisms identified

Background Information

There are four *Plasmodium* species. Humans become infected by the parasite via the bite from an infected *Anopheles* mosquito. Once the fertilized eggs penetrate the skin, they migrate to the liver within 1 hour. After 8 days of gestational development in the liver, the merozoite form enters the blood and penetrates the erythrocytes 2 days later. Depending on the species, the merozoites can cause the erythrocytes to become enlarged and distorted in shape. Additionally, each species causes distinct inclusions or markings within the cytoplasm. The organisms grow readily within the erythrocytes until they fill the red blood cells. With the simultaneous rupture of many infected erythrocytes, the patient spikes a fever.

All *Plasmodium* species can be seen on thin or thick stained blood films. The thin films are used to observe the change in characteristics of the infected erythrocytes and to identify the changes in cytoplasm that are characteristic of each species. The thick film is used when there is a low level of infection with fewer parasites or when the erythrocytes have already lysed and it is difficult to differentiate among the species.

Purpose of the Test

The peripheral smear is used to detect and identify the specific *Plasmodium* species that has caused malaria.

Procedure

A fingerstick or earlobe puncture is used to obtain peripheral blood. Two or three of each of the thick and thin slides are prepared at the bedside.

As an alternative, a lavender-topped tube with ethylene diaminetetraacetic acid (EDTA) is used to collect 7 ml of venous blood.

Findings

ABNORMAL VALUES

Plasmodium vivax	*Plasmodium falciparum*
Plasmodium ovale	*Plasmodium malariae*

Interfering Factors

• Clotting of the specimen

Nursing Implementation

Pretest

To establish the pattern of fever, monitor the temperature every 4 hours and document the results. Instruct the patient to tell you if chills and fever begin.

Notify the laboratory to draw the blood immediately before the time of the next anticipated fever spike.

QUALITY CONTROL

In malaria, the cycle of fever occurs about every 48 hours, depending on the species. In the time just prior to the onset of fever, the erythrocytes are full of merozoites and have not yet caused hemolysis. More than one blood test may be needed to verify the diagnosis.

Posttest

On the requisition form, write any history of travel in endemic areas of the world, particularly in subtropical and tropical countries.

MICROFILARIA SMEAR

(PERIPHERAL BLOOD)

Synonyms:

blood smear for *Trypanosoma* or Filaria parasites, blood smear for parasites

——————————————— **NORMAL VALUES** ———————————————

No parasites visualized

Background Information

Filarial worms of different species infect humans by insect bite from infected flies or mosquitoes. These parasites survive in warm climates, particularly in Africa, Mexico, Asia, India, Central and South America, the Philippines, and a few of the Caribbean islands. Once the filariae have infected a human, the ova mature to adult worms, reproduce, and reside in various tissues, including lymph glands and subcutaneous tissues.

The microfilariae are the larval stage of the parasite. They reside within erythrocytes and in the peripheral blood of the infected person. Their presence can be detected and the species identified by microscopic examination of the blood. Thick and thin blood films are prepared and stained to enhance the visualization.

The microparasites are often found in greater quantities in the blood in a diurnal rhythm. The optimal yield is often at noon and midnight, depending on the species and the geographic region. One negative result may not be conclusive because it is difficult to isolate the microfilariae. They may or may not be in the blood at the time the blood sample is obtained. Biopsy of the skin or subcutaneous mass may also be needed.

Purpose of the Test

A peripheral blood smear for filariae is performed in the diagnosis of elephantiasis, trypanosomiasis, or parasitic infection of the blood.

Procedure

A fingerstick or earlobe puncture is used to obtain a peripheral blood sample for thick and thin films or smears.

As an alternative, a lavender-topped tube with EDTA may be used to collect 7 ml of venous blood.

Findings

ABNORMAL VALUES

Wuchereria bancrofti   *Brugia malayi*
Loa loa   *Dipetalonema perstans*
Mansonella ozzardi

Interfering Factors

• None

Nursing Implementation

Pretest

Schedule the tests for 12 noon and midnight to 2 A.M. because these are the best hours for the diurnal rhythms of the parasites. If the patient spikes a fever, this is also an optimal time for the blood sample to be obtained.

Question the patient about any recent travel or residence in a tropical country or primitive region of the world. If there is a positive history, include the date or dates of travel and the geographic exposure on the requisition slip.

Posttest

Arrange for prompt transport of the slides or blood to the laboratory.

QUALITY CONTROL

For effective visualization, the blood or films must be fresh. As the microfilariae move around or flagellate, they will move the erythrocytes and can be located more easily.

NEUTROPHIL ALKALINE PHOSPHATASE

Synonyms:

NAP, leukocyte alkaline phosphatase

───────────── **NORMAL VALUES** ─────────────

40–130 (Teitz, 1990)

Background Information

Chronic myeloproliferative diseases are hematologic malignancies that produce rapid, excessive cloning of a multipotential cell of the bone marrow. The cloning can proceed along different granulocytic, erythroid, or megakaryocytic lines, producing excessive neutrophils, erythrocytes, platelets, or other related cells derived from progenitors. The four chronic myeloproliferative diseases are chronic myelogenous leukemia, polycythemia vera, myelofibrosis, and essential thrombocytopenia.

The neutrophil alkaline phosphatase test produces a characteristic chemical reaction that helps to differentiate among these myeloproliferative disorders. Neutrophil alkaline phosphatase is an enzyme located in neutrophils. The enzyme is detected in an alkaline medium and in the presence of dye.

In the test method, 100 stained neutrophils are given a rating score of 0 to 4, based on the intensity of the color of the reaction. Thus, the range is 0 to 400, and the reference range or normal range is 40 to 130. The scoring is somewhat subject to color interpretation, and the reference range varies among laboratories.

Among the myeloproliferative disorders, chronic myelogenous leukemia tends to produce low scores regardless of the total white cell count. The other myeloproliferative disorders have higher scores.

Purpose of the Test

This test helps differentiate chronic myelogenous leukemia from leukemoid reaction and other myeloproliferative diseases. It is also useful in the evaluation of Hodgkin disease and its response to therapy.

Procedure

Fingerstick or earlobe puncture is used to make six slides with smears of the peripheral blood. As an alternative, a green-topped tube with heparin or oxalate anticoagulant is used to collect 7 ml of venous blood.

Findings

ELEVATED VALUES

Polycythemia vera
Myelofibrosis
Leukemoid reactions
Acute lymphoblastic leukemia

Hairy cell leukemia
Down syndrome
Hodgkin disease
Neutrophilia, secondary to infection

DECREASED VALUES

Chronic myelogenous leukemia
Acute myeloid leukemia
Sideroblastic anemia
Thrombocytopenic purpura
Acute monocytic leukemia
Collagen disease

Cirrhosis of the liver
Congestive heart failure
Gout
Diabetes mellitus
Hereditary hypophosphatemia

Interfering Factors

- Pregnancy
- Acute stress
- Neutropenia
- Delay in the final preparation of slides

Nursing Implementation

Pretest

To ensure a valid test, verify that the recent peripheral blood neutrophil count is greater than $1000/mm^3$.

Posttest

Arrange for immediate transport of the slides or blood specimen to the laboratory.

QUALITY CONTROL

To avoid rejection of the specimen, the slides must be fixed in preservative within 30 minutes.

OSMOTIC FRAGILITY

(WHOLE BLOOD)

Synonyms:

OF, erythrocyte fragility, RBC fragility

─────────────── **NORMAL VALUES** ───────────────

INITIAL HEMOLYSIS OF ERYTHROCYTES:	0.45% sodium chloride (NaCl) *or* SI 4.5 g/L NaCl
COMPLETE HEMOLYSIS OF ERYTHROCYTES:	0.3% NaCl *or* SI 3 g/L NaCl

Background Information

Osmotic fragility refers to the ability of erythrocytes to absorb water without lysis of the cell membrane. The variation of time in the results is based on the surface area and cell volume. Abnormal erythrocytes, such as spherocytes, have greater than normal volume. They demonstrate lysis in the presence of a hypotonic saline solution because of increased osmotic fragility. Abnormal erythrocytes, such as hypochromic cells, have a greater than normal surface area. They resist lysis in the presence of a hypotonic saline solution because of decreased osmotic fragility.

Purpose of the Test

Osmotic fragility is used in the evaluation of immunohemolytic conditions, including hemolytic anemia and hereditary spherocytosis.

Procedure

A purple- or green-topped tube with EDTA or heparin is used to collect 5 ml of venous blood.

QUALITY CONTROL

The tourniquet must not be applied tightly or kept in place long. Venipuncture technique must be smooth, with a blood flow that fills the vacuum tube readily. If the blood has excessive turbulence because of flawed venipuncture technique, the hemolysis of the erythrocytes alters the test results.

Findings

ELEVATED VALUES
Hereditary spherocytosis
Acquired immune hemolytic anemia with spherocytosis
Hereditary stomatocytosis

DECREASED VALUES

Iron deficiency anemia
Hemoglobinopathy
Leptocytosis

Microcytic anemia
Thalassemia

Interfering Factors

- Hemolysis
- Clotting of the blood sample
- Delay in analysis of the blood

Nursing Implementation

Pretest

No special patient instructions or interventions are needed.

Posttest

Arrange for prompt transport of the specimen to the laboratory.

QUALITY CONTROL
The results are most accurate when the test is performed on fresh cells. A delay of more than 6 hours before analysis or the clotting of the specimen results in an invalid test.

PARIETAL CELL ANTIBODY

(SERUM)

Synonyms:
PCA, antiparietal cell antibody

NORMAL VALUES

Negative; no parietal cell antibodies are present

Background Information

The parietal cells of the gastric mucosa manufacture intrinsic factor, the glycoprotein that promotes intestinal absorption of cobalamin (vitamin B_{12}). When the parietal cells are destroyed, cobalamin deficiency and pernicious anemia develop. Parietal cell antibodies can be detected in most cases of pernicious anemia and atrophic gastritis. The two conditions often coexist and are characterized by the absence of parietal and chief cells in the gastric mucosa.

The presence of parietal cell antibodies and intrinsic factor antibodies suggests that pernicious anemia and some cases of atrophic gastritis are autoimmune disorders. The autoantibodies may be the cause of atrophic gastritis, which then leads to pernicious anemia, but the exact relationship has not yet been proved (Tietz, 1990). Additionally, other known autoimmune disorders can demonstrate parietal cell antibody, with or without atrophic gastritis or pernicious anemia.

Purpose of the Test

The parietal cell antibody test is useful in the diagnosis of pernicious anemia and some cases of atrophic gastritis.

Procedure

A red-topped tube is used to collect 7 ml of venous blood.

Findings

ELEVATED VALUES

Pernicious anemia	Atrophic gastritis
Hashimoto thyroiditis	Addison disease
Myasthenia gravis	Juvenile diabetes
Gastric ulcer	Iron deficiency anemia
Sjögren syndrome	

Interfering Factors

• None

Nursing Implementation

Pretest

No specific patient instruction or intervention is needed.

Posttest

Arrange for prompt transport of the specimen to the laboratory.

QUALITY CONTROL

The cells must be separated from the serum without delay. The serum is stored at −20° C until it is analyzed.

SCHILLING TEST

(URINE)

Synonyms:

Vitamin B_{12} absorption test, radioactive vitamin B_{12} absorption test with (without) intrinsic factor

NORMAL VALUES	
STAGE 1:	10–40% cobalt-58–labeled vitamin B_{12} excretion/24-hour urine collection *or* SI 0.10–0.40 (fraction of dose excreted) (Mettler and Guiberteau, 1991)
STAGE 2:	0–42% cobalt-57–labeled vitamin B_{12} + intrinsic factor excretion/24-hour urine collection *or* SI 0.00–0.42 (fraction of dose excreted)
COBALT-57:	Cobalt-58 Ratio: 0.7–1.3

Background Information

Critical Thinking: The patient has an abnormal Schilling test and is diagnosed with pernicious anemia. After effective treatment, what changes in nursing outcomes do you anticipate?

When vitamin B_{12} is poorly absorbed from the small intestine, pernicious anemia, a megaloblastic anemia, develops gradually. The poor absorption of vitamin B_{12} can be caused by malabsorption in the small intestine or by a defect of intrinsic factor. The Schilling test measures the ability of the small intestine to absorb vitamin B_{12} and also identifies the source of the problem.

In normal physiology, vitamin B_{12} is absorbed in the terminal segment of the small intestine in the presence of intrinsic factor. Once vitamin B_{12} enters the blood stream, it is bound to plasma proteins or is stored by the liver. It is an essential ingredient for normal hematopoiesis.

In stage 1 of the test, a measured oral dose of radiolabeled cobalt-58–vitamin B_{12} is absorbed. It has been blocked from the liver and plasma proteins, so it must be excreted in the urine. In the 24-hour urine collection, the normal excretion is 10 to 40% of the oral dose of cobalt-58–labeled vitamin B_{12}. The normal value indicates that intrinsic factor is sufficient and the intestine is functional for the absorption of vitamin B_{12}. When the stage 1 urine value is less than 7%, the results indicate there is pernicious anemia or malabsorption. Stage 2 of the test is used to distinguish between these two causes.

In stage 2, the process is repeated, but the radiolabeled vitamin B_{12} contains intrinsic factor (cobalt-57–labeled vitamin B_{12} + intrinsic factor). In the 24-hour urine collection, the normal excretion is 10 to 42% of the oral dose of cobalt-57–labeled vitamin B_{12} plus intrinsic factor. When the result remains lower than normal, the problem is malabsorption. Low values in the presence of intrinsic factor imply that the problem has to do with the structure and integrity of the intestinal mucosa.

It is also possible to perform both stages of this test at the same time. The radionuclides in the urine can be measured separately because of the different energies of cobalt-57 and cobalt-58. The results are expressed as the ratio cobalt-57:cobalt-58. In normal function, they are absorbed and excreted in almost equal amounts. When the value of cobalt-57–labeled vitamin B_{12} plus intrinsic factor is normal, but the value of cobalt-58–labeled vitamin B_{12} without intrinsic factor is low, the cause is pernicious anemia. In this case, the cobalt-57:cobalt-58 ratio is greater than 1.7. This alternative method requires only one test period and minimizes the opportunity for error that results from incomplete collection of urine.

Purpose of the Test

The 24-hour urine test measures vitamin B_{12} absorption before and after the administration of intrinsic factor to differentiate between pernicious anemia and malabsorption of the small intestine.

Procedure

Traditional method, stage 1: After administration of an oral dose of cobalt-58–labeled vitamin B_{12} and an intramuscular dose of unlabeled vitamin B_{12}, urine is collected for 24 hours.

Traditional method, stage 2: Five days later, after administration of an oral dose of cobalt-57–labeled vitamin B_{12} plus intrinsic factor and an intramuscular dose of unlabeled vitamin B_{12}, urine is collected for 24 hours.

Combined method: After oral administration of cobalt-58– and cobalt-57–labeled vitamin B_{12} plus intrinsic factor, urine is collected for 24 hours.

Findings

DECREASED VALUES

Pernicious anemia	Abnormality of the small intestine
Severe ileal disease	Chronic pancreatitis
Crohn disease	Giardiasis
Total gastrectomy	Radiotherapy
Celiac disease	

Interfering Factors

- Failure to maintain pretest nothing-by-mouth status
- Failure to administer vitamin B_{12} intramuscularly
- Incomplete urine collection
- Renal dysfunction

- Recent vitamin B$_{12}$ injection
- Recent radioisotope scan
- Fecal contamination of urine specimen
- Pregnancy and lactation

Nursing Implementation

Pretest

Schedule the bone marrow examination, serum folate determination, and serum vitamin B$_{12}$ determination before the Schilling test because the administered vitamin B$_{12}$ will alter the bone marrow and serum levels of these other tests.

Schedule the Schilling test before any radioactive scans because the radioactive materials of the scans will alter the count of the radiolabeled vitamin B$_{12}$.

Instruct the patient to discontinue food intake at midnight before the test (Jacobs, 1990). Water is permitted.

Explain the procedure to the patient, including the need to save all urine for each 24-hour collection period.

QUALITY CONTROL

No fecal material can be mixed in with the urine. The unabsorbed radiolabeled vitamin B$_{12}$ is excreted in the feces. If fecal contamination occurs, the urine will have a falsely elevated result.

During the Test

Stage 1

Before the vitamin B$_{12}$ is given to start the test, have the patient void to empty the bladder in preparation for the 24-hour urine collection.

Administer the oral dose of cobalt-58–labeled vitamin B$_{12}$. At the same time or within 2 hours, administer the "flushing dose" of vitamin B$_{12}$, 1000 µg intramuscularly.

Instruct the patient to resume food and beverage intake 1 to 2 hours after the oral dose of radiolabeled vitamin B$_{12}$ is given. Encourage extra water and fluids throughout the test to ensure the production of at least 1 L of urine in the 24-hour period.

Collect all urine for 24 hours, starting with the time of the oral dose of radiolabeled vitamin B$_{12}$.

Stage 2

Five days later, begin the second stage of the test. Instruct the patient to void and empty the bladder in preparation for the 24-hour collection of urine.

Administer the oral dose of cobalt-57–labeled vitamin B$_{12}$ with 60 mg of active hog intrinsic factor to the fasting patient.

At the same time or within 2 hours, administer the flushing dose of unlabeled vitamin B$_{12}$, 1000 μg intramuscularly.

Instruct the patient to collect all urine for 24 hours, starting at the time of the oral dose of radiolabeled vitamin B$_{12}$ and intrinsic factor.

Instruct the patient to resume food and beverage intake 1 to 2 hours after the oral dose of radiolabeled vitamin B$_{12}$ and intrinsic factor is given. Encourage sufficient extra fluids to produce at least 1 L of urine in the collection period.

Combined Method

Instruct the patient to void and empty the bladder in preparation for the 24-hour collection of urine.

Administer the capsule of cobalt-58–labeled vitamin B$_{12}$ simultaneously with the cobalt-57–labeled vitamin B$_{12}$ plus intrinsic factor to the fasting patient. At the same time or within 2 hours, administer the flushing dose of unlabeled vitamin B$_{12}$, 1000 μg intramuscularly.

Instruct the patient to collect all urine for 24 hours, resume food and fluid intake, and drink extra fluids, as described previously.

Posttest

Ensure that the urine container and requisition slip have the patient's name and the dates and times of the start and finish of the collection period.

Arrange for prompt transport of the urine specimen to the laboratory.

SICKLE CELL TESTS

(BLOOD)

Synonyms:

dithionite test, itano solubility test; metabisulfate test, sickle cell solubility test, Sickledex

───────────────────────── **NORMAL VALUES** ─────────────────────────

Negative

Background Information

The normal adult forms of hemoglobin are identified as HbA, HbA$_2$, and HbF. Common variant hemoglobins are identified as HbS, HbC, HbD, and HbE, but sickle cell hemoglobin (HbS) is the most common of the abnormal hemoglobins.

HbS is synthesized because there is a single amino acid substitution in the structure of a particular gene. As a result of this genetic structural change, the hemoglobin is altered in stability and solubility. The term "sickled" is used

TABLE 16–4
SICKLE CELL DISEASES WITH ABNORMAL VARIANT HEMOGLOBINS

Sickle cell anemia
HbSC disease
Sickle beta-thalassemia
$HbSD_{Punjab}$
HbSE disease
$HbSO_{Arab}$
HbS_{Lepore}

because in deoxygenated states, HbS converts the erythrocytes into sickle or crescent shapes.

The homozygous (pure) form of HbS produces sickle cell anemia. The infant inherits the HbS from both parents and the erythrocytes have only HbS, with no HbA or HbA_2 present. Other forms of sickle cell anemia are inherited when one parent has HbS and the other parent has beta-thalassemia or an abnormal hemoglobin (Table 16–4). The heterozygous (mixed) form of HbS produces sickle cell trait, and each erythrocyte has some HbA and some HbS. In the trait condition, the proportion of normal hemoglobin is always greater than that of HbS, usually in the 55 to 65% range.

Because all infants are born with 100% HbF, sickle cell anemia may not be detected by these test methods until the baby is 6 months of age. By this time, affected infants have replaced the HbF with HbS, and the test result is positive. These various sickle cell tests should not be used to screen the newborn or young infant (Smith and Kinney, 1993).

There are a number of limitations to these tests. Polycythemia or hyperglobulinemia may produce a false-positive result. Patients who have severe anemia will have a false-negative result. When the test result is positive, there is no differentiation between sickle cell anemia and sickle cell trait. With suspicious findings, the test should be repeated. Hemoglobin electrophoresis is the preferred method to confirm the diagnosis and differentiate between sickle cell disease and sickle cell trait.

Critical Thinking:
When genetic screening for sickle cell carriers is performed, what additional health care services should be provided to the patients and families who have positive results?

Purpose of the Test

The sickle cell test is a screening test that is used to detect HbS, the sickling hemoglobin; to evaluate hemolytic anemia; and to help identify the cause of hereditary anemia.

Procedure

A purple- or green-topped tube is used to collect 7 ml of venous blood. As an alternative method, a fingerstick or earlobe puncture can be performed to obtain a capillary specimen.

QUALITY CONTROL

With venipuncture, the tourniquet must not be applied tightly or for a prolonged time. The venipuncture should be smooth, with a blood flow that fills the tube readily. If the blood has excessive turbulence because of flawed venipuncture technique, the hemolysis of the erythrocytes will alter the test results.

Findings

POSITIVE VALUES

Sickle cell anemia
Sickle cell trait
Other sickling disorders

Interfering Factors

- Hemolysis
- Coagulation of the specimen
- Blood transfusion within the past 3 to 4 months

Nursing Implementation

Pretest

No specific patient instruction or intervention is needed.

Posttest

Provide support to the parents who become upset when they learn of the abnormal findings. Additional testing must be performed before any diagnosis is confirmed. With a positive test result, assist with the scheduling of additional tests that will determine the exact diagnosis.

TOTAL BLOOD VOLUME

(BLOOD)

Synonym:
plasma blood volume

Background Information

The total blood volume test consists of the red cell volume test and the plasma volume test. The normal amounts of red cells and plasma fluid vary with the individual's body surface, weight, height, gender, and age. There are many

——————— **NORMAL VALUES** ———————

RED CELL VOLUME
Male: 25–35 ml/kg
Female: 20–30 ml/kg
PLASMA CELL VOLUME: 40–50 ml/kg
TOTAL BLOOD VOLUME: 60–80 ml/kg

pathophysiologic conditions that also alter the number of red cells or the fluid volume of the plasma, or both.

Polycythemia vera is caused by an increase in red cell volume or red cell mass. It is indicated by laboratory test results showing elevated hemoglobin, hematocrit, and red blood cell count. An elevation of the red cell volume can be caused by polycythemia vera or relative polycythemia. In severe, absolute polycythemia, there is an increase in the red cell volume, plasma volume, and total blood volume. In relative polycythemia, there is a decrease in plasma volume and total blood volume. Although there is a relative increase in the red cell volume, it is due to hemoconcentration and not to an increase in the number of erythrocytes.

The red cell volume test may also be used in the assessment of anemia. In moderate to severe anemia, there is a decrease in the red cell volume, with normal to decreased total blood volume. The decrease of the red cell volume is due to smaller, thinner, or fewer erythrocytes, or a combination of these factors, in a stable plasma volume.

Red cell volume or red cell mass is measured by radioactive sodium chromate (chromium-51) bound to erythrocytes. The plasma volume is measured by radioactive iodine (iodine-125 or iodine-131) bound to albumin. In both tests, the radiolabeled tracers are injected intravenously and blood is drawn at timed intervals. A scintillation counter is used to measure the test values.

Purpose of the Test

The three tests of red cell volume, plasma cell volume, and total blood volume are used to distinguish between absolute polycythemia vera and relative polycythemia vera. Red cell volume is used to help assess anemia and the effect of cancer chemotherapy or radiation. The plasma volume or total blood volume, or both, can be used to help evaluate complicated fluid and electrolyte problems.

Procedure

Red Cell Volume: Two green-topped, heparinized tubes are used to obtain 8 ml of venous blood. Chromium-51 radioisotope is added to the erythrocytes and the cells are diluted in saline. The radioisotope-tagged erythrocytes are injected intravenously into the patient. After 10 minutes, a green-topped, heparinized tube is used to obtain 8 ml of venous blood from the opposite arm. A scintillation counter measures the radioactive erythrocyte count, and the red cell volume is calculated.

Plasma Volume: Two green-topped, heparinized tubes are used to obtain 8 ml of venous blood. In the laboratory, radiolabeled albumin is added to the patient's plasma. This plasma preparation is injected intravenously into the patient. Using green-topped, heparinized tubes, blood samples of 5 ml each are drawn 10, 20, and 30 minutes later. In some laboratory methods, only one posttest sample is drawn after 10 minutes. A scintillation counter measures the radioactive albumin count, and the plasma volume is calculated.

Total Blood Volume: The total volume of the blood is calculated by adding the test values for the red cell volume plus the plasma volume.

Findings

ELEVATED VALUES

TOTAL BLOOD VOLUME

Absolute polycythemia vera
Pulmonary diseases
Starvation
Acidosis
Renal insufficiency

Cardiac failure
Overhydration
Thyrotoxicosis
Pregnancy
Congenital cardiac abnormality

RED CELL VOLUME

Absolute polycythemia vera
Relative polycythemia vera
Hemoglobinopathy

Pulmonary diseases
Neoplasm
Congenital cardiac abnormality

PLASMA VOLUME

Anemia
Splenomegaly
Vasodilation
Cardiac failure
Acidosis
Pregnancy

Absolute polycythemia vera
Macroglobulinemia
Overhydration
Cirrhosis
Renal insufficiency

DECREASED VALUES

TOTAL BLOOD VOLUME

Severe anemia
Hemorrhage
Burns
Chronic renal failure

Vomiting, diarrhea
Diabetes mellitus
Dehydration
Starvation

RED CELL VOLUME

Anemia
Acute and chronic blood loss
Pheochromocytosis

Chronic infection
Starvation
Chronic renal failure

PLASMA VOLUME

Dehydration	Chronic infection
Preeclampsia	Vomiting, diarrhea
Acute hemorrhage	Radiation
Tissue hypoxia	

Interfering Factors

- Recent radioactive isotope scan
- Bleeding or edematous tissue
- Time delay in obtaining second blood specimens

Nursing Implementation

Pretest

Schedule this test before any other radioisotope tests.

Obtain the patient's accurate weight and height and record them in the chart.

Because of the administration of radioisotopes, a written consent may be needed.

Explain to the patient that there will be several sets of blood samples drawn before and after the administration of the radioisotopes.

During the Test

Ensure that the patient is present and available for the second set of blood tests, which are carried out on a timed basis.

Posttest

Write the patient's height, weight, and age on the requisition slip.

If the health condition permits it, encourage the patient to drink extra fluids and to void. The half-life of the radioisotopes is only a few hours, so exposure to low-dose radiation is minimal. The radioisotopes are excreted in the urine.

TYPE AND CROSSMATCH

(BLOOD)

Synonyms:

blood compatibility testing, crossmatch

─────────────────── **NORMAL VALUES** ───────────────────

Not applicable

Background Information

Human blood is typed by group, based on the presence or absence of A,B, AB, O, and Rh antigens. Blood group A has A antigens on the erythrocytes and anti-B antibodies in the serum. Blood group B has B antigens on the erythrocytes and anti-A antibodies in the serum. Blood group AB (universal receiver) has the double set of antigens on the erythrocytes and no antibodies in the serum, whereas blood group O (universal donor) has no antigens on the erythrocytes and a double set of antibodies in the serum (Table 16–5). When Rh antigens are also present on the erythrocytes, the person is classified as Rh-positive. With no Rh antigens on the erythrocytes, the person is classified as Rh-negative.

In preparation for blood transfusion, the intended recipient's blood is tested for ABO/Rh$_o$ (D) type and antibody screening. In the crossmatch part of the test, the donor's blood type is determined and the blood is screened to identify antibodies. In selecting a donor's blood that matches that of the recipient, there must be a compatibility of antigens and antibodies so that the transfusion is safe for the recipient. Incompatibility results in agglutination and hemolysis of the erythrocytes. Incompatible blood must not be administered to the patient.

The process of typing and crossmatching the blood provides a probable compatibility between the blood of the donor and that of the recipient. Despite careful work, there is some incidence of transfusion reaction. The process of typing and crossmatch cannot detect all possible antibodies and it cannot detect reactions to components other than erythrocytes. Most cases of severe transfusion reaction are due to clerical error, including administration of the wrong unit of blood to the patient or identification of the wrong patient. Complications of a severe transfusion reaction include a shortened life span or hemolysis of the erythrocytes, anaphylaxis, or sudden death.

TABLE 16–5
ERYTHROCYTE ANTIGENS AND ANTIBODIES—ABO SYSTEM

Blood Group	Erythrocyte Antigens	Serum Antibodies
A	A	Anti-B
B	B	Anti-A
AB	AB	None
O	None	Anti-A, anti-B

Purpose of the Test

In preparation for transfusion, these tests are performed to determine the major blood groups, to screen for antibodies, and to determine the compatibility of the blood of the recipient and the potential donor.

Procedure

Intended Recipient's Blood: Two red-topped tubes and a lavender-topped tube are used to collect 7 ml of venous blood in each tube.

> **QUALITY CONTROL**
>
> To prevent hemolysis of the erythrocytes, the tourniquet must be tied lightly and for a brief time only. Venipuncture technique must be smooth, with a blood flow that fills the vacuum tube readily. If the blood has excessive turbulence because of flawed venipuncture technique, hemolysis will alter the test results.

Findings

POSITIVE CROSSMATCH

Incompatibility between the donor's and recipient's blood

NEGATIVE CROSSMATCH

Probable compatibility between the donor's and recipient's blood. The donor unit of blood is considered safe for transfusion to the recipient.

Interfering Factors

- Hemolysis
- Inadequate identification procedure

Nursing Implementation

Critical Thinking: The patient calls you over and shows you that her transfusion identification wristband has the wrong name and information on it. What are the potential complications of this error? How can you intervene so that this error is not repeated?

Pretest

Ask the intended recipient if there is history of a blood transfusion in the past 3 months. Antibodies from a previous transfusion may be present. Additional testing is needed when there is a positive antibody screen.

During the Test

When blood is to be drawn, the intended recipient must be identified with absolute certainty by the person who draws the blood:

- The intended recipient must state his or her name.
- The hospital wristband is compared with the verbal identification.

• A transfusion wristband is also applied to the recipient's wrist. This wristband contains the recipient's name, hospital identification number, and the date and initials of the phlebotomist. In some institutions, additional information includes the patient's birth date and sex, the physician's name, and the room and bed number.

• The specimen tubes and the requisition form are also labeled with the same identification information.

• The requisition form is signed by the phlebotomist, indicating that all identification information has been verified on the two wristbands and by the intended recipient.

Posttest

Once the type and crossmatch is completed, the donor blood units are available for the recipient. Donor crossmatched blood is usually held for no more than 24 hours.

Use the same, careful identification procedure when the blood is to be administered. The consequences of an error in identification are profound and can result in the death of the patient.

DIAGNOSTIC PROCEDURES

BONE MARROW EXAMINATION

(MICROSCOPY)

Synonyms:

marrow aspiration biopsy, bone marrow aspiration and biopsy

NORMAL VALUES

Normal bone marrow

Background Information

The bone marrow is responsible for hematopoiesis—the formation of blood cells. Shortly after birth, the entire medullary cavity is occupied by hematopoietic red marrow. With physical growth, the bones and the medullary spaces also increase in size, and the excess space in the medullary cavities fills with fat cells or yellow marrow. By later childhood and throughout adulthood, the only bones

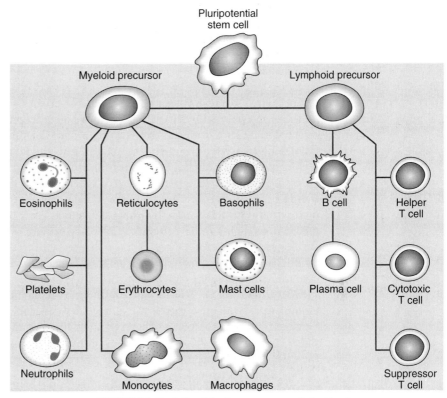

Pluripotential
stem cell

Myeloid precursor

Lymphoid precursor

Eosinophils   Reticulocytes   Basophils   B cell   Helper
T cell

Platelets   Erythrocytes   Mast cells   Plasma cell   Cytotoxic
T cell

Neutrophils   Monocytes   Macrophages   Suppressor
T cell

FIGURE 16–5. Cells of the bone marrow and the blood.

that have red marrow are the flat bones of the skull, vertebrae, shoulder, pelvis, sternum, rib cage, and proximal ends of long bones.

In the marrow, it is believed that a pluripotential cell is capable of producing more differentiated stem cells for hematopoiesis (Fig. 16–5). The lymphoid stem cells and hematopoietic stem cells evolve into a variety of committed precursor cells, based on microenvironmental factors and the presence of colony-stimulating factors (Haueber and DiJulio, 1989). Once the precursor cells are committed, blood cells proliferate and mature along specific lines. In their mature forms, cells are released from the marrow and enter the blood.

Most of the formed cells of the blood originate from hematopoietic stem cells. The hematopoietic line further differentiates into particular groups of cells of a particular line, including the granulocyte, erythroid, monocyte, and megakaryocyte lines. The mature forms of blood cells include the erythrocytes, leukocytes, and platelets.

The lymphoid stem cell and its lymphoid precursor cells produce the B lymphocytes and plasma cells. The lymphocytes are small white blood cells that carry out the activities of the immune system. In the blood, there are other cells of the immune system, but they are produced by the thymus and secondary lymphoid tissue rather than by the bone marrow.

EXAMINATION OF THE MARROW. The aspirated cells of the bone marrow are used to investigate hematologic disorders. A small sample of the cells is often representative of the whole marrow. Microscopic examination of the cells provides information about the cause, type, and extent of the abnormality. A peripheral blood smear is performed on the same day to compare and incorporate pertinent findings.

The marrow cells are examined for characteristics of the tissue. *Cellularity* indicates the proportion of aspirate that is hematopoietic cells rather than fat cells. *Distribution* provides an estimate or count of the number of each type of cell found in the marrow specimen. The marrow cells should be in proper proportion to each other, without excessive or diminished cells of a particular type. The *maturation* of the cells is also observed. Nuclear and cytoplasmic development should be in balance, without deficiency or impairment in either stage. Bizarre maturation can be caused by some leukemias and by toxicity from some medications. Some forms of anemia cause impairment of nuclear or cytoplasmic development. *Abnormal cells* refer to the presence of irregular or abnormal cells in the marrow. These include mast cells, osteoblasts, osteoclasts, and metastatic neoplastic cells (Henry, 1990).

IRON STAINING OF THE MARROW. In microcytic anemia, the bone marrow examination evaluates the iron stores and sideroblasts that are present. Sideroblasts are early forms of marrow cells that contain iron pigment. As the slides of the marrow are prepared, iron stain is applied. When iron is present in the cytoplasm, Prussian blue, a dark blue precipitate, emerges. About one third of the rubricytes should be iron-positive sideroblasts.

When the amount of iron stain in the cells is abnormally high, it is caused by excess iron storage or excess formation of sideroblasts. The underlying diseases include hemolytic or sideroblastic anemia, the anemia associated with decreased erythropoiesis, ineffective erythropoiesis, or chronic inflammatory disease. When the iron stores or number of sideroblasts is decreased, it may be due to iron deficiency anemia or the anemia of chronic disease.

ANEMIAS. In addition to microcytic anemia, the examination of the marrow can demonstrate a megaloblastic process that is associated with macrocytic anemia. In macrocytic anemia, the erythrocytes are enlarged in diameter or cell volume, or both. In normocytic anemia, without an increase in the reticulocytes in the peripheral blood, the marrow is assessed for abnormal or deficient erythropoiesis.

CYTOPENIA. When the peripheral blood demonstrates deficiencies of cells, the examination of the marrow is performed to identify the presence and quality of precursor cells. In the blood, neutropenia is the deficiency of neutrophils, thrombocytopenia is the deficiency of platelets, and pancytopenia is the overall lack of blood cells. The possible causes include decreased production, impaired maturation, or increased destruction of one or more types of precursor cell. The examination of the marrow sometimes identifies leukemia or another hematologic malignancy as the cause.

IMMUNOGLOBULINS. The infiltration of abnormal plasma cells or lymphocytes in the marrow can cause immunoglobulin abnormality. These abnormal changes in the marrow are the cause of plasma cell myeloma or macroglobinemia.

Purpose of the Test

The bone marrow aspiration and biopsy, with microscopic examination of the tissue, is used to evaluate hematopoiesis, including erythroid, myeloid, megakaryocyte, and lymphoid processes. It diagnoses malignancy of primary and metastatic origin and determines the cause of infection. The examination of the marrow also is used to evaluate the progression of some hematologic diseases or the response of the marrow to chemotherapy treatment, such as in Hodgkin disease.

Procedure

A local anesthetic is used for the procedure. In bone marrow aspiration, a bone marrow needle is inserted into the medullary cavity of a bone. Fluid and marrow cells are aspirated into a syringe. When a bone marrow biopsy is required, the biopsy needle removes a core of marrow tissue. Slides are prepared and tissue specimens are collected. When indicated, culture specimens are obtained.

The aspiration sites include the sternum, iliac crest, spinous process of the vertebrae, and proximal tibia (Fig. 16–6). In adults, the posterior iliac crest is the most common site. In infants and young children, the proximal tibia is used.

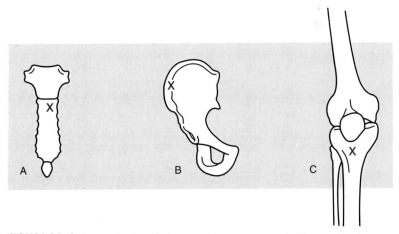

FIGURE 16–6. Anatomic sites for bone marrow aspiration. *A*, The sternum between the second and third intercostal spaces. *B*, The iliac crest on the rim or upper posterior surface. *C*, The proximal tibia about 1 to 2 inches below the patella of the infant or small child.

Findings

ABNORMAL VALUES

Iron deficiency anemia
Sideroblastic anemia
Anemia of chronic disease
Megaloblastic anemia
Macroglobulinemia
Myelofibrosis
Leukemia
Multiple myeloma
Hodgkin disease
Lymphoma
Metastatic bone cancer

Infection
  histoplasmosis
  miliary tuberculosis
  infectious mononucleosis
Agammaglobulinemia
Aplastic anemia
Collagen disease
Parasitic disease
  malaria
  leishmaniasis

Interfering Factors

• Failure to obtain an adequate specimen

Nursing Implementation

Pretest

Assess the patient for anxiety or the need for additional information. Common sources of anxiety are fear of the procedure and fear of the possible diagnosis.

Obtain a signed consent from the patient or the person who is legally responsible for the patient's health care decisions.

During the Test

Position the patient according to the site that will be biopsied. For a sternal or tibial biopsy, the supine position is used. Biopsy of the iliac crest requires a lateral recumbent or prone position. Vertebral biopsy is performed with the patient in a seated position.

Prepare the skin by shaving (as needed) and cleansing it with an antiseptic solution.

Provide support and reassurance as the local anesthetic is instilled. The patient feels brief discomfort as the needle and anesthetic solution penetrate the skin and infiltrate the periosteum.

Caution the patient to remain immobile as the biopsy needle is inserted into the marrow. Some pain is felt as the marrow is aspirated.

Assist with the preparation and labeling of the slides. The clot and biopsy tissue are placed in a sterile specimen jar that contains fixative (formalin or Zenker solution).

Once the needle is removed, apply pressure to the site, using a small sterile gauze. Once bleeding has stopped, apply a small sterile dressing. The patient with a low platelet count is prone to prolonged bleeding.

Posttest

Arrange for prompt transport of the specimens and slides to the laboratory. Reassure the patient that for a few days, mild discomfort at the biopsy site is expected. Any signs of persistent bleeding or infection should be reported to the physician.

BONE MARROW SCAN

(NUCLEAR SCAN)

The bone marrow scan uses technetium sulfur colloid (techetium-99m) to image the reticuloendothelial system of the bone marrow. Once the radioisotope is injected intravenously, it moves to the marrow because the colloid particles undergo phagocytosis by the reticuloendothelial system. In a whole body scan, the images demonstrate the presence of hematologic malignancy, bone marrow infarct, aplastic anemia, myelofibrosis, or abnormal distribution of the marrow. The scan also locates active sites of marrow tissue for biopsy purposes and identifies extramedullary sites of hematopoiesis such as the liver or spleen. When erythroid studies are desired, most procedures use radioactive indium-111 chloride isotope bound to transferrin. Active erythropoietic marrow cells absorb these tracers, and the scanning process is performed 24 to 48 hours later. Indium scans are useful in identifying aplastic anemia, myelofibrosis, and other hematologic disorders (Aburano et al., 1992).

A complete discussion of nuclear scans is presented in Chapter 10.

REFERENCES

Aburano, T., et al. (1992). Tc-99m HMPAQ-labeled leukocytes for hematopoietic marrow imaging-comparison with In-111 chloride. *Clinics in Nuclear Medicine, 17*, 938–944.

Alkire, K., et al. (1990). Physiology of blood and bone marrow. *Seminars in Oncology Nursing, 6*, 99–108.

Balaban, E.P., et al. (1993). Evaluation of bone marrow iron stores in anemia associated with chronic disease: A comparative study of serum and red cell ferritin. *American Journal of Hematology, 42*, 177–181.

Brigden, M.L. (1993). Iron deficiency anemia. Every case is instructive. *Postgraduate Medicine, 93*, 181–182, 185–192.

Bushnell, F.K.L. (1992). A guide to primary care of iron deficiency anemia. *The Nurse Practitioner, 17*, 68–74.

Campbell, T.M. (1991). Hyperleukocytosis in leukemia. *Dimensions in Oncology Nursing, 5*, 11–15.

Haeuber, D., & DiJulio, J.E. (1989). Hematopoietic colony stimulating factors: An overview. *Oncology Nursing Forum, 16*, 247–255.

Hays, K. (1990). Physiology of normal bone marrow. *Seminars in Oncology Nursing, 6*, 3–8.

Henry, J.B. (Ed). 1991. *Clinical diagnosis and management by laboratory methods* (18th ed.). Philadelphia: W.B. Saunders.

Jacobs, D.S., et al. (Eds.). (1990). *Laboratory test handbook* (2nd ed.). Baltimore: Williams & Wilkins.

Kantarjian, H.M., et al. (1992). Prognostic significance of elevated serum beta 2-microglobin levels in adult lymphocytic leukemia. *American Journal of Medicine, 93,* 599–604.

Means, R.T. (1992). Anemia: when—and how aggressively—to work it up. *Hospital Medicine 10,* 87–90, 96.

Mettler, F.A., & Guiberteau, M.J. (1991). *Essentials of nuclear medicine imaging* (3rd ed.). Philadelphia: W.B. Saunders.

Nickoloff, E. (1988). Schilling test: Physiologic basis for and use as a diagnostic test. *Critical Review Clinical Laboratory Science, 26,* 263–276.

Ranney, H.M. (1992). The spectrum of sickle cell disease. *Hospital Practice, 27,* 133–137.

Sanfillipo, F. (1991). The influence of HLA and ABO antigens on graft rejection and survival. *Clinics in Laboratory Medicine, 11,* 537–550.

Schindler, L.W. (1988). *Understanding the immune system* (NIH publication No. 88-529). Washington, D.C.: U.S. Department of Health and Human Services, Public Health Service, National Institutes of Health.

Sears, D.A. (1992). Anemia of chronic disease. *Medical Clinics of North America, 76,* 567–579.

Smith, J.A., & Kinney, T.R. (1993). Sickle cell disease: Screening and management in newborns and infants. *American Family Physicians, 48,* 95–102.

Tabbara, I.A. (1992). Hemolytic anemia. Diagnosis and management. *Medical Clinics of North America, 16,* 649–668.

Teitz, N.W. (Ed.). (1990). *Clinical guide to laboratory tests* (2nd ed.). Philadelphia: W.B. Saunders.

Unkle, D., et al. (1991). Blood antibodies and uncrossmatched type O blood. *Heart Lung, 20,* 284–286.

Workman, M.L. (1993). The immune system: Your defense partner and offensive foe. *AACN Clinical Issues in Critical Care Nursing, 4,* 453–470.

CHAPTER 17

Gastrointestinal Function

This chapter discusses the laboratory tests and diagnostic procedures that identify abnormalities in the structure and function of the alimentary canal. The organs include the esophagus, stomach, small bowel, and large bowel. Additionally, this chapter includes the tests that assess the peritoneum and peritoneal cavity.

The laboratory tests measure the specific aspects of secretion, digestion, absorption, and elimination as functions performed by the gastrointestinal tract. Additionally, tissue biopsy, culture, and microscopic examination of the secretions and fecal matter provide data about the disease process and cause of tissue damage.

Many of the diagnostic procedures use endoscopic or x-ray studies with barium to visualize the intestinal lumen and its mucosal lining. Nuclear scans also provide visualization of the alimentary tract and its function. Because these diagnostic procedures visualize segments of the intestinal tract, more than one test may be required for a complete assessment of the intestinal problem.

In addition to a diagnosis, the examiner provides descriptive data about the pathologic condition, including specific information about the length, depth, and location of the abnormality, as well as any alteration of function that is observed.

The extent of involvement is described by a specific vocabulary. A *diffuse process* involves the entire alimentary canal or an entire organ, such as the colon. A *regional process* involves a complete portion of an organ, such as the ileum of the small bowel. A *focal process* involves a small area, such as a single lesion in the cecum.

The depth of the pathologic condition refers to the penetration of the disease process into the various layers of intestinal tissue. The alimentary tract consists of four layers of tissue. From the lumen outward, the layers are the mucosa, submucosa, muscularis, and adventitia or serosa. A lesion, therefore, may involve only the mucosal layer or may penetrate more deeply into the submucosal or muscularis layers. A *transmural lesion* involves all four layers of the tissue wall.

The diameter of the lumen of the alimentary tract can be altered by a pathologic condition. Narrowing or obstruction of the lumen may be caused by inflammation, edema, strictures, stenosis, adhesions, or twisting (volvulus) of the intestinal tissue. Altered neuromuscular function can dilate or relax tissue walls, with a resultant widening of a portion of the bowel and loss of peristaltic activity. Depending on the extent of the disease process, alteration of the size of the lumen affects the passage of food, fluid, gas, and fecal matter through the intestinal tract.

Malignant growths in the intestinal tract incorporate all these dimensions. Cancerous tumors tend to grow inward, narrowing the lumen. As they grow, they also extend in length. Additionally, the depth of tissue involvement increases and the tumor may become a transmural lesion or even break out beyond the tissue border to spill into the peritoneal cavity or extend into a contiguous organ.

LABORATORY TESTS

CA 19-9

(SERUM)

Synonym:
carbohydrate antigen 19-9

NORMAL VALUES

Adult: <37 U/ml *or* SI <37 kU/L

Background Information

Determination of CA 19-9, an oncofetal antigen, is a new test that is potentially useful as a tumor marker. This antigen appears in the serum of adults when (1) the cells of particular organs undergo healing and regeneration and (2) there is proliferation of malignant cells in tumors that are known to produce the antigen. In benign disease, the serum value rises mildly and is usually less than 100 U/ml. In malignant conditions, the level is much higher.

Purpose of the Test

CA 19-9 is a tumor marker that monitors the course of the disease and the success of therapy and predicts the recurrence of stomach, liver, pancreatic, and colorectal cancer. Because of its low sensitivity and specificity, CA 19-9 is not used as a screening tool for asymptomatic patients.

Procedure

A red-topped tube with a serum separator is used to obtain 5 to 10 ml of venous blood.

Findings

ELEVATED VALUES

Malignancy	Benign Conditions
Intraabdominal cancer	Inflammatory bowel disease
Cancer of the pancreas	Acute pancreatitis
Cancer of the stomach	Hepatobiliary disease
Cancer of the colon	
Hepatobiliary cancer	

Interfering Factors

• None

Nursing Implementation

No specific patient instruction or intervention is needed.

CARCINOEMBRYONIC ANTIGEN

(SERUM, EFFUSION FLUID)

Synonym:
CEA

NORMAL VALUES

Adult Nonsmoker: <2.5 ng/ml *or* SI 2.5 µg/L
Adult Smoker: up to 5 ng/mL *or* SI 5 µg/L

Background Information

Carcinoembryonic antigen is an oncofetal antigen that is present in the fetus. In the adult circulation, however, it is present only in minute amounts. When the antigen appears in the adult circulation, it indicates (1) a response to healing and regeneration of cells of particular tissues or (2) malignancy. In cancer, necrosis of the malignant tissue permits the antigen to escape through damaged cell membranes.

In benign disorders, the serum value rarely rises to greater than 10 ng/ml, whereas in malignant conditions, the serum value is greater than 10 ng/ml. Smokers have elevated values without necessarily having a benign or malignant condition.

This test has low specificity regarding the site of disease and the differentiation between benign and malignant growth. It cannot, therefore, be used as a screening tool. In patients who do have a malignancy that secretes carcinoembryonic antigen, sequential determinations are useful to provide early detection of recurrent disease. The carcinoembryonic antigen levels rise months to years before there is clinical evidence of metastasis.

Purpose of the Test

Carcinoembryonic antigen is a tumor marker used to (1) monitor the success of cancer therapy, (2) stage colorectal cancer, and (3) monitor for recurrence of cancer in the gastrointestinal tract, particularly colorectal cancer (Massoni, 1990). The increase in values serves as an indicator for further diagnostic testing.

Procedure

A red-topped or lavender-topped tube is used to collect 5 to 10 ml of venous blood. There should be no heparin or ethylenediaminetetraacetic acid in the tube.

The schedule for testing and monitoring the patient's condition follows: presurgery, 4 weeks postoperatively, monthly for 1 to 2 years, and at regular intervals thereafter for a total testing time of 5 years.

QUALITY CONTROL

Venipuncture technique must be smooth, with a blood flow that fills the vacuum tube readily. If the blood has excessive turbulence because of flawed venipuncture technique, the hemolysis of the erythrocytes will alter the test results.

The serum must be chilled immediately and radioimmunoassay analysis performed within 24 hours. If there is a delay, the serum must be frozen to −20° C immediately.

Findings

ELEVATED VALUES

Malignant Conditions	Benign Conditions
Colorectal cancer	Ulcerative colitis
Stomach cancer	Crohn disease
Pancreatic cancer	Hepatitis
Breast cancer	Cirrhosis
Lung cancer	Pulmonary infection
Thyroid medullary cancer	
Ovarian cancer	
Metastatic disease (liver, bone, lung)	

Interfering Factors

- Recent administration of radioisotopes
- Smoking
- Heparin
- Hemolysis

Nursing Implementation

Pretest

Schedule any radioisotope study shortly after this test is performed.
If the patient is a smoker, indicate this information on the requisition slip.

Posttest

The serum sample is packed in a container with ice and is sent directly to the laboratory.

D-XYLOSE ABSORPTION TEST

(WHOLE BLOOD, URINE)   *Synonym:*

xylose tolerance test

Background Information

Malabsorption and steatorrhea may originate from two different sources of pathophysiologic change. One is a luminal defect of the small bowel. This source of malabsorption may involve pancreatic disease, loss of bile salts, or Crohn disease. The other category is a disorder caused by a defect in the epithelium or membrane of the small bowel. This source of malabsorption may involve

━━━━━━━━━━━━ **NORMAL VALUES** ━━━━━━━━━━━━

Urine
Child: 16–33% of ingested dose/5 hours *or* SI 0.16–0.33 (fraction of ingested dose)
Adult (5-g dose): >1.2 g/5 hours *or* SI >8.00 mmol/L/5 hours
Adult (25-g dose): >4 g/5 hours *or* SI >26.64 mmol/L
Adult >65 years: 3.5 g/5 hours *or* SI >23.31 mmol/L
Whole Blood
Child (1 hour): >30 mg/dl *or* SI >2.0 mmol/L
Adult (2 hours, 5-g dose): >20 mg/dl *or* SI >1.33 mmol/L
Adult (2 hours, 25 mg/dl): >25 mg/dl *or* SI >1.67 mmol/L

gluten-sensitive enteropathy, celiac disease, or Whipple disease. The D-xylose absorption test is used to investigate the cause of malabsorption and steatorrhea and helps to determine the origin of the problem.

D-Xylose is a carbohydrate (a pentose sugar) that does not require pancreatic enzymes for its absorption. In normal patients and in those with a lumen disorder such as pancreatic disease, a portion of ingested D-xylose is absorbed by the duodenum and jejunum and can be recovered later in the blood and urine.

When the amount of recovered D-xylose is less than normal, the most likely cause is malabsorption caused by an epithelial or membrane disorder of the upper small bowel. Since there is more than one disease that may cause this change, a follow-up endoscopic biopsy of small bowel tissue will be needed to make the diagnosis.

PHYSIOLOGIC BASIS OF THE TEST. Following a measured dose of D-xylose ingested orally, a portion should be absorbed by the duodenum and jejunum. The sugar reaches the blood stream in 30 to 60 minutes and the blood level is sustained for up to 2 hours. Thereafter, this sugar is filtered from the blood by the kidney. Within 5 hours, 16 to 23% of the initial dose should appear in the urine (Jacobs et al., 1990).

The D-xylose test is most accurate when both serum and urine specimens are analyzed at timed intervals. The accuracy of the test is dependent on the rate of absorption by the intestine and the rate of excretion by the kidneys. These and numerous other variables can interfere with the accuracy of the test results.

Purpose of the Test

This test is used to investigate the cause of steatorrhea, to diagnose malabsorption syndrome, and to evaluate the functional ability of the duodenum and jejunum in the digestion of carbohydrates.

Procedure

Critical Thinking: The D-xylose test is underway. The 4-year-old patient had the morning blood tests, but she is now so upset that she will not drink the D-xylose solution. How can the nurse obtain the cooperation of the child?

To verify adequate renal function, blood specimens for blood urea nitrogen and creatinine determinations are drawn, and a urinalysis is obtained in the early morning before the D-xylose test begins.

The recommended dose of D-xylose for adults and children older than 12 years of age is 25 g mixed in 250 ml of water. For children younger than 12 years of age, the recommended dose is 5 g or 0.5 g/kg of body weight.

A red-topped tube is used to collect 5 to 10 ml of venous blood for each specimen. In most institutions, a single blood sample is obtained 1 hour after the D-xylose is ingested. In some institutions, serial samples are obtained at 30, 60, and 120 minutes after the D-xylose is ingested.

For adults and children older than 12 years of age, all urine is collected for 5 hours.

For geriatric patients, those with some renal insufficiency, and infants or children younger than 12 years of age, the test may be limited to a single blood sample after 1 hour, with no urine collection.

QUALITY CONTROL

The full 25-g dose of D-xylose for adults is preferred because it will help detect less severe conditions. This dose, however, can cause diarrhea and vomiting. Hypermotility of the intestine interferes with absorption and results in lower than normal values.

Findings

DECREASED VALUES

Malabsorption Syndromes

Tropical sprue
Nontropical sprue (celiac disease, gluten-sensitive enteropathy)
Whipple disease
Amyloidosis
Scleroderma
Small bowel ischemia

Lymphoma
Parasitic disease (hookworm, schistosomiasis, *Giardia lamblia*)
Gastroenteritis
Zollinger-Ellison syndrome
Radiation enteritis

Interfering Factors

• Failure to maintain pretest dietary restrictions
• Physical activity during the test
• Poor renal function
• Ascites
• Vomiting or diarrhea
• Rapid or delayed gastric emptying
• Hypomotility or intestinal stasis
• Dehydration and hypovolemia

Nursing Implementation

Pretest

Instruct the patient of the following regarding preparation for the test:

- The patient should discontinue all foods that contain pentose sugar (fruits, jellies, jams) for 24 hours before the test.
- The patient should discontinue all medications for 24 hours before the test (if possible).
- Adults should refrain from ingestion of all food for 8 hours (children for 4 hours) before the test. Water intake is permitted and encouraged.

Ensure that early morning blood urea nitrogen, creatinine, and urinalysis results are posted in the patient's chart.

During the Test

At 8 A.M., the patient drinks the prescribed dose of D-xylose mixed in 250 ml of water. This is followed by another 250 ml of water. At 9 A.M., a third 250 ml of water is taken, with water intake as desired thereafter.

Instruct the patient to maintain bed rest in a supine position throughout the test period.

The patient voids at 8 A.M., and this specimen is discarded. For the next 5 hours, all urine specimens are collected, using a brown or dark container. The urine is kept refrigerated.

After ingestion of the D-xylose, observe for vomiting or diarrhea. Notify the physician and laboratory of the problem.

QUALITY CONTROL

Hypermotility of the intestinal tract, physical activity, vomiting, and failure to collect all urine specimens can result in invalid test results.

Posttest

All blood specimens are labeled, including the time and date of each sample.

The refrigerated urine container is also labeled, including the time and date of the start and finish of the collection period.

The specimens are sent to the laboratory immediately. This prevents warming by the temperature of the room.

GASTRIC ANALYSIS

(GASTRIC SECRETION)

Synonyms:

tube gastric analysis, pentagastrin stimulation test, gastric acid stimulation test

━━━━━━━━━━━━━━━━━━ **NORMAL VALUES** ━━━━━━━━━━━━━━━━━━

pH:	<2 *or* SI <2
Basal Acid Output (BAO):	**Male:** 4.2 mEq/hour *or* SI 4.2 mmol/hour **Female:** 1.8 mEq/hour *or* SI 1.8 mmol/hour
Maximal Acid Output (MAO):	**Male:** 22.6 mEq/hour *or* SI 22.6 mmol/hour **Female:** 15.2 mEq/hour *or* SI 15.2 mmol/hour
Peak Acid Output (PAO):	**Male:** 35 mEq/hour *or* SI 35 mmol/hour **Female:** 25 mEq/hr *or* SI 25 mmol/hour
BAO:MAO Ratio:	<0.4 (40%) *or* SI <0.4 (40%)

Background Information

Gastric analysis is a laboratory measurement of the acid content of gastric secretions. The secretions are obtained by aspiration of the stomach contents via a nasogastric tube. There are two phases of the test: basal acid output (BAO) and maximal acid output (MAO). The BAO is obtained with the patient in a resting state. Four 15-minute collections of gastric secretions are carried out in the first hour of the test. The patient is then given an injection of pentagastrin to stimulate the secretory flow of the gastric acids. Following the injection, the MAO is obtained from four 15-minute collections of gastric secretions. The MAO represents gastric acid collection while the stomach is at maximal ability to secrete acid.

The peak acid output (PAO) is a mathematical calculation based on the analysis of the two 15-minute specimens with the highest acid values. The BAO:MAO ratio is a numeric comparison of the results obtained at rest and after stimulation.

Because of different methods of collection and analysis, there is a rather wide range of normal values. Males, however, have higher acid values than do females, and aging results in lower acid values.

Patients who have marginal ulcers or duodenal ulcers tend to have higher than normal acid output. Patients who have gastric cancer or gastric ulcers tend to have lower than normal acid output. Gastric analysis is used to support the diagnosis but cannot be used as the sole measure to confirm the diagnosis.

In Zollinger-Ellison syndrome (gastrinoma), there is massive acid hypersecretion. Additionally, the BAO:MAO ratio is elevated beyond 0.6 (60%). These patients have a continuously high BAO, causing the ratio to rise. The MAO does not rise after stimulation because the gastric secretory cells are already producing at maximal capacity.

The normal pH of gastric secretions ranges from 1.5 to 3.5 as the measure of acidity. When the pH value is greater than 6 after maximal stimulation, the condition is called *anacidity*. This is a supportive finding in the diagnosis of pernicious anemia.

The gastric analysis test with pentagastrin stimulation replaces the nocturnal acid output gastric analysis test, the histamine analysis test, and the tubeless gastric analysis test.

The gastric analysis test has its own problems associated with accuracy in the technique of specimen collection and the methods of analysis. Because of these problems, the gastric analysis test is rarely performed today. Gastric biopsy specimens using a fiberoptic gastroscope and serum gastrin radioimmunoassay techniques are reliable and accurate alternatives.

Purpose of the Test

Gastric analysis is used to evaluate the ability of the stomach to produce acid secretions in a resting state and after maximal stimulation.

Procedure

Critical Thinking: The nasogastric tube is in place, but at the start of the procedure no gastric secretions are aspirated by intermittent intestinal suction. What can the nurse do to investigate and correct the problem?

The nasogastric tube is passed into the stomach until the tip of the tube rests in the distal portion of the stomach. Secretion removal is performed by manual aspiration with a Toomey syringe or machine aspiration with intermittent intestinal suction.

BASAL ACID OUTPUT PHASE. Secretions are removed during four 15-minute consecutive intervals. The secretions of each collection interval are stored in separate containers and labeled correspondingly, as "BAO 1," "BAO 2," and so on. On completion of the first hour of specimen collection, the MAO phase begins.

MAXIMAL ACID OUTPUT. The patient is given a subcutaneous injection of pentagastrin (Peptavlon), 6 mcg/kg of body weight. The medication stimulates gastric acid secretion. In the next hour, four more specimens are collected for 15-minute intervals each. The containers are labeled correspondingly, as "MAO 1," "MAO 2," and so forth.

QUALITY CONTROL

The proper placement of the tip of the nasogastric tube in the distal portion of the stomach may be confirmed by fluoroscopy. This helps ensure complete collection of gastric acids and avoids inadvertent collection of bile from the duodenum.

Findings

ELEVATED VALUES

Zollinger-Ellison syndrome
Retained antrum syndrome
G cell hyperplasia
Duodenal ulcers

Vagal hyperfunction
Basophilic leukemia
Systemic mastocytosis

DECREASED VALUES

Pernicious anemia
Cancer of the stomach
Myxedema

Gastric ulcer
Chronic gastritis
Postsurgical antrectomy or vagotomy

Interfering Factors

- Failure to maintain a nothing-by-mouth status
- Failure to collect a complete sample of secretions
- Esophageal disease, aortic aneurysm
- Gastric hemorrhage

Nursing Implementation

Pretest

Explain the procedure to the patient so that fear and apprehension are minimized.

Obtain an informed consent from the patient or the person designated to make health care decisions for the patient.

For 24 hours before the test, alcohol, tobacco, and medications that affect gastric acid secretion are discontinued.

Food is discontinued for 12 hours and water is discontinued for 8 hours before the test. Until the test is completed, the sight and smell of food is avoided.

QUALITY CONTROL

Psychologic, physiologic, and environmental stimuli are reduced to avoid additional gastric acid secretion and to improve the reliability of the test results.

During the Test

To collect the secretions with a Toomey syringe, aspirate gently every 5 minutes.

After administration of pentagastrin, assess for side effects of nausea, dizziness, headache, tachycardia, palpitations, and diaphoresis. If they occur, they should be mild and of short duration.

Posttest

Remove the nasogastric tube and allow the patient to resume eating.

Ensure that each specimen container has a lid and is labeled appropriately.

GASTRIN

(SERUM)

Synonyms:

—————————————— **NORMAL VALUES** ——————————————

Male Adult (16–60 Years):	<100 pg/ml or SI <100 ng/L
Female Adult (16–60 Years):	<75 pg/ml or SI <75 ng/L
Adult (>60 Years):	>100 pg/ml or SI >100 ng/L
Child:	<10–125 pg/ml or SI <10–125 ng/L
Infant (0–4 Days):	120–183 pg/ml or SI 120–183 ng/L

Background Information

The two forms of gastrin in the blood are G-34 (big gastrin) and G-14 (little gastrin). They are also called gastrin I and gastrin II, respectively. The gastrins are small but powerful peptides that stimulate gastric and pancreatic secretion.

The gastrins are produced primarily by the G cells in the antrum of the stomach. Once manufactured, the gastrins are first secreted into the blood stream and then return to the body of the stomach where they stimulate gastric acid production, antral motility, and the secretion of pepsin and intrinsic factor. The gastrins also stimulate pancreatic acinar and ductular cell secretions.

Gastrin secretion is increased by vagal stimulation and inhibited by the presence of hydrochloric acid. The normal gastrin levels fluctuate daily in a circadian rhythm cycle and in relationship to meals.

Purpose of the Test

The radioimmunoassay of serum gastrin is a helpful adjunctive test to diagnose Zollinger-Ellison syndrome and pernicious anemia.

Procedure

A red-topped tube, without anticoagulant, is used to collect 5 to 10 ml of venous blood.

Findings

ELEVATED VALUES

Zollinger-Ellison syndrome   Chronic atrophic gastritis
Pernicious anemia   Gastric ulcer
Antral G cell hyperplasia   Vagotomy without gastric resection
Pyloric obstruction   Chronic renal failure
Gastric cancer

DECREASED VALUES

Antrectomy with vagotomy   Hypothyroidism

Interfering Factors

- Failure to maintain a nothing-by-mouth status
- Recent radioisotope administration
- Gastroscopy
- Heparin anticoagulant in the vacuum tube

Nursing Implementation

Pretest

Schedule this test before gastroscopy and any radioisotope procedures. Instruct the patient to discontinue all food intake for at least 12 hours before the test.

QUALITY CONTROL

Recent ingestion of protein causes an elevation of the serum gastrin level.

Posttest

Ensure that the specimen is sent to the laboratory without delay.

QUALITY CONTROL

Gastrin is unstable at room temperature, and delay will cause invalid results. In the laboratory, the serum is separated out by refrigerated centrifuge and the specimen is frozen immediately.

5-HYDROXYINDOLEACETIC ACID, QUANTITATIVE

(URINE)

Synonyms:

5-HIAA; 5-HIAA, quantitative, urine

NORMAL VALUES

Adult: 1–7 mg/24 hours *or* SI 5–37 µmol/24 hours

Background Information

5-Hyroxyindoleacetic acid (5-HIAA) is a urinary metabolite of serotonin. The elevated value serves as a marker for malignancy. The parent hormone, serotonin, and this urinary metabolite are produced by most carcinoid tumors.

TABLE 17–1
CLASSIFICATION OF CARCINOID TUMORS

Intestinal Classification	Anatomic Location
Foregut carcinoid tumors	Bronchus, stomach, duodenum, pancreas
Midgut carcinoid tumors	Jejunum, ileum, ascending colon
Transverse carcinoid tumors	Transverse colon, descending colon, rectum

Carcinoid tumors are neuroendocrine tumors that arise from neural crest cells. During fetal development, these neural crest cells migrate to many organs throughout the body. If they become malignant in later life, they are classified as neuroendocrine tumors because they secrete hormones. In addition to serotonin secretion, carcinoid tumors of the foregut may also secrete adrenocorticotropic hormone, insulin, growth hormone, calcitonin, and gastrin.

One method of classifying carcinoid tumors is by their anatomic location in the intestinal tract (Table 17–1). Some of these tumors remain small, and although they secrete serotonin and the 5-HIAA metabolite, they cause no problems. Others, however, become aggressive. They increase in size, hormone output, and 5-HIAA output; they can metastasize to distant sites of the bone, brain, cervical nodes, and liver.

Purpose of the Test

The quantitative measure of 5-HIAA in the urine is used to diagnose carcinoid tumor and provide ongoing evaluation of the stability of the tumor mass.

Procedure

For a 24-hour period, all urine is collected in a large container.

QUALITY CONTROL

The bottled specimen is cooled in the refrigerator during the collection period. Once a preservative is added, the specimen can be stored in the laboratory for 2 weeks at 4° C.

Findings

ELEVATED VALUES

Midgut carcinoids
Foregut carcinoids
Ovarian carcinoids
Tropical sprue
Celiac disease

Whipple disease
Oat cell carcinoma of the bronchus
Cystic fibrosis
Chronic intestinal obstruction

DECREASED VALUES

Mental depression
Mastocytosis
Hartnap disease

Small bowel resection
Phenylketonuria

Interfering Factors

- Numerous foods that contain serotonin
- Numerous medications that react with the laboratory reagent

Nursing Implementation

Pretest

Instruct the patient to avoid all foods that are high in serotonin for 48 hours before the test. These foods falsely elevate the test results and include avocados, tomatoes, bananas, plums, walnuts, pineapples, and eggplant. For 48 hours before the test, discontinue all medications that interfere with the analysis procedure because they falsely elevate the results.

QUALITY CONTROL

The specific medication list depends on the method of laboratory analysis. To identify these medications, the nurse should call the laboratory beforehand.

During the Test

For the 24-hour period of urine collection, the container is kept in the refrigerator.

Posttest

Arrange for transport of the cooled specimen immediately.

LACTOSE TOLERANCE TEST

(BLOOD, URINE, FECES)

Synonym:
oral lactose tolerance test

Background Information

Lactose is a disaccharide that is present in milk and milk products. For absorption to occur, the lactose is hydrolyzed in the small intestine by the enzyme lactase. As a result, the lactose disaccharide is split into the monosaccharides

──────────── **NORMAL VALUES** ────────────

Adult
Blood Glucose: 20–30 mg/dl *or* SI 1.1–1.7 mmol/L
Urine Lactose (24-hour): 12–40 mg/dl *or* SI 0.7–2.2 mmol/L
Feces: pH 7–8; glucose <1+
Child
Urine Lactose (24-hour): <1.5 mg/100 dl

glucose and galactose. These simple sugars are then absorbed through the microvilli and pass into the portal venous system by diffusion.

In the normal physiology of lactose metabolism, the absorption results in a slight rise in blood glucose, with small amounts of lactose present in the urine and small amounts of glucose present in the feces. The feces are normal in consistency and color; they are neutral or alkaline in pH measurement.

When lactase is deficient, the lactose disaccharide cannot be absorbed and this sugar remains in the intestine. The sugar attracts water into the bowel lumen, causing osmotic diarrhea. Bacterial fermentation causes bloating, cramps, gas formation, and abdominal distention.

Lactose intolerance–lactase deficiency may be congenital and can affect the neonate as soon as the ingestion of milk begins. It also may be an acquired condition that develops in later life, or it can be caused by intestinal disease that damages the tissue integrity of the microvilli in the small bowel.

Critical Thinking: The Korean patient has lactose intolerance as verified by the laboratory results. In your nutritional teaching, which alternative foods can be substituted for milk? Are cultural food preferences included in your plan?

The basis of the lactose tolerance test is to provide an oral source of lactose to the fasting patient. In lactose tolerance–lactase deficiency, the serial blood samples will show a flat glucose curve rather than the mild elevation that is expected. Higher levels of lactose appear in the urine within 24 hours. The fecal matter changes to watery, greenish yellow diarrhea, and the feces are acidic and positive for glucose.

This test has a 20% incidence of error, with findings that are either falsely positive or falsely negative. Additionally, some lactose-intolerant patients demonstrate normal test findings (Jacobs et al., 1990).

Purpose of the Test

This test identifies lactose intolerance–lactase insufficiency. It is used in the work-up for abdominal distention, chronic diarrhea, and abdominal cramps associated with the ingestion of milk. It is also used to investigate the cause of malabsorption syndrome.

Procedure

The fasting patient takes an oral dose of lactose with 200 to 300 ml of water. The usual dose is 50 g or 0.75 to 1.5 g/kg of body weight, but a smaller dose is used for children or for patients suspected of having severe disease. Diagnostic results are obtained from the analysis of serial blood samples, a 24-hour urine collection, or a sample of feces. In some cases, the blood test may be combined with either the urine test or the stool test.

Blood: Gray-topped (fluoride) tubes or capillary tubes are used to collect small venous samples that include the fasting, baseline specimen and additional specimens at timed intervals (30, 60, 120, 180, and 240 minutes).

Urine: After ingestion of the lactose, all urine specimens are collected in a glass container for 24 hours.

Feces: Five hours after ingestion of lactose, a stool sample is collected in a clean, dry container.

Findings

POSITIVE VALUES

Lactose intolerance–lactase insufficiency
Ulcerative colitis
Jejunitis
Giardiasis
Whipple disease
Viral or bacterial bowel infection
Crohn disease
Small bowel resection
Nontropical sprue
Tropical sprue
Cystic fibrosis
Abetalipoproteinemia

Interfering Factors

- Failure to maintain dietary and exercise restrictions
- Delayed emptying of the stomach
- Vomiting
- Diabetes mellitus

Nursing Implementation

Pretest

Instruct the patient regarding the following pretest restrictions:

- No food intake for 8 hours before or during the test
- No smoking or gum chewing before or during the test

QUALITY CONTROL

Alterations in gastric motility and gastric emptying will affect the rate of absorption and alter test results.

During the Test

Assess for any signs of watery diarrhea, abdominal cramps, or nausea because the lactose dosage can exacerbate symptoms.

Notify the physician of any vomiting, since this could affect the amount and rate of lactose absorption.

Some laboratories require activity restriction during the test. This can be verified by the laboratory personnel.

Posttest

After 4 hours, when the blood work is completed, the patient can resume activity and diet.

Remind the patient to continue with collection of the urine for 24 hours and to collect a fecal specimen in the fifth hour of the test, as prescribed.

QUALITY CONTROL

All tubes and containers must be labeled and include the date and time of each specimen collection. This is because the blood glucose levels will vary during the test period. The laboratory slip should indicate the time of lactose administration as well as the times of specimen collection.

OCCULT BLOOD

(FECES)

Synonyms:

blood, occult, stool; Colo-Rect; Colo-Screen; Hema-Check; Hemoccult II; Quick-Cult

—————————————— **NORMAL VALUES** ——————————————

Negative for occult blood

Background Information

Occult blood refers to blood that is present in the feces but is not visible. The feces are unchanged in color and consistency despite the presence of blood. In some cases, the blood is occult because the amount is too small to be seen. In other cases, there is a slow but steady leakage of blood that mixes with the feces. Generally, the source of occult bleeding is somewhere within the proximal gastrointestinal tract, rather than outlet bleeding from rectal or anal tissue.

In contrast to occult bleeding, a loss of 50 to 75 ml or more of blood in the lumen of the upper gastrointestinal tract changes the color and consistency of feces to a dark red or black, tarry stool. Approximately the same quantity of bleeding in the lower intestinal tract changes the feces to black with a tarry quality, or streaked with bright red blood. In both cases, the larger amount of blood is visible and the term "occult blood" does not apply.

Whenever blood enters the lumen of the intestinal tract, it will ultimately appear in the feces. Slightly more than one half of the bleeding sites are in the upper gastrointestinal tract, including the esophagus, stomach, and duodenum. Just less than one half of the sites are in the lower gastrointestinal tract, including the colon and rectum. Few bleeding episodes originate in the jejunum or ileum (Henry, 1991).

There are a number of commercial tests available to detect occult blood, but there are problems with validity of the results. One source of the high incidence of false-positive and false-negative results is that normal individuals lose up to 2 to 2.5 mg/g of blood in the feces daily. Tests that are sensitive enough to detect small quantities of blood have a higher incidence of false-positive results. Tests that are less sensitive to small amounts of blood have a higher incidence of false-negative results. Other factors that affect the accuracy of the test results are the proportion of blood per volume of stool, the water content of the stool, flawed technique of stool collection, and the pretest dietary regimen (Jacobs et al., 1990).

Most of the tests of fecal occult blood are based on chemical detection of the enzyme activity of peroxidase or pseudoperoxidase present in erythrocytes, hemoglobin, and myoglobin. Dietary intake of meat will cause false-positive results because it contains both hemoglobin and protein. Ascorbic acid (vitamin C) depresses peroxidase activity; dietary intake of this vitamin causes false-negative results. Some medications and alcohol irritate the intestinal mucosa and cause their own source of occult blood. The fecal occult blood test replaces the outdated stool for guaiac test.

Despite the difficulties with fecal occult blood tests, positive results are taken seriously. If any one of the three specimens contains occult blood, the test is considered positive. Because of the potential risk of cancer, particularly in the colon, physicians recommend that a positive fecal occult blood test be followed up with a routine colonoscopy or barium enema. As illustrated in Figure 17–1, benign polyps, arteriovenous malformations, and cancer are among the more common causes of occult blood in the lower gastrointestinal tract (Church, 1992).

Purpose of the Test

This test detects fecal occult blood from a gastrointestinal source and is used as a screening tool for an early diagnosis of bowel cancer.

Procedure

Three different stool specimens are collected in plastic containers.

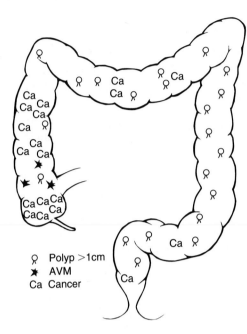

♀ Polyp >1cm
✱ AVM
Ca Cancer

FIGURE 17–1. Sites of occult bleeding in the colon. Cancer, benign polyps, and arteriovenous malformations are three causes of occult bleeding. Their location and characteristic pathologic features are identified in follow-up colonoscopy. (Reproduced with permission from Church, J.M. [1992]. Colonoscopy for the diagnosis and treatment of colorectal bleeding. *Seminars in Colon and Rectal Surgery, 3,* 43.)

Findings

POSITIVE VALUES

Esophageal varices
Mallory-Weiss tears
Hiatal hernia
Gastritis
Peptic ulcer
Crohn disease
Kaposi sarcoma

Dysentery
Parasitic disease
Diverticular disease
Benign polyps of the colon
Arteriovenous malformation of the colon
Hemorrhagic disease
Intussusception

Interfering Factors

- Dietary: recent intake of animal protein, vegetable peroxidase, and vitamin C
- Failure to refrigerate the specimen

Nursing Implementation

Pretest

Instruct the patient to avoid the following foods for 2 to 3 days before the test and during the test period: red meat, chicken, fish, turnips, and horseradish. Citrus juice can be taken in limited quantity only.

Inform the patient to discontinue aspirin, nonsteroidal antiinflammatory drugs, and alcohol until the test is completed.

QUALITY CONTROL

The animal protein and vegetables add to the peroxidase measured in the test. The ascorbic acid inhibits the peroxidase activity. These alterations falsely affect test results.

Instruct the patient regarding correct collection procedure (see also Chapter 2). Three separate stool specimens are placed in plastic containers with lids. The specimens are refrigerated until taken to the laboratory.

SEROTONIN

(BLOOD)

Synonym:

5-Hydroxytryptamine, blood

NORMAL VALUES

50–175 ng/ml *or* SI 0.28–0.99 µmol/L (Tietz, 1992)
Values vary among laboratories, depending on the method of analysis.

Background Information

Serotonin is a hormone that is normally present in many tissues of the body. When it is present in the blood, the serotonin is concentrated in platelets and is released during coagulation processes. Specific cells in the gastrointestinal mucosa provide one source of serotonin production.

Carcinoid tumors are malignant growths that secrete excess serotonin. They cause carcinoid syndrome, with symptoms of flushing, diarrhea, cardiac valvular disease, bronchoconstriction, and hepatomegaly. Primary carcinoids are usually located in the ileum or stomach, but they may also be located in the pancreas, duodenum, bronchus, and ovary. These malignancies may also grow aggressively and metastasize to the liver, brain, bone, and cervical glands.

Purpose of the Test

The blood level of serotonin is used to diagnose carcinoid syndrome and to detect carcinoid tumor in patients who have normal or borderline 5-HIAA laboratory values.

Procedure

A chilled vacuum tube that contains ethylenediaminetetraacetic acid and sometimes ascorbic acid is used to collect 5 to 10 ml of venous blood. Laboratory policy will determine the specific tube and preservative, based on the method of analysis used.

Findings

ELEVATED VALUES
Carcinoid syndrome
Abdominal carcinoid tumor with metastases
Dumping syndrome
Acute intestinal obstruction
Cystic fibrosis
Acute myocardial infarction
Celiac disease

DECREASED VALUES

Down syndrome
Phenylketonuria (untreated)
Parkinson disease
Severe mental depression

Interfering Factors

- Monoamine oxidase inhibitors
- Radioisotopes
- Foods rich in serotonin

Nursing Implementation

Pretest

Schedule this test before any scans or other tests that use radioisotopes. The radioisotopes would interfere with the radioimmunoassay method of analysis.

Monoamine oxidase inhibitors should be discontinued for 1 week before the test because they elevate the serum level of serotonin.

Some laboratory methods require several days of avoidance of foods that are rich in serotonin (avocado, banana, eggplant, and tomato).

Posttest

Pack the blood sample in ice and arrange for immediate transport of the specimen to the laboratory.

QUALITY CONTROL

Because serotonin is unstable, the collection tube must contain the proper preservative and be chilled on ice before and after the test.

In the laboratory, the blood sample will be analyzed immediately or frozen for storage within 4 hours.

DIAGNOSTIC PROCEDURES

BARIUM ENEMA

(RADIOLOGY)

Synonyms:

NORMAL VALUES

No lesions, deficits, or abnormalities of the colon are noted.

Background Information

Barium enema is a basic radiographic test that is performed when disease of the large bowel is suspected. It is used to investigate the cause of a change in elimination patterns, melena, obstruction of the colon, or the presence of an abdominal mass that has a suspected location in the colon.

Barium serves as an excellent contrast medium because it is radiopaque, has a different density than body tissue, and can be instilled into hollow organs such as the colon (Fig. 17–2). It coats the mucosa with a thin layer of contrast medium so that x-rays provide a clear view of the interior surfaces. In a barium enema, the entire colon and the distal portion of the ileum can be visualized.

When barium is the only contrast material used, the technique is called a single-contrast study. A double-contrast technique uses barium in conjunction with air as the contrast medium. After barium is instilled, the air is introduced

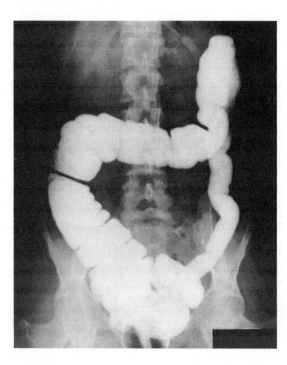

FIGURE 17–2. Barium enema. Radiopaque barium sulfate fills the colon in this lower gastrointestinal study. (Reproduced with permission from Adler, A.M., & Carlton, R.R. [1994]. *Introduction to radiography and patient care* [vol. 1, Slide 200]. Philadelphia: W.B. Saunders.)

by insufflation. The air dilates the lumen and provides a clearer view of the mucosal surface. During the barium enema procedure, fluoroscopy is used to monitor filling by the contrast medium and guide the selection of areas that require x-ray filming.

If it is suspected that colonic perforation or fistula exists, this test is either contraindicated or is performed cautiously using a water-soluble contrast medium. Ulcerative colitis, severe diverticulitis, acute bloody diarrhea, or pneumatosis cystoides intestinalis all have potential complications, such as perforation of the bowel. If barium enters the venous circulation via ulcerated mucosa, cardiac arrest will occur.

Purpose of the Test

The barium enema is used to investigate and identify pathologic conditions that change the structure or function of the colon.

Procedure

After the colon is completely emptied of feces, the contrast medium is instilled. The patient's positional changes (supine, prone, lateral) are used to enhance the gravity flow of the contrast material throughout the entire colon. Fluoroscopic and x-ray images are taken to identify the abnormalities. The procedure takes approximately 45 minutes to 1 hour to complete.

Findings

ABNORMAL VALUES

Adenocarcinoma	Diverticulitis
Sarcoma	Hirschsprung disease
Carcinoma	Idiopathic megacolon
Saccular or villous polyps	Gastroenteritis
Chronic amebic dysentery	Intestinal structural change
Ulcerative colitis	Sigmoid torsion
Crohn disease	Intussusception

Interfering Factors

- Upper gastrointestinal series within 3 days before this test
- Inability to retain barium
- Incomplete cleansing of the colon

Nursing Implementation

Pretest

Schedule the barium enema before any other barium studies. Residual barium from the upper gastrointestinal tract will interfere with visualization of the colon.

Provide a complete explanation of the procedure for bowel cleansing. When the patient is very young or very old and the procedure is to be performed in an outpatient setting, the caregiver or a second person should be present and included in the teaching. Written instructions will help ensure thorough bowel preparation.

Obtain a signed consent from the patient or the person legally responsible for the patient's health care decisions.

Bowel Preparation: The exact cleansing procedure is defined by the radiologist or by hospital protocol. Since there is variation in procedure, the common methods of preparation are presented here.

A clear liquid diet begins 12 to 24 hours before the test to reduce the amount of fecal matter.

A cathartic such as castor oil, magnesium citrate or senna extract (X-Prep) is taken on the afternoon before the test. Bisacodyl (Dulcolax) tablets are taken on the evening before the test and a bisacodyl (Dulcolax) suppository is inserted on the morning of the test.

A warm tap water enema (2 L for adults) is given on the night before the test or at 6 A.M. on the day of the test. When all fecal matter has been removed, the enema returns will be clear.

Extra oral fluids are taken in the pretest period to prevent dehydration or excess absorption from the barium contrast medium in the colon. Some

Critical Thinking: An elderly patient is scheduled for a barium enema to be done as an outpatient procedure. When you provide the pretest instruction, the patient tells you that she lives alone and her severe arthritis prevents her from administering the cleansing enema. What alternatives can you suggest to her?

protocols require extra fluids in the afternoon and evening, but a complete nothing by mouth status is started by midnight before the test.

For children younger than 4 years, the bowel preparation is prescribed on an individualized basis.

QUALITY CONTROL

To obtain a clear and accurate visualization of the lumen, all fecal matter, residual gas, and mucus must be removed.

Posttest

The patient is assisted to the toilet or in the use of a commode or bedpan to evacuate the contrast medium.

A laxative is prescribed to eliminate the residual barium and to prevent the constipation caused by the barium. Residual barium changes the feces to a gray or whitish color for 24 to 72 hours after the test.

Encourage the patient to rest for the remainder of the day because this test is tiring. Elderly patients are vulnerable to weakness and may experience a fall. They also may become mentally confused because of dehydration, so restoration or an increase in fluid intake is important.

BARIUM SWALLOW

(RADIOLOGY)

Synonym:

esophagography

--- **NORMAL VALUES** ---

No structural or functional abnormalities are visualized.

Background Information

The barium swallow procedure may be performed as a separate barium study or as a routine part of the upper gastrointestinal series. Dysphagia is the most common problem investigated by the barium swallow. The cause can be an obstruction in a part of the esophagus or a neuromuscular deficit that interferes with swallowing and slows the transit time for the passage of food to the stomach. The normal transit time from the oropharynx to the stomach is 6 to 15 seconds.

Purpose of the Test

The barium swallow is used to identify abnormalities in the structure or function of the esophagus.

Procedure

The patient takes repeated swallows of barium liquid to provide views of the passage of contrast during swallowing and peristaltic movement of the esophagus. Fluoroscopy and x-rays are used for visualization as the patient is in vertical, semivertical, and horizontal positions on the tilting x-ray table.

Findings

ABNORMAL VALUES

Swallowed foreign body
Stricture
Hiatal hernia
Polyps, tumors, carcinoma
Ulcers or peptic esophagitis
Varices

Achalasia (neuromuscular incoordination)
Esophageal spasm
Pharyngeal neuromuscular weakness
Plummer-Vinson syndrome

Interfering Factors

• Failure to maintain a nothing-by-mouth status

Nursing Implementation

Pretest

Provide an explanation of the procedure and obtain written consent from the patient or the person legally responsible for the patient's health care decisions.
Instruct the patient to fast from all food and liquids for 12 hours before the test.
At the radiology setting, have the patient remove all clothes, jewelry, and metallic objects. A surgical gown is worn.

Posttest

A laxative is given to help eliminate the barium from the intestinal tract.
Inform the patient that the feces will appear gray or whitish for 24 to 72 hours until all barium is expelled.

COMPUTED TOMOGRAPHY OF THE GASTROINTESTINAL TRACT

(SCAN)

Synonyms:
CT scan, CAT, computerized axial tomography

The computed tomography scan uses x-rays to provide multidimensional scanning of the body tissue. This test is used to detect intraabdominal masses, including abscess, tumor, or metastases. It is also useful in the staging of abdominal malignancy and is the best test to assess a tumor of the salivary gland. A complete discussion of computed tomography is presented in Chapter 12.

ENDOSCOPIC ULTRASONOGRAPHY

(ENDOSCOPY-ULTRASOUND)

Synonym:
EUS

Background Information

Endoscopic ultrasonography is an imaging technique that uses a special endoscope that is fitted with an ultrasound transducer (Spada et al., 1990). Endoscopy, without ultrasound, examines the mucosal lining and lumen of the intestinal tract. With endoscopic ultrasound, the instrument provides images of the submucosal and muscle layers of the intestinal walls.

The examination of the upper gastrointestinal (GI) tract includes the esophagus, stomach, and duodenum. The examination of the lower GI tract includes the tissue of the colon. Using this technique, it is possible to identify submucosal tumor, invasion of lymph nodes, leiomyoma or other tumor invasion of muscle tissue, vascular lesions, cystic growths, and pressure from an abnormality or tumor mass in a contiguous organ. The procedure can provide data for the staging of a malignant tumor.

Sonographic examination can also provide imaging of the organs that surround the upper or lower GI tract. In the upper GI tract, the endoscope with ultrasound uses the high-resolution sound waves that pass through the GI tract walls. The images view the mediastinum and heart, the liver, bile ducts, pancreas, hepatic renal angle, and splenic renal angle (Sivac, 1987). In colonic ultrasonography, parts of the liver, pancreas, and kidneys can be seen. With endorectal ultrasound, the uterus, vagina, bladder, prostate gland, and seminal vesicles are observed (Rosch and Classen, 1992).

The patient preparation and nursing care for endoscopic ultrasonography are the same as for the endoscopic procedure used. This information is presented in the section on esophagogastroduodenoscopy, flexible sigmoidoscopy, and lower panendoscopy. Additional information on ultrasound procedure is presented in Chapter 8.

ESOPHAGEAL FUNCTION TESTS

(MANOMETRY)

Synonyms:
esophageal manometry, Tuttle test (pH probe for reflux or esophageal acidity test), Bernstein test (acid perfusion test)

--- **NORMAL VALUES** ---

Esophageal Manometry (Drossman, 1987)	
Lower Esophageal Sphincter	
(LES) Pressure:	mean value of 19.2 ± 6.9 mm Hg
% LES Relaxation	
(wet swallows):	96% ± 10%
Primary Peristalsis Esopha-	mean amplitude 65–71 mm Hg
geal Body (wet swallow):	mean duration 3.3–6.2 seconds
Primary Peristalsis Esopha-	mean amplitude 45 mm Hg
geal Body (dry swallow):	mean duration 4.7–4.8 seconds
Esophageal Body	present (frequently to infrequently)
(tertiary contractions):	mean amplitude 12 ± 3 mm Hg
	mean duration 2.9–3.1 ± 0.4–0.5 sec
Tuttle Test:	alkaline (esophageal pH of 6 or higher)
Bernstein Test:	negative

Background Information

The esophagus is a muscular segment of the alimentary tract that propels food from the pharynx to the stomach by peristalsis. In peristaltic activity, smooth muscle contraction causes the intraluminal pressure to rise, and smooth muscle relaxation causes the intraluminal pressure to fall. The alternating waves of contraction and relaxation continuously move the bolus of food downward from high-pressure to low-pressure areas.

The final portion of the esophagus is called the lower esophageal segment (LES). Its functions are to accept the bolus of food, transport it to the stomach, and prevent regurgitation of gastric contents back into the esophagus. When at rest, the LES pressure is higher than that of the stomach. The combination of the pressure gradient and the LES sphincter or sphincter-like function prevents gastroesophageal reflux.

ESOPHAGEAL MANOMETRY. The pressure within the body of the esophagus and at the lower esophageal segment can be measured at rest and during swallowing to provide information about peristalsis. The measures of the amplitude, frequency, and duration of the pressure define the effectiveness of esophageal motor function.

Patients who require this test have a history of unexplained dysphagia and chronic heartburn. The cause of the dysphagia may be progressive systemic sclerosis or esophageal motor dysfunction. The origin of the heartburn may be hiatal hernia. The manometry test helps rule out angina or other cardiac problems as the source of chest pain.

TUTTLE TEST. During manometry testing, the Tuttle test is used to measure the pH within the esophagus. The normal esophageal pH is 6 or higher, an alkaline environment. The normal pH of the stomach is 1 to 3, an acidic reading. A lower than normal esophageal pH is caused by the regurgitation of gastric acids into the esophagus. The regurgitation is called gastroesophageal reflux and is caused by an incompetent LES.

BERNSTEIN TEST. During manometry testing, the Bernstein test may be performed to identify the patient's subjective response to heartburn pain in the presence of dilute hydrochloric acid. In a positive result, the patient's esophagus is the source of the pain; it is sensitive to the presence of gastric acid.

Purpose of the Test

Esophageal manometry is used to diagnose and evaluate esophageal motor disorders, including the evaluation of dysphagia. It is also used to evaluate pre- or postoperative esophageal surgery designed to improve esophageal motility and prevent esophageal reflux. During manometry, drug provocation can be used to evaluate chest pain that is presumed to be of esophageal origin. When the patient has drug-provoked chest pain at the same time that the pressure readings are abnormal, the esophagus is identified as the source of the pain (Maber et al., 1990).

The Tuttle test is used to document gastroesophageal reflux or to evaluate the results of medical-surgical antireflux treatment. The Bernstein test is used to determine that the heartburn is of esophageal rather than cardiac origin.

Procedure

In *esophageal manometry*, a triple-lumen catheter is passed into the esophagus via the nose or mouth. The patient is then put into a supine position with a swallowing sensor attached to the neck. All channels of the catheter record pressures from the esophagus during a series of wet swallows (5 ml of water delivered by syringe) and dry swallows. The pressure readings give data about LES pressure, LES relaxation, peristalsis, and spontaneous contractions of the esophagus (Fig. 17–3).

Provocative testing is performed to clarify the source of the dysphagia or chest pain, or both. A cholinergic drug, edrophonium chloride (Tensilon) is given intravenously, and the pressure readings are repeated.

QUALITY CONTROL

Prior to the start of the procedure, the entire system of components must be connected and checked for accurate function. This includes calibration of the recording system and accuracy of the pressure transducers and pressure response rates.

In the *Tuttle test*, the pH probe is attached to the esophageal manometer tube so that the tip can obtain a pH reading in the esophagus and stomach. Acidity readings from the esophagus are taken after swallowing, Valsalva maneuvers, straight leg-raising maneuvers, and abdominal compressions. If necessary, an infusion of 300 ml of 0.1 N hydrochloric acid is instilled into the stomach and the preceding maneuvers are repeated.

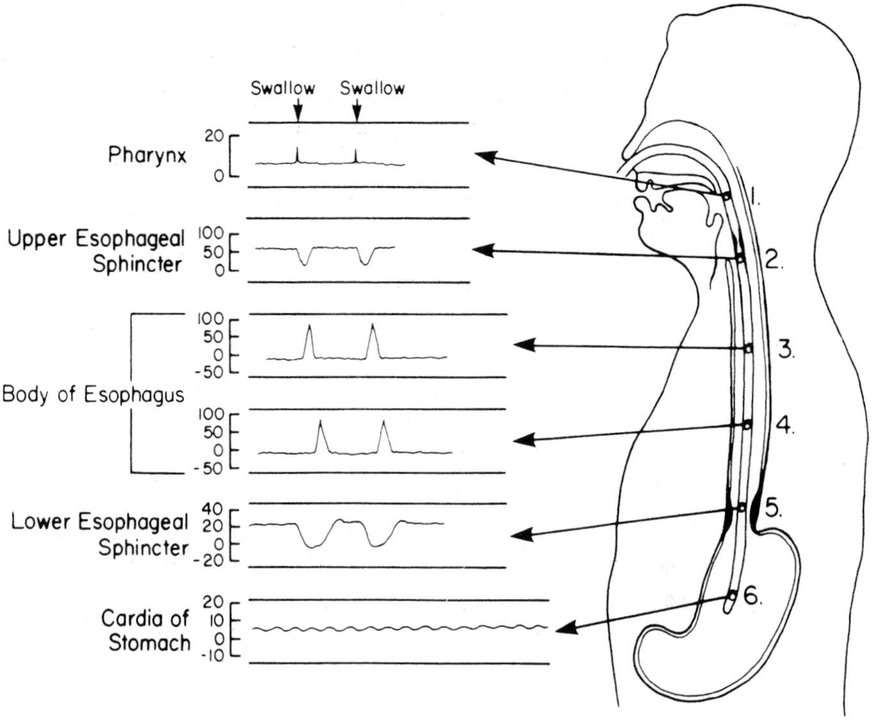

FIGURE 17–3. Esophageal manometry. Schematic representation of the intraluminal pressure events obtained at various points at rest and during swallows in a healthy subject. Pressure scales are in millimeters of mercury (mm Hg). (Reproduced with permission from Drossman, D.A. [Ed.]. [1987]. *Manual of gastroenterologic procedures* [2nd ed.]. New York: Raven Press.)

QUALITY CONTROL

Prior to the start of the procedure, the pH probe and reference electrode must be connected to the pH meter, with calibration for accurate pH readings.

In the *Bernstein test*, a drip of 0.1 N hydrochloric acid is instilled through the esophageal manometry catheter or a nasogastric tube until the patient complains of heartburn or until 30 minutes have passed without symptoms. The solution is alternated with normal saline flow to confirm that the heartburn occurs in the presence of hydrochloric acid and disappears in the presence of normal saline.

Findings

ABNORMAL VALUES

Achalasia
Progressive systemic sclerosis
(scleroderma)

Esophageal spasm
Gastroesophageal reflux
Hiatal hernia

Interfering Factors

TABLE 17–2	
COMPLICATIONS OF ESOPHAGEAL MANOMETRY TESTS	
Complication	**Nursing Assessment**
Vasovagal response	Bradycardia (pulse <60 beats per minute) Hypotension Cold, clammy skin
Cholinergic reaction (side effects of edrophonium chloride)	Dizziness Diaphoresis Flushing Nausea and vomiting Muscle cramps Urinary urgency Bradycardia (pulse <60 beats per minute)

- Unstable cardiac status
- Uncooperative patient

Nursing Implementation

Pretest

Instruct the patient to maintain a fasting state for 8 hours prior to the start of the test.

Inform the patient about the procedure and obtain a written consent from the patient or the person legally responsible for the patient's health care decisions.

Complications

Patients who have an unstable cardiac status, particularly with poor tolerance to vagal stimulation, should not undergo this test. A vasovagal reflex can occur, and atropine sulfate should always be on hand during the test.

When provocation testing is carried out with edrophonium chloride, side effects can occur. Atropine sulfate must be on hand for the reversal of the side effects and to counteract the cholinergic effect of the drug. The nursing assessment of complications of esophageal manometry is presented in Table 17–2.

ESOPHAGOGASTRODUODENOSCOPY

(ENDOSCOPY)

Synonyms:

EGD, upper gastrointestinal endoscopy

─────────────── **NORMAL VALUES** ───────────────

> No abnormal structures or functions are observed in the esophagus, stomach, or duodenum.

Background Information

In upper gastrointestinal endoscopy, the fiberoptic endoscope provides visualization of the lumen and mucosal lining of the esophagus, stomach, and upper duodenum.

The flexible fiberscope is a long tube filled with tens of thousands of thin glass fibers. By refraction and reflection, the fibers transmit light and the visualized image from the distal lens to the examiner's eyepiece, even when the tube is curved or flexed. Because of the ability to bend and rotate its distal segment, the fiberscope can be directed to view each segmented area until the entire lumen of each organ has been seen (Fig. 17–4). Within the instrument, there are columns to irrigate, suction, instill air or gas, and insert instruments.

In the diagnostic uses of esophagogastroduodenoscopy, tissue abnormalities are observed for their location, size, contour, shape, position, mobility, and surface appearance. Tissue or secretion samples are obtained by biopsy, scrapings, or aspiration and are sent for laboratory analysis.

Purpose of the Test

The many purposes of upper gastrointestinal endoscopy include (1) identification and biopsy of tissue abnormality, (2) determination of the exact site and cause of upper gastrointestinal bleeding, (3) evaluation of the healing of gastric ulcers, (4) evaluation of the stomach and duodenum after gastric surgery, and (5) investigation for the cause of dysphagia, dyspepsia, gastric outlet obstruction, or epigastric pain.

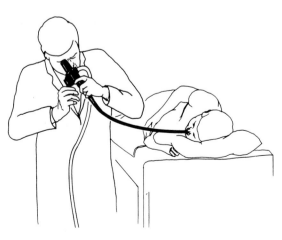

FIGURE 17–4. Esophagogastroduodenoscopy. Once the endoscope is inserted, the tube is moved around and rotated to obtain visualization of the lumen of the upper intestine. (Reproduced with permission from Sivak, M.V. [1987]. *Gastrologic endoscopy*. Philadelphia: W.B. Saunders.)

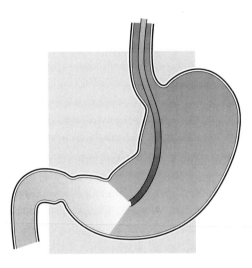

FIGURE 17–5. Endoscopic visualization of the upper gastrointestinal tract. The flexible tube, fiberoptic filaments, and a light are used to examine the mucosal surface of the esophagus, stomach, and duodenum for inflammation, erosion, ulceration, bleeding sites, stricture, and abnormal tissue.

Procedure

Virtually all patients have the procedure performed under intravenous sedation, although infants and small children may require general anesthesia (Ellett, 1991).

Once the throat is anesthetized, the endoscope is passed through the mouth into the esophagus. As the tube is advanced distally and then withdrawn, the esophagus, stomach, pylorus, and upper duodenum are visualized. As the scope is moved around, and with 360-degree rotation and flexion of the tip, the surface of the entire lumen is visualized (Fig. 17–5). Tissue or cell samples are obtained for cytologic studies, as indicated.

QUALITY CONTROL

The endoscope and accessory parts must be mechanically cleansed and then disinfected or sterilized after each procedure. The goals are to remove organic matter and infectious agents, thus minimizing the potential for transmission of infection (Schaffner, 1990; Bottrill, 1991).

Findings

ABNORMAL RESULTS

Ulcers, acute or chronic, gastric or duodenal
Tumors, benign or malignant
Diverticula
Stenosis, esophageal or pyloric
Hiatal hernia
Esophageal rings

Inflammation (esophagitis, gastritis, duodenitis)
Mallory-Weiss syndrome
Varices, esophageal or gastric

Interfering Factors

- Failure to maintain a nothing-by-mouth status
- Unstable or life-threatening cardiac or pulmonary condition
- Known or suspected perforation of the stomach or intestine
- Shock
- Recent myocardial infarction

Nursing Implementation

Pretest

Schedule this test at least 2 days after an upper GI series so that the barium will not interfere with visualization.

Inform the patient about the procedure and obtain written consent from the patient or the person legally designated to make health care decisions for the patient.

Provide written posttest instructions because temporary memory loss will occur after sedative administration.

Critical Thinking: When a 7-year-old child must have an EGD, what pretest nursing actions can be utilized to minimize fear and anxiety in the child?

When the procedure is to be performed in an ambulatory setting, someone must accompany the patient and provide transportation after discharge.

Instruct the patient to take nothing by mouth for 6 to 8 hours before the procedure.

Obtain the pretest coagulation profile, which includes prothrombin time, partial thromboplastin time, bleeding time, and platelet count. Place the results in the patient's chart.

On the morning of the test, obtain and record the vital signs, including blood pressure, pulse, and respirations.

Assist the patient with the removal and storage of eyeglasses, dentures, jewelry, hairpins, and clothing. A surgical gown is worn.

During the Test

Position the patient on the examination table in the left lateral recumbent position.

Intravenous medication is given for relaxation and analgesia. Meperidine (Demerol), 25 to 50 mg, is often followed by diazepam (Valium), 1 to 3 mg, or midazolam (Versed), 1 mg in adults and 0.5 mg in elderly patients. To prevent apnea, respiratory depression, or cardiac arrest, these medications are given slowly over a period of 1 to 2 minutes. Naloxone (Narcan) is kept on hand to reverse any respiratory depressive effect of meperidine, but it is ineffective against diazepam.

Oxygen delivered by nasal cannula will increase the patient's oxygen reserves and help prevent hypoxia (Aker, 1990).

Monitor vital signs at frequent intervals throughout the procedure. In most hospitals, automated blood pressure, pulse oximetry, and cardiac monitoring are used for all endoscopy patients or for selected patients who are more vulnerable. These are elderly patients and those with a history of cardiac disease (Kidwell, 1991).

Assist with the collection of specimens obtained by biopsy, brush technique, or washing technique (see also Gastrointestinal Cytologic Studies). Tissue samples are placed in a jar with preservative and labeled appropriately. The requisition slip includes the source of the tissue, the procedure, and the date.

Posttest

Continue to assess the vital signs and level of consciousness until the patient is stable.

Review the posttest instructions, including the following:

• Throat lozenges or saline gargle to relieve the discomfort in the throat
• No driving for 12 hours
• Resumption of oral fluids and food, once the gag reflex and sensation in the throat have returned

Complications

The incidence of overall complications in esophagogastroduodenoscopy is quite low, and the procedure is considered reasonably simple. Potential complications can occur, however, and require ongoing assessment during and after the procedure (Taffet et al., 1991; Sivak, 1987).

Infection is the most common complication. Aspiration pneumonia associated with oversedation and transient bacteremia are the most likely infections. Bacteremia may result from a variety of microorganisms from the patient's intestine or from contaminated instruments; the bacteria are introduced into the blood stream during the procedure.

Mild hypoxemia and hypoventilation occur fairly often during the procedures. The respiratory insufficiency is attributed to a combination of premedication with sedative-narcotics, the presence of the endoscope in the hypopharynx, and aspiration of fluids into the trachea. Elderly patients and those with chronic obstructive pulmonary disease are most vulnerable.

Serious cardiac complications are rare, but about one third of all patients will exhibit arrhythmias during the procedure. The triggering factors are not fully understood, but hypoxia and anxiety are contributing factors. Elderly patients and those with a history of cardiac or chronic lung disease are most vulnerable.

Perforation of the pharynx, esophagus, or stomach can occur with uncooperative patient behavior or because of anatomic abnormality. Bleeding may be the

TABLE 17–3
COMPLICATIONS OF ESOPHAGOGASTRODUODENOSCOPY

Complication	Nursing Assessment
Infection	Fever Malaise Shaking chills Elevated white blood cell level Cough Dyspnea
Respiratory depression	Respiratory rate <12 breaths per minute Shallow breathing Pallor, cyanosis Tachycardia
Cardiac arrhythmia	Irregular pulse Premature ventricular contractions Premature atrial beats Atrial fibrillation
Perforation, bleeding	Hematemesis Melena Persistent pain in the esophagus, mediastinum, or epigastric area Persistent dysphagia Fever

result of perforation, a dislodged clot, or a coagulation disorder. The nursing assessments for complications of esophagogastroduodenoscopy are presented in Table 17–3.

GALLIUM SCAN

(RADIONUCLIDE SCAN)

Synonyms:

gallium-67 imaging, total body scan

───── **NORMAL VALUES** ─────

No anatomic or functional abnormalities are visualized

Background Information

When the radiopharmaceutical gallium-67 is injected into the blood stream, it will bind to transferrin and other plasma proteins. As the gallium-67 is transported through the blood stream, it will concentrate in neoplastic tumors and sites of inflammation. The uptake mechanism is not fully understood but may be related to transferrin receptor sites in malignant tissue and an attraction to neutrophils, bacteria, and purulent matter contained in inflamed or infected tissue.

Gallium-67 is a radioactive isotope that emits gamma rays. The radiopharmaceutical is detected by the rectilinear scanner or scintillation scanner and camera as it circulates throughout the plasma and concentrates in areas of abnormality. The nuclear scan may be performed as a total body scan or may concentrate on spot imaging of a particular body region, or both.

The gallium-67 radioisotope has a half-life of 78 hours. It is partially excreted from the body by the kidneys and colon over a period of 3 days.

Purpose of the Test

The gallium scan is used to locate malignancy, metastases, and sites of inflammation and abscess formation.

Procedure

The radionuclide is injected intravenously. Four to 6 hours later, images are taken to identify infectious or inflammatory disease; 24 hours later, images are taken to identify tumors. Additional images may be taken at 24-hour intervals for up to 72 hours. A single body region requires 45 minutes, and a total body scan takes 90 minutes for completion.

Since gallium-67 will accumulate in the colon, the presence of feces can interfere with the visualization of the abdominal region. Some nuclear medicine protocols require an enema removal of the fecal matter in the pretest period or in the interval between the injection and the start of the scanning process. The nurse should consult with the nuclear medicine department for specific instructions (Plankey and Plankey, 1990).

Findings

ABNORMAL VALUES

Peritonitis
Abdominal abscess
Osteomyelitis
Granulomatous disease
Pneumonia
Pneumocystis carinii
Sarcoidosis

Malignancy of the head-neck, bronchus, thorax, liver, genitourinary tract, and lymphatic system
Metastatic disease
Amebiasis

Interfering Factors

- Barium in the intestinal tract
- Recent lymphangiography
- Pregnancy

Nursing Implementation

Pretest

Schedule this test before any barium studies or lymphangiography.

QUALITY CONTROL

The gamma rays of the gallium-67 scan cannot penetrate the retained barium. Recent lymphangiography will increase the gallium uptake in the lungs, giving a false-positive reading.

Explain the procedure to the patient and obtain an informed consent from the patient or the person legally responsible for the patient's health care decisions.

Instruct the patient regarding the specific bowel preparation required.

Posttest

Use gloves to dispose of fecal matter and wash hands immediately after removing gloves.

Teach the patient to flush the toilet promptly after evacuation and to wash the hands promptly.

QUALITY CONTROL

The radioactive dosage is small and the exposure is minimal for 72 hours. Nevertheless, the fecal matter contains the excreted radioisotope. Handwashing and hygiene measures prevent additional radiation contact with the skin.

GASTRIC EMPTYING SCAN

(RADIONUCLIDE SCAN)   *Synonyms:*

Background Information

In normal physiology of gastric emptying, solid foods first undergo churning and grinding activity until the solids consist of small particles. Strong contractions by the antral portion of the stomach cause emptying of the solid matter through the pylorus into the duodenum. Liquids are emptied from the stomach by gravity, with some assistance from peristalsis.

The rate of gastric emptying depends partially on the quality of muscle tone (reflected by the number and intensity of peristaltic waves) and the opening of the pylorus. The emptying rate is also influenced by the foods that have been

═══════════════════════════ **NORMAL VALUES** ═══════════════════════════

There is no delay in gastric emptying.
Half-Time Emptying of Liquid Phase: 40 minutes (range: 12 to 65 minutes)
Half-Time Emptying of Solid Phase: 90 minutes (range 45 to 110 minutes)

ingested. Large meals will slow the emptying rate, as will high-calorie or fatty meals. In addition, body posture and gravity will alter the rate. When the person lies on the right side, the rate of emptying accelerates because the food moves closer to the pyloric outlet.

The stomach empties at a faster rate when peristalsis increases, as in response to inflammation or fibrosis. Delay in emptying can be caused by a structural abnormality or a functional change in the muscle tissue that weakens muscle contractility.

Purpose of the Test

The gastric emptying scan uses a radionuclide, a scintiscanner, and computer analysis to measure the precise rate of emptying of the stomach. This test is particularly helpful in monitoring the effect of therapy in patients who have abnormal gastric motility.

Procedure

When the "solid phase" of the radiopharmaceutical is used, the patient ingests a measured portion of cooked chicken liver, scrambled egg, or egg white, labeled with technetium-99m sulfur colloid as the radionuclide. When the "liquid phase" of the radiopharmaceutical is used, the patient drinks indium-111 DPTA mixed with orange juice or water. When the patient is given the radiopharmaceutical mixed with food or fluid, the total amount must be ingested as quickly as possible.

 ┌───┐
QUALITY CONTROL
└───┘
The accuracy of the test is dependent on the exact dose of the radiopharmaceutical entering the stomach promptly.

On conclusion of the meal, the first scan of the stomach and small bowel is taken with the patient in an upright position. Thereafter, the patient is in a supine position for images taken every 15 minutes and sits up in the nonimaging intervals. The test usually requires 3 hours to complete (Fig. 17–6).

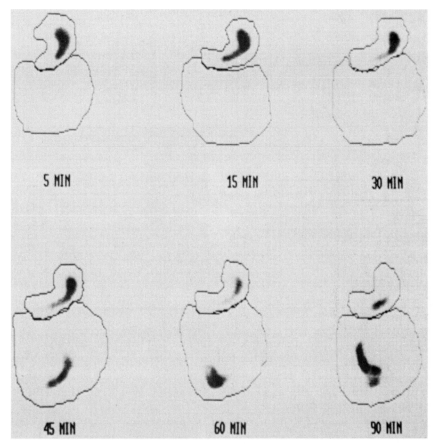

FIGURE 17–6. Gastric emptying scan. Sequential images of normal gastric emptying are shown with a computer region of interest around the stomach and small bowel. By 45 minutes the stomach is beginning to empty, and by 90 minutes more than half the activity is in the small bowel. (Reproduced with permission from Mettler, F.A., & Guiberteau, M.J. [1991]. *Essentials of nuclear medicine imaging* [3rd ed., p. 206]. Philadelphia: W.B. Saunders.)

Findings

ELEVATED VALUES

Gastric peptic ulcer
Zollinger-Ellison syndrome
Malabsorption syndromes

DECREASED VALUES

Diabetes mellitus (diabetic gastroparesis)
Low intracellular concentrations of potassium
Gastroesophageal reflux
Duodenal peptic ulcer
Anorexia nervosa

Idiopathic intestinal obstruction
Postoperative gastric surgery
Gastric outlet obstruction
Scleroderma
Amyloidosis

Interfering Factors

- Failure to maintain a nothing-by-mouth status
- Pregnancy, lactation

Nursing Implementation

Pretest

Teach the patient about the procedure and obtain an informed consent from the patient or person legally designated to make health care decisions for the patient.

Reassure the patient that the test is painless and easily tolerated. No special radiation precautions are needed because the dose of the radioisotope is small and the half-life is short.

Instruct the patient to fast from food and liquids for 8 hours prior to the start of the test.

Posttest

No specific patient instruction or intervention is needed.

GASTROESOPHAGEAL REFLUX SCAN

(RADIONUCLIDE SCAN)

Synonym:
GE reflux scan

─────── **NORMAL VALUES** ───────

The gastroesophageal reflux is 3% or less.

Background Information

Gastroesophageal reflux is the passive backflow of gastric juices into the esophagus. When the gastric acids are in contact with the esophageal mucosa of adults, they cause reflux esophagitis with ulcers, stricture, or shortening of the esophagus. The patient experiences the symptom of heartburn. In children, the consequences are much more significant. The reflux can rise up the esophagus and enter the trachea. The child can develop failure to thrive, aspiration pneumonia, esophageal stricture, or esophagitis.

Normally, the pressure gradient, sphincter activity, and anatomic angle at which the esophagus connects with the stomach all act to prevent the regurgitation of acid into the esophagus. The abnormal reflux of gastric acids occurs when (1) the pressure of the LES is lower than that of the stomach, (2) the sphincter activity is impaired, or (3) the esophagogastric angle is wider or more open. Under these conditions, gastroesophageal reflux occurs when the body is in a supine position or there is increased intraabdominal pressure.

This nuclear scan is more precise than esophageal barium studies in the diagnosis of gastroesophageal reflux. Unlike esophageal manometry tests, it does not require intubation. A gastroesophageal reflux result that is 4% or higher is considered abnormal.

Purpose of the Test

This scan uses a radionuclide and computer-assisted scintigraphy to identify and measure gastroesophageal reflux. It can also be used to measure the response to treatment, including the surgical repair of a hiatal hernia.

Procedure

An abdominal binder with an inflatable cuff is applied to the patient's abdomen. The adult patient drinks the radiopharmaceutical technetium-99m sulfur colloid mixed in a solution of orange juice and dilute hydrochloric acid. When the patient is an infant or small child, the radiopharmaceutical may be mixed in the formula or administered by nasogastric tube. An additional ounce of water is then given to clear the esophagus of any residual radiopharmaceutical.

The gamma camera takes pictures while the patient is in a supine position and as the binder is gradually tightened by the inflatable cuff. Body position, abdominal pressure, and the presence of acid are used to aggravate the reflux. Images of the reflux of the radiopharmaceutical are taken and the computer linkage provides graphic data to measure the degree of gastroesophageal reflux (Fig. 17–7). The procedure requires 2 hours of imaging time.

Findings

ELEVATED VALUES
Gastroesophageal reflux caused by
   hiatal insufficiency
   hiatal hernia
   systemic progressive sclerosis (scleroderma)
   idiopathic chalasia
   failed antireflux surgery

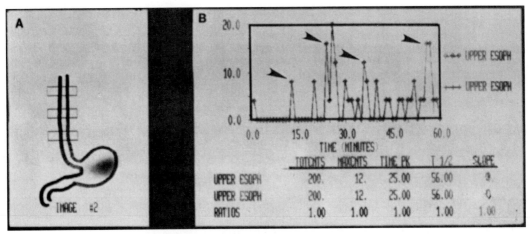

FIGURE 17–7. Gastroesophageal reflux scan. *A*, Anterior view of the chest and upper abdomen shows activity within the stomach and three computer regions of interest. *B*, A computer-generated graph of activity over the upper esophagus shows multiple spikes indicating significant reflux. (Reproduced with permission from Mettler, F.A., & Guiberteau, M.J. [1991]. *Essentials of nuclear medicine imaging* [3rd ed., p. 205]. Philadelphia: W.B. Saunders.)

Interfering Factors

- Failure to maintain a nothing-by-mouth status

Nursing Implementation

Pretest

Inform the patient about the procedure and obtain written consent from the patient or person legally designated to make the health care decisions for the patient.

Instruct the patient to discontinue all foods and fluids for 8 hours before the test. An alternative protocol is a fast from food for 8 hours and from fluids for 2 hours before the test (Mettler and Guiberteau, 1991).

Posttest

No special patient instruction or intervention is needed.

GASTROINTESTINAL BLEEDING SCAN

(RADIONUCLIDE SCAN)   *Synonyms:*

gastrointestinal scan to investigate blood loss, GI scintigraphy

─────────── **NORMAL VALUES** ───────────

> No evidence of a focal area of increased activity

Background Information

The source of GI bleeding (melena) is sometimes difficult to locate, particularly in the small bowel or colon. Endoscopic examination is often used but is not always successful. Heavy bleeding obscures the viewing tip of the endoscope, intermittent bleeding may not be active at the time, and the small bowel is too narrow and long for endoscopic visualization.

The GI bleeding scan uses nuclear imaging to identify the location of the bleeding. The intravenous radionuclide circulates through the vasculature until it reaches the site of the bleeding. There, it leaks through the break in the vascular wall and intestinal mucosa and accumulates in the intestinal lumen. The pooled blood and radionuclide is called a "focal area of increased activity." The nuclear imaging process records the image of the pooled blood and the start of its peristaltic flow in the intestinal tract. This test is sensitive to small amounts of bleeding; it can detect a bleeding rate of 0.2 ml/minute. The usual time required for this procedure is 30 to 45 minutes.

Purpose of the Test

Technetium-99m sulfur colloid or technetium-99m–labeled red blood cells are administered to the patient intravenously. When tagged red blood cells are used, the source is the patient's own blood.

Using a scintillation camera, images of the abdomen and pelvis are taken at 5-minute intervals for 45 minutes and at 15- to 60-minute intervals thereafter, as needed. With technetium-99m–labeled red blood cells, reimaging can be performed for up to 24 hours. The prolonged study time is used when early results are negative and bleeding is intermittent.

Findings

ABNORMAL VALUES

Diverticula	Ulcers
Angiodysplasia	Inflammatory bowel disease
Neoplasm	Polyps
Meckel diverticulum	Intussusception

Interfering Factors

- Recent upper GI series or barium enema
- Pregnancy
- Hemodynamic instability due to blood loss

Nursing Implementation

Pretest

Schedule this test before any barium studies are performed.

Explain the procedure to the patient. Except for the venipuncture, the procedure is painless.

Obtain a written consent from the patient or person legally designated to make health care decisions for the patient.

Take the vital signs and record the data in the patient's chart.

Posttest

On return to the unit, take the patient's vital signs and assess for shock. There is the potential for acute bleeding while the patient is in the nuclear medicine unit or during transport back to the nursing unit.

GASTROINTESTINAL CYTOLOGIC STUDIES

(CYTOLOGY)

Synonyms:

─────────────────────── **NORMAL VALUES** ───────────────────────

Within normal limits; no evidence of abnormal cells or infectious organisms

Background Information

Cytologic examination of tissue from the GI tract is dependent on the ability to collect cells from a specific lesion or precise area. Once the cells are collected, cytologic study and microscopic analysis provide information about cellular changes. Specimens of the GI tract for cytologic study are usually obtained during an endoscopic procedure, including esophagogastroduodenoscopy, endoscopic retrograde cholangiopancreatography, and colonoscopy.

Purpose of the Test

Cytologic study identifies benign or malignant growth that is evident in the biopsy specimen. It helps identify particular infections that cause characteristic cell changes. In some cases, the result is nonspecific. These results describe new epithelial tissue, also called "epithelial repair." The presence of healing or repair implies that the new cellular activity is in response to an injury to the tissue.

Procedure

During the endoscopic examination, specimens of tissue can be obtained by biopsy, brush technique, or washing technique. The specific methods of handling the biopsy tissue, exfoliative cytologic specimen, and type of fixative can vary from one hospital to another. Generally, the endoscopy personnel coordinate the activity and procedure with the laboratory so that the tissue is not damaged or destroyed.

> **QUALITY CONTROL**
>
> To avoid confusion from mislabeling, the laboratory requisition, the slides, and the specimen containers must include the patient's name and the source of the tissue.

BIOPSY TECHNIQUE. This is performed by passing a forceps through the endoscope and obtaining several small samples of suspicious tissue. The tissue samples are placed on a filter paper and the paper is placed into a specimen jar with fixative solution.

BRUSH TECHNIQUE. This involves the use of a disposable brush that is sent through the endoscope and passed over a suspicious area of tissue to obtain a sample of cells. The brush, with its cells and exudate, is placed in a jar of fixative solution. An alternative method is to pass the brush over a slide that is moistened with normal saline. The slide is then placed in preservative in a container, or it is sprayed with fixative.

WASHING TECHNIQUE. This involves the use of the endoscope to inject 25 ml of normal saline onto the lesion, with subsequent aspiration of the fluid, cells, and exudate into a specimen cup.

> **QUALITY CONTROL**
>
> This specimen must be placed in ice and sent to the laboratory immediately. Since no fixative is used, heat or time delay would result in lysis of the cells.

Findings

ABNORMAL VALUES

Esophagus	Stomach	Colon
Herpes simplex virus	*Candida albicans*	Cytomegalovirus
Candida albicans	Intestinal metaplasia	Herpes simplex virus
Cytomegalovirus	Epithelial cell repair	Adenocarcinoma
Barrett metaplasia	Large cell malignant lymphoma	Squamous cell dysplasia
Epithelial repair		Infectious colitis
Squamous cell carcinoma		
Adenocarcinoma		
Large cell malignant lymphoma		

Interfering Factors

- Barium study within 2 to 3 days before endoscopy
- Failure to properly label or transport the specimen
- Food or particulate matter near the lesion

Nursing Implementation

Nursing measures are the same as those for the particular endoscopic procedure used.

LOWER PANENDOSCOPY

(ENDOSCOPY)

Synonym:

colonoscopy

───────────── **NORMAL VALUES** ─────────────

No abnormalities of structure or mucosal surface are observed in the colon or terminal ileum.

Background Information

The familiar synonym of colonoscopy refers only to the endoscopic visualization of the colon. With improvement in the equipment and the newer technique of lower panendoscopy, the endoscope can now explore the total colon and 20 to 30 cm of the ileum. The patient may have a colonoscopy only or may require the more extensive lower panendoscopy. Currently, the endoscopic examination is preferred over barium enema for examination of the colon.

The flexible fiberscope is a long tube filled with thousands of ultrathin glass fibers. By reflection and refraction, these fibers transmit the light and visualized image from the distal lens to the viewer's eyepiece, even when the tube is curved. The flexibility of the tube enables it to be passed beyond each flexure of the colon (Fig. 17–8). The distal segment of the tube can be rotated through 360 degrees so that all aspects of the lumen are observed. There are columns within the instrument for irrigation, suction, instrumentation, and instillation of air or gas.

Purpose of the Test

The purpose of lower panendoscopy is to identify and biopsy abnormal tissue in the colon and terminal ileum, investigate the cause of chronic diarrhea, locate the source of GI bleeding, and evaluate the colon for recurrent polyps or malignant growth.

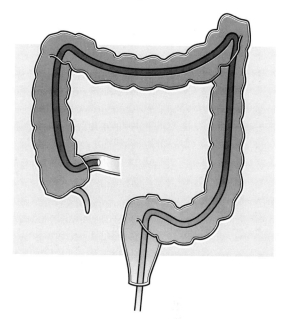

FIGURE 17–8. Lower panendoscopy. The endoscopic instrument is passed through the entire colon and into the distal segment of the ileum. The combination of the flexible tube, fiberoptics, and the light enables the examiner to visualize the entire mucosal surface, identifying sites of bleeding, inflammation, tissue irregularity, or abnormal tissue.

Procedure

Virtually all patients have the procedure performed under intravenous sedation, although infants and small children may require general anesthesia (Ellett, 1991). The tip of the endoscope is inserted into the rectum and passed through the sigmoid, descending, transverse, and ascending colon. In the cecum, the ileocecal valve is visualized; the tip of the instrument is passed through and advanced into the distal ileum.

QUALITY CONTROL

The colonoscope and accessory parts must be mechanically cleansed and then disinfected or sterilized after each procedure. The goals are to remove the organic matter and infectious agents, thus minimizing the potential transmission of infection (Schaffner, 1990; Bottrill, 1991).

Findings

ABNORMAL VALUES

Diverticulitis
Granulomatous disease
Polyps
Site of lower intestinal bleeding
Proctitis
Gay bowel syndrome

Crohn disease
Ulcerative colitis
Carcinoma
Colitis (radiation, ischemia, infectious)
Pneumatosis cystoides intestinalis

Interfering Factors

- Massive bleeding in the colon
- Toxic colitis
- Inflammatory bowel disease or stricture
- Peritonitis or bowel perforation
- Acute diverticulitis
- Recent myocardial infarction, pulmonary embolus, or acute cardiopulmonary disease
- Recent pelvic or colon surgery
- Large aortic or iliac aneurysm
- Pregnancy, second or third trimester
- Uncooperative behavior
- Poor bowel preparation
- Retained barium
- Failure to maintain pretest dietary restrictions

Nursing Implementation

Critical Thinking: An elderly patient has a lower panendoscopy procedure scheduled. In your care plan, what nursing measures will help ensure the safety of the patient before, during, and after the procedure?

Pretest

Schedule this test before any barium studies.

Explain the procedure to the patient and obtain written consent from the patient or the person legally responsible for the patient's health care decisions.

Provide instructions about bowel cleansing. Since the protocol varies among institutions, follow the endoscopist's particular requirements. General guidelines follow.

- Clear liquid diet for 48 hours before the test, to reduce the amount of feces
- Milk of Magnesia, 2 oz. taken 2 nights before the test and magnesium citrate, 10 oz., taken on the night before the test
- A tap water enema administered on the night before the test and tap water enemas administered at 6 A.M. until the enema returns are clear and free of fecal matter

On the morning of the test, take baseline vital signs and record the results in the patient's chart.

During the Test

Premedicate the patient with intravenous meperidine (Demerol), 25 to 50 mg, for analgesia and relaxation. This may be followed by intravenous diazepam (Valium), 1 to 3 mg or intravenous midazolam (Versed), 1 mg for adults and 0.5 mg for the elderly patient. To prevent apnea, respiratory depression, or cardiac arrest, these medications must be given slowly over a period of 1 to 2 minutes.

Naloxone (Narcan) is kept on hand to reverse the respiratory depressive effect of meperidine, but it is ineffective against diazepam.

Oxygen by nasal cannula increases the patient's oxygen reserves and helps prevent hypoxia (Aker, 1990).

Monitor the vital signs at frequent intervals throughout the procedure. In hospitals, automated blood pressure, pulse oximetry, and cardiac monitoring may be used for all endoscopy patients or for selected patients who are more vulnerable. This group includes elderly individuals and those with a history of cardiac disease (Kidwell, 1991).

Monitor for the vasovagal reflex that can occur during the procedure. Atropine sulfate is kept on hand to overcome the effects of sudden bradycardia.

Provide comfort and emotional support to help reduce anxiety and promote relaxation. The patient can be restless or uncomfortable during insufflation and manipulation of the endoscope and may require additional medication.

Assist with the collection of tissue specimens, as described in Gastrointestinal Cytologic Studies, earlier.

Posttest

Monitor vital signs every 15 minutes or continue automated monitoring until the results are stable.

Check the rectal area for signs of blood.

Send the properly identified tissue specimens to the laboratory without delay.

As soon as the patient is more responsive, the intake of food and liquids can resume.

On discharge from an ambulatory care setting, the patient must be accompanied by a responsible person who will provide transportation home. Because of the effects of the intravenous medication, the patient cannot drive a car for 8 to 12 hours, until thinking is clear and memory is restored.

Complications

During the procedure, the patient can experience respiratory depression or respiratory arrest because of the sedative anesthetics or narcotic analgesics. Intravenous diazepam can cause thrombophlebitis in the small vein used for administration of medication.

The vasovagal reflex is thought to be caused by the stretching of the mesentery as the endoscope is advanced through the colon. Up to 40% of the patients will demonstrate electrocardiographic abnormality during colonoscopy (Sivac, 1987). Serious arrhythmia or myocardial infarction can occur during or just after the procedure.

Hemorrhage and perforation are serious but infrequent complications. They are caused by manipulation of the endoscope and the use of force when advancing

TABLE 17–4
COMPLICATIONS OF LOWER PANENDOSCOPY

Complication	Nursing Assessment
Respiratory depression, apnea	Infrequent, irregular, shallow breathing Respiratory rate <12 breaths per minute Hypotension Bradycardia Hypoxemia Diaphoresis Nausea, vomiting
Vasovagal reflex	Bradycardia (pulse <60 beats per minute) Hypotension Cold, clammy skin
Cardiac arrhythmia	Premature atrial contractions Premature ventricular contractions Sinus tachycardia ST-T depression Chest pain Hypotension Atrial or ventricular fibrillation Cardiac arrest
Hemorrhage, perforation	Rectal bleeding Abdominal distention Persistent abdominal pain Abdominal tenderness on palpation Malaise Elevated hematocrit Hypotension Tachycardia

the endoscope. Patients with diverticular disease, adhesions, stricture, or severe inflammatory disease are most vulnerable. The nursing assessment of complications of lower panendoscopy are presented in Table 17–4.

PARACENTESIS

(PERITONEAL FLUID)

Synonyms:

peritoneal fluid analysis, abdominal paracentesis, abdominal tap

Background Information

Normal patients have less than 50 ml of peritoneal fluid and no distention of the abdominal cavity. Peritoneal fluid is an ultrafiltrate of plasma; the amount is in homeostatic balance between formation and reabsorption.

——————————— NORMAL VALUES ———————————

Appearance:	clear, odorless, pale yellow, scanty
Ammonia:	<50 µg/dl
Amylase:	138–404 amylase units/L
Bacteria-fungi:	None present
Cells:	No malignant cells present
Glucose:	70–90 mg/dl *or* SI 3.89–4.99 mmol/L
Protein:	0.3–4.1 g/dl *or* SI 3–41 g/L
Red Blood Cells:	None
White Blood Cells:	<300 per µl *or* SI

One cause of ascites is when plasma fluid leaves the circulation and becomes deposited in the peritoneal cavity. The fluid may leave the circulation because of a change in the hydrostatic or oncotic pressure in capillaries, or there is altered permeability of the capillaries. The other cause of fluid accumulation in the peritoneal cavity is the failure of the lymphatic system to reabsorb the fluid in sufficient amounts.

The peritoneal fluid can be aspirated by the paracentesis procedure. The fluid will undergo laboratory analysis, including cytologic study, chemistry analysis, and microbiologic examination, as requested.

On gross examination of an abnormal specimen, the fluid can appear bright red and bloody, indicating rupture of an organ from blunt trauma. Cloudy fluid is often due to infection, strangulated bowel, or organ rupture. Greenish fluid can result from perforation of the duodenum or gallbladder, causing bile peritonitis. Milky fluid may be the result of blockage of the thoracic duct from causes such as malignancy, hepatic cirrhosis, adhesions, and infection from tuberculosis or parasites. When the ascites is advanced, the fluid volume can increase to 750 to 1500 ml or more.

Purpose of the Test

Abdominal paracentesis is used to examine the peritoneal fluid as part of the investigation of ascites, the effect of blunt abdominal trauma, or the cause of an acute abdomen when perforation is suspected.

Procedure

Under local anesthesia, a long, thin needle or trochar and stylet is inserted through the skin and into the abdominal cavity. The insertion site is midline, about 1 to 2 in. below the umbilicus. Either a syringe or a three-way stopcock with polyethylene tubing is used to draw off the fluid. For cytologic examination, 50 to 250 ml of fluid is needed (Ehya, 1991). The procedure takes about 30 to 45 minutes to complete.

Findings

ABNORMAL VALUES

Peritonitis, bacterial
Traumatic rupture of the bowel,
    gallbladder, spleen, liver, bladder
Pancreatitis
Strangled, infarcted bowel
Appendicitis
Tumor (benign, malignant)

Duodenal ulcer, perforated
Perforated intestine
Chyle from a blocked thoracic duct
Hepatic cirrhosis
Hypoproteinemia
Infectious peritonitis (tuberculous,
    fungal, parasitic)
Congestive heart failure

Interfering Factors

- Contamination of the fluid by urine, feces, blood, or bile
- Pregnancy
- Coagulation disorder
- Intestinal obstruction
- Abdominal wall infection
- Uncooperative behavior
- History of multiple abdominal surgical procedures
- Portal hypertension

Nursing Implementation

Pretest

Within 48 hours of the test, obtain the hematocrit, prothrombin time, partial thromboplastin time, and platelet values because of the risk of bleeding in the posttest period.

Explain the procedure to the patient and obtain written consent from the patient or person legally responsible for making health care decisions for the patient.

Record baseline vital signs, temperature, weight, and measure of the abdominal girth.

When removal of a large volume of fluid is anticipated, the installation of a central venous pressure (CVP) line may be indicated. Record baseline CVP readings.

Just prior to the procedure, have the patient void to completely empty the bladder to help prevent an inadvertent puncture of the organ.

Position the patient in a full Fowler position. There may be some modification of position according to the physician's preference.

During the Test

Reassure the patient to alleviate fear. Some pain or a jolting sensation is felt when the needle or trochar penetrates the peritoneum. Encourage the patient to remain immobile during the procedure.

Assist with the collection of the fluid specimens.

Monitor vital signs every 15 minutes. Observe for pallor, dizziness, diaphoresis, or other signs of impending shock.

On removal of the needle, an adhesive bandage is applied to the puncture site. On removal of the trochar, a suture or two are used to close the abdomen, and a small dressing is applied to the incision.

Posttest

Vital signs, a CVP reading, and abdominal girth measurement are recorded. Thereafter, the vital signs and the CVP readings are taken every hour for 6 hours or until the patient is stable (Drossman, 1987). The dressing is checked for excessive drainage or blood.

The nurse's note about the procedure describes the patient's tolerance of the test, the amount of fluid removed, and the color, odor, and characteristics of the fluid. The amount of peritoneal fluid is also recorded as output on the input-output sheet.

All specimens are appropriately labeled, including identification as a paracentesis specimen. The requisition slip states the specific laboratory analyses to be performed. The specimen bottles, slides, and tubes are all sent to the laboratory without delay.

Complications

The two complications of diagnostic paracentesis are hemorrhage and perforation of the bowel. Additionally, patients who have severe liver disease are at risk for the development of hepatic coma. A summary of the complications of paracentesis and the associated nursing assessments are found in Table 17–5.

PERCUTANEOUS PERITONEAL BIOPSY

(CYTOLOGY)

Synonyms:

The peritoneal biopsy is used to help evaluate unexplained ascites. It provides a tissue sample of the peritoneum and helps rule out tuberculosis, fungal infection, and metastatic carcinoma. The procedure used to obtain the sample is essentially the same as that of paracentesis. The specimen is obtained using a Cope needle that consists of a trochar, biopsy shaft, and snare. Once the biopsy shaft is in the peritoneal cavity, the snare is introduced down the shaft and is then drawn back until it touches the inner lining of the peritoneum. With rotation of

TABLE 17–5
COMPLICATIONS OF ABDOMINAL PARACENTESIS

Complication	Nursing Assessment
Hemorrhage	Hypotension Tachycardia Dyspnea Diaphoresis and pallor Acute abdomen or abdominal distress Ecchymosis Elevated hematocrit Decreased CVP
Perforation of the bowel	Acute abdominal pain Abdominal distention Board-like abdomen Shock (hypotension, tachycardia) Sepsis (fever)
Hepatic coma	Mental confusion Lethargy Drowsiness, stupor Elevated serum ammonia

CVP = central venous pressure.

the shaft, the snare removes a small scraping of tissue. This is repeated in several directions to obtain three to four tissue samples.

After withdrawal of the trochar, the tissue samples are placed in a jar with formalin preservative. The jar is labeled appropriately, including the tissue source and procedure used. The specimen is sent to the laboratory without delay (see also Gastrointestinal Cytologic Studies).

Following the test, the patient remains on bedrest for 6 hours. The vital signs are taken every hour for the 6 hours or until the signs are stable. The abdomen and dressing are assessed for swelling, ecchymosis, or leakage of peritoneal fluid.

ROENTGENOGRAPHY OF THE ABDOMEN

(RADIOLOGY)

Synonyms:
abdominal flat plate, flat plate of the abdomen

Background Information

Plain radiographs of the abdomen provide information about the gas patterns, air fluid levels in the GI tract, possible free air in the peritoneal cavity or retroperitoneal space, and areas of calcification.

Tumors, swelling of the mucosa, abscess formation, and fluid in the intestinal lumen can be identified by gas patterns. Air fluid levels can indicate intestinal obstruction. Calcifications inside or outside the intestinal tract are usually due to parasites or infections such as *Echinococcus cysticercus*, tuberculosis, and *Brucella*. Some tumors are calcified, such as Wilms tumor, mucinous carcinoma of the stomach, and colloid carcinoma of the colon.

Other calcifications can be visualized in the kidneys, bladder, genital tract, and abdominal wall. Calcium salt deposits are visible in chronic inflammation of the gallbladder, pancreatitis, and myoma of the uterus. Additional discussion of plain roentgenography is presented in Chapter 9.

SIGMOIDOSCOPY

(ENDOSCOPY)

Synonyms:

flexible sigmoidoscopy, rigid sigmoidoscopy, proctosigmoidoscopy, proctoscopy, anoscopy

─────────────── **NORMAL VALUES** ───────────────

No tissue abnormalities are seen in the distal colon or rectum.

Background Information

Sigmoidoscopy uses a flexible or rigid sigmoidoscope to examine the sigmoid colon and rectum. The flexible instrument can be inserted to a somewhat greater depth than can the rigid instrument. Rigid sigmoidoscopy, also called *proctoscopy* or *proctosigmoidoscopy*, uses a plastic disposable, or metal nondisposable, sigmoidoscope to examine the distal sigmoid colon and rectum. *Anoscopy* uses a short, blunt anoscope to examine the anus and rectum. Anoscopy is usually performed in conjunction with sigmoidoscopy or colonoscopy.

Purpose of the Test

Sigmoidoscopy is used as a screen for cancer of the colon in individuals older than 45 to 50 years of age. It is also used to investigate the source of unexplained rectal bleeding, to evaluate the postoperative anastomosis of the colon, and to diagnose or monitor inflammatory bowel disease. Anoscopy is used to investigate anal symptoms such as bleeding, pain, discomfort, or prolapse.

Procedure

The patient is placed in a lateral or knee-chest (jackknife) position (Fig. 17–9). Generally, no sedative anesthetic is needed. The well-lubricated instrument is

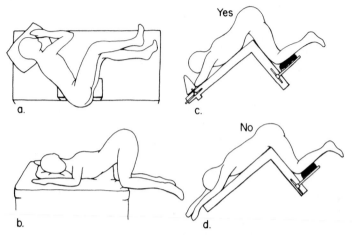

FIGURE 17–9. Three major positions for anoscopy and sigmoidoscopy. *a*, Left lateral (Sims) position. *b*, Knee-chest position. *c*, Prone, inverted jackknife position. *d*, An improper jackknife position is shown; the knee rest is too low, and no elbow rest is provided. (Reproduced with permission from Drossman, D.A. [1987]. *Manual of gastrointestinal procedures* [2nd ed., p. 128]. New York: Raven Press.)

inserted into the anus and advanced to the desired depth. A tissue biopsy specimen, culture specimen, or sample of fecal matter may be obtained during the procedure. The time needed for the examination is 5 to 10 minutes.

QUALITY CONTROL

The nondisposable instruments and accessory parts must be mechanically cleansed and disinfected or sterilized after each procedure. The goals are to remove organic matter and infectious agents, thus minimizing the potential transmission of infection (Schaffner, 1990; Bottrill, 1991).

Findings

ABNORMAL VALUES

Sigmoidoscopy	**Anoscopy**
Colitis (acute, pseudomembranous, ulcerative, following radiation therapy)	Hemorrhoids
	Fissure
	Fistula in ano
Polyps	Crohn disease
Colorectal cancer	Pilonidal sinus with abscess
Gay bowel syndrome	Abscess formation
Irritable bowel syndrome	Anal herpes
Sigmoid volvulus	Squamous cell carcinoma
Crohn disease	Anal condylomas
Intestinal ischemia	Perianal hematoma

Parasitic disease

Prolapsed rectum
Adenomatous polyps

Interfering Factors

- Uncooperative patient behavior
- Severe bleeding
- Suspected bowel perforation
- Peritonitis
- Toxic megacolon
- Acute diverticulitis
- Paralytic ileus

Nursing Implementation

Pretest

Explain the procedure to the patient and obtain a written consent from the patient or person legally responsible for making the patient's health care decisions.

Since bowel preparation varies among individuals, the examining physician should be consulted for specific instructions. The preparation usually consists of a combination of laxative and one or two Fleet enemas. The goal is to empty the lower colon of fecal matter.

During the Test

Position and drape the patient.

Provide reassurance and promote relaxation during the procedure. A few deep breaths help to relax sphincter muscles.

Assist with the collection of tissue or other specimens.

Posttest

Inform the patient that flatulence and mild gas pain may be experienced from the air that was put into the colon during the examination. When a biopsy is performed, it is normal to see a small amount of blood in the stool. Both of these aftereffects are temporary.

Label any specimen containers, including the name of the procedure and the tissue source. Send it to the laboratory without delay.

UPPER GASTROINTESTINAL AND SMALL BOWEL SERIES

(RADIOLOGY)

Synonyms:

upper GI series, small bowel follow-through

―――――――――――――――――――― **NORMAL VALUES** ――――――――――――――――――――

No structural or functional abnormalities are found.

Background Information

The upper GI series involves a radiologic examination from the oral part of the pharynx to the duodenojejunal junction. When the small bowel requires examination, the small bowel series directly follows the upper GI series.

The barium liquid is a chalky contrast medium that is taken orally. Because it is radiopaque, it outlines the size, shape, and contour of the intestinal lumen. Fluoroscopy and spot x-ray films are used to obtain the gastrointestinal images.

The common sources of abnormality in the upper GI tract are caused by stricture, inflammation, swelling, ulcers, tumors, motility disorders, or structural changes in the wall of the intestine.

The normal rate of gastric emptying is 4 hours, with an average rate of 2 hours. Gastric retention rates of 6 to 8 hours are very abnormal (Plavsik et al., 1992).

Purpose of the Test

The upper GI series detects disorders of structure or function of the esophagus, stomach, and duodenum. One week postoperatively, it is used to evaluate the results of gastric surgery, particularly when an anastomotic leak is suspected. As an extension of the upper GI series, the small bowel series detects disorders of the jejunum and ileum.

Procedure

The patient drinks a barium solution to provide contrast views during swallowing and peristaltic action in the esophagus. As the barium coats the mucosal lining of the stomach, additional films are taken to outline the shape and contour of the organ. The patient's postional changes (vertical, supine, prone, and lateral) help to coat the mucosa and identify gastroesophageal reflux and hiatal hernia.

When a small bowel series is included in this radiologic study, the transit time of the barium can be from 30 minutes to 6 hours before it reaches the colon. At the start of the small bowel series, additional barium is taken orally. The transit time can be shortened by having the patient drink 200 ml of iced water or eat a light meal after all the additional barium has left the stomach. Fluoroscopic views are taken three times in the first hour and every 30 minutes thereafter. Radiographic films are taken of any abnormality.

When the small bowel series is performed separately, enteroclysis, also known as a small bowel enema, may be used to instill the barium. A radiopaque catheter is passed through the nose or mouth and advanced to the distal duodenum or jejunum. Barium is then instilled by the catheter route directly into the small bowel. Excellent views of the total small bowel can be completed in 20 to 30 minutes.

Findings

ABNORMAL VALUES

Esophagus	Small Bowel
See section on barium swallow	Malabsorption
Stomach-Duodenum	Crohn disease
Peptic ulcer (gastric, duodenal)	Chronic appendicitis
Cancer (stomach, duodenum)	Stricture
Pyloric obstruction	Hodgkin disease
Benign tumor	Lymphosarcoma
Gastric inflammatory disease	Diffuse sclerosis
Perforation	Surgical resection
Diverticula	Disaccharidase deficiency
	Intussusception
	Perforation
	Congenital abnormality

Interfering Factors

- Failure to maintain the nothing-by-mouth status
- Excess air in the small bowel

Nursing Implementation

Pretest

Explain the procedure to the patient and obtain a written consent from the patient or the person legally responsible for making health care decisions for the patient.

Instruct the patient to fast from all food for 8 hours and all liquids for 4 hours before the test.

Most oral medications are withheld in the 8 hours before the test. Narcotics and anticholinergics are withheld for 24 hours before the test because they slow the motility of the intestinal tract.

During the Test

The hospitalized patient may return to the nursing unit for an interval before the small bowel filming begins. Obtain instructions from the radiology department about the nothing by mouth status or eating a prescribed meal.

Posttest

A laxative is given to help evacuate the barium promptly. Retained barium can cause constipation, obstruction, or fecal impaction.

Inform the patient that the feces will be gray or whitish for 24 to 72 hours until all barium has been evacuated.

The patient should plan to rest for the remainder of the day because the test is tiring.

REFERENCES

Ahlquist, D.A., et al. (1993). Accuracy of fecal occult blood screening for colorectal neoplasia. *Journal of the American Medical Association, 269,* 1262–1267.

Aker, J. (1990). Review of current research on midazolam and diazepam for endoscopic medication. *Gastroenterology Nursing, 13,* 245, 255, 265, 275, 285.

Bailey, E. (1992). Office endoscopy. *Gastroenterology Nursing, 14,* 237–239.

Bertagnolti, M.E., et al. (1989). Use of endoscopic ultrasound in patients with esophageal motility disorders. *Gastroenterology Nursing, 12,* 98–99.

Boatwright, D.N., et al. (1991). Preparing children for endoscopy and manometry. *Gastroenterology Nursing, 13,* 142–145.

Bottrill, P. (1991). Gastrointestinal endoscopy—A guideline for safe clinical practice. A British perspective. *Gastroenterology Nursing, 13,* 234–238.

Church, J.M. (1992). Colonoscopy for the diagnosis and treatment of colorectal bleeding. *Seminars in Colon and Rectal Surgery, 3,* 42–46.

Collins, P.M. (1990). Tumor markers and screening tools in cancer detection. *Nursing Clinics of North America, 25,* 283–290.

Datz, F.L. (1988). *Handbooks in radiology. Nuclear medicine.* Chicago: Year Book Medical.

Drossman, D.A. (Ed.). (1987). *Manual of gastroenterologic procedures* (2nd ed.). New York: Raven Press.

Ehya, H. (1991). Effusion cytology. *Clinics in Laboratory Medicine, 11,* 443–468.

Ellett, M.L. (1991). General anesthesia: An alternative to sedation for pediatric endoscopic procedures. *Gastroenterology Nursing, 13,* 166–168.

Geisinger, K.R., et al. (1991). Gastrointestinal cytology. *Clinics in Laboratory Medicine, 11,* 403–441.

Harty, R.F., & Leibach, J.R. (1985). Immune disorders of the gastrointestinal tract and liver. *Medical Clinics of North America, 69,* 675–704.

Henry, J.B. (1991). *Clinical diagnosis and management by laboratory methods* (18th ed.). Philadelphia: W.B. Saunders.

Jacobs, D.S., et al. (Eds.). (1990). *Laboratory test handbook* (2nd ed.). Baltimore: Williams & Wilkins.

Ingoldby, C.J.H., et al. (1987). Endoscopic needle aspiration cytology: A new method for the diagnosis of upper gastrointestinal cancer. *Gut, 28,* 1142.

Kidwell, J.A. (1991). Nursing care for patients receiving conscious sedation during gastrointestinal endoscopic procedures. *Gastrointestinal Nursing, 13,* 134–139.

Maber, K.A., et al. (1990). Intraesophageal balloon distension in the manometric evaluation of chest pain. *Gastrointestinal Nursing, 13,* 4–8.

Massoni, M. (1990). Nurses' GI handbook . . . gastrointestinal. *Nursing, 20,* 65–80.

Mettler, F.A., & Guiberteau, M.J. (1991). *Essentials of nuclear medicine imaging* (3rd ed.). Philadelphia: W.B. Saunders.

Monroe, D. (1989). Patient teaching for x-ray and other diagnostics. *RN, 52,* 36–40.

Moss, A.A., et al. (Eds.). (1992). *Computed tomography of the body with magnetic resonance imaging* (vol. 3, Abdomen and pelvis). Philadelphia: W.B. Saunders.

Plankey, E.D., & Plankey, M.W. (1990). A nuclear approach to cancer detection. *American Journal of Nursing, 90,* 107–108.

Plavsic, B.M., et al. (1992). *Gastrointestinal radiology.* New York: McGraw-Hill.

Rosch, T., & Classen, M. (1992). Colonoscopic ultrasonography. *Seminars in Colon and Rectal Surgery, 3,* 49–56.

Schaffner, M. (1990). Infection control issues in the gastrointestinal endoscopy unit. *Gastroenterology Nursing, 12,* 279–284.

Shoat, B.A., et al. (1990). Intraoperative endoscopy of the small bowel: Treatment for occult hemorrhage. *AORN Journal, 51,* 776–777, 779, 781–782.

Sivak, M.V. (1987). *Gastroenterologic endoscopy.* Philadelphia: W.B. Saunders.

Spada, I., et al. (1990). Endoscopic ultrasonography. *Gastroenterology Nursing, 13,* 24–30.

Sweeney, J.A.P. (1990). Endoscopy assessment tool—A new approach. *Gastroenterology Nursing, 13,* 71–76.

Sweeney, J.P. (1992). Assessing the patient undergoing GI endoscopy. *Gastroenterology Nursing, 14,* 266–269.

Taffet, S.L., et al. (1991). Esophageal and gastric endoscopy in critically ill patients: How can it help you? *Postgraduate Medicine, 89,* 123–126, 265–268.

Tietz, N.W., et al. (1992). *Applied laboratory medicine.* Philadelphia: W.B. Saunders.

Wright, T.L., & Heyworth, M.F. (1989). Maldigestion and malabsorption. In M.H. Sleisenger, & J.S. Fortran (Eds.). *Gastrointestinal disease* (pp. 263–282). Philadelphia: W.B. Saunders.

CHAPTER 18

Hepatic, Biliary, and Pancreatic Function

This chapter discusses the laboratory tests and diagnostic procedures used to identify dysfunction or abnormality in the liver, gallbladder, and pancreas. These organs are in close proximity to each other in the upper abdomen. Additionally, they share the biliary tree for drainage of bile and they interact with the intestinal tract and the portal vein system for the digestion and metabolism of food. Because of the common location and shared structure, abnormalities can start in one organ and directly extend to the others. Usually, several laboratory tests and diagnostic procedures are needed to identify the specific source of the problem and to detect any expansion of disease.

The laboratory tests generally measure the metabolic functions of the liver, exocrine functions of the pancreas, the effects of cholestasis in the liver or biliary system, and the presence of cellular damage or necrosis. There is no one laboratory test that gives a specific diagnosis, for example, cirrhosis of the liver; however, a combination of tests and a pattern of abnormal results provide strong indicators of organ damage and its cause. In addition to diagnostic information, many of these laboratory tests are used to screen for abnormality or to monitor the course of the disease and response to treatment.

The diagnostic procedures provide visualization of the structure and function of the liver, biliary system, and pancreas. With the use of radiography, radionuclide scanning, endoscopy, and ultrasound, the size, shape, and contour of the organs and their ducts are revealed. Microscopic analysis of tissue samples also provides data about the quality of the cells, their ability to function, and the cause of abnormality.

LABORATORY TESTS

ALANINE AMINOTRANSFERASE

(SERUM)

Synonyms:

ALT, glutamic-pyruvic transaminase, SGPT, GPT, transaminase

NORMAL VALUES

Average Adult Range:	10–35 IU/L at 37° C
Male >60 Years:	13–40 IU/L at 37° C
Female >60 Years:	10–28 IU/L at 37° C
Male Infant–Adult <60 Years:	15–35 IU/L at 37° C
Female Infant–Adult <60 Years:	15–35 IU/L at 37° C
Male Newborn–1 Year:	13–45 IU/L at 37° C
Female Newborn–1 Year:	15–45 IU/L at 37° C

Background Information

Alanine aminotransferase (ALT) is a transaminase enzyme that is found predominantly in the liver and to a lesser extent in the kidneys, heart, skeletal muscle, and pancreas. There is always some ALT present in the blood. Within the liver cells, the ALT is located in the cytoplasm of each hepatocyte.

When there is injury or necrosis of the liver cells, the ALT leaves the cytoplasm, passes through the damaged cell membrane, and enters the serum. When acute hepatitis occurs, the serum level can rise to 20 times or more the normal value. In cases of obstructive jaundice, cirrhosis, and liver tumor, the ALT values will be mildly to moderately elevated, or from two to four times the normal value.

The ALT enzyme value also rises slightly as a result of myocardial infarction, congestive heart failure, and shock. It is believed that in these conditions, there is an impaired blood supply and lack of adequate oxygenation to the liver, causing some liver damage and a rise in the hepatic source of the transaminase enzyme (Raphael, 1983). The ALT test replaces the old cephalin flocculation, isocitric dehydrogenase, and thymol turbidity tests.

Purpose of the Test

The ALT test is used to detect heptocellular injury. It is the most specific of the transaminase enzyme tests in the detection of acute hepatitis from viral, toxic, or drug-induced causes. ALT values are usually compared to aspartate aminotransferase (AST) values (ALT:AST ratio) to help differentiate among the different forms of liver disease.

Procedure

A red-topped, sterile tube is used to collect 5 to 10 ml of venous blood.

QUALITY CONTROL

Venipuncture technique must be smooth, with a blood flow that fills the vacuum tube readily. If the blood has excessive turbulence because of flawed venipuncture technique, the hemolysis of the erythrocytes will alter the test results.

Findings

ELEVATED VALUES

Acute or chronic hepatitis	Myocardial infraction
Liver cell necrosis of any cause	Shock
Acute pancreatitis	Dermatomyositis
Cirrhosis	Infectious mononucleosis
Obstructive jaundice	Muscular dystrophy
Biliary obstruction	Muscle trauma
Liver tumor	Recent surgery
Fatty liver	Preeclampsia
Reye syndrome	Hemolytic anemia
Chronic alcohol abuse	

Interfering Factors

- Hemolysis

Nursing Implementation

Pretest

Many medications cause an elevated test result. If they cannot be discontinued for 12 hours, list the medications on the requisition slip.

ALKALINE PHOSPHATASE

(SERUM)

Synonyms:

ALP, total alkaline phosphatase, T-ALP

NORMAL VALUES	
Adult:	4.5–13 King-Armstrong units/dl *or* SI 32–92 U/L
	1.4-4.4 Bodansky units
Child:	15–30 King-Armstrong units/dl *or* SI 107–213 U/L
	5–14 Bodansky units
Infant:	10–30 King-Armstrong units/dl *or* SI 71–213 U/L

Background Information

Serum alkaline phosphatase (ALP) is an enzyme that functions in an alkaline environment (with an optimum pH of 10). The ALP enzymes are located in the osteoblast cells of bone, in liver cells, and also in the intestines, kidney, and placenta. This enzyme is excreted via the biliary tract.

The function of any enzyme is to activate or catalyze particular chemical reactions of cells in the region in which the enzyme is located. A high level of any enzyme usually means that there is an increased synthesis or manufacture of the enzyme by a specific organ or tissue. Thus, the ALP enzyme will rise with increased osteoblast activity in bones during the healing of a fracture. The normal high level in children and adolescents is related to vigorous bone growth.

In the presence of a lesion or disease in tissue that contains the ALP enzyme, the level will also rise. Thus, the serum value of ALP will rise with biliary tract obstruction or hepatic malignancy as the affected tissue synthesizes additional ALP enzymes.

Purpose of the Test

Serum ALP provides a nonspecific indicator of liver disease, bone disease, or hyperparathyroidism. It is part of a battery of tests that evaluate liver function. It also serves as a nonspecific tumor marker, indicating rapid cell growth or accelerated function due to malignancy of the liver or bone.

Procedure

A red-topped sterile tube is used to collect 5 to 10 ml of venous blood.

QUALITY CONTROL

The serum must be kept refrigerated until analyzed, since heat or warmth will falsely elevate the results. The specimen should be analyzed within 4 hours because the value will rise during the storage period.

Findings

ELEVATED VALUES

Cancer of the liver
Biliary obstruction (gallstones or
   pancreatic cancer)
Cholestasis
Sclerosing cholangitis
Cirrhosis
Acute fatty liver
Infectious mononucleosis
Infiltrating liver disease (abscess,
   sarcoid, tuberculosis, amyloidosis)
Tumors (such as hypernephroma)

Paget disease
Osteogenic sarcoma
Bone metastases
Osteomalacia
Rickets
Leukemia
Myelofibrosis
Healing bone fracture
Acromegaly
Hyperthyroidism
Hyperparathyroidism

DECREASED VALUES

Malnutrition (protein or magnesium deficiency, or both)
Hypophosphatemia
Hypothyroidism

Interfering Factors

- Pregnancy
- Healing bone fracture
- Fatty food intake 2 to 4 hours before the test

Nursing Implementation

Pretest

Instruct the patient to discontinue food intake for 12 hours before the test if this is laboratory policy. Foods in general, and fatty foods in particular, can elevate the test results in some individuals (Jacobs, 1990).

ALKALINE PHOSPHATASE ISOENZYMES

(SERUM)

Synonym:

I-ALP

	NORMAL VALUES	
ISOENZYMES	PERCENT INACTIVATION AFTER 16 MINUTES AT 55° C	FRACTIONAL INACTIVATION AFTER 16 MINUTES AT 55° C
Liver	50–70	0.50–0.70
Bone	90–100	0.90–1.00
Intestine	50–60	0.50–0.60
Placenta	0	0
Regan	0	0

Background Information

The isoenzymes of ALP are measurements of the components of the liver, bone, intestinal, placental, and Regan isoenzymes to the total ALP. The tests are not fully developed for clinical use, since interpretation is difficult and better methodology is under development (Tietz, 1990).

The value of each isoenzyme is expressed as the percentage of isoenzyme that is inactivated after 16 minutes of exposure to heat at 55° C. Thus, the remainder of the total ALP is attributed to one of the other isoenzymes. This heat method is combined with serum electrophoresis to attain more specific results without overlap of values. In the older adult, the total ALP is composed of 40% bone isoenzymes and 60% liver isoenzymes.

Purpose of the Test

When the total ALP level is elevated, the alkaline phosphatase isoenzymes help identify the source of the pathologic change in enzyme activity. Generally, the goal is to distinguish between liver and bone pathology.

Procedure

A red-topped sterile tube is used to collect 5 to 10 ml of venous blood. There is no need for the patient to fast before the test.

> **QUALITY CONTROL**
>
> The specimen is kept refrigerated until the analysis is performed. The temperature control must be set at exactly 55° C to obtain results by the heat inactivation technique. Any variation in temperature control will affect the quality of the test and its results.

Findings

ELEVATED VALUES

Bone isoenzyme: Increased osteoblastic activity
Liver I isoenzyme: Hepatic congestion, pregnancy
Liver II isoenzyme: Parenchymal cell damage
Biliary ALP: Cholestasis
Intestinal ALP: Intestinal disease, patients with type O or type B blood
Placental ALP: Third trimester of pregnancy
Unidentified isoenzymes (Regan, Nagao): Neoplasm

Interfering Factors

• Exposure of serum sample to heat

Nursing Implementation

Pretest

No specific preparation or intervention is needed.

ALPHA$_1$-FETOPROTEIN

(SERUM, AMNIOTIC FLUID)

Synonyms:

AFP, α_1-fetoprotein

NORMAL VALUES

Adult:	2–16 ng/ml *or* SI 2–16 µg/L
Normal Pregnancy:	550 ng/ml *or* SI 550 µg/L
(Result rises to this maximum value in third trimester of pregnancy)	

Background Information

Alpha₁-fetoprotein (AFP) is synthesized by the fetal yolk sac and fetal liver. During pregnancy, it is found in fetal plasma, amniotic fluid, and maternal circulation. The normal value rises as the pregnancy progresses to term.

In normal, nonpregnant adults, AFP exists at low levels. The value will rise in liver disorders because of hepatocyte regeneration. Thus, some elevations are due to healing activity after trauma to the liver, exposure to hepatotoxins, or exposure to the hepatitis virus.

Purpose of the Test

In nonpregnant adults, this test serves as a tumor marker. AFP provides a strong indication of the diagnosis of primary hepatocellular carcinoma (hepatoma). In this condition, the value will rise to greater than 1000 ng/ml (SI = 1000 µg/L) or even dramatically higher. Additionally, the test is diagnostic for testicular germinal carcinoma, including endodermal sinus tumor (yolk sac tumor), embryonal carcinoma, teratocarcinoma, and choriocarcinoma. These tumors can exist in nongonadal sites, as in the retroperitoneum and mediastinum. Additional procedures such as scanning or biopsy will be needed to confirm the diagnosis.

In patients who are being treated for hepatoma or germinal tumor, AFP values will be used to monitor the response to antineoplastic medications. A rising AFP level indicates increased tumor growth, and a falling value indicates a favorable response to the medications.

Critical Thinking: An infant is born with anencephaly. What are the ethical considerations and legal parameters in the parent's decision to donate the infant's organs for transplant purposes?

In the pregnant female, AFP is used for intrauterine screening, optimally in the 16th to 18th week of pregnancy. Abnormally elevated values are often present in cases of open neural tube deficits, which include spina bifida, myelomeningocele, and anencephaly. Other congenital defects may also cause an elevation of AFP.

Because this test can have false-positive results in pregnancy, the abnormal elevation is considered to be only suggestive of abnormality in the fetus. Other tests such as ultrasound of the fetal spine and analysis of the amniotic fluid are needed to provide additional data.

Procedure

A red-topped, sterile tube is used to collect 5 to 10 ml of venous blood. There is no need for the patient to fast for this test.

If amniotic fluid is to be analyzed, 2 ml of the fluid is collected during the amniocentesis.

QUALITY CONTROL
The specimen is kept refrigerated until the analysis is performed.

Findings

ELEVATED VALUES

Nonpregnant State	**Pregnant State**
Liver cancer	Spina bifida
Gonadal germinal tumor	Myelomeningocele
Cancer of the pancreas	Fetal death
Cancer of the stomach	Anencephaly
Cancer of the gallbladder	Oligohydramnios
Cancer of the bile ducts	Esophageal atresia
Necrosis of the liver	Congenital nephrosis
Hepatitis	Multiple pregnancy
Cirrhosis	Preeclampsia
Liver trauma	Abruptio placentae

Interfering Factors

- Recent radioisotope scan

Nursing Implementation

Pretest

On the requisition slip, include the following data: gestational age, maternal weight, race, and diabetic status.

QUALITY CONTROL

These are variables that affect the interpretation of normal values.

AMMONIA

(SERUM)

Synonym:

NH_3

NORMAL VALUES

Adult:	15–45 µg/dl *or* SI 11–22 µmol/L
Child:	29–70 µg/dl *or* SI 21–50 µmol/L
Neonate:	90–150 µg/dl *or* SI 64–107 µmol/L

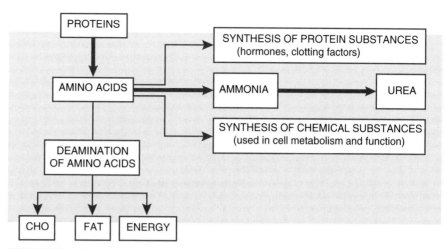

FIGURE 18–1. The synthesis of proteins by the liver. Ammonia is a toxic chemical by-product created by the utilization of amino acids. Ammonia should be converted to urea by the liver and the urea excreted in urine. When ammonia is retained, the level rises in the blood. After it crosses the blood-brain barrier, the elevated ammonia level affects cerebral function and results in hepatic encephalopathy.

Background Information

Critical Thinking: The patient with hepatic encephalopathy has a serum ammonia level of 70 µg/dl (SI: 50 µmol/L). At the time of the next blood test, he refuses to be tested and states, "I want no more tests or treatments. I want to die." How can the nurse respond?

Ammonia, a by-product of protein catabolism, is manufactured during the process of deamination of amino acids. It is made by the metabolizing tissues of the body and by bacterial activity that acts on protein in the intestine. As ammonia enters and circulates in the blood stream, the liver pulls it out of the portal vein circulation. In hepatic metabolic function, the ammonia is used in the urea synthesis cycle and is converted to urea. The kidneys remove the urea from the circulation and excrete it in the urine. The two most common causes of an elevated ammonia level are the failure of hepatic cells to function in the conversion of ammonia to urea and the impairment of the portal vein circulation, which prevents ammonia from reaching the liver tissue (Fig. 18–1).

Purpose of the Test

The ammonia level is used to evaluate or monitor severe liver failure, hepatoencephalopathy, and the effects of impaired portal vein circulation. It is used in the preliminary identification of rare types of inborn errors of metabolism that affect the urea synthesis cycle of the neonate (aminoaciduria). It is also used to help diagnose Reye syndrome, a childhood disorder that results in an acute fatty liver and encephalopathy.

Procedure

A gray-, lavender-, or green-topped sterile tube is used to collect 3 to 5 ml of venous blood.

> **QUALITY CONTROL**
>
> The vacuum tube must be completely filled and then kept sealed to prevent a false-positive result. Once the blood is drawn, the vial must be placed on ice and and rotated immediately to chill the specimen.

Findings

ELEVATED VALUES

Liver failure (hepatic necrosis, terminal cirrhosis)
Hepatoencephalopathy
Portal hypertension
Portacaval shunting of the blood
Inborn errors of metabolism that affect the urea synthesis cycle
   (some aminoaciduria)
Reye syndrome

Interfering Factors

- Tobacco smoke
- High protein intake
- Gastrointestinal hemorrhage
- Hyperalimentation (total parenteral nutrition)
- Ureterosigmoidostomy

Nursing Implementation

Pretest

Instruct the patient to fast from food for 8 hours prior to the test, since protein intake will raise the ammonia level. Water intake is permitted. Instruct the patient not to smoke before the test, since the smoke itself will alter the results.

Posttest

Ensure that the vial of blood is kept on ice and is sent to the laboratory immediately.

> **QUALITY CONTROL**
>
> The blood must be delivered to the laboratory in its ice container. To avoid false-positive results, the tube will be centrifuged and the serum analyzed or frozen for storage within 20 minutes.

AMYLASE

(SERUM)

Synonyms:

NORMAL VALUES

Adults:	60–180 Somogyi units *or* 25–125 U/L
Children:	>1 year: same as adult values
Neonates:	5–65 U/L

Background Information

Amylase is a group of enzymes manufactured in the exocrine pancreas and parotid glands. The digestive function is to hydrolyze starch and convert it to maltose. The alpha-amylase that is present in saliva converts some of the starch, but the vast majority of the activity results from pancreatic amylase. The lack of pancreatic amylase results in poor digestion of dietary starch. Thus, the fecal matter becomes bulky and undergoes increased bacterial fermentation.

When the acinar cells of the pancreas produce the amylase, the enzymes normally flow out through the pancreatic ducts, common bile duct, and ampulla of Vater to empty into the duodenum. Inflammation or obstruction in any part of the drainage system will cause regurgitation of the amylase back into pancreatic tissue. The amylase is then absorbed into the blood stream via the pancreatic venules and the lymphatics.

With inflammation of the parotid glands, as in parotitis (mumps), there is serum absorption of the salivary amylase. Pancreatic inflammation and ductal obstruction appear to be the cause of hyperamylasemia in intestinal diseases such as perforated peptic ulcer, intestinal obstruction, mesenteric infarct, and other serious intestinal disorders.

Mucoviscidosis is a congenital pancreatic disease that causes dysfunction of mucus-secreting glands. Thick, viscid mucus obstructs the pancreatic ductal system, causing acinar cell atrophy and cystic fibrosis of the pancreas. In children who have advanced cystic fibrosis, the serum amylase levels are decreased.

Purpose of the Test

Serum amylase is used to investigate the cause of abdominal pain or epigastric pain, with the goal of differentiating between acute pancreatitis and a surgical emergency such as perforation of the stomach or infarct of the bowel. It helps in the diagnosis of acute pancreatitis, traumatic injury to the pancreas or a surgical complication that affects the pancreas.

Procedure

A red-topped, sterile tube is used to collect 5 to 10 ml of venous blood.

QUALITY CONTROL

Personnel should not talk, sneeze, or cough near an open collection tube. Their saliva will add to the amylase content of the specimen.

Findings

ELEVATED VALUES

Acute pancreatitis
Obstruction of the ampulla of Vater
Obstruction of the common bile duct
Pancreatic cancer
Pancreatic pseudocyst
Pancreatic ascites
Pancreatic abscess

Trauma to the pancreas
Parotitis (mumps)
Intestinal obstruction
Perforated peptic ulcer
Aortic aneurysm
Traumatic shock

DECREASED VALUES

Chronic pancreatitis
Cirrhosis
Hepatitis

Pancreatic cancer
Toxemia of pregnancy
Cystic fibrosis

Interfering Factors

- Ingestion of alcohol prior to the test
- Recent use of morphine, which closes the sphincter of Oddi

Nursing Implementation

Pretest

Instruct the patient not to ingest alcohol for 24 hours before the test. Alcohol stimulates the secretion of salivary amylase. No other fasting measures are required.

Prior to the test, morphine, codeine, meperidine (Demerol), and other drugs that affect amylase levels may be omitted.

AMYLASE

(URINE)

Synonyms:

─────────────── **NORMAL VALUES** ───────────────

| Adult: | 4–30 IU/2 hours (2-hour test) |
| | Up to 3000 U/24 hours (24-hour test) |

Background Information

Amylase is excreted or cleared from the body in the urine. When the serum amylase level is elevated, the glomerular filtration rate increases and a greater amount of amylase clearance occurs. The amount of amylase clearance is measured in units per volume in a specified period.

Purpose of the Test

In acute pancreatitis, the elevation of serum amylase lasts for only 3 to 4 days. It may be missed because of the timing of the blood work. Urine amylase levels remain elevated for up to 2 weeks after an episode of acute pancreatitis. Thus, urine amylase can help diagnose acute pancreatitis when the serum levels are borderline or normal.

Procedure

Urine is collected in a clean container for a specific period. The most common time span is 2 hours, but 6-, 8-, or 24-hour collection periods are sometimes used. During the test, the specimen is kept refrigerated or on ice.

Findings

ELEVATED VALUES
Acute pancreatitis
Cancer of the head of the pancreas
Pancreatic pseudocyst
Gallbladder disease
Obstruction (pancreatic ducts, intestine, salivary glands)
Parotitis (mumps)

DECREASED VALUES
Alcoholism
Chronic pancreatitis
Cancer of the liver
Hepatitis
Hepatic abscess
Cirrhosis

Interfering Factors

- Heavy menstrual flow
- Bacterial contamination of the urine
- Salivary amylase contamination of the specimen
- Omission of any voided specimen
- Failure to cool the specimen

Nursing Implementation

Pretest

Instruct the patient not to ingest alcohol for 24 hours before the test. Alcohol stimulates the secretion of salivary amylase.

Just before the start of the test, instruct the patient to void and discard the specimen. This urine has been in the bladder for an unknown period.

All subsequent specimens are collected and added to the clean urine container, including the final voided urine of the period.

During the test, refrigerate the container of urine or place the container in a basin of ice. Amylase is unstable in acidic urine.

On the specimen label and the requisition slip, write the date and time for the start and finish of the test.

ASPARTATE AMINOTRANSFERASE

(SERUM)

Synonyms:

AST; glutamate oxaloacetate transaminase, serum; SGOT; GOT; transaminase

NORMAL VALUES

Average Adult Range:	8–20 U/L
Male Adult >60 Years:	11–26 U/L
Female Adult >60 Years:	10–20 U/L
Child <5 Years:	19–28 U/L
Infant:	16–72 U/L
Newborn:	16–72 U/L

Background Information

AST is a transaminase enzyme found predominantly in the heart, but it is also highly concentrated in the liver. It is present to a lesser extent in skeletal muscle, kidney, brain, pancreas, spleen, and lungs. There is always some concentration in the blood. Most of the AST within the liver cells is located in the mitochondria of hepatocytes. The discussion of AST as a laboratory test in heart disease is presented in Chapter 14.

When there is mild injury, inflammation, or necrosis of liver cells, the AST is released through damaged cell membranes and results in rising levels within the serum. With severe damage, the mitochondria of the hepatocytes are destroyed, and greater amounts of AST are released. In severe or fulminant viral hepatitis, the AST value can rise to 20 to 100 times the normal value.

Since AST is also present in skeletal muscle tissue and other organs, the serum AST value will rise because of inflammation, injury, or necrosis of those tissues. Generally, these elevations are slight to moderate, although shock, acute pancreatitis, and infectious mononucleosis occasionally cause a severe elevation of the serum value. This test replaces the old cephalin flocculation and thymol turbidity tests.

Purpose of the Test

AST is an indicator of inflammation, injury, or necrosis of the tissues that contain the enzyme. It shows moderate elevation for a timed interval after myocardial infarction. In liver disease, it is an indicator of hepatocellular damage from any cause.

AST is also used to monitor liver function in patients who receive medication that is potentially hepatotoxic. When the value rises to more than three times the upper limit of normal, the physician should be notified. This is generally the indication to discontinue the medication.

Comparisons of AST to ALT are sometimes used to differentiate among the causes of hepatocellular damage. The results are expressed as a ratio of AST to ALT. Since the amounts of each enzyme are about equal, the ratio is expressed as AST = ALT or AST:ALT = 1. In alcoholic hepatitis, the AST value is greater than the ALT value (AST > ALT) or the ratio is expressed numerically. For example, AST:ALT = 3:1 means that the AST value is three times greater than the ALT value. It is proposed that alcohol is toxic to the mitochondria of the hepatocytes and therefore the AST level rises to more than the ALT level. Conversely, the ALT value can rise to greater than the AST value (ALT > AST). This is often true in viral hepatitis.

Procedure

A red-topped sterile tube is used to collect 5 to 10 ml of venous blood.

QUALITY CONTROL

Venipuncture technique must be smooth, with blood flow that fills the tube readily. If the blood has excessive turbulence because of flawed venipuncture technique, the hemolysis of erythrocytes will alter the results.

Findings

ELEVATED VALUES

Myocardial infarction
Pericarditis
Cardiac arrhythmias
Following cardiac surgery, catheterization
Heart failure
Hepatitis (viral, toxic)
Hemochromatosis
Cirrhosis
Hepatic congestion
Hepatic tumor (primary or metastatic)
Obstructive jaundice
Infectious mononucleosis
Shock

Renal infarction
Pulmonary infarction
Legionnaires disease
Acute pancreatitis
Cerebral necrosis (trauma, cerebrovascular accident, surgery)
Dermatomyositis
Polymyositis
Trichinosis
Muscular dystrophy
Delirium tremens
Gangrene
Severe injury to skeletal muscle tissue

DECREASED VALUES

Pregnancy

Interfering Factors

- Hemolysis
- Failure to maintain a nothing by mouth status
- Intense exercise prior to the test

Nursing Implementation

Pretest

Instruct the patient to fast for 12 hours before the test (overnight). The ambulatory patient should avoid strenuous exercise before the test.

BILIRUBIN, TOTAL, DIRECT, INDIRECT, NEONATAL

(SERUM)

Synonyms:

total bilirubin, blood bilirubin; serum bilirubin; plasma bilirubin
direct bilirubin; conjugated bilirubin
indirect bilirubin; unconjugated bilirubin, free bilirubin
neonatal bilirubin, total bilirubin, neonatal; baby bilirubin; microbilirubin

━━━━━━━━━━━━━━ **NORMAL VALUES** ━━━━━━━━━━━━━

TOTAL BILIRUBIN	
Adult:	0.3–1 mg/dl *or* SI 5–17 μmol/L
Child:	0.2–0.8 mg/dl *or* SI 3.4–13.6 μmol/L
Full-term Neonate	
(By 72 Hours After Birth):	6–10 mg/dl *or* SI 103–171 μmol/L
Premature Neonate:	up to 12 mg/dl *or* SI up to 205 μmol/L
	Note: The values for premature neonates vary according to the degree of prematurity
Direct Bilirubin (Adult):	0–0.4 mg/dl *or* SI <5 μmol/L
Indirect Bilirubin (Adult):	0.2–0.8 mg/dl *or* SI 3.4–13.6 μmol/L

Background Information

PRODUCTION. Bilirubin is produced in the reticuloendothelial cells, primarily the Kupffer cells of the liver. It is also produced in the reticuloendothelial cells of the spleen, bone marrow, and lymph nodes. Most bilirubin is formed from the hemoglobin as the reticuloendothelial cells break down senescent erythrocytes that have reached the end of their 120-day life span. The remainder of bilirubin formation is from the enzymes that contain heme and from the destruction of damaged, abnormal erythrocytes that have a short life span.

TRANSPORT. Once bilirubin is produced, it is transported in plasma to the liver. In this transport process, bilirubin is bound to molecules of albumin and is called indirect or unconjugated bilirubin. A small amount of the unconjugated bilirubin remains in the plasma circulation, but the rest of it is acted on by the liver to convert it to direct, conjugated bilirubin.

CONJUGATION. Within the liver cells, indirect bilirubin is first separated from the albumin. It is then acted on by the enzyme glucuronyltransferase, is conjugated with glucuronic acid, and is transformed into direct, conjugated bilirubin. The conjugated bilirubin is a water-soluble, yellow-green pigment that can now cross the cell membrane and enter bile canaliculi. As it mixes with fluid, the conjugated bilirubin becomes a component of bile.

EXCRETION. The excreted bile flows from canaliculi and hepatic ducts within the liver to the biliary ductal system. Bile and its conjugated bilirubin component are concentrated and then stored in the gallbladder. The bile exits to the duodenum via the cystic and common ducts (Fig. 18–2). About 300 mg of bilirubin is released into the duodenum daily (Raphael, 1983). The physiologic basis for the bilirubin diagnostic tests is presented in Table 18–1.

JAUNDICE. This is a clinical term that describes the yellow discoloration of the skin and sclera caused by excess bilirubin in the blood and body tissues. The jaundice becomes visible when the total serum bilirubin level rises to greater than 2 mg/dl. The elevated serum bilirubin level is called hyperbilirubinemia.

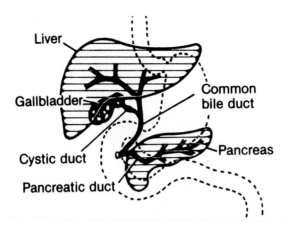

FIGURE 18–2. Anatomy of the gallbladder and its ducts. (Reproduced with permission from *Gallstones.* [1987]. [NIH publication No. 87-2897, p. 1]. Washington, D.C.: U.S. Department of Health and Human Services, Public Health Service, National Institutes of Health.)

TABLE 18–1
PHYSIOLOGIC BASIS FOR BILIRUBIN DIAGNOSTIC TESTS

Anatomic Sites	Physiology of Bilirubin Formation, Transport, and Excretion	Diagnostic Tests
Reticuloendothelial system	Hemolysis of senescent and abnormal erythrocytes	
	Formation of unconjugated bilirubin	
Circulation	Transport of unconjugated bilirubin to the liver	Indirect serum bilirubin
Liver	Conversion of unconjugated to conjugated bilirubin	Total serum bilirubin and direct serum bilirubin
	Excretion of bilirubin in bile salts and bile	
Biliary ductal system	Concentration, transport, storage, and excretion of bile	
Intestine	Conversion of direct bilirubin to urobilinogen	Fecal urobilinogen
	Excretion of urobilinogen	
Kidney	Filtration and excretion of urobilinogen and bilirubin	Urine urobilinogen and urine bilirubin

One method of classification of jaundice is based on the predominant type of elevation of bilirubin in the blood. A rise in the *unconjugated bilirubin* is usually due to excessive hemolysis of red blood cells and is sometimes called *hemolytic jaundice.* A rise in the *conjugated bilirubin* is usually due to obstruction in the flow of bile and is sometimes referred to as *cholestasis.* The obstruction can occur at any level from bile canaliculi to the ampulla of Vater or from intrahepatic to extrahepatic sites.

A second method of classification is based on three possible locations of the problem. They are the prehepatic, hepatic, and posthepatic categories of jaundice.

Prehepatic Jaundice. This means that the problem occurs before the bilirubin reaches the liver. The causes are all hemolytic, and more erythrocytes are hemolyzed than can be transported or conjugated. Thus, the elevation of bilirubin is due to the rise in the indirect or unconjugated component.

Hepatic Jaundice. This means that the origin of the problem is within the liver. Some of the abnormalities are due to an inability to transport or conjugate bilirubin within hepatocytes, resulting in an elevation of indirect, unconjugated bilirubin. Other abnormalities are due to blockage in the excretion of the bile within the liver, and the problem is referred to as intrahepatic cholestasis. The blockage can occur at the cell level when injured or diseased hepatocytes cannot permit conjugated bilirubin from crossing the cell membranes or exiting from the bile canaliculi and hepatic ducts. When conjugated bilirubin cannot be excreted, there is a resultant rise in the serum values.

Posthepatic Jaundice. This means that the origin of the problem is outside or beyond the liver and it is sometimes called extrahepatic cholestasis. The bile flow is obstructed somewhere in the biliary ductal system, including at the head of the pancreas, within the ampulla of Vater, and in the common bile duct. In these cases, there is also a rise in the direct, conjugated bilirubin value. A summary of the classifications of jaundice is presented in Table 18–2.

TABLE 18–2
CLASSIFICATION OF JAUNDICE

Category of Jaundice	Origin of the Problem	Type of Bilirubin Elevation
Prehepatic	Excessive hemolysis of erythrocytes Hemolytic jaundice	Indirect (unconjugated)
Hepatic	Defect in transport or conjugation in hepatocytes Physiologic or neonatal jaundice	Indirect (unconjugated)
Hepatic	Injury to or disease of hepatocytes Blockage of intrahepatic bile canaliculi Intrahepatic cholestasis	Direct (conjugated)
Posthepatic	Blockage in the biliary ductal system Extrahepatic cholestasis	Direct (conjugated)

Critical Thinking: A 2-day-old neonate is to be discharged from the newborn nursery. The value of the neonate's total bilirubin has risen to 14 mg/dl (SI: 239 μmol/L). In your discharge plan, what do you teach the mother about follow-up assessment and care for the baby?

Neonatal Jaundice. Newborn infants experience varying levels of elevated bilirubin in the first few days of life. The condition is called *physiologic jaundice.* It is not clear why this condition occurs, but it is temporary. The condition may be due to excess hemolysis of red blood cells, a transient defect in glucuronyl transferase enzyme activity, or a reabsorption of unconjugated bilirubin from the intestine. If the bilirubin level rises to more than 15 mg/dl or remains at greater than 10 mg/dl for longer than 14 days, the jaundice is considered pathologic.

Other causes of neonatal jaundice are considered abnormal or pathologic, including ABO or Rh incompatibility that causes a big rise in unconjugated bilirubin. If the unconjugated bilirubin rises to more than 20 mg/dl, there is potential for kernicterus. In this state, bilirubin is deposited in the brain, and permanent damage can occur. The multiple causes of kernicterus include hemolysis of erythrocytes, impaired ability of the liver to conjugate bilirubin, impairment of the unconjugated bilirubin to bind to albumin for transport, and possible impairment of the glucuronyl transferase activity in the conjugation of bilirubin.

If the infant is born with biliary atresia, the extrahepatic biliary ducts are blocked. There will be a rapid, severe rise in conjugated bilirubin.

Purpose of the Test

Total serum bilirubin is the sum total of indirect unconjugated bilirubin and direct conjugated bilirubin in the blood. The purpose of the total bilirubin test is to evaluate liver function, diagnose jaundice, monitor the progression of jaundice, and determine whether an infant needs treatment to prevent kernicterus. The purpose of the indirect and direct bilirubin tests is to help identify the underlying cause of hyperbilirubinemia.

Procedure

Adult: A red-topped, sterile tube is used to collect 5 to 10 ml of venous blood.

Infant: A blue capillary tube is used to draw drops of blood from the heel, which has been pricked by a sterile lancet.

Neonatal bilirubin generally is used for infants less than 10 days of age. Thereafter, total serum bilirubin is requested, the capillary tubes remain in use for collection of the specimen.

In the laboratory analysis, the total bilirubin and direct bilirubin are measured directly. The indirect bilirubin is calculated by subtracting the value for the direct bilirubin from the value for the total bilirubin.

Total bilirubin − direct bilirubin = indirect bilirubin

QUALITY CONTROL

Venipuncture technique must be smooth with a blood flow that fills the vacuum tube readily. If the blood flow has excessive turbulence because of flawed venipuncture technique, hemolysis of the erythrocytes will alter the test results.

Findings

ELEVATED VALUES

Total Serum Bilirubin

Hepatocellular damage (toxic or neoplastic)
Biliary tree obstruction (intra- or extrahepatic)
Neonatal (physiologic jaundice)
Hemolytic diseases
Gilbert disease (familial hyperbilirubinemia)
Dubin-Johnson syndrome

Direct Bilirubin

Hepatotoxins causing necrosis
Neoplasm (primary or metastatic)
Dubin-Johnson syndrome
Sclerosing cholangitis
Cancer of the ampulla of Vater
Parasites
Pregnancy
Lymphoma
Infection of liver

Cirrhosis
Medications
Cholangiocarcinoma
Primary biliary cirrhosis
Biliary atresia
Biliary stones
Acute pancreatitis
Cancer of the pancreas

Indirect Bilirubin

Familial defects of erythrocytes (spherocytosis, sickle cell disease)
Traumatic tissue injury with hemorrhage of hematoma
Malaria
Hodgkin disease
Familial enzyme disorders (glucuronyl transferase deficiency,
   Gilbert disease)
Neonatal jaundice (physiologic jaundice)
Rh or ABO incompatibility
Blood transfusion reaction due to incompatibility
Medications

Interfering Factors

- Sunlight
- Hemolysis
- Failure to maintain a nothing by mouth status (adults only)

Nursing Implementation

Pretest

Instruct the patient to fast from food for 8 to 12 hours (overnight), since
   serum lipids will alter results.

Posttest

Ensure that the vial of blood or microcapillary tube is covered and sent to the laboratory without delay.

QUALITY CONTROL

Since bilirubin is photosensitive, the blood sample must be protected from exposure to light or prolonged time in a lighted environment.

CAROTENE

(SERUM)

Synonym:

carotene, beta

NORMAL VALUES

Adult:	40–200 µg/dl *or* SI 0.7–3.7 µmol/L
Infant:	up to 60 µg/dl *or* SI up to 1.52 µmol/L

Background Information

Beta-carotene is a fat-soluble provitamin, a precursor of vitamin A. It is found in fresh yellow fruits and vegetables. In humans, the highest levels are found in food faddists who restrict their diet to these foods only. The excessive intake is not toxic but it will cause high serum carotene levels and yellow coloring of the skin. Carotenoderma appears in the nasolabial folds, hands, and feet and can be confused with jaundice. Unlike jaundice, however, the yellow coloring does not affect the sclera.

The absorption of carotene is dependent on normal absorption of dietary fat in the intestine. Either the lack of carotene in the diet or disturbances in the intestinal absorption of fat will result in low levels of serum carotene.

Purpose of the Test

Serum carotene is used to screen for fat malabsorption. It is also used to diagnose carotenoderma, caused by the high intake of carotene-rich foods.

Procedure

A red-topped, sterile tube is used to collect 5 to 10 ml of venous blood.

QUALITY CONTROL

After centrifuge, the specimen must not be exposed to light.

Findings

ELEVATED VALUES

Excessive intake of carotene
Carotenoderma
Liver disease
Diabetes mellitus
Hypothyroidism
Hyperlipidemia

Pregnancy
Subacute thyroiditis
Hyperlipoproteinemia (types I, IIA, IIB)
Myxedema
Nephrotic syndrome

DECREASED VALUES

Fever
Liver disease
Small bowel disease

Enteritis
Malabsorption (with loss of fat and vitamin A)

Interfering Factors

- Failure to maintain a nothing by mouth status
- Exposure of specimen to sunlight

Nursing Implementation

Pretest

Instruct the patient to fast from food for at least 8 hours (overnight).

CERULOPLASMIN

(SERUM)

Synonyms:

Background Information

Ceruloplasmin, an alpha$_2$-globulin, is a copper-binding protein that is synthesized by the liver. Its exact function is unknown, but the serum ceruloplasmin contains most of the total plasma copper. As an enzyme, it may be important in the regulation of oxidation of metallic ions, including iron.

Because it is one of a group of serum proteins categorized as acute-phase reactants, the serum ceruloplasmin level rises in conditions of inflammation,

——————————— **NORMAL VALUES** ———————————

Adult:	20–40 mg/dl *or* SI 200–350 mg/L
Neonate–3 Months:	5–18 mg/dl *or* SI 50–180 mg/L

infection, surgery, trauma, and malignancy. The acute-phase reactants are part of the body's response designed to handle extensive insult or injury.

The decreased response or low level of ceruloplasmin is associated with malabsorption, protein loss, and advanced liver disease that results in inadequate manufacture of all serum proteins. The low ceruloplasmin level is specifically associated with Wilson disease, an autosomal recessive disease that results in the deposit of copper in all body tissues. The most common organ sites are the brain and liver, and the high level of copper deposits in the liver results in the onset of cirrhosis. The effect of a high copper level in the brain includes a loss of coordination, spasticity, rigidity, difficulty in speaking, and dysphagia.

Purpose of the Test

Ceruloplasmin is used to evaluate chronic active hepatitis, cirrhosis, and other liver diseases. Because the low levels can indicate Wilson disease, the test is also used to help diagnose unexplained central nervous system disorders that affect coordination.

Procedure

A red-topped, *chilled*, sterile tube is used to collect 5 to 10 ml of venous blood.

QUALITY CONTROL

Venipuncture technique must be smooth, with a blood flow that fills the vacuum tube readily. If the blood has excessive turbulence because of flawed venipuncture technique, the hemolysis of the erythrocytes will alter the results.

Findings

ELEVATED VALUES

Inflammation
Tissue necrosis
Trauma
Primary biliary cirrhosis
Rheumatoid arthritis

Leukemias
Hodgkin disease
Malignancy
Systemic lupus erythematosus

DECREASED VALUES

Wilson disease
Nephrotic syndrome
Hepatocellular disease

Menke disease
Malabsorption syndrome

Interfering Factors

- Pregnancy
- Hemolysis
- Failure to maintain a nothing by mouth status

Nursing Implementation

Pretest

Instruct the patient to fast from food and fluids for 12 hours before the test. High levels of serum lipids (lipemia) will affect the results.

Inform the physician or laboratory, or both, if the patient is pregnant or taking oral contraceptives. High levels of estrogen will cause high levels of ceruloplasmin.

Posttest

Ensure that the vial of blood is placed on ice and sent to the laboratory immediately.

QUALITY CONTROL

Prolonged exposure to room temperature will result in a falsely depressed value. Once the chilled specimen reaches the laboratory, it is centrifuged immediately. The fresh serum will be analyzed without delay, or it is frozen until the test can be performed.

FECAL FAT

(FECES)

Synonyms:

fecal lipids; fat, quantitative; 72-hour stool collection; stool fat, quantitative.

Background Information

In normal digestive processes, dietary fats undergo digestion and absorption in the small intestine. The first stage is emulsification of the neutral fats or triglycerides by bile acids and bile salts. In this emulsification process, the bile acts as a detergent and breaks the globules of fat into tiny droplets. This provides a large surface for lipolytic activity by the pancreatic enzyme lipase.

```
━━━━━━━━━━━━━━━━━━  NORMAL VALUES  ━━━━━━━━━━━━
┌──────────────────────────────────────────────────────────────┐
│  Adult:                        <7 g/24 hours                   │
│  Adult (Fat-free Diet):        <4 g/24 hours                   │
│  Child (Newborn–6 Years):      <2 g/24 hours                   │
│  Infant (Breast-fed):          <1 g/24 hours                   │
└──────────────────────────────────────────────────────────────┘
```

Critical Thinking: When the patient brings the fecal fat specimen to the clinic, she admits that she left the specimen on the back porch during the collection period. "I don't want it in my refrigerator," she adds. How can you resolve this problem?

In the second stage, the pancreatic lipase splits the fat molecule into free fatty acids, glycerol, and glycerides (monoglycerides and diglycerides), the end products of fat digestion. Bile salts then surround some of these end products and carry them to the mucosal cell membranes for absorption by the small intestine. The free fatty acids and monoglycerides are soluble and are absorbed directly into the small intestine without the assistance of the carrier mechanism.

In normal digestion, virtually all fatty acids, monoglycerides, and triglycerides are absorbed. The normal adult excretes only a small portion of fat in the feces. When there is malabsorption of fat, a high level of fat appears in the feces and is called steatorrhea. The possible causes are (1) a lack of bile flow into the intestine, (2) pancreatic insufficiency, and (3) damage to the mucosal cells of the small intestine.

Purpose of the Test

Fecal fat is the definitive test to identify steatorrhea. It does not define the cause of the problem but rather evaluates the ability to digest fat from dietary intake. Abnormal results support evidence of hepatobiliary, pancreatic, or small intestinal disease.

Procedure

For 3 days preceding the test and during the 3 days of specimen collection, the patient eats a standard, high-fat diet (100 g of fat per day). The 72-hour collection of feces is performed on days 4, 5, and 6 of the diet. All fecal matter in the 72-hour period is collected in a clean, heavy plastic, screw-capped container. The specimen is refrigerated during the collection period.

Findings

ELEVATED VALUES

Pancreatic insufficiency	Regional enteritis
Pancreatic obstruction	Celiac disease
Pancreatic resection	Tropical sprue
Whipple disease	Radiation enteritis
Cystic fibrosis	Gastroduodenal fistula
Chronic pancreatitis	Extensive small bowel resection

Biliary tract obstruction	Scleroderma
Liver cirrhosis	Intestinal tuberculosis
Impaired hepatic function	Dumping syndrome
Thyrotoxicosis	Psoriasis
Addison disease	Lymphomas

Interfering Factors

- Use of improper collection container
- Contamination of the sample
- Failure to follow the dietary prescription
- Incomplete collection—omission of any specimen
- Alcohol ingestion before or during the test
- Ingestion of mineral oil before or during the test

Nursing Implementation

Pretest

Instruct the patient to follow the prescribed diet for 3 days before and 3 days during the test. Ingestion of alcohol is omitted for 24 hours before collection and during the 3 days of collection.

Instruct the patient about proper collection procedure, including the correct type of container (see Chapter 2).

QUALITY CONTROL

Improper containers include coffee cans, paper cartons, waxed containers, or plastic bags. The specimen must be free of urine, toilet paper, tongue depressors, and plastic spoons.

During the Test

Ensure that the specimen is refrigerated for the entire collection period and until it is transported to the laboratory.

Posttest

Write the time and date for the start and finish of the collection period on the container label and on the requisition slip.

GAMMA-GLUTAMYLTRANSFERASE

(SERUM)

Synonyms:

γ-glutamyltransferase, γ-glutamyltranspeptidase, GGT, GGTP, GTP, GT

─────────────── **NORMAL VALUES** ───────────────

Average Adult Range:	5–40 IU/L
Male Adult:	22.1 ± 11.7 IU/L
Female Adult:	15.4 ± 6.58 IU/L
Children >4 Years:	same as adult values

Background Information

Gamma-glutamyltransferase is a biliary enzyme that is present in cell membranes and microsomes of cells. It is most predominant in the kidney, but it is also amply present in the liver and pancreas. The enzyme's probable functions are to assist in the transport of amino acids across cell membranes and in glutathione metabolism.

The serum level of gamma-glutamyltransferase rises when there is intrahepatic or posthepatic biliary obstruction. This laboratory value will rise early and remain elevated as long as the dysfunction persists. This test replaces the old sulfobromophthalein sodium test.

Purpose of the Test

The gamma-glutamyltransferase test is used to detect hepatobiliary disease. The gamma-glutamyltransferase values will rise in parallel to the values of ALP, leucine aminopeptidase, and 5′-nucleotidase in conditions of posthepatic jaundice and in diseases of the liver and pancreas.

In the presence of elevated ALP, the gamma-glutamyltransferase level is used to differentiate between hepatobiliary and bone sources of abnormality.

The gamma-glutamyltransferase is also used to diagnose and evaluate chronic alcoholic liver disease. It can detect the resumption of drinking in the alcoholic patient.

Procedure

A red- or green-topped sterile tube is used to collect 5 to 10 ml of venous blood.

Findings

ELEVATED VALUES

Obstructive biliary disease
Obstructive liver disease
Acute liver disease (hepatitis, cirrhosis)
Acute pancreatitis
Hepatoma
Cancer of the pancreas

Infectious mononucleosis
Hyperthyroidism
Systemic lupus erythematosus
Myocardial disease
Following renal transplantation

DECREASED VALUES

Hypothyroidism

Interfering Factors

- Intake of alcohol within 60 hours before the test
- Use of medications: barbiturates, phenytoin, and oral contraceptives
- Failure to maintain a nothing by mouth status

Nursing Implementation

Pretest

Instruct the patient to abstain from alcohol for 72 hours prior to the test. Inform the patient to fast from food and fluids for 12 hours before the test. Inform the physician or laboratory of the use of medications that interfere with the results. Patients who must continue to take these medications should not suspend the dosage schedule. An alternative test such as leucine aminopeptidase or 5'-nucleotidase may be preferable.

HEPATITIS VIRUS TESTS

Acute viral hepatitis is an infection that causes systemic illness and in-flammation of liver cells. There are different causative agents of the disease, based on the antigen properties of each virus. Although these viruses are different in their characteristics and modes of transmission, they produce clinically similar forms of disease.

Hepatitis A is caused by the hepatitis A virus. Hepatitis B is caused by the hepatitis B virus. Non-A, non-B hepatitis is caused by at least two viruses, type C (parental transmission) and type E (enteric transmission). Recently, a blood test to detect the antibody to the hepatitis C virus was developed. To date, however, the virus that causes hepatitis C has not been isolated, and there is no laboratory test for its antigen. Delta hepatitis is caused by the delta virus. The hepatitis E virus has been recovered from the sera of patients with non-A, non-B hepatitis. Although research testing for the hepatitis E virus antibody is under way, there is no commercial test available to detect hepatitis E virus infection at this time (Favorov, 1992; Abbott Laboratories, 1992).

The diagnosis of hepatitis is usually based on the clinical manifestations and liver function tests. The hepatitis virus tests are used to determine which of the viruses has caused the infection. Once the specific virus is identified, the patient's treatment and epidemiologic interventions are more accurate.

The hepatitis virus tests are all performed on blood samples, with analysis by either radioimmunoassay or enzyme immunoassay (enzyme immunoassay or enzyme-linked immunosorbent assay). These tests identify the antigens or antibodies related to the specific virus. An antigen is the substance that provokes the production of a specific immune response. An antibody is an immunoglobulin that is produced in response to the antigen, with specific binding affinity to that antigen.

The series of hepatitis B tests can be confusing because more than one component of the virus is tested. The hepatitis B virus is a DNA virus with a protein surface coat and a nucleic acid core. There is also an e component that is thought to be a degradation product of the core of the virus. The surface coat of the hepatitis B virus is an antigen, the hepatitis B surface antigen, with a corresponding antibody response, the hepatitis B surface antibody. The core is an antigen called the core antigen or the hepatitis B core antigen, with a corresponding antibody response, the hepatitis B core antibody. It is also possible to detect the e antigen and the corresponding e core antibody.

HEPATITIS A ANTIBODY

(SERUM)

Synonyms:
HAV, Ab; HAVAb; anti-HAV

NORMAL VALUES ---

Hepatitis A Antibody:	negative
IgM Type:	negative
IgG Type:	negative

Background Information

The hepatitis A virus is transmitted by the fecal-oral route, primarily after ingestion of virus-contaminated water, food, milk, or shellfish. Although the antigen has been found in fecal matter, the serologic diagnosis is based on the presence of hepatitis A antibodies in the blood. There are two types of hepatitis A antibodies: the IgM type and the IgG type.

The IgM type, also called anti-HAV IgM, appears early. It is present in the blood within 1 week after symptoms begin. It peaks within 3 months and subsides in 4 to 6 months during convalescence. The IgG type, also called anti-HAV total or hepatitis A antibody IgG, begins to rise after 4 weeks of infection and persists for life (Fig. 18–3).

Purpose of the Test

The hepatitis A virus antibodies identify the hepatitis A virus as the cause of infection. The specific antibody type distinguishes between current and past infection.

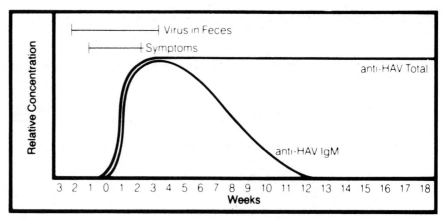

FIGURE 18–3. Hepatitis A diagnostic profile. (Reproduction of *Hepatitis A diagnostic profile taken from "Principles in Practice: Testing for Viral Hepatitis"* has been granted with approval of Abbott Laboratories, all rights reserved by Abbott Laboratories.)

Procedure

A red-topped, sterile tube is used to collect 5 to 10 ml of venous blood.

QUALITY CONTROL

Venipuncture is always performed with gloves and careful use and disposal of needles. When hepatitis is suspected, extra attention to technique should help prevent needlestick or contact with blood from splashes. A note regarding suspected hepatitis should be written on the requisition slip to alert the laboratory personnel.

Findings

ELEVATED VALUES

Hepatitis A virus antibody: hepatitis A infection
IgM: current hepatitis A infection, acute or convalescent stage
IgG: old hepatitis A infection with permanent immunity to reinfection by the hepatitis A virus

Interfering Factors

• Recent administration of radioisotopes

Nursing Implementation

Pretest

No specific patient instruction or intervention is needed.

HEPATITIS B CORE ANTIBODY

(SERUM)

Synonyms:

anti-HBc, AHBC, antibody to hepatitis B core antigen, antihepatitis B core, core antibody HBcAb

---

NORMAL VALUES

Hepatitis B Core Antibody:	negative
Type IgM:	negative
Type IgG:	negative

Background Information

The hepatitis B core antibody is either a marker of hepatitis B infection in the acute or chronic phase of illness or a marker of past illness. This hepatitis B core antibody appears after 1 to 2 weeks of infection, before symptoms appear. It rises during the acute stage, with a peak and plateau during convalescence several months later. It remains elevated for months to years and is considered a lifetime marker of past infection (Fig. 18–4). When the subtypes are tested, a positive IgM result indicates an acute infection and a positive IgG result indicates a chronic infection or carrier state.

The hepatitis B core antibody provides additional opportunity to obtain diagnostic information during the convalescent phase of a hepatitis B infection. After 3 months of infection, the hepatitis B surface antigen disappears, and the hepatitis B surface antibody will not appear until 6 months after the onset of infection. The 3-month interval between these occurrences is called the "core

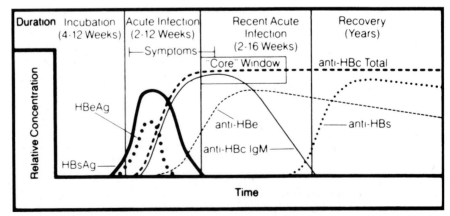

FIGURE 18–4. Hepatitis B serologic profile. (Reproduction of *Hepatitis B serologic profile taken from "Principles in Practice: Testing for Viral Hepatitis"* has been granted with approval of Abbott Laboratories, all rights reserved by Abbott Laboratories.)

window." The hepatitis B core antibody (type IgM) is the only substance to indicate a positive value during that time frame.

The hepatitis B core antibody may also be present because of passive immunity. The patient can acquire the passive immunity through blood transfusion, after administration of hepatitis B immune globulin injection, or as an infant born of a mother who had hepatitis B in the recent past. The passive antibodies disappear within 2 to 4 months.

Purpose of the Test

Hepatitis B core antibody is used to assess the stage of hepatitis B infection.

Procedure

A red-topped, sterile tube is used to collect 5 to 10 ml of venous blood.

QUALITY CONTROL

Venipuncture is always performed with gloves and careful use and disposal of needles. When hepatitis is suspected, extra attention to technique helps prevent needlestick injury or contact with splashing blood. A note regarding suspected hepatitis should be included on the requisition slip to alert the laboratory personnel.

Findings

ELEVATED VALUES

Hepatitis B core antibody: hepatitis B infection
IgM: acute or convalescent stage
IgG: chronic stage or past infection

Interfering Factors

* Recent administration of radioisotopes

Nursing Implementation

Pretest

No specific patient instructions or intervention is needed.

HEPATITIS B e ANTIBODY

(SERUM)

Synonyms:
anti-HBe, HBeAb

─────────────────── **NORMAL VALUES** ───────────────────

| **Anti-HBe:** | negative |

Background Information

In hepatitis B infection, the hepatitis B e antibody indicates reduced infectivity with lower potential for the transmission of infection to others. The antibody usually appears after the hepatitis B e antigen disappears, or about 3 months after the onset of infection (Fig. 18–4). This antibody to the HB e antigen can persist for years but by itself is not considered a marker for hepatitis B infection.

Purpose of the Test

The hepatitis B e antibody helps stage the course of the illness and is a prognostic indicator.

Procedure

A red-topped, sterile tube is used to collect 5 to 10 ml of venous blood.

QUALITY CONTROL
Venipuncture is always performed with gloves and careful use and disposal of needles. When hepatitis is suspected, extra attention to technique should help prevent needlestick or contact with the blood from splashing. A note regarding suspected hepatitis should be written on the requisition slip to alert the laboratory personnel.

Findings

ELEVATED VALUES

Reduced infectivity in convalescence
Reduced infectivity in a carrier state
Reduced infectivity in chronic infection

Interfering Factors

• Radioactive scan in the preceding week

Nursing Implementation

No specific patient instruction or intervention is needed.

HEPATITIS B e ANTIGEN

(SERUM)

Synonym:

HBeAg

___

NORMAL VALUES

Hepatitis B e Antigen:	negative

Background Information

The hepatitis B e antigen is found in patients infected with the hepatitis B surface antigen. The hepatitis B e antigen appears in the serum about 1 week after the hepatitis B surface antigen appears, persists for 3 to 6 weeks, and disappears about 1 week before the hepatitis B surface antigen disappears (Fig. 18–4).

In the acute stage of hepatitis B infection, the hepatitis B e antigen indicates the period of greatest infectivity and ability to transmit the infection to others. The presence of the hepatitis B e antigen beyond 12 weeks is an indication of a chronic carrier state with potential for chronic liver disease.

Purpose of the Test

The hepatitis B e antigen determination is used in the diagnosis and prognosis of hepatitis B infection. It is also used as a test for pregnant women who are hepatitis B surface antigen–positive. If the mother is also positive for the hepatitis B e antigen, the probability is high that she will transmit the virus to her newborn child.

Procedure

A red-topped sterile tube is used to collect 5 to 10 ml of venous blood.

QUALITY CONTROL

Venipuncture is always performed with gloves and careful use and disposal of needles. When hepatitis is suspected, extra attention should be paid to technique so that needlestick or contact with blood from splashes is avoided. A note regarding suspected hepatitis should be written on the requisition slip to alert the laboratory personnel.

Findings

ELEVATED VALUES

Increased infectivity in acute stage
Increased infectivity and chronic carrier of hepatitis B
Chronic liver disease

Interfering Factors

• Radioactive scan in the preceding week

Nursing Implementation

Pretest

No special patient instruction or intervention is needed.

HEPATITIS B SURFACE ANTIBODY

(SERUM)

Synonyms:

HBsAb; anti-HBs, antibody to hepatitis B surface antigen, HBsAgAb, hepatitis B s antibody

--------------------------- **NORMAL VALUES** ---------------------------

Hepatitis B Surface Antibody:	negative

Background Information

The hepatitis B surface antibody appears several weeks to several months after the hepatitis B surface antigen has disappeared. It remains during convalescence and may or may not disappear after recovery (Fig. 18–4). The presence of this antibody usually, but not always, indicates that recovery is complete and that there is now immunity to any recurrent hepatitis B infection. If this antibody and the hepatitis B core antibody are present simultaneously, immunity to recurrent hepatitis B infection is definite. The hepatitis B surface antibody test replaces the old Australian antigen antibody test.

Purpose of the Test

The hepatitis B surface antibody test is used to evaluate possible immunity or the need for vaccination in individuals at high risk for the development of hepatitis B infection. It is also used to evaluate the need for hepatitis B immune globulin after a needlestick incident.

Procedure

A red-topped, sterile tube is used to collect 5 to 10 ml of venous blood.

QUALITY CONTROL
Venipuncture is always performed with gloves and careful use and disposal of needles. When hepatitis is suspected, extra attention to technique should help prevent needlestick or contact with splashing blood. If hepatitis is suspected, a note should be written on the requisition slip to alert the laboratory personnel.

Findings

ELEVATED VALUES

Convalescent stage of hepatitis B infection
Clinical recovery from hepatitis B infection

Interfering Factors

• Recent administration of radioisotopes

Nursing Implementation

Pretest

No specific patient instruction of intervention is needed.

HEPATITIS B SURFACE ANTIGEN

(SERUM)

Synonyms:
HBsAg, HAA, hepatitis-associated antigen

———————————————————— **NORMAL VALUES** ————

Hepatitis B Surface Antigen:	negative

Background Information

The hepatitis B virus is transmitted by a parenteral route, for example, exposure to infected blood or blood products, sexual transmission, and perinatal exposure. The best markers indicating the presence of hepatitis B infection are the hepatitis B surface antigen and the hepatitis B e antigen.

The hepatitis B surface antigen is present 2 to 4 weeks before liver enzyme levels become elevated and up to 5 weeks before the patient demonstrates clinical symptoms. During the course of the illness, the values of the hepatitis B surface antigen rise, peak, and then decline steadily over a 12-week period as the infection resolves (Fig. 18–4). In a different pattern, if the hepatitis B surface antigen rises to a plateau and remains elevated for 4 to 6 months or more, the patient is probably a carrier of hepatitis B virus or has a chronic hepatitis B infection (Hollinger, 1991). This diagnostic test replaces the old Australian antigen test.

Purpose of the Test

The hepatitis B surface antigen is used to identify the specific type of hepatitis and to diagnose the infection in its acute or chronic stage. It is used to screen blood donors, resulting in the rejection of any donor who is positive. It is also used to evaluate risk in needlestick incidents involving health care personnel.

Procedure

A red-topped tube is used to obtain 5 to 10 ml of venous blood.

QUALITY CONTROL

Venipuncture is always performed with gloves and careful use and disposal of needles. When hepatitis is suspected, extra attention to technique helps prevent contact with the blood from a needlestick injury or splashing. The requisition slip should contain a note regarding suspected hepatitis to alert the laboratory personnel.

Findings

ELEVATED VALUES

Active acute hepatitis B infection
Active chronic hepatitis B infection
Chronic carrier of hepatitis B surface antigen

Interfering Factors

• Recent administration of radioisotopes

Nursing Implementation

Pretest

No specific patient instruction or intervention is needed.

HEPATITIS C ANTIBODY

(SERUM)

Synonym:

anti-HCV

NORMAL VALUES

Hepatitis C Antibody:	negative

Background Information

Non-A, non-B hepatitis is responsible for almost all cases of posttransfusion hepatitis. One causative agent is now identified as the hepatitis C virus. The virus is spread via a blood transfusion from an infected donor or parenterally through the use of contaminated needles.

A recently approved enzyme-linked immunoadsorbent assay can identify the hepatitis C antibody. The antibody appears from 16 to 24 weeks up to 1 year after transaminase enzyme levels become elevated. The antibody will disappear in patients who are fully recovered but will persist at an elevated level when the infection is chronic.

Purpose of the Test

The hepatitis C antibody determination is used to diagnose hepatitis and the specific virus involved. The test is also used to screen the blood of potential donors, with rejection of those with positive results.

Procedure

A red-topped, sterile tube is used to collect 5 to 10 ml of venous blood.

QUALITY CONTROL

Venipuncture is always performed with gloves, being careful in the use and disposal of contaminated needles. When hepatitis is suspected, one should be especially careful to prevent needlestick injury or contact with splashing blood. A note should be included on the requisition slip to alert the laboratory personnel of suspected hepatitis.

Findings

ELEVATED VALUES

Hepatitis C

Non-A, non-B hepatitis

Interfering Factors

- Recent administration of radioisotopes

Nursing Implementation

Pretest

No specific patient instruction or intervention is needed.

HEPATITIS DELTA ANTIBODY

(SERUM)

Synonym:

anti-delta, anti-HD

NORMAL VALUES

Anti-delta:	negative
Type IgM:	negative
Type IgG:	negative

Background Information

The hepatitis delta virus is an incomplete RNA virus that cannot survive alone. This virus is transmitted primarily by the parenteral route and coinfects or superinfects a liver that is already infected with the hepatitis B virus. The hepatitis delta virus depends on the synthesis of the hepatitis B surface antigen surface coat to infect and multiply within the individual. When the hepatitis delta virus coinfects with the hepatitis B virus, the infection is more severe or relapsing. When the hepatitis delta virus is a superinfection, it occurs in the chronic carrier stage of hepatitis B. This leads to a chronic delta hepatitis infection, with severe acute illness.

There is a positive reaction to the hepatitis delta antibody and its subtypes, which appear 5 to 7 weeks after the onset of infection. A positive IgM result indicates acute illness by the hepatitis delta virus. A positive IgG result indicates the chronic carrier stage of hepatitis delta.

Purpose

The purpose of the test is to diagnose hepatitis delta and the stage of infection (acute, chronic, or recurrent).

Procedure

A red-topped, sterile tube is used to collect 5 to 10 ml of venous blood.

QUALITY CONTROL

Venipuncture is always performed with gloves and careful use and disposal of needles. When hepatitis is suspected, extra attention should be paid to technique, avoiding needlestick injury or splashing blood. A note regarding suspected hepatitis should be included on the requisition slip to alert the laboratory personnel.

Findings

ELEVATED VALUES

Hepatitis delta
Type IgM: acute hepatitis delta
Type IgG: chronic carrier, hepatitis delta

Interfering Factors

• Recent administration of radioisotopes

Nursing Implementation

Pretest

No specific patient instruction or intervention is needed.

LACTATE DEHYDROGENASE

(SERUM)

Total lactate dehydrogenase and its isoenzyme LDH5 will be mildly elevated in the presence of primary hepatic disease. The most common causes are hepatitis, cirrhosis, congestion of the liver, and hepatic anoxia. These tests are costly to perform and are not part of a liver function screen. A complete discussion of lactate dehydrogenase and its isoenzymes is presented in Chapter 14.

LEUCINE AMINOPEPTIDASE

(SERUM)

Synonym:
LAP

━━━━━━━━━━━━━━━━━━━ **NORMAL VALUES** ━━━━━━━━━━━━

Adult Male:	80–200 U/ml Goldberg-Rutenberg units *or* SI 19.2–48 U/L
Adult Female:	75–185 U/ml Goldberg-Rutenberg units *or* SI 18.0–44.0 U/L

Background Information

Leucine aminopeptidase is a proteolytic enzyme that is produced for further breakdown of peptides and amino acids. The enzyme is produced in the cells of virtually all human tissue, but there is a larger concentration in the biliary epithelium of the liver, biliary tract, pancreas, and mucosa of the intestine. The source of the serum level of leucine aminopeptidase is probably liver tissue.

During pregnancy, the serum value rises progressively, peaks at the end of the third trimester, and subsides in the postpartum period. In this instance, the origin of the leucine aminopeptidase enzyme appears to be the placenta.

Leucine aminopeptidase is not widely used, but it is part of the group of tests that evaluate hepatobiliary disease. In purpose, it is similar to ALP, GGP, and 5'-nucleotidase, but it is more specific than ALP because it does not become elevated in bone disorders.

Purpose of the Test

Leucine aminopeptidase is used to detect hepatobiliary disease and biliary obstruction. It also helps differentiate hepatobiliary disorders from bone disease.

Procedure

A red-topped, sterile tube is used to collect 5 to 10 ml of venous blood.

Findings

ELEVATED VALUES

Obstructive hepatobiliary disease
Severe preeclampsia
Hepatitis
Cirrhosis
Biliary atresia

Metastatic cancer of the liver and pancreas
Acute intoxication
Chronic alcohol abuse

Interfering Factors

• Pregnancy

Nursing Implementation

Pretest

When fasting is required by an individual laboratory, instruct the patient to discontinue all food and fluids for 12 hours before the test.

LIPASE

(SERUM)

Synonyms:

NORMAL VALUES

Adult: <200 U/L

Background Information

Lipase is an enzyme manufactured primarily by the pancreas. The function of this digestive enzyme is to hydrolyze fatty acids. Lipolysis by lipase increases in the presence of bile salts because the bile emulsifies the fat and creates a greater surface area for the lipase activity. If bile is not present, the lipase is ineffective.

In pancreatic disorders, the serum value of lipase is usually parallel and complementary to amylase, but clinically, lipase is considered to be more sensitive and specific in the diagnosis of acute pancreatitis.

Purpose of the Test

Serum lipase is used to diagnose pancreatitis and pancreatic disease.

Procedure

Critical Thinking: During the venipuncture, the blood flow into the vacuum tube is very slow. After the blood undergoes centrifuge, the serum is pink instead of clear. How can the venipuncture technique be improved to minimize or eliminate hemolysis of the erythrocytes?

A red-topped, sterile tube is used to collect 5 to 10 ml of venous blood.

QUALITY CONTROL

Venipuncture must be smooth, with a blood flow that fills the vacuum tube readily. If the blood has excessive turbulence because of flawed venipuncture technique, the hemolysis of the erythrocytes will alter the test results.

Findings

ELEVATED VALUES

Acute pancreatitis
Pancreatic cyst or pseudocyst
Pancreatic ductal obstruction
Peritonitis

Colic from gallstone
Primary biliary cirrhosis
Strangulated or perforated bowel

Interfering Factors

- Heparin
- Narcotics
- Hemolysis
- Failure to maintain a nothing by mouth status

Nursing Implementation

Pretest

In dialysis patients, ensure that the lipase blood sample is obtained prior to a dialysis treatment. The heparin used during dialysis would cause a false rise in the lipase value.

Instruct the patient to discontinue all food and fluid for 12 hours before the test.

5'-NUCLEOTIDASE

(SERUM)

Synonyms:
5'-N; 5'-NT

─────────────── NORMAL VALUES ───────────────

Adults:	2–17 IU/L

Background Information

5'-Nucleotidase is an enzyme found in the plasma membranes of all cells; its function is to assist in the catabolism of nucleic acids. The enzyme is active in the liver because of the multiple metabolic functions of that organ. 5'-Nucleotidase is mostly inactive in bone tissue because bone cells are relatively stable and undergo few metabolic changes. This test replaces the sulfobromophthalein sodium test.

Purpose of the Test

5'-Nucleotidase demonstrates a dramatic rise in the presence of extrahepatic or intrahepatic biliary obstruction and cancer of the liver. It parallels the values of glutamyltransferase, leucine aminopeptidase, and ALP in the presence of hepatobiliary disease. Unlike ALP, it remains at normal levels in the presence of bone disease.

Procedure

A red-topped, sterile tube is used to collect 5 to 10 ml of venous blood.

QUALITY CONTROL

Venipuncture technique must be smooth, with a blood flow that fills the vacuum tube readily. If the blood has excessive turbulence because of flawed venipuncture technique, the hemolysis of the erythrocytes will elevate the test results.

Findings

ELEVATED VALUES

Common bile duct obstruction
Hepatic cirrhosis
Biliary cirrhosis
Metastatic cancer of the liver

Lymphoma of the liver
Hepatitis (viral, toxic)
Pregnancy (third trimester)

Interfering Factors

• Failure to maintain a nothing-by-mouth status
• Hemolysis

Nursing Implementation

Pretest

Since lipemia will elevate the serum value, instruct the patient to fast from food and fluids for 12 hours before the test.

PROTEIN ELECTROPHORESIS

(SERUM)

Synonym:

serum protein electrophoresis

─────────── **NORMAL VALUES** ───────────

Adult:	albumin: 3.5–5 g/dl *or* SI 35–50 g/L
	alpha₁-globulin: 0.1–0.3 g/dl *or* SI 1–3 g/L
	alpha₂-globulin: 0.6–1 g/dl *or* SI 6–10 g/L
	beta globulin: 0.7–1.1 g/dl *or* SI 7–11 g/L
	gamma globulin: 0.8–1.6 g/dl *or* SI 8–16 g/L
Children:	albumin: 3.6–5.2 g/dl *or* SI 36–52 g/L
	alpha₁-globulin: 0.1–0.4 g/dl *or* SI 1–4 g/L
	alpha₂-globulin: 0.5–1.2 g/dl *or* SI 5–12 g/L
	beta globulin: 0.5–1.2 g/dl *or* SI 5–11 g/L
	gamma globulin: 0.5–1.7 g/dl *or* SI 5–17 g/L

Background Information

Total serum consists of albumin and globulins. The process of electrophoresis uses an electric field to separate out the fractional protein components in greater detail and to measure the quantity of each component. It is possible to quantify more than 100 plasma proteins by electrophoresis.

ALBUMIN. This is the largest component and constitutes up to two thirds of the total plasma proteins (Henry, 1991). The functions of albumin are to (1) maintain oncotic pressure (the pressure that holds water within vascular walls), (2) sustain a reserve nitrogen pool for tissue growth and repair, and (3) serve as a transport or carrier protein for numerous substances such as medications, lipids, bilirubin, hormones, minerals, and fat-soluble vitamins.

GLOBULINS. There are three main subgroups of globulins: alpha, beta, and gamma globulins. In each of these subgroups, there are numerous component fractions with distinct functions. The main fractions are presented here, but there are numerous additional fractions present in the blood.

The largest of the *alpha₁-globulins* is alpha₁-antitrypsin, a protease inhibitor that inactivates trypsin in the blood.

Alpha₂-globulins consist of two important plasma proteins: haptoglobin and alpha₂-macroglobulin. Haptoglobin binds the hemoglobin that has been released from the lysis of erythrocytes. This hemoglobin-binding capacity preserves iron and additional protein. Alpha₂-macroglobulin is a protease inhibitor. Because of its large size relative to other globulins, it cannot pass into glomerular filtrate. In nephrotic syndrome, when other smaller globulins are lost via the glomerular filtrate, the concentration of alpha₂-macroglobulin will increase dramatically and allow the serum globulins to rise to a level that equals or exceeds the albumin level. Alpha₂-globulin can also sustain the oncotic pressure within the vascular system.

BETA₁-GLOBULINS. These globulins consist mainly of transferrin, the iron-transporting protein. It carries ferric ions from intracellular storage to the bone marrow.

BETA$_2$-GLOBULINS. These globulins consist primarily of the low-density lipoprotein that transports cholesterol to the cells. Other beta globulins are fibrinogen and complement factors.

GAMMA GLOBULINS. These globulins consist of the immunoglobulins G,A,D,E, and M. They are usually identified as IgG, IgA, IgD, IgE, and IgM. Each of these plasma proteins is designed to carry out antibody activity by binding with and neutralizing specific antigens.

Purpose of the Test

Serum protein electrophoresis is used in the detection of hepatobiliary disease, in the evaluation of nutritional status, and to detect monoclonal gammopathy. The latter refers to the presence of a pattern of spikes of the M protein in the densitometer tracing that indicates myeloma, amyloidosis, macroglobulinemia, and occasionally lymphoma.

Procedure

A red-topped, sterile tube is used to collect 5 to 10 ml of venous blood.

QUALITY CONTROL

Once the blood has been centrifuged in the laboratory, the serum is kept refrigerated until the analysis is performed.

Findings

ELEVATED VALUES

Albumin
Dehydration
Alpha$_2$-Globulins
Nephrotic syndrome
Neoplasm
Rheumatic fever
Acute infection
Gamma Globulins
Polyclonal gammopathies
Chronic liver diseases (hepatitis, cirrhosis)
Collagen diseases (systemic lupus erythematosus, rheumatoid arthritis)
Infection
Inflammation (sarcoidosis)
Neoplasm
Monoclonal gammopathies
Myeloma
Macroglobulinemia

Alpha$_1$-Globulins
Inflammatory disease
Neoplastic disease
Beta Globulins
Hyperlipoproteinemia
Monoclonal gammopathies

DECREASED VALUES

Albumin

See section on serum albumin

Alpha$_2$-Globulin

Hemolysis

Hepatocellular damage

Gamma Globulins

Response to cytoxic or immuno-
　suppressive medication

Lymphocytic leukemia

Lymphosarcoma

Multiple myeloma

Immunodeficiency syndrome

Alpha$_1$-Globulin

Hereditary alpha$_1$-antitrypsin deficiency

Beta Globulins

Hypobetalipoproteinemia

Interfering Factors

• None

Nursing Implementation

Pretest

No specific patient instruction or preparation is necessary.

SERUM PROTEINS, TOTAL, ALBUMIN, GLOBULIN

(SERUM)

Synonyms:

total protein: TP, serum total protein; albumin: Alb; globulin: globulins, calculated; albumin: globulin ratio, A:G ratio

Background Information

The parenchymal cells of the liver are responsible for the manufacture of the serum proteins: albumin, fibrinogen and other coagulation factors, and most of the alpha and beta globulins. The exceptions to hepatic synthesis of globulins are the immunoglobulins (gamma globulins) that are manufactured by the reticuloendothelial system.

Plasma proteins are amino acids that are linked together by peptide bonds to form polypeptide chains. The plasma proteins function to (1) maintain oncotic pressure within the walls of blood vessels; (2) provide a reserve source of protein for tissue growth and repair; (3) provide transport for lipids, lipid-soluble substances, iron, copper, and calcium; (4) act as immunologic agents; (5) provide factors for coagulation; and (6) provide numerous enzymes for a variety of activities (Raphael, 1983).

—————————————— **NORMAL VALUES** ——————————————

TOTAL PROTEIN	
Adult, Ambulatory:	6.4–8.2 g/dl *or* SI 64–83 g/L
Adult, Recumbent:	6–7.8 g/dl *or* SI 60–78 g/L
Child >3 Years:	6–8 g/dl *or* SI 60-80 g/L
Newborn:	4–7 g/dl *or* SI 40–70 g/L
ALBUMIN	
Adult, >60 Years:	3.4–4.8 g/dl
Adult, 18–60 Years:	3.5–5 g/dl
Child:	3.2–5.4 g/dl
Newborn:	2.8–4.4 g/dl
GLOBULIN:	2.8–4.4 g/dl
ALBUMIN:GLOBULIN RATIO:	>1

Critical Thinking: The patient with liver damage has decreased serum values for total protein, albumin, and globulin. Create a care plan that identifies potential problems caused by these deficiencies. What types of nursing interventions could prevent or minimize the problems?

TOTAL SERUM PROTEIN. The blood chemistry analysis of total serum protein provides a broad indicator of the quantity and concentration of all plasma proteins except fibrinogen. The total serum protein test is nonspecific in that it does not provide detailed information regarding the individual globulin components. This information is obtained from a serum protein electrophoresis test.

ALBUMIN. This is the largest component of the plasma proteins and is responsible for about 75% of the colloidal osmotic pressure within the blood. Albumin also serves as a reserve nitrogen source for tissue growth and healing, and it is a transport vehicle for many substances.

GLOBULIN. This refers to the group of globulin proteins: alpha, beta, and gamma globulins. Each component globulin has a specific function, but generally the globulins are either enzymes or immunologic agents. The two globulins affected by liver disease are the alpha$_1$-globulin (antitrypsin) and gamma globulin.

Purpose of the Test

A total serum protein determination generally is performed as part of a blood chemistry screen to provide information regarding the aggregate value or concentration of proteins in the plasma. The total does not, however, provide information about the component parts or indicate the cause of abnormal values. Liver disease is one source of abnormal values, but there are many other nonhepatic reasons for the protein values to rise or fall.

The measurement of serum albumin is useful in the evaluation of nutritional status, since a major source of protein is dependent on the intake of protein foods. The albumin level helps evaluate the oncotic pressure within the vasculature and the effects of renal and other chronic diseases. It is not possible for the body to produce excess albumin, but high albumin levels are produced from the loss of vascular fluid, as in dehydration. The albumin level rises because of the high concentration of the albumin in a smaller volume of plasma fluid.

Loss of albumin occurs because of decreased synthesis of protein, as in liver disease or malnutrition, or because of acute or chronic inflammatory disease. When albumin cannot be retained within the vasculature, there will be severe loss of this protein. The albumin can be excreted in urine because of damage to glomeruli of the kidney. It can also be lost through the skin, as in burns, and through inflammatory damage to the intestinal tract. Lastly, albumin may be decreased because of a rapid consumption of proteins in a hypermetabolic disorder.

In the blood chemistry profile, globulin is calculated by subtracting the value of albumin from the total protein value.

$$\text{total serum protein} - \text{albumin} = \text{globulin}$$

Because the globulin component consists of a group of distinct globulins, an abnormal value indicates the need for specific valuations, provided by protein electrophoresis or immunoassay.

The albumin:globulin ratio is a calculation that measures the proportion of the albumin and globulin components. Thus, the ratio is obtained by dividing the albumin value by the globulin value.

$$\text{albumin/globulin} = \text{albumin:globulin ratio}$$

In normal health, the result is greater than 1 because there is more albumin than globulin in the blood. In a disease condition that causes the albumin level to fall and the globulin level to rise, the albumin:globulin ratio will be less than 1. The albumin:globulin ratio is used to demonstrate the severity and progression of the disease and to indicate the need for specific data from serum electrophoresis.

Procedure

A red-topped, sterile tube is used to collect 5 to 10 ml of venous blood. A capillary tube is used for newborns.

QUALITY CONTROL

Venipuncture technique must be performed skillfully, since prolonged application of a tourniquet and hemolysis will give a false elevation of the total protein value. If intravenous fluids are being administered, the blood sample is drawn from the opposite arm. This avoids local hemodilution and a false decrease in all protein values.

Findings

ELEVATED VALUES
Total Protein
Dehydration

Hyperimmunoglobulinemia
Polyclonal or monoclonal gammopathies
Albumin
Dehydration
Globulin
Inflammatory conditions
Macroglobulinemia of Waldenström
Multiple myeloma
Collagen diseases
Sarcoidosis
Cirrhosis
Chronic active hepatitis

DECREASED VALUES

Total Protein
Protein-losing gastroenteropathies
  (Crohn disease, ulcerative colitis,
  intestinal fistula)
Acute burns (thermal injury)
Nephrotic syndrome
Severe protein deficiency
Chronic liver disease
Malabsorption syndrome
Agammaglobulinemia
Pregnancy (third trimester)
Globulin
Agammaglobulinemia
Hypogammaglobulinemia
Protein-losing enteropathies
Lymphomas
Multiple myeloma

Albumin
Rapid hydration or overhydration
  with intravenous fluids
Malnutrition
Cirrhosis
Chronic alcoholism
Nephrotic syndrome
Malignancy
Protein-losing enteropathies (Crohn
  disease, ulcerative colitis, burns)
Severe skin disease
Draining fistula
Thyroid disease
Peptic ulcer
Collagen diseases
Infection and fever
Heart disease
Albumin:Globulin Ratio
Cirrhosis and other liver diseases
Chronic glomerulonephritis
Nephrotic syndromes
Macroglobulinemia of Waldenström
Sarcoidosis
Collagen diseases
Severe infections
Severe or chronic inflammatory
  diseases
Ulcerative colitis
Cachexia
Multiple myeloma
Burns

Interfering Factors

- Hemolysis
- Prolonged bed rest
- Massive intravenous infusion
- Venous stasis
- Peripheral vascular collapse
- Hyperlipidemia
- Hyperbilirubinemia

Nursing Implementation

Pretest

No specific patient instruction or intervention is needed.

PROTHROMBIN TIME

(SERUM)

The prothrombin time is a measure of clotting ability. Severe liver disease results in depressed values of plasma prothrombin and factors II, VII, IX, and X. The injured hepatocytes are unable to use fat-soluble vitamin K to manufacture the clotting factors. When these clotting factors are inadequate or depressed, the serum prothrombin time is prolonged and it takes longer for a clot to form. Liver diseases that can cause a prolonged or elevated prothrombin time include advanced cirrhosis, infectious hepatitis, liver failure, Wilson disease, hemochromatosis, and hepatoma.

Conditions that impair the absorption of fat-soluble vitamin K from the intestine also cause a prolonged prothrombin time. The reason is that there is a deficiency in the supply of vitamin K for the liver to use in the manufacture of clotting factors. Conditions that inhibit the absorption of vitamin K include obstructive jaundice, biliary cirrhosis, and cancer of the head of the pancreas. A full discussion of this test is presented in Chapter 6.

SWEAT TEST

(SWEAT)

Synonyms:
chloride, sweat; cystic fibrosis sweat test; iontophoresis

──────────── **NORMAL VALUES** ────────────

Adults and Children:	5–40 mEq/L *or* SI 5–40 mmol/L

Background Information

Cystic fibrosis (mucoviscidosis) of the pancreas is an autosomal recessive disease that is characterized by abnormal secretion of pancreatic exocrine glands and the other distinct exocrine glands of the body. In cystic fibrosis, there is increased sodium and chloride content in the sweat gland secretions.

In children up to the age of 20 years, a sweat chloride concentration greater than 60 mEq/L on at least two test results is considered diagnostic for cystic fibrosis. In adults, values up to 70 mEq/L may be normal.

This test can produce false results because of poor technique. The diagnosis of cystic fibrosis, therefore, is based on at least two positive sweat test results, a genetic or family history, and the presence of clinical manifestations that include chronic obstructive pulmonary disease or pancreatic exocrine insufficiency.

Purpose of the Test

The chloride sweat test is used to diagnose cystic fibrosis in children.

Procedure

Sweat is obtained by stimulating skin sweat production with pilocarpine and low-voltage electric current in a process called iontophoresis. The pads of pilocarpine and sodium chloride are placed on cleansed skin of the right arm or right leg and the electrodes are strapped on over the pads. Over a period of 45 minutes to 1 hour, mild electric shocks transmit small amounts of pilocarpine into the skin. Pilocarpine is a cholinergic drug that evokes a sweat response. On removal of the electrodes, the sweat is collected on sterile gauze pads or filter paper, weighed, and then analyzed for chloride content.

Findings

ELEVATED VALUES

Cystic fibrosis
Adrenal insufficiency
Ectodermal dysplasia
Renal insufficiency
Nephrogenic diabetes insipidus

Hypothyroidism
Malnutrition
Fucosidosis
Glucose-6-phosphate deficiency
Mucopolysaccharidosis

DECREASED VALUES

Edema
Hypoproteinemia

Interfering Factors

• Dermatitis or skin lesion
• Improper placement of electrodes

- Inadequate sweat collection
- Salt depletion in the body
- Excessive sweating with fever or exercise just before the test

Nursing Implementation

Pretest

Explain the procedure to the parents and the child.

Reassure them that the electrodes produce a mild tingling sensation but do not cause shock or pain.

Encourage the parents to accompany the child during the test and to bring a book or favorite toy for the child. These distractions will help pass the time and minimize the child's apprehension.

Prior to placement of the electrodes, the skin area must be cleansed with soap and water and dried thoroughly.

QUALITY CONTROL

Earlier deposits of salt and perspiration must be removed to ensure that results are valid. Only the right arm or thigh is used; the palm of the hand is never used as a site for electrode placement. The electrodes must be placed correctly to avoid burning the skin.

During the Test

At the start of the test, ask the child to tell you if there is any burning sensation. If this occurs, the test is stopped and the electrodes are checked and repositioned.

Posttest

The skin may appear reddened at the site of the electrodes. Reassure the patient and the parents that the redness will disappear in a few hours.

UROBILINOGEN

(FECAL)

Synonym:

fecal urobilinogen

NORMAL VALUES

Adult:	40–280 mg/day *or* 75–275 Ehrlich units/100 g

Background Information

Conjugated bilirubin becomes a component of bile and enters the duodenum via biliary tract drainage. In the intestine, the bilirubin is converted to urobilinogen by the action of bacterial flora. Most of the urobilinogen is excreted from the body in the fecal matter.

Excess urobilinogen in the feces usually is caused by excess production of bilirubin and bile pigment. The excess production occurs because of a rapid, abnormal rate of erythrocyte hemolysis. Laboratory analysis may demonstrate a dramatic excess of more than 400 mg/day.

Diminished urobilinogen in the feces is usually due to severe biliary tract obstruction or hepatocellular damage. Laboratory analysis may demonstrate a marked decrease to less than 5 mg/day.

Purpose of the Test

Fecal urobilinogen is used to help detect disorders of erythrocytes and helps confirm the diagnosis of liver disease or biliary tract obstruction.

Procedure

The procedure may be based on a single stool specimen, several consecutive daily stool specimens, or a pooled 4-day specimen. Since the amount of urobilinogen in feces is not always consistent from one day to the next, multiple specimens are often required (see also Chapter 2).

Findings

ELEVATED VALUES

Hemolytic anemia
Thalassemia
Hemorrhage into body tissues

Sickle cell anemia
Pernicious anemia

DECREASED VALUES

Cirrhosis with hepatocellular jaundice
Hepatitis
Depressed erythropoiesis as in aplastic anemia
Choledocholithiasis
Tumors (head of the pancreas, ampulla of Vater, bile duct)

Interfering Factors

- Exposure of specimen to sunlight or warmth
- Antibiotic reduction of intestinal flora
- Contamination of the specimen

Nursing Implementation

Pretest

Instruct the patient to place all the stool in one or more special darkened containers, as required by the particular method of collection.

The stool specimen must not be contaminated with toilet paper or urine.

QUALITY CONTROL

When it is exposed to sunlight or the warmth of room temperature urobilinogen will convert to urobilin. All specimens are kept refrigerated in dark containers, until they are transported to the laboratory.

Posttest

The requisition slip and container or containers for pooled or multiple specimens are labeled with the dates of specimen collection.

The single, fresh specimen is sent to the laboratory immediately. Refrigeration is required when there is a delay in transport of 30 minutes or more.

UROBILINOGEN

(URINE)

Synonyms:

urinary urobilinogen, 2-hour urine urobilinogen

--- **NORMAL VALUES** ---

Male:	0.3–2.1 mg/2 hours *or* SI 0.5–3.6 µmol/2 hours
Female:	0.1–1.1 mg/2 hours *or* SI 0.2–1.9 µmol/2 hours

Background Information

Conjugated bilirubin exits from the liver as a component of bile. It passes through the biliary ductal system and enters the intestinal tract at the duodenum. In the intestine, bilirubin is converted to urobilinogen by the action of bacterial flora.

Most of the urobilinogen is excreted from the body in the fecal matter. The small remainder is absorbed by the portal vein system. From this circulatory portion, most will return to the liver via the enterohepatic circulation and will be recycled in bile. The remainder of the circulatory portion is filtered out of the blood by the kidney and is excreted in the urine (Fig. 18–5).

Urinary urobilinogen increases when there is (1) excessive bilirubin formation

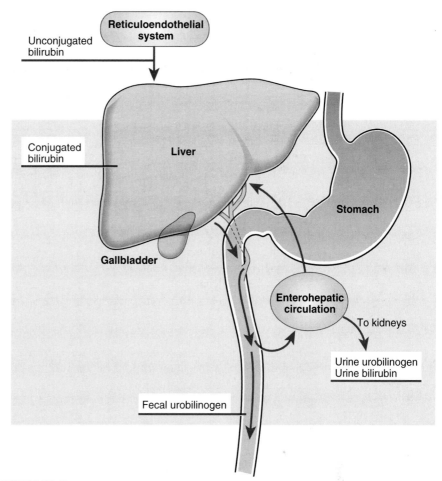

FIGURE 18–5. Pathways for bilirubin metabolism. Several organs and organ systems make different forms and amounts of bilirubin and urobilinogen.

as occurs in excessive hemolysis of erythrocytes, (2) constipation that increases the time that urobilinogen is in contact with bacterial flora, (3) bacterial intestinal infection, and (4) liver disease that interferes with the enterohepatic circulation.

Urobilinogen decreases when there is (1) obstruction or impairment of the flow of bile into the intestine, (2) reduction in the intestinal flora, (3) rapid intestinal transit time, and (4) renal insufficiency.

Purpose of the Test

The test is used to screen for evidence of hemolytic anemia or as an early indicator of moderate damage to the liver parenchymal cells. In both cases, the values are elevated. When the values are decreased, the most common causes are intrahepatic or extrahepatic obstruction.

Procedure

The 2-hour urine collection is scheduled in the afternoon, between noon and 4 P.M., because there is a diurnal pattern of excretion of urine urobilinogen.

Findings

ELEVATED VALUES

Moderate hepatocellular damage (hepatitis, hepatotoxicity from drugs or toxins, hepatic hypoxia)
Portal vein cirrhosis
Congestive heart failure

Hemolytic anemia
Hemorrhage into tissues
Intravascular hemolysis
Pernicious anemia
Constipation

DECREASED VALUES

Biliary tract obstruction
Massive hepatocellular damage
Renal insufficiency

Interfering Factors

- Failure to collect all specimens in the time allotted
- Exposure of the specimen to light or warmth
- Recent or current use of antibiotics

Nursing Implementation

Pretest

Explain the procedure to the patient to maximize cooperation and accuracy in the collection of the specimen

Schedule the test from 2 to 4 P.M. The patient voids just before 2 P.M., and this specimen is discarded because the urine has been in the bladder for an unknown period.

Give the patient 500 ml of water to drink all at once.

From 2 to 4 P.M., place all voided urine in a dark-colored, sterile urine container. As an alternative, a clear container can be covered with aluminum foil to protect the urine from light. Keep the urine in the refrigerator during the test period.

QUALITY CONTROL

The urine specimen must not be exposed to sunlight or remain at room temperature. Urobilinogen is unstable and will convert to urobilin in the presence of sunlight, fluorescent light, or warmth.

Posttest

On completion of the test, send the urine container to the laboratory immediately. The analysis will be performed within 30 minutes or the specimen will be frozen for longer storage.

DIAGNOSTIC PROCEDURES

CHOLANGIOGRAPHY, INTRAOPERATIVE OR POSTOPERATIVE

(RADIOGRAPHY)

Synonym:

T-tube cholangiogram

NORMAL VALUES

The bile ducts are patent with no evidence of retained gallstones, obstruction, or other abnormality.

Background Information

When there are stones in the gallbladder, it is also possible to have one or more small calculi in the biliary tract. During surgery to remove the gallbladder, it is essential to locate any ductal stone so that it can be removed. In the surgical exploration of the cystic and common ducts, the calculus can move around easily and elude contact with the surgeon's probe. The stone can, however, be identified by radiographic contrast medium and x-ray study.

Because of the higher rate of accuracy in locating ductal stones through radiology, the intraoperative cholangiography is often a routine part of cholecystectomy surgery. During the surgery, a small catheter is placed in the cystic duct, and radiographic contrast medium is instilled into the cystic and common ducts.

Alternatively, if the cholangiogram is performed in the immediate postoperative period, the contrast medium is injected into the common bile duct by way of the T tube. X-ray visualization confirms the presence or absence of ductal stones. If the patient experiences obstructive jaundice or a fistula in the postoperative period, the postoperative cholangiogram is performed before the T tube is removed, usually within 7 to 10 days after surgery.

Purpose of the Test

During or after cholecystectomy, the cholangiogram is used to locate any ductal stone and evaluate the biliary tract for any other problems that would obstruct the flow of bile.

Procedure

About 20 ml of radiopaque contrast medium is injected slowly into the T tube, which is located in the common bile duct. X-ray films are then taken to visualize the lumen of the duct.

Findings

ABNORMAL FINDINGS

Biliary duct calculus
Neoplasm
Fistula

Interfering Factors

- Obesity
- Pregnancy (first trimester)
- Failure to maintain a nothing by mouth status
- Gas in the intestine overlying the biliary ducts

Nursing Implementation

Pretest

Question the patient about any history of allergy to iodine or seafood or previous allergic reaction to iodine-based contrast medium.

An informed consent must be signed by the patient or the person legally responsible for the patient's health care decisions.

Instruct the patient to discontinue all oral fluids and food for 12 hours before the test.

TABLE 18-3

COMPLICATIONS OF CHOLECYSTOGRAPHY AND CHOLANGIOGRAPHY

Complication	Nursing Assessment
Moderate allergic reaction	Urticaria (hives)
	Angioedema (diffuse swelling of the skin)
	Edema of the larynx and oropharynx
	Wheezing and coughing
	Apprehension
	Nausea and vomiting
Severe allergic reaction (anaphylaxis)	Urticaria
	Angioedema
	Pallor or cyanosis
	Bronchospasm
	Respiratory failure
	Tachycardia
	Hypotension
	Shock
	Seizures
	Coma
	Death

Posttest

Reapply a sterile dressing on the wound area of the T tube. Reconnect the T tube to its drainage collection system.

Complications

Occasionally, a reaction can occur because of allergy to the iodinated contrast medium. The severity of the reaction can range from mild itching and swelling to anaphylaxis, respiratory arrest, and death. Depending on the patient's sensitivity to iodine, the reaction can be mild and delayed in onset or sudden, intense, and potentially catastrophic within minutes after the contrast medium is injected. The medical and nursing personnel of the radiology department remain observant for any signs of allergic response so that immediate intervention can be initiated. A summary of the complications and the appropriate nursing assessments are provided in Table 18–3.

CHOLANGIOGRAPHY, INTRAVENOUS

(RADIOGRAPHY)

Synonyms:

intravenous cholangiogram, IVC

————————————— **NORMAL VALUES** —————————————

The hepatic, cystic, and common bile ducts are patent, with no evidence of stones, obstruction, or other abnormality.

Background Information

Intravenous cholangiography provides a clear view of the biliary ductal system. This test may be used for patients who have had a cholecystectomy and now have a possible stone in the cystic or common duct. It is also used for patients who cannot undergo an oral cholecystogram because of intestinal disease, inflammation, or poor tolerance of the oral contrast medium.

The radiopaque iodine contrast medium is injected intravenously. Within 15 to 20 minutes, the contrast material is in the intrahepatic, hepatic, cystic, and common ducts. It takes much longer for the gallbladder to concentrate the contrast medium, and this organ may not be visualized on x-ray film for 1 to 2 hours.

Intravenous cholangiography is not used often because other tests are more accurate and reliable in the detection of biliary ductal abnormality. Today, computed tomography (CT), ultrasound, percutaneous transhepatic cholangiography, and endoscopic retrograde cholangiopancreatography (ERCP) are preferable methods.

Purpose of the Test

The intravenous cholangiogram is used to visualize the biliary ductal system in an effort to identify calculi and other causes of obstruction of bile.

Procedure

To begin to clear the bowel of fecal matter and gas, the patient takes two bisacodyl (Ducolax) tablets on the morning of the day before the test and has nothing by mouth after midnight on the night before the test. On the morning of the test, a saline enema may be given.

In the radiology department, an intravenous dose of radiopaque iodine-based dye is administered to the patient. Starting about 20 minutes later, x-rays films are taken at intervals until the visualization of the ducts is completed in 1 to 2 hours.

If visualization of the gallbladder is desired, the patient is given a fatty meal to stimulate contraction of the gallbladder. An additional series of x-ray films is then taken. The total time for the intravenous cholangiography is 1 to 8 hours, depending on the extent of the study and filming that is desired.

Findings

ABNORMAL VALUES

Stone in the cystic or common duct
Gallbladder stones
Inflammatory disease of the gallbladder
Nonfunctional gallbladder
Polyps or benign tumors of the biliary ducts

Interfering Factors

* Retained barium in the intestine
* Impaired hepatic function
* Jaundice from biliary obstruction
* Pregnancy (first trimester)

Nursing Implementation

Pretest

Schedule the intravenous cholangiogram before any intestinal barium studies are performed.

QUALITY CONTROL

Retained barium will obscure the view of the gallbladder and biliary tree.

Question the patient about any history of allergy to iodine or seafood or allergic reaction to a previous diagnostic test that used an iodine-based contrast medium.

An informed consent must be signed by the patient or the person legally responsible for the patient's health care decisions.

Instruct the patient in pretest preparation, including bowel cleansing and the discontinuation of all food and fluid after midnight on the night before the test.

Advise the patient that a sensation of warmth and flushing of the skin may be felt at the time of the injection. Reassure the patient that this is common and will last for only a short while.

Complications

Occasionally, a reaction can occur because of allergy to the iodinated contrast medium. The severity of the reaction can range from mild itching and swelling to anaphylaxis, respiratory arrest, and death. Depending on the patient's sensitivity to iodine, the reaction can be mild and delayed in onset or sudden, intense, and potentially catastrophic within minutes after the contrast medium is injected. The medical and nursing personnel of the radiology department are observant for any sign of allergic response so that immediate intervention can be initiated. A summary of the complications and the appropriate nursing assessments are provided in Table 18–3.

CHOLECYSTOGRAPHY, ORAL

(RADIOGRAPHY)

Synonyms:

gallbladder series, GB series, oral cholecystogram

─────────── **NORMAL VALUES** ───────────

The gallbladder and biliary ductal system are able to fill, concentrate, contract, and empty, with no evidence of stone, obstruction, or other abnormality.

Background Information

Bile is manufactured in the liver and excreted via the intrahepatic ducts, the hepatic ducts, and the cystic duct. It is then stored and concentrated in the gallbladder. As ingested fat reaches the duodenum, the gallbladder is stimulated to contract and expel the bile. The bile flows back out the cystic duct, through the common duct, and into the duodenum where it will emulsify fats in digestive processes.

Stones can form in the gallbladder and sometimes lodge in the cystic or common duct (Fig. 18–6). Most stones are made of bile pigment and cholesterol and some are made of calcium carbonate. Stones in the gallbladder cause acute pain as the gallbladder contracts and squeezes down on them. Stones in the ducts will obstruct the flow of bile and cause posthepatic jaundice.

Oral cholecystography uses a radiopaque, iodine-based contrast medium and a series of x-ray films to demonstrate the storage and excretion ability of the gallbladder and biliary tree. Once ingested, the contrast medium is absorbed by the intestine and enters the blood stream. The liver clears it from the blood and excretes it into the hepatic and biliary ducts. About 16 hours after ingestion, the gallbladder should be filled with concentrated contrast material. Initial x-ray films demonstrate a well-filled gallbladder and identify the presence of any stones.

After x-ray verification of contrast medium in the gallbladder, the patient is given a fatty meal to stimulate the contraction of the gallbladder and the excretion of the contrast material through the cystic duct and common duct and into the duodenum. X-ray films provide visualization of this phase and identify any ductal stones or other abnormalities.

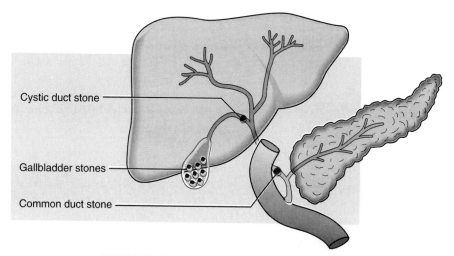

FIGURE 18–6. Common anatomic locations of gallstones.

Critical Thinking: The Latino patient speaks minimal English. His oral cholecystogram could not be completed because the undissolved ionopaque (Telepaque) tablets were wrapped in their foil papers in his stomach. How can the nurse and radiology personnel communicate more effectively with non–English-speaking patients?

The oral cholecystogram is not always precise because of a number of problems that can occur. Visualization of the gallbladder is dependent on an adequate amount of contrast medium reaching these areas. The patient may not ingest the complete amount of the contrast material. Additionally, vomiting, diarrhea, or malabsorption will interfere with the intestinal absorption of the contrast medium. Severe liver disease or biliary obstruction will impair the uptake and excretion of the contrast medium, and an inflamed gallbladder cannot concentrate the contrast medium sufficiently to provide for radiographic visualization. When nonvisualization occurs, the test must be repeated with a double dose of contrast medium.

This test is used less widely today because of the better diagnostic alternatives available. CT and ultrasound are more sensitive and consistent in the detection of gallstones.

Purpose of the Test

The oral cholecystogram is used to visualize the gallbladder and biliary ductal system in an effort to identify stones and other causes of obstruction.

Procedure

The patient eats a fat-free meal on the evening before the test and thereafter ingests nothing by mouth (no food or fluids except water). Two or 3 hours after eating, the patient takes the prescribed number of tablets of iopanoic acid (Telepaque) or other prescribed iodinated contrast medium. In some radiology settings, a saline enema may be required in the early morning of the test to remove any gas or feces that can obscure the view.

During the test, the patient will undergo a series of initial x-ray studies over a period of 45 to 60 minutes. These films will identify the gallbladder filled with contrast material and any stones that are present. The patient is then given a fatty meal or a synthetic fat substance (Bilevac) that causes the gallbladder to contract within 10 to 30 minutes. A second series of x-ray films demonstrates the contrast material in the cystic and common ducts and its entry into the duodenum. This second phase of the test takes an additional 1 to 2 hours to complete.

QUALITY CONTROL

The cholecystogram should be scheduled before any barium tests; retained barium in the intestine will prevent a view of the biliary tract. Since the test is dependent on the patient's compliance with pretest instructions, adequate explanations are important.

Findings

ABNORMAL VALUES

Gallstones
Nonfunctioning gallbladder
Polyp or benign tumor of biliary duct
Cholecystitis

Interfering Factors

- Failure to maintain a fat-free diet and a nothing-by-mouth status before the test
- Failure to take all the contrast tablets
- Intestinal loss of contrast material
- Pregnancy (first trimester)
- Retained barium in the intestine
- Impaired hepatic function
- Biliary obstruction and jaundice

Nursing Implementation

Pretest

Schedule this test before any required barium tests.

QUALITY CONTROL

Retained barium in the intestinal tract will obscure the view of the gallbladder and biliary tree.

Question the patient about any history of allergy to iodine or seafood or a previous allergic reaction during a diagnostic test that used an iodine-based dye.

Obtain an informed consent signed by the patient or the person legally responsible for the patient's health care decisions.

Instruct the patient regarding pretest procedure:

- The patient must eat a fat-free meal the night before the test, with no further intake of food or beverages, except water.
- Two or 3 hours after dinner, the patient begins to take the six tablets of iopanoic acid with 8 oz. of water. One tablet is taken every 5 minutes until all six have been ingested. The patient may continue to drink water as desired until midnight and follows a completely nothing by mouth protocol thereafter.

A saline enema in the morning may be required.

After the ingestion of the contrast medium, any vomiting or diarrhea must be reported to the physician and radiologist.

QUALITY CONTROL

The patient must understand the pretest instructions and be willing to comply. Failure to take the iopanoic acid as prescribed results in inadequate visualization of the gallbladder and ducts.

Posttest

If a repeat test must be performed on the next day, instruct the patient to maintain a low-fat diet until the pretest procedure begins again.

Complications

Occasionally, a reaction can occur because of allergy to the iodinated contrast medium. The severity of the reaction can range from mild and delayed in onset to sudden, intense, and potentially catastrophic. The medical and nursing personnel remain observant for any sign of allergic response so that immediate intervention can be initiated. See Table 18–3 for a summary of the complications and the appropriate nursing assessments.

COMPUTED TOMOGRAPHY OF THE LIVER, BILIARY TRACT, AND PANCREAS

(TOMOGRAPHY)

Synonym:

CT scan

Images of the liver, gallbladder, and pancreas are clearly demonstrated by CT scan. In liver disease, the CT scan is used to detect tumor, abscess, cyst, or bleeding in the liver. It also can help identify the source of jaundice due to liver disease or obstruction of the biliary ducts. In pancreatic disease, the CT scan identifies tumors, cysts, and pseudocysts. An enlarged, edematous pancreas is an indication of acute pancreatitis. A complete discussion of CT scanning is presented in Chapter 12.

ENDOSCOPIC RETROGRADE CHOLANGIOPANCREATOGRAPHY

(ENDOSCOPY)

Synonym:
ERCP

─────────────── **NORMAL VALUES** ───────────────

> The anatomy of the ductal systems of the gallbladder, liver, and pancreas are patent, with no evidence of obstruction from stone, stricture, or tumor.

Background Information

Bile is manufactured in the liver and normally exits via intrahepatic ducts, the common hepatic duct, and the cystic duct and is stored in the gallbladder. The bile is released from the gallbladder and flows back through the cystic duct to the common duct and through the ampulla of Vater to exit into the duodenum.

Pancreatic enzyme secretions are manufactured in the pancreas and normally drain from multiple small ducts into the main pancreatic duct within the organ. The pancreatic duct joins with the common bile duct at the ampulla of Vater, and the pancreatic secretions exit into the duodenum.

When there is obstruction of the ductal system in any part of the biliary tree or at the head of the pancreas, bile flow is impeded and obstructive jaundice is evident. If there is obstruction of the pancreatic ductal system, pancreatitis occurs. Pancreatic obstruction that extends into the ampulla or the common duct, or both, also will cause jaundice.

Purpose of the Test

ERCP is performed to examine the anatomic structure of the biliary and pancreatic ductal systems and to identify the cause and location of obstruction. The endoscope permits direct visualization of the duodenum, papilla, and ampulla of Vater. Once the cannula is inserted into each main duct, radiopaque dye is instilled and multiple x-ray views are used to demonstrate the filling of that duct. Cytologic examination can be performed on the pancreatic secretions.

Diagnostic ERCP is used to investigate the cause of obstructive jaundice or persistent abdominal pain, or both, associated with a biliary or pancreatic disorder. The most common findings are a retained stone in the common bile duct, chronic pancreatitis, and cancer.

Therapeutic ERCP is used to provide treatment of pancreatobiliary disorder and may follow as a direct extension of the diagnostic test (Irani, 1990). Common therapeutic interventions include sphincterotomy with the removal of a retained stone, balloon catheter dilation of a stricture, or placement of a stent to relieve the obstruction and reestablish patency of the duct.

Procedure

A side-viewing duodenoscope or other type of fiberoptic endoscope is passed through the mouth, esophagus, and stomach, and into the duodenum. At the ampulla of Vater, a small cannula is inserted into the ampulla and then, in turn, into the common duct and pancreatic duct (Fig. 18–7). An intravenous bolus of glucagon may be given for its antispasmodic effect on the intestine and the sphincter of Oddi. Fluoroscopic views are used to guide the placement of the instrument. Once the cannula is in the common duct, radiopaque contrast is instilled and multiple x-rays films are taken. To enhance the gravity flow of the contrast medium, the patient is assisted in changing positions, and the table is tilted so that all branches of the biliary tree are filled and visible. Once the biliary duct examination is completed, the cannula is relocated to the pancreatic duct and the radiographic procedure with contrast medium is repeated.

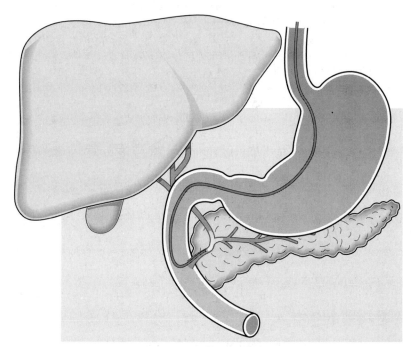

FIGURE 18–7. Endoscopic retrograde cholangiopancreatography. At the level of the duodenum, the papilla is located and the cannula is inserted through it. Once the cannula is in the ampulla of Vater, it is passed into the common bile duct. Once that phase of the examination is completed, the cannula is passed into the pancreatic duct.

PANCREATIC CYTOLOGY. When cytologic examination of the pancreatic secretions is indicated, it is performed during endoscopic retrograde pancreatography phase of the procedure. The patient is given an intravenous bolus of secretin to stimulate the flow of pancreatic secretions. A sample of the secretion is aspirated from the duct and is sent to the laboratory for cytologic analysis.

QUALITY CONTROL

The endoscope and its accessories must be cleaned, disinfected, and dried meticulously to reduce the number of microorganisms. ERCP is a deeply invasive endoscopic procedure that can easily result in sepsis (Schaffner, 1990).

Before the examination starts, the nurse tests all equipment for correct mechanical function and proper illumination. The imaging systems must also be fully operational. Back-up equipment is kept available to prevent or rectify malfunction (Vennes, 1987).

Two vials of pancreatic secretions are collected for cytologic examination. The first is discarded because the initial flow of secretions also contain diatrizoate meglumine (Renografin), the contrast medium. The second specimen is the one to be identified, labeled, packed in ice, and sent to the laboratory quickly. The cooling process minimizes the deterioration of any cells within the fluid. The laboratory analysis of the fresh, cooled specimen is carried out as quickly as possible.

Findings

ABNORMAL VALUES

Biliary	Pancreatic
Biliary stone	Acute, recurring pancreatitis
Papillary stenosis	Chronic pancreatitis
Fibrosis or stricture	Cancer, adenocarcinoma
Sclerosing cholangitis	Pseudocyst
Cholangiocarcinoma	Fistula
Caroli disease (cystic dilation of the ducts)	Abscess
Primary biliary cirrhosis	
Lymphoma	
Liver metastases	

Interfering Factors

- Uncooperative behavior
- Severe, acute pancreatitis
- Acute biliary obstruction

- Septic cholangitis (unless biliary drainage is performed)
- Acute myocardial infarction
- Pancreatic pseudocyst
- Esophageal or gastric outlet obstruction
- Hepatitis B infection

Nursing Implementation

Pretest

Provide preprocedure teaching so that the patient can relax during the 1-hour examination. Because ERCP is uncomfortable, intravenous medication will provide relaxation and analgesia. The patient will be aware enough to assist in changing from a lateral to a prone position and to remain immobile during the viewing process.

An informed consent must be signed by the patient or the person legally responsible for the patient's health care decisions.

Baseline vital signs are taken and recorded.

Question the patient regarding any history of allergy to iodine or seafood or during a previous diagnostic study that used iodine. Inform the physician and radiologist of any positive history so that steroids can be prescribed in the pretest period or plans can be made to use a noniodide contrast medium.

Instruct the patient to discontinue all foods and fluids for 12 hours before the test.

One hour before the start of the procedure, an intravenous infusion is started in the arm or hand. When cholangitis or infection is suspected, systemic antibiotics are started and continued into the postprocedure period.

Intravenous diazepam (Valium), meperidine, and atropine are used to provide relaxation, analgesia, and reduced motility of the intestinal tract. Alternatively, a bolus dose of midazolam (Versed) exerts a powerful, rapid enhancement of the narcotic. It also provides sedation and amnesia.

The side effects of diazepam and midazolam are central nervous system and respiratory depression (Aker, 1990). Once the administration of medication begins, the nurse monitors the vital signs and respiratory status frequently. Since there is a high risk of apnea, a hand-held resuscitator (Ambu bag) and crash cart must be present at all times (Urban, 1989). In many endoscopy units, automated blood pressure, pulse oximetry, and cardiac monitoring are used for all endoscopy patients.

Prior to insertion of the endoscope, the patient's mouth and throat are anesthetized with a topical spray. After that, the tongue feels thick, and it is hard to swallow. An oral brace is inserted into the mouth to keep it open; a suction catheter is inserted to remove saliva.

The patient wears a lead shield over the thyroid gland. Personnel in the room must wear a lead body shield and thyroid shield because of repeated exposure to radiation during the procedure.

During the Test

Continue to assess the patient's cardiovascular and respiratory status frequently. Oxygen administered by nasal cannula will increase the patient's oxygen reserves and help prevent hypoxemia (Aker, 1990). Sudden bradycardia from a vasovagal reflex can also occur.

QUALITY CONTROL

To prevent respiratory depression or cardiac arrest, intravenous analgesics are given slowly over a 1- to 2-minute period. Naloxone (Narcan) is kept on hand to reverse the respiratory depressive effect of meperidine, but it is ineffective against diazepam. Atropine sulfate is kept on hand to overcome the effects of bradycardia.

Assist the patient with positioning and relaxation.

Posttest

Critical Thinking: After an ERCP, the patient complains of drowsiness, dry mouth, and abdominal pain. Which of these problems takes priority?

The nurse monitors the cardiovascular and respiratory status at 15-minute intervals until the patient is stable.

The patient ingests nothing by mouth until the gag reflex and swallowing ability return at which point clear fluids are started; a light meal can follow shortly thereafter. In the first hour or so, colicky abdominal pain can occur because of the air that was inserted during the test. It is a temporary discomfort and will disappear as soon as the patient returns to a normal eating pattern (Urban, 1989).

The nurse teaches the patient to use throat lozenges or warm saline gargles to relieve soreness in the throat.

Discharge teaching includes informing the patient to notify the physician of any severe or prolonged symptoms of abdominal pain, fever, nausea, or vomiting.

Complications

Tissue manipulation in ERCP and the already compromised state of the patient's health can result in complications. Sometimes, a complication begins within hours and other times it takes a day or two to develop. Sepsis is the greatest problem, affecting either the biliary tract or pancreas. Pancreatitis occurs most frequently, and research studies describe a 0.7 to 7% incidence after ERCP (Bozymski, 1987). Table 18–4 provides a summary of the complications and the appropriate nursing assessments.

TABLE 18–4
COMPLICATIONS OF ENDOSCOPIC
RETROGRADE CHOLANGIOPANCREATOGRAPHY

Complication	Nursing Assessment
Pancreatitis	Acute epigastric pain
	Abdominal distention
	Ecchymosis of the skin in the left flank or periumbilical area
	Board-like abdomen
	Nausea and vomiting
Cholangitis (bacterial infection of the biliary tree)	Moderate abdominal pain
	Leukocytosis and abnormal liver function test results
	Fever and chills
	Jaundice
Cardiovascular change:	Hypotension
arrhythmia	Tachycardia
angina	Cardiac arrhythmia
shock	Tachypnea or dyspnea
	Diaphoresis
	Chest pain
Perforation	Acute epigastric pain
	Abdominal distention
	Board-like abdomen
	Shock
	Sepsis
Bleeding	Hypotension
	Tachycardia
	Dyspnea
	Diaphoresis and pallor
	Acute abdomen or abdominal distention
	Ecchymosis
	Melena

LIVER-BILIARY SCAN

(RADIONUCLIDE
IMAGING)

Synonyms:

biliary tree scan, hepatobiliary imaging, hepatobiliary scintigraphy, DISDA
scan, HIDA scan

─────── **NORMAL VALUES** ───────

There is a homogeneous uptake of the radionuclide throughout the liver,
with excretion into the biliary tree and gallbladder, and emptying into the
duodenum. The liver and biliary tract are normal in structure and
function.

Background Information

Technetium-99m sulfur colloid is bonded with an IDA imaging agent for the radionuclide imaging of the liver and biliary tract. For this scan, the technetium derivative is usually technetium-DISDA or technetium-HIDA. After the intravenous injection of the radionuclide imaging agent, the hepatocytes clear the agent from the blood and concentrate it within the liver. Shortly thereafter, there is clearance of the radionuclide agent from the liver. It will enter hepatic ducts, biliary ducts, and the gallbladder, and finally exit via the duodenum.

When the gallbladder is inflamed, the radiopharmaceutical cannot enter. With obstruction in the biliary tract, there is good visualization of the liver and part of the biliary tree, but there is no radiopharmaceutical beyond the point of obstruction. The patient who is scheduled for this test is usually jaundiced and has an elevated serum bilirubin level.

Purpose of the Test

The liver-biliary scan is used for visualization of the biliary ductal system for the purpose of diagnosis of an acute or chronic biliary tract disorder.

Procedure

After the intravenous dose of the radiopharmaceutical is administered, a gamma camera takes serial images of the abdomen at 5- to 10-minute intervals. In a normal hepatobiliary system, the gallbladder and biliary tree are visible within 30 minutes, and the radiopharmaceutical enters the duodenum within 60 minutes. If the common bile duct and the duodenum are not visualized within 1 hour, delay images are taken every hour for 4 hours.

The uptake and excretion of the isotope is recorded on x-ray film, video screen, or photographic film. The procedure takes from 1 to 4 hours.

Findings

ABNORMAL VALUES

Cholecystitis, acute or chronic
Obstruction of the biliary tract
Biliary atresia
Stenosis of the ampulla of Vater

Interfering Factors

- Failure to maintain a nothing-by-mouth status
- Prolonged fasting or hyperalimentation
- Pregnancy
- Hepatocellular disease

Nursing Implementation

Pretest

Obtain informed consent from the patient or the person legally responsible for the patient's health care decisions.

For an elective procedure, instruct the patient to discontinue all food and fluids for 8 hours before the test. When this test is performed on an urgent basis, a minimum of a 2-hour fast is desirable.

QUALITY CONTROL

The patient must fast before the test to prevent food stimulation of the gallbladder. When there is food in the stomach, the gallbladder contracts intermittently and will not fill with the radiopharmaceutical. This causes a false-positive result.

Paradoxically, prolonged fasting can also cause a false-positive result, so the maximum time for the patient to fast is 8 hours.

LIVER BIOPSY

(TISSUE BIOPSY)

Synonym:

percutaneous liver biopsy

──────────────────── **NORMAL VALUES** ────────────────────

The liver cells are normal with no evidence of inflammation, scarring, degeneration, tumor, or other pathologic condition.

Background Information

The liver biopsy is performed by percutaneous needle aspiration or needle excision of a small sample of liver tissue. Microscopic examination of the stained tissue provides specific and detailed information about the tissue cells, structure, and any pathologic change that is identified.

Some diagnostic data have already been obtained, and the abnormal results are indicators that a liver biopsy is needed. The abnormal findings often include an unexplained enlargement of the liver, persistent elevation of liver function test results, jaundice, or a history of infiltrating disease that commonly affects the liver.

Purpose of the Test

The biopsy is used to diagnose pathologic changes in the liver and to help evaluate the extent of the disease process.

Procedure

Liver biopsy is performed by using needle aspiration to obtain a small sample of liver tissue for microscopic examination. After administration of local anesthesia, the aspirating needle is placed between the anterior and midaxillary lines, usually in the sixth or seventh intercostal space (Fig. 18–8). While the patient holds his or her breath on expiration, the needle is inserted quickly and a 10-ml syringe is used to aspirate a small sample of liver tissue. Once the needle is removed, the patient resumes breathing.

Once the aspiration is completed, the tissue is placed in a specimen container filled with formalin or saline. The specimen is labeled and sent to the pathology laboratory for microscopic examination.

QUALITY CONTROL

The aspiration must be coordinated with breathing because during expiration the liver and diaphragm are at their highest position.

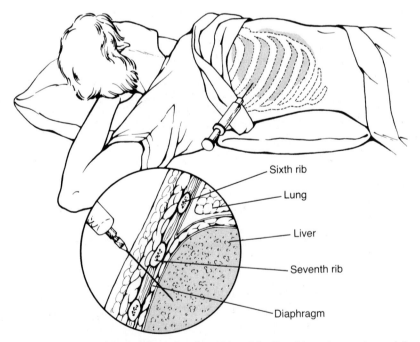

FIGURE 18–8. Liver biopsy. The patient is positioned for liver biopsy in a supine or left lateral position with the right arm abducted. (Reproduced with permission from Burden, N. [1993]. *Ambulatory surgical nursing* [p. 576]. Philadelphia: W.B. Saunders.)

When the patient holds his or her breath, the liver tissue is immobile. Both of these factors help prevent laceration of the liver and diaphragm.

Findings

ABNORMAL VALUES

Cirrhosis	Hemochromatosis
Alcoholic liver disease	Sarcoidosis
Chronic hepatitis B	Amyloidosis
Hepatoma	Wilson disease
Metastatic cancer	Miliary tuberculosis
Cyst of the liver	

Interfering Factors

- Obesity
- Infection in right pleural cavity or right upper quadrant of the abdomen
- Noncooperative behavior
- Abnormal clotting ability

Nursing Implementation

Pretest

Obtain a signed consent from the patient or the person legally responsible for the patient's health care decisions.

Provide pretest teaching about the procedure, positioning, breathing instructions, and posttest instructions. Since patients tend to experience anxiety about this test, provide reassurance and support as needed.

Instruct the patient to discontinue all food and fluids for 8 hours before the test.

Check that a recent prothrombin time; partial thromboplastin time, and platelet count have been obtained and that the results are within safety guidelines for this procedure. The laboratory reports are placed in the chart and the physician is notified of abnormal values.

QUALITY CONTROL

Patients with liver disorders may also have poor clotting ability. The prothrombin time should not be more that 3 seconds greater than the control time, and the platelet count should be greater than 100,000 cells/mm^3.

Take baseline vital signs and record them in the patient's chart.

Critical Thinking: After a liver biopsy, the patient with hepatoencephalopathy is very restless and tries repeatedly to get out of bed. How can the nurse intervene to help him remain quiet and in the proper position?

Administer any prescribed pretest medication about 1 hour before the test. Meperidine, 50 mg, or diazepam, 10 mg is commonly used for analgesia and relaxation.

Position the patient on the left side or in the supine position, with the arm under the head. The skin is cleansed with antiseptic and draped with a sterile cloth.

During the Test

Stand beside the patient to provide reassurance and help in remaining immobile. Despite the use of local anesthesia, the patient feels some pain in the side and top of the shoulder as the needle passes through phrenic nerves and into the liver.

Assist with the placement of the tissue into the specimen container and label it appropriately.

Cover the aspiration site with a sterile dressing, take vital signs, and position the patient on the right side. Record assessment data and a note about the procedure in the patient's chart.

Posttest

For 1 to 2 hours, the patient remains positioned on the right side with a pillow pressing on the waist area. This helps the liver remain somewhat compressed against the rib cage and will help promote clotting.

Vital signs are monitored frequently until they are stable. It is customary to take them every 15 minutes for 1 hour, every hour for 4 hours, and every 4 hours thereafter.

The nurse observes for signs of bleeding on a frequent or regular basis. The dressing is not removed, however. If bleeding occurs, it is likely to flow into the peritoneal cavity or appear as ecchymosis on the lateral rib cage.

The patient can resume food and fluid intake as soon as desired. Bed rest, however, remains in effect for 12 to 24 hours.

Complications

Usually, complications do not occur, but there is potential for bleeding, pneumothorax, and peritonitis. If a small blood vessel is punctured inadvertently during the procedure, blood loss will be greater than normal. Because coagulation may not occur properly, ongoing blood loss can be considerable to severe. If a bile duct is punctured inadvertently, bile will leak into the peritoneal cavity and cause severe peritonitis. If the needle was angled too high, the diaphragm or lung can be punctured or lacerated, resulting in pneumothorax. A summary of the complications and the appropriate nursing assessments are presented in Table 18–5.

TABLE 18–5
COMPLICATIONS OF LIVER BIOPSY

Complication	Nursing Assessment
Bleeding	Tachycardia
	Hypotension, shock
	Pallor and diaphoresis
	Dyspnea
	Distended abdomen
	Board-like abdomen
	Ecchymosis
	Decreased hematocrit
	Abdominal pain
Peritonitis	Persistent, severe pain in the abdomen or shoulder
	Board-like abdomen
	Fever
	Tachycardia
	Hypotension, shock
Pneumothorax	Dyspnea
	Cyanosis
	Hypotension
	Restlessness, apprehension

LIVER-SPLEEN SCAN

(RADIONUCLIDE IMAGING)

Synonym:

liver scan

--- **NORMAL VALUES** ---

There is a homogeneous uptake of the radionuclide throughout the liver and spleen. The organs are normal in their structure and function.

Background Information

Technetium-99m sulfur colloid is a radioactive nuclide used to scan the liver and spleen. Each of these organs contains reticuloendothelial cells. Because of their phagocytosis capability, the reticuloendothelial cells accumulate the isotope and allow simultaneous imaging of both organs.

Space-occupying lesions such as tumor, abscess, hematoma, or scarring do not fill with radioisotope. The image created by the radioisotope reveals the deficit and demonstrates the decreased activity in a particular area. The abnormal finding is called a filling defect or "cold spot." Additional information about nuclear scanning is found in Chapter 10.

The liver and spleen are evaluated for size, shape, position, homogeneity of activity, the presence of defects, and the distribution of radionuclide in the liver and spleen (Mettler and Guiberteau, 1991).

Purpose

The liver-spleen scan is used to confirm and evaluate suspected hepatocellular disease or enlargement of the liver and to detect space-occupying lesions.

Procedure

After the technetium-99m sulfur colloid is injected intravenously, it is cleared from the blood by the liver within minutes. The liver will absorb 80 to 90% of the radionuclide, and the spleen will absorb most of the remainder. Once the radionuclide is concentrated in the organ, it emits impulses that are converted into images. Within 15 to 30 minutes after injection, a rotating gamma camera or scintillation scanner is used to obtain anterior, posterior, and lateral views of the liver and spleen. The images are recorded on x-ray film, video screen, or photographic film. The procedure takes 1 to 2 hours to complete.

Findings

ELEVATED VALUES

Hepatomegaly, splenomegaly
Hepatitis
Cirrhosis
Metastatic liver cancer
Cyst formation

Abscesses
Tumor of liver or spleen
Hematoma of liver or spleen
Hemangioma

Interfering Factors

- Pregnancy
- Breast-feeding

Nursing Implementation

Pretest

Obtain an informed consent from the patient or the person legally responsible for the patient's health care decisions.
Ask the female patient if she is pregnant or breast-feeding. The radiation from the radionuclide would transmit to the infant via the breast milk; the radiation from x-rays can harm the fetus.

Posttest

The radionuclide is eliminated from the body in the urine within 24 hours. Instruct the patient to flush the toilet and wash the hands immediately after voiding to minimize exposure to the small amount of radiation present in the urine.

PERCUTANEOUS TRANSHEPATIC CHOLANGIOGRAPHY

(RADIOGRAPHY)

Synonyms:

transhepatic cholangiography, PTC, PTHC

──────────────── **NORMAL VALUES** ────────────────

The biliary ducts are patent and demonstrate normal anatomic structure. There is no evidence of tumor, stone, or stricture.

Background Information

Once ultrasound has identified dilated biliary ducts, percutaneous transhepatic cholangiography is used to evaluate the cause and location of the biliary tract obstruction. It is also used when ERCP is incomplete or when the patient cannot tolerate endoscopy.

When obstructive jaundice is demonstrated, the location of the obstruction can be intrahepatic or extrahepatic. The underlying cause of the obstruction is usually gallstone, parasites, or tumor. Percutaneous transhepatic cholangiography allows contrast medium to be instilled into the biliary tree via percutaneous needle insertion into the hepatic ducts of the liver. Fluoroscopy and x-ray films assist the physician in the placement of the needle and in obtaining multiple views of obstruction in the biliary ductal system.

Purpose of the Test

Percutaneous transhepatic cholangiography is used to diagnose the cause of obstructive jaundice, visualize the anatomic structure of intrahepatic and extrahepatic ducts, and evaluate changes in the biliary tree that are caused by pancreatic disease (Drossman, 1987).

Procedure

Percutaneous transhepatic cholangiography is performed in a fluoroscopy room that contains emergency equipment needed in case of an allergic reaction

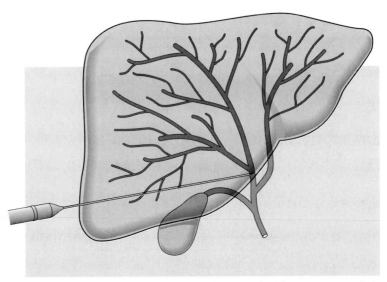

FIGURE 18–9. Percutaneous transhepatic cholangiography. The aspirating needle is passed through the patient's skin and liver tissue until the tip penetrates one of the hepatic ducts. Radiopaque medium is then instilled into the biliary tree to enhance radiographic visualization.

to the contrast medium. The patient is sedated with intravenous diazepam and placed in a supine position on the fluoroscopy table.

The skin is prepared, draped, and anesthetized locally. The site of the needle insertion is in the lower right lateral surface or angled toward the dorsal surface at the level of the eighth or ninth intercostal space. The patient is instructed to inhale deeply, exhale fully, and hold his or her breath on expiration. At that point, the needle is inserted into the liver near the hepatic ducts. As the patient resumes shallow breathing, the needle is repositioned until its tip is well into one of the hepatic ducts (Fig. 18–9). The placement of the needle is guided by visualization with fluoroscopy, but many passes may be needed until the position is correct.

Contrast medium is injected slowly into the duct until all of the biliary tree is filled with contrast material. If there is excess bile present in dilated ducts, the bile is aspirated slowly and and is gradually replaced with an equal amount of contrast medium. A specimen of bile is sent to the laboratory for culture and cytologic analysis.

A tilt table is used to take multiple x-ray films of the patient in various positions until the total biliary tree is visualized. At the end of the procedure, the biliary ducts are aspirated of contrast medium, and the dilated ducts are decompressed. The entire procedure takes 45 minutes to 1 hour.

QUALITY CONTROL

The presence of gas, fecal matter, or residual barium overlying the biliary tract will obscure the view. This test must be scheduled before any barium studies. The patient must be in a fasting state, and an enema is used to clear out the gas and feces before the test is performed.

Findings

ABNORMAL VALUES

Gallstones
Cancer of the pancreas
Hepatitis

Biliary tract obstruction
Nonobstructive jaundice
Cirrhosis

Interfering Factors

- Obesity
- Ascites
- Gas in the intestinal tract
- Failure to maintain a nothing by mouth status
- Bleeding abnormalities
- Sepsis, peritonitis
- Allergy to iodine-based contrast medium

Nursing Implementation

Pretest

Schedule this test before any barium studies are performed.

QUALITY CONTROL

The presence of residual barium, gas, or fecal matter overlying the biliary tract will obscure the view.

Question the patient about any history of allergy to iodine or seafood or a previous allergic reaction to iodine-based contrast medium.

An informed consent must be signed by the patient or person legally responsible for the patient's health care decisions.

To prevent sepsis, antibiotics may be prescribed in the pretest period and continued into the posttest period.

Instruct the patient to take the prescribed laxative on the night before the test and a cleansing enema on the morning of the test.

The patient is instructed to discontinue all food and fluids for 12 hours before the test.

Additional pretest instructions include information about the procedure. The patient is informed that pain control is provided by intravenous medication and a local anesthetic to numb the skin. The patient will be asked to remain absolutely still during the procedure; the tilting of the table is used to help the dye flow into all ducts. The breathing instructions of deep inspiration, expiration, and holding the breath should be practiced.

The nurse assesses and records baseline vital signs, including blood pressure, pulse, respiratory rate, and temperature. Any elevation of the temperature is reported to the physician and radiologist, since sepsis and peritonitis are absolute contraindications to performing the test.

Recent prothrombin time and complete blood count reports should be in the patient's chart, since poor clotting ability is an absolute contraindication and moderate to severe anemia may be a contraindication to performance of this test.

QUALITY CONTROL

The prothrombin time should be no more than 3 seconds greater than the control time, and the platelet count should be more than 100,000 cells/mm^3.

Posttest

The nurse takes vital signs regularly and frequently because of the risk of hemorrhage or hypotension. Generally, the pattern is every 15 minutes for 1 hour, every hour for 4 hours, and every 4 hours thereafter, until the patient is stable. The temperature is taken initially and every 4 hours thereafter because of the risk of sepsis and cholangitis.

Place the patient on his or her right side, with a pillow or sandbag pressed against the lower ribs and abdomen. The gentle pressure and immobility help promote clotting. Bed rest is maintained for 6 hours after the test.

Since hemorrhage or biliary leakage could require surgery, the nothing by mouth status is maintained until the patient is stable.

The nurse observes the lower right area of the rib cage for signs of bleeding, hematoma formation, ecchymosis, or leakage of bile. Some small leakage of blood is expected.

Complications

Complications from percutaneous transhepatic cholangiography occur more from dilation of the biliary ducts than from the number of passes with the needle. Sometimes, bleeding complications begin during the test, and emergency surgery will be required to control or correct it. Other complications tend to appear within hours after the test is completed. Cholangitis and sepsis often occur when the underlying problem is gallstones, cancer of the bile duct, or cancer of the pancreas. A summary of the complications and appropriate nursing assessments are presented in Table 18–6.

TABLE 18–6
COMPLICATIONS OF PERCUTANEOUS TRANSHEPATIC CHOLANGIOGRAPHY

Complication	Nursing Assessment
Cholangitis (bacterial infection of the biliary tree)	Moderate abdominal pain Leukocytosis Abnormal liver function test results Fever and chills Jaundice
Peritonitis	Acute abdominal pain Abdominal distention Board-like abdomen Hypotension, shock Fever
Bleeding	Hypotension, shock Tachycardia Dyspnea Diaphoresis and pallor Acute abdomen Localized ecchymosis in the lower right lateral area of the ribs or side of the abdomen just below the ribs

ULTRASOUND OF THE LIVER, GALLBLADDER, BILIARY TRACT, AND PANCREAS

(ULTRASONOGRAPHY)

Synonyms:

Ultrasound uses high-frequency sound waves to visualize the size and structure of internal organs. When the sound waves pass through skin and muscle and then reach an organ or tissue surface of a different texture, the sound waves are reflected back. The echoes are changed, amplified, and demonstrated on a cathode ray tube.

Ultrasound is a major diagnostic tool for the examination of the hepatobiliary and pancreatic organs. It can detect a liver cyst, abscess, hematoma, primary neoplasm, and metastatic disease. In the biliary system, gallstones are visible, and dilation of the biliary tract is well demonstrated. An enlarged or edematous pancreas is measurable. Pancreatic abscess, pseudocyst, and pancreatic tumor are readily identified. A complete discussion of ultrasound is presented in Chapter 8.

REFERENCES

Abbott Laboratories. (1992). Principles in practice: Testing for viral hepatitis. North Chicago, Illinois: Abbott Laboratories.

Aker, J. (1990). Review of current research on midazolam and diazepam for endoscopic premedication. *Gastroenterology Nursing, 13*, 245, 255, 265, 285.

AORN Journal. (1991). Proposed recommended practices: Care of instruments, scopes, and powered surgical instruments. *AORN Journal, 54*, 316, 318–320, 322+.

Black, M. (1988). Drug induced hepatitis. *Emergency Medicine, 20*, 131–132.

Bozymski, E.M. (1987). Endoscopic retrograde cholangiopancreatography. In D.A. Drossman (Ed.), *Manual of gastroenterologic procedures* (2nd ed., pp. 103–109). New York: Raven Press.

Drossman, D.L. (Ed.). (1987). *Manual of gastroenterologic procedures* (2nd ed.). New York: Raven Press.

Dublin, A.B. (1989). *Outpatient invasive radiologic procedures: Diagnostic and therapeutic.* Philadelphia: W.B. Saunders.

Favorov, M.O. (1992). Serological diagnosis of hepatitis E infection. *Journal of Medical Virology, 36*, 246–250.

Griffith, H.W. (1989). *Instructions for patients. Medical tests and diagnostic procedures.* Philadelphia: Lea & Febiger.

Henry, J.B. (1991). *Clinical diagnosis and management by laboratory methods* (18th ed.). Philadelphia: W.B. Saunders.

Hollinger, F.B. (1991). Viral hepatitis. Antibodies and antigens furnish many answers. *Consultant 31*, 33–36, 41–42.

Hospital Infection Control. (1990). Testing underway for HCV; upsurge in HAV under study. *Hospital Infection Control, 17*, 107–108.

Howard, V. (1989). Endoscopic retrograde cholangiopancreatography. *Nursing Times, 85*, 49, 51.

Irani, S.K. (1990). Endoscopic management of pancreatic disorders. *Gastroenterology Clinics of North America, 19*, 975–993.

Jacobs, D.S., et al. (Eds.). (1990). *Laboratory test handbook* (2nd ed.). Baltimore: Williams & Wilkins.

Keith, J.S. (1985). Hepatic failure: Etiologies, manifestations, and management. *Critical Care Nurse, 5*, 60–86.

Kidwell, J.A. (1991). Nursing care for the patient receiving conscious sedation during gastrointestinal endoscopic procedures. *Gastroenterology Nursing, 13*, 134–139.

Kirby, D.F. (1990). Antibiotic prophylaxis: The who, when, where, why, and with what! *Gastroenterology Nursing, 13*, 9–12.

Lail, L.M., & Cotton, P.B. (1990). Risks of endoscopic retrograde cholangiopancreatography and therapeutic applications. *Gastroenterology Nursing, 12*, 239–245.

Li, K.C.P., et al. (1990). MR imaging of the liver. Technique considerations. *Applied Radiology, 19*, 10–15.

McConnell, E.A. (1991). Diagnosing rectal bleeding. *Nursing 91, 21*, 102–103.

Mettler, F.A., & Guiberteau, M.J. (1991). *Essentials of nuclear medicine imaging* (3rd ed.). Philadelphia: W.B. Saunders.

Monroe, D. (1990). Patient teaching for x-ray and other diagnostics. *RN, 53*, 52–56.

Raphael, S.S. (1983). *Lynch's medical laboratory technology* (4th ed.). Philadelphia: W.B. Saunders.

Schaffner, M. (1990). Infection control issues in the gastrointestinal endoscopy unit. *Gastroenterology Nursing, 12*, 279–284.

Sivak, M.J. (1987). *Gastroenterologic endoscopy.* Philadelphia: W.B. Saunders.

Soloway, H.B. (1990). The advent of hepatitis testing. *Medical Laboratory Observer, 22*, 33–34, 36.

Spada, I., et al. (1990). Endoscopic ultrasonography. *Gastroenterology Nursing, 13*, 24–30.

Sundaram, S.G., et al. (1992). Alpha-fetoprotein and screening markers of congenital disease. *Clinics in Laboratory Medicine, 12*, 481–492.

Sweeney, J.A.P. (1990). Endoscopic assessment tool—A new approach. *Gastroenterology Nursing, 13*, 71–76.

Theriem, S. (1990). Educating patients on the run. *Gastroenterology Nursing, 13*, 54–56.

Tietz, N.W. (Ed.). (1990). *Clinical guide to laboratory tests.* (2nd ed.). Philadelphia: W.B. Saunders.

Todays OR Nurse. (1991). Cleaning products may cause analytical equipment errors. *Today's OR Nurse 13*, 39.

Urban, M.H. (1989). Endoscopic retrograde cholangiopancreatography: A diagnostic outpatient procedure. *AORN Journal, 50*, 572–573, 576–577, 579–581.

Vennes, J.A. (1987). Technique of ERCP. In M. Sivak (Ed.), *Gastroenterologic Endoscopy* (pp. 562–580). Philadelphia: W.B. Saunders.

Wilkinson, M.M. (1990). Nursing implications after endoscopic retrograde cholangiopancreatography. *Gastroenterology Nursing, 13*, 105–109.

CHAPTER **19**

Endocrine Function

Since the endocrine system influences all body systems, one of the most difficult diagnostic problems is recognizing clinical manifestations as possible endocrine dysfunction. Once symptoms are recognized as a potential endocrine disorder, the clinician must select from a wide variety of specific and nonspecific tests. Some of the tests are invasive, and others present no potential danger for the client. Other tests may have potential side effects that would be harmful to the patient unless assessed by the nurse, with appropriate action taken.

The endocrine system is confusing, as hormones often have more than one name and therefore more than one abbreviation. Also, with the new scientific and medical technology available, something new is being learned every day about human hormones. The way hormones interact does not make clinical differentiation or learning easy.

Radioimmunoassay (RIA) techniques have revolutionized the diagnostic evaluation of patients with endocrine problems. These techniques have replaced older tests, which lacked specificity and reliability. Computed tomography (CT) and magnetic resonance imaging (MRI) have permitted more confidence in the diagnostic evaluation of many patients with endocrine system dysfunction. Even today, however, most tests confirm rather than make a diagnosis. Many test results will support a diagnosis but do not rule it out.

There are myriad tests available to assess endocrine function. This chapter focuses on common tests used clinically today. Some classic tests are no longer performed and are not included in this chapter. Although some tests are no longer performed in research institutions, they are performed in community hospitals and will be included in this chapter.

Table 19–1 provides an easy reference for the varied laboratory tests, based on the endocrine gland involved.

TABLE 19–1
LABORATORY TESTS ACCORDING TO ORGAN INVOLVEMENT

Endocrine Organ	Endocrine Test
Adrenal gland	ACTH, plasma
	ACTH stimulation test
	Aldosterone, serum
	Aldosterone, urinary
	Catecholamines, plasma
	Catecholamines, urinary
	Cortisol, plasma
	Dexamethasone suppression test
	Free cortisol
	Metyrapone
	17-Hydroxycorticosteroids
	17-Ketogenic steroids
	17-Ketosteroids, urinary
Kidney	Osmolality, plasma
	Osmolality, urinary
	Renin, plasma
Pancreas	Fasting blood glucose
	Glucagon
	Glucose, capillary
	Glucose, urinary
	Glycosylated hemoglobin assay
	2-Hour postprandial glucose
	Insulin, blood
	Insulin tolerance test
	Ketones, serum
	Ketones, urinary
	Oral glucose tolerance test
	Tolbutamide stimulation test
Parathyroid gland	Calcium, ionized
	Parathyroid hormone
	Vitamin D, activated
Pituitary gland	Growth hormone
	Growth hormone stimulation test
	Growth hormone suppression test
	Osmolality, serum
	Osmolality, urinary
	Vasopressin, plasma
	Water deprivation test
	Water-loading test
Thyroid gland	Calcitonin
	Free thyroxine
	Free triiodothyronine
	Long-acting thyroid stimulation
	Resin triiodothyronine
	Thyroglobulin autoantibodies
	Thyroid microsomal autoantibodies
	Thyrotropin

ACTH = adrenocorticotropic hormone

TABLE 19–1
LABORATORY TESTS ACCORDING TO ORGAN INVOLVEMENT—*Continued*

Endocrine Organ	Endocrine Test
Thyroid gland—cont'd	Thyrotropin-releasing hormone
	Thyroxine, serum
	Thyroxine-binding globulin
	Triiodothyronine

LABORATORY TESTS

ADRENOCORTICOTROPIC HORMONE

(PLASMA)

Synonym:

ACTH

───────────── **NORMAL VALUES** ─────────────

In A.M.:	25–100 pg/ml *or* SI 25–100 ng/L
In P.M.:	0–50 pg/ml *or* SI 0–50 ng/L

Background Information

Adrenocorticotropic hormone (ACTH) is produced and secreted by the anterior pituitary gland. Its secretion is under the control of the hypothalamus and the central nervous system by neurotransmitters and corticotropin-releasing hormone (CRH). ACTH, in turn, regulates the secretion of the glucocorticoids and androgens from the adrenal cortex.

The mechanism of regulation of CRH, ACTH, and the adrenal hormones are multiple, and patterns of secretion of these hormones vary within the individual and among individuals. CRH and ACTH are excreted episodically and by circadian rhythm. Increases in ACTH levels cause increased levels of the glucocorticoids and androgens in the blood within minutes. Generally, CRH, ACTH, and cortisol (the major glucocorticoid) levels are low in the evening and continue to decline for the first few hours of sleep. After 3 to 5 hours of sleep, the levels of the hormones increase, and then peak after 6 to 8 hours of sleep. On waking, the hormone levels begin to decline. Superimposed on this circadian rhythm are episodic secretions. The hormone levels increase with exercise, eating, and stress.

Multiple factors may interfere with the circadian rhythm of CRH, ACTH, and cortisol, including changes in one's sleep pattern, meal times, and emotional or physical stress as well as central nervous system disorders, hepatic disorders, and renal failure.

Stress will cause an increase in CRH levels and thus an increase in ACTH, which will stimulate an increase in plasma cortisol levels. The stress may be physical, such as serious illness, hypoglycemia or surgery, or psychologic, such as severe anxiety. The episodic secretion of the hormones may abolish their circadian rhythm if the stress response is chronic. When high-dose exogenous glucocorticoid therapy is administered, the hormonal stress response of CRH and ACTH is suppressed.

A feedback mechanism also regulates the hypothalamus-pituitary-adrenal hormonal responses. As the cortisol level increases in the plasma, it inhibits both ACTH secretion by the pituitary gland and CRH secretion by the hypothalamus (Fig. 19–1). It is this feedback inhibition of CRH and ACTH, which occurs with prolonged exogenous administration of glucocorticoids, that can cause atrophy of the adrenal glands.

An increase or decrease in the production of ACTH will cause an increase or decrease in the glucocorticoid levels. A deficiency of ACTH will cause secondary adrenal insufficiency. An increase in ACTH will cause Cushing disease (Cushing syndrome is a primary adrenal disorder).

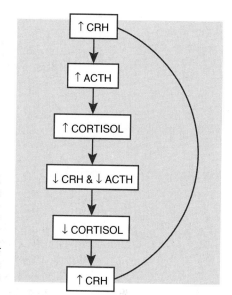

FIGURE 19–1. Hypothalamic-pituitary-adrenal axis. Hypothalamic control of adrenal hormone secretion occurs through release of corticotropin-releasing hormone (CRH), which stimulates the secretion of adrenocorticotropic hormone (ACTH) by the pituitary. ACTH stimulates the adrenals to increase their secretion of cortisol. By a negative feedback mechanism, the increase in serum cortisol level suppresses the release of CRH and ACTH.

Purpose of the Test

A plasma ACTH determination is obtained to diagnose Cushing disease and differentiate primary and secondary adrenal insufficiency.

Procedure

Venipuncture is required to obtain 7 ml of venous blood in a heparinized green-topped tube. The plasma ACTH is measured by RIA.

Findings

Increase	Decrease
Primary adrenal insufficiency	Primary adrenal hypersecretion
Cushing disease	Cushing syndrome
Congenital adrenal hyperplasia	
Ectopic ACTH syndrome	

Tumors of the adrenal gland may suppress the ACTH level if they produce glucocorticoids; however, not all adrenal tumors do.

Interfering Factors

• Noncompliance with medication, diet, or activity restrictions
• Administration of radioactive scans within 7 days
• Pregnancy

Critical Thinking: How will the ingestion of exogenous glucocorticoids affect the results of an ACTH Level?

- Ingestion of
    Alcohol
    Amphetamines
    Calcium gluconate
    Corticosteroids
    Estrogen
    Lithium
    Spironolactone

Nursing Implementation

Pretest

Explain to the patient about the need to obtain two specimens of blood, one in the early morning (6 to 8 A.M.) and one in the evening (6 to 11 P.M.). The early morning specimen reflects the peak secretion time and the evening specimen the low secretion period for ACTH.

Instruct the patient to ingest nothing by mouth for 12 hours before the test. Some physicians recommend a low-carbohydrate diet for 2 days before the test.

Obtain a medication history and question prescriber if any interfering drugs should be withheld.

Inquire and note on requisition slip if the patient is pregnant, as this may affect test results.

During the Test

Have a glass heparinized syringe and ice available.

After blood is obtained by venipuncture, place the specimen on ice and immediately send to the laboratory.

Notify laboratory personnel that the specimen is being transported, as it should be frozen until an RIA can be performed.

Posttest

The patient resumes a normal diet, activity, and medication regimen.

ADRENOCORTICOTROPIC HORMONE STIMULATION TEST

(PLASMA)

Synonyms:

ACTH stimulation test, rapid ACTH testing, cosyntropin test, Cortrosyn stimulating test

─────────────── **NORMAL VALUES** ───────────────

> Within 30–60 minutes there is an increase of plasma cortisol to
> ≥ 18 µg/dl or SI ≥ 497 mmol/L

Background Information

Critical Thinking: The patient has been ill for many weeks, during which multiple intravenous injections and lines have been necessary. When it is time for the second blood collection for the ACTH stimulation test, the patient refuses. How can the nurse help?

ACTH is secreted by the pituitary gland. Its target organ is the adrenal cortex, where it stimulates the secretion of the glucocorticoids, aldosterone, and androgens. Synthetic ACTH, known as cosyntropin (Cortrosyn), will normally have the same effect—an increase in adrenal cortex hormones. A normal response will exclude the diagnosis of primary adrenocorticoid insufficiency, since the gland was able to respond. A normal response will also rule out complete ACTH deficiency (secondary adrenocorticoid failure) because complete lack of ACTH would cause adrenal atrophy and the gland would be unable to respond.

In an abnormal response, primary or secondary adrenal insufficiency may be present. To distinguish between the two forms, aldosterone levels may be measured (see pp. 602–605). If no change occurs in the aldosterone levels after cosyntropin is given, primary adrenal insufficiency is present. With secondary adrenal insufficiency, aldosterone levels will increase by more than 4 µg/dl.

Purpose of the Test

The ACTH stimulation test is performed to diagnose primary and secondary adrenal insufficiency.

Procedure

Baseline plasma cortisol levels are obtained. Cosyntropin, 0.25 mg, is given intravenously. Cosyntropin may be given intramuscularly if the patient is not hypotensive (Jurney et al., 1987). After 30 to 60 minutes, another plasma cortisol level is obtained.

Findings

Increase	**No Change**
Normal response	Addison disease
	Adrenal atrophy

Interfering Factors

• See discussion of plasma cortisol (pp. 614–616).

Nursing Implementation

See section on plasma cortisol (pp. 614–616).

Pretest

Explain to the patient the need for more than one venipuncture procedure.

ALDOSTERONE, SERUM

(SERUM)

Synonyms:

NORMAL VALUES

ADULT, (AVERAGE SODIUM DIET)
  Peripheral Blood, Supine Position: 3–10 ng/dl *or* SI 0.08–0.27 nmol/L
  Peripheral Blood, Upright Position: 5–30 ng/dl *or* SI 0.14–0.83 nmol/L
  After fludrocortisone acetate (Florinef) Suppression or Intravenous Saline Infusion: <4 ng/dl *or* SI <0.11 nmol/L
  Adrenal Vein: 200–800 ng/dl *or* SI 5.54–22.16 nmol/L
CHILD
  11–15 Years: <5–50 ng/dl *or* SI less than 0.14–1.39 nmol/L
  3–11 Years: <5–80 ng/dL *or* SI less than 0.14–2.22 nmol/L
  1–3 Years: 5–60 ng/dl *or* SI 0.14–1.7 nmol/L
  1 Week–1 Year: 1–160 ng/dl *or* SI 0.03–4.43 nmol/L

Background Information

Aldosterone is a mineralocorticoid produced by the adrenal cortex and controlled primarily by the renin-angiotensin system (Fig. 19–2). Renin secreted by the kidneys acts on angiotensinogen to convert it to angiotensin I. Later, angiotensin I is converted to angiotensin II. Angiotensin II stimulates the adrenal cortex to produce and secrete aldosterone. The aldosterone acts on the renal tubules to (1) increase sodium retention and thus increase fluid retention, which increases plasma fluid volume and blood pressure, and (2) increase potassium excretion in the urine.

Another stimulant for aldosterone secretion is the serum potassium level. When serum potassium levels are elevated, there is an increased secretion of aldosterone, promoting greater urinary excretion of potassium.

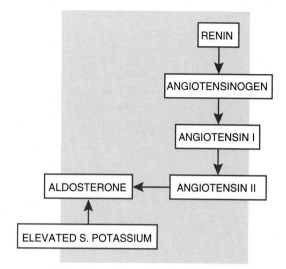

FIGURE 19–2. Primary regulation of aldosterone secretion.

The presence of high levels of aldosterone is called aldosteronism. Primary aldosteronism often is caused by adrenal adenoma (Conn syndrome). The condition is characterized by hypertension with hypokalemia and urinary potassium loss. Secondary aldosteronism is caused by nonadrenal disease that stimulates the adrenal cortex to produce and secrete excessive aldosterone.

In testing for serum aldosterone levels, there are a number of variables that must be controlled to provide accurate results. A low-salt diet, upright position, and stress all produce increased levels of aldosterone. A high-salt diet and supine position decrease the serum levels. With the administration of fludrocortisone acetate or intravenous saline, the secretion of aldosterone is suppressed in normal patients or in patients with secondary aldosteronism, but serum levels rise in patients with primary aldosteronism.

Purpose of the Test

The aldosterone level is used in the work-up for hypertension and in the diagnosis of aldosteronism.

Procedure

A red-topped or green-topped heparinized tube is used to collect 7 to 10 ml of venous blood. The vascular site may be any peripheral vein. The patient may be in a supine or upright position. A blood sample from the adrenal vein may be needed to confirm the diagnosis of adrenal adenoma.

Other diagnostic methods include the administration of 2 L of normal saline in 4 hours prior to the blood test or drawing the blood on the third day after the administration of fludrocortisone acetate, a synthetic mineralocorticoid.

Findings

ELEVATED VALUES

Primary Aldosteronism	**Secondary Aldosteronism**
Adrenal adenoma (Conn syndrome)	Laxative abuse
Adrenal hyperplasia	Excessive diuretic therapy
	Nephrotic syndrome
	Renal juxtaglomerular hyperplasia
	Renin-producing renal tumor
	Bartter syndrome
	Toxemia of pregnancy

DECREASED VALUES

Addison disease	Turner syndrome
Aldosterone deficiency	Diabetes mellitus
Renin deficiency	Acute alcoholic intoxication

Interfering Factors

- Licorice
- Uncontrolled sodium intake
- Postural changes
- Warming of the specimen
- Recent radioisotope administration

Nursing Implementation

Pretest

Critical Thinking: As the night nurse, you note an empty pepperoni pizza box at the bedside of a patient scheduled for a serum aldosterone level in the morning. What should you do?

Instruct the patient to follow a normal sodium intake (3 g/day) for 2 to 4 weeks if not contraindicated by clinical status.

Instruct the patient to discontinue all diuretics, antihypertensives, cyclic progesterone, estrogens, and licorice for 2 to 4 weeks as ordered.

Administer potassium replacement, as needed.

Schedule any radioactive scans after the aldosterone level is obtained.

During the Test

Supine Position

On the morning of the test, instruct the patient to remain flat in bed until the specimen is drawn.

Upright Position

On the morning of the test, instruct the patient to remain seated in a chair for 2 hours until the blood is drawn.

Posttest

Ensure that the requisition slip contains the following information:

- The time and date of the test
- the venous source of the blood
- the patient's position
- the pretest diet
- the time and date of administration of fludrocortisone acetate or intravenous saline infusion

Place the blood specimen on ice and arrange for its immediate transport to the laboratory.

ALDOSTERONE, URINARY

(URINE)

Synonyms:

NORMAL VALUES

2–26 µg/24 hours *or* SI 6–72 nmol/24 hours

Background Information

Aldosterone is a mineralocorticoid produced by the adrenal cortex. Its synthesis and release is controlled primarily by the renin-angiotensin system. Aldosterone acts on the renal tubules to resorb greater quantities of sodium, and therefore water, and increases the excretion of potassium into the urine. Elevated levels of urinary aldosterone may be caused by excess secretion of aldosterone by the adrenal glands, excessive secretion of renin, or conditions that result in decreased kidney perfusion.

The normal value for this test varies among laboratories.

Purpose of the Test

The main use of the urine aldosterone test is to help identify primary hyperaldosteronism caused by adrenal adenoma.

Procedure

A 24-hour urine specimen is collected in a clean plastic container. Some laboratories add a measured quantity of preservative (boric, acetic, or hydrochloric acid) to the container before the start of the collection period.

Findings

ELEVATED VALUES

Aldosterone-producing adrenal adenoma (Conn syndrome)
Adrenal hyperplasia
Nephrotic syndrome
Renin-producing renal hyperplasia or tumor
Renal hypertension
Bartter syndrome
Preeclampsia

DECREASED VALUES

Addison disease
Aldosterone deficiency
Renin deficiency
Diabetes mellitus
Acute alcoholic intoxication

Interfering Factors

- Excess salt intake
- Recent administration of radioisotopes
- Licorice
- Failure to collect all urine
- Warming of the specimen

Nursing Implementation

Pretest

Critical Thinking: While you are attempting to collect a 24-hour urine specimen, your teenage patient keeps "forgetting" and voids in the toilet. What approach would be most effective in gaining the patient's cooperation?

Instruct the patient to follow a normal (3 g/day) sodium diet for 2 to 4 weeks. Excessive sodium intake suppresses sodium secretion and causes a false decrease in the aldosterone value.

Administer prescribed potassium to correct any deficiencies that may be present.

Instruct the patient to discontinue all diuretics, antihypertensives, and oral contraceptives for 2 weeks as ordered. These medications interfere with the test results.

Schedule any radioisotope scan after the urine test is completed.

During the Test

At the start of the test, instruct the patient to void at 8 A.M. and discard this urine. The collection period starts at this time and the patient collects all the urine for 24 hours, including the 8 A.M. specimen of the following morning.

On the requisition slip and specimen label, write the patient's name and the time and date of the start and finish of the test period.

Keep the urine refrigerated or on ice throughout the collection period.

Posttest

On the requisition slip, write the pretest sodium diet.

Arrange for prompt transport of the cooled specimen to the laboratory.

CALCITONIN

(SERUM OR PLASMA)

Synonyms:

CT, thyrocalcitonin

NORMAL VALUES	
SERUM	**Adult Male:** <40 pg/ml *or* SI <40 ng/L
	Adult Female: <25 pg/ml *or* SI less than 25 ng/L
	Infant:
	Cord blood: 30–240 pg/ml *or* SI 30–240 ng/L
	7 days old: 77–293 pg/ml *or* SI 77–293 ng/L
PLASMA	**Male:** ≤19 pg/ml *or* SI ≤19 ng/L
	Female: ≤14 pg/ml *or* SI ≤14 ng/L

Background Information

Calcitonin is a hormone produced and secreted by the parafollicular cells (C cells) of the thyroid gland. It may also be produced and secreted by ectopic sites such as the lungs, intestines, pituitary gland, and bladder. The action of calcitonin is to inhibit bone reabsorption, inhibit calcium absorption in the gastrointestinal tract, and increase calcium and phosphate excretion from the kidneys. It is believed that calcitonin is not secreted until plasma calcium levels reach 9.3 ng/dl.

Purpose of the Test

A calcitonin determination is usually performed to diagnose medullary carcinoma of the thyroid gland.

Procedure

Venipuncture is performed to obtain 7 ml venous blood in a heparinized green-topped tube. Calcitonin is measured using RIA. To assess familial medullary cancer in relatives of patients with the cancer, a provocation test may be performed. Calcium chloride, 150 mg, is given intravenously over 10 minutes or pentagastrin, 0.5 mg, is given intravenously over 5 to 10 minutes. Patients with medullary cancer will respond to these stimulants with excessive secretion of calcitonin.

Findings

INCREASE
Cancer of the thyroid
Chronic renal failure
Ectopic secretion by malignant tumors
Endocrine tumors of the pancreas
Pernicious anemia
Subacute Hashimoto thyroiditis
Parathyroid adenoma or hyperplasia
Pregnancy

Interfering Factors

• Noncompliance with fasting requirement

Nursing Implementation

Nursing actions are similar to those in other venipuncture procedures.

Pretest

Instruct the patient not to eat or drink anything but sips of water for 8 hours before the blood is drawn.

Posttest

Inform the laboratory personnel that a calcitonin level is being obtained, as the blood sample must be separated immediately.
The blood sample must be sent to the laboratory immediately after it is drawn.
The patient may resume a normal diet.

CALCIUM, IONIZED

(SERUM)

Synonyms:
dialyzable calcium, free calcium

─────────────── **NORMAL VALUES** ───────────────

45–55 of total serum calcium *or* SI 0.45–0.55 (fraction of total serum calcium)
Adult, Serum: 4.65–5.28 mg/dl *or* SI 1.16–1.32 mmol/L
Child, Serum: 4.80–5.52 mg/dl *or* SI 1.20–1.38 mmol/L

Background Information

Review the discussion of serum calcium (pp. 696–700).

Serum calcium levels consist of ionized or free calcium and calcium bound to protein. It is the free calcium that is used by the body. Total calcium levels are influenced by serum albumin levels, but ionized calcium levels are not.

Purpose of the Test

This test is used to assess primary hyperparathyroidism, especially in patients with low albumin levels.

Procedure

Venipuncture is performed to fill a red-topped tube. Exposure to air is prevented by using a vacuum tube.

Findings

Since ionized calcium in blood increases and decreases with blood pH, any condition that causes a variation in the blood pH will cause a change in the free calcium level. The following, therefore, is a partial listing.

Increase	Decrease
Acidosis	Alkalosis
Acromegaly	Acute pancreatitis
Addison disease	Blood transfusions, multiple
Ectopic neoplasms	Diarrhea
Hyperparathyroidism	Hypomagnesemia
Prolonged immobility	Hypoparathyroidism
Osteoporosis	Malabsorption syndrome
Paget disease	Osteomalacia
Pheochromocytoma	Renal failure
	Starvation
	Vitamin D deficiency

Interfering Factors

- Diet high in calcium
- Diet deficient in vitamin D
- Multiple drugs, including
  Antacids
  Anticonvulsants
  Aspirin
  Barbiturates
  Gentamicin
  Insulin
  Lithium
  Steroids
  Thiazide diuretics
  Thyroid hormones

Nursing Implementation

The nurse provides actions similar to those of other venipuncture techniques.

Pretest

The patient maintains bed rest in a supine position for 30 minutes before the blood is drawn.

Posttest

Refrigerate specimen or send to the laboratory on ice immediately.

CATECHOLAMINES, PLASMA

(PLASMA)

Synonyms:

catecholamine fractionalization, plasma

NORMAL VALUES

CATECHOLAMINE:	SUPINE	STANDING
Epinephrine:	<50 pg/ml *or*	<900 pg/ml *or*
	SI <273 pmol/L	SI <4914 pmol/L
Norepinephrine:	110–410 pg/ml *or*	125–700 pg/ml *or*
	SI 650–2423 pmol/L	SI 739–4137 nmol/L
Dopamine:	<87 pg/ml *or*	<87 pg/ml *or*
	SI <475 pmol/L	SI <475 pmol/L

Background Information

The catecholamines are three hormones produced and secreted by the adrenal medulla. This structure is the inner core of the adrenal glands, which lie at the superior pole of each kidney. The catecholamines are epinephrine, norepinephrine, and dopamine (a precursor of norepinephrine). The adrenal medulla will secrete the catecholamines when stimulated by preganglionic neurons. The result mimics the effect of a mass discharge of the sympathetic nervous system. Their secretion is part of the "fight or flight" response. The catecholamines help maintain serum glucose levels by promoting liver glycogenolysis, stimulating the secretion of insulin and glucagon, and by lipolysis. The catecholamines stimulate the reticular activating system, making the person more alert.

Purpose of the Test

Plasma catecholamines are usually assessed to diagnose pheochromocytoma or to identify extraadrenal tumors after abdominal surgery. Pheochromocytomas are tumors developing in the sympathetic nervous system. These tumors usually secrete epinephrine or norepinephrine, or both, sometimes dopamine.

Procedure

Plasma catecholamines are measured using radioenzymatic technique. A venous sampling of 10 ml of blood is drawn into a green-topped tube with ethylenediaminetetraacetic acid (EDTA), once while the patient is lying down and then with the patient standing. The normal values vary among laboratories. Results may not reveal a tumor that secretes intermittently, so the test may be ordered for when the patient is symptomatic. To localize small tumors, percutaneous venous catheterization may be needed.

A *clonidine suppression test* may be performed to differentiate between pheochromocytoma and essential hypertension. With this test, clonidine, 0.3 mg, is given 2 to 3 hours before a venous blood sample is taken. Clonidine suppresses neurogenic catecholamine release. If suppression occurs, the test result is consistent with the diagnosis of essential hypertension. If the catecholamines remain elevated, the diagnosis of pheochromocytoma is supported.

Findings

Increase
Pheochromocytoma
Ganglioneuroma
Neuroblastoma

Interfering Factors

- Noncompliance with diet and relaxation requirements

- Amine-rich foods and drinks
- Cold environment
- Medications
    - Amphetamines
    - Decongestants
    - Epinephrine
    - Levodopa
    - Phenothiazines
    - Reserpine
    - Sympathomimetics
    - Tricyclic antidepressants

Nursing Implementation

Pretest

Critical Thinking: The patient with newly diagnosed hypertension appears agitated as a heparin lock is about to be inserted for catecholamine levels. When questioned, the patient says that the test is unnecessary and implies distrust of his physician. How should the nurse respond?

Instruct the patient to avoid amine-rich foods and drinks for 48 hours before the test (e.g., avocados, bananas, beer, cheese, chianti wine, cocoa, coffee, and tea).

Instruct the patient not to smoke for 24 hours before the test.

Explain to the patient that a venous catheter (heparin lock) is inserted 24 hours before the blood sample is drawn, as venipuncture may increase catecholamine levels).

Instruct the patient to lie down and relax for an hour before the blood is drawn.

During the Test

The nurse carries out duties similar to those of other venipuncture procedures, except that blood is drawn through the heparin lock.

After the first sample is drawn, the patient stands for 10 minutes, and a second sample is drawn.

Include on the requisition slip the position of the patient when the blood was drawn.

Posttest

The patient may resume pretest diet and activity. Notify the laboratory that the specimen is coming, since it must be frozen immediately.

CATECHOLAMINES, URINARY

(URINE)

Synonyms:

NORMAL VALUES	
Norepinephrine:	15–56 µg/24 hours *or* SI 88.6–331 nmol/24 hours
Epinephrine:	<15 pg/ml *or* SI <82 nmol/24 hours
Dopamine:	100–400 pg/ml *or* SI 625–2750 nmol/24 hours
Vanillylmandelic Acid:	2–7 mg/24 hours *or* SI 10–35 µmol/24 hours
Metanephrine:	24–96 µg/24 hours
Normetanephrine:	75–375 µg/24 hours

Background Information

Catecholamines are excreted in the urine in conjugated and unconjugated (free) forms. Together these forms make up the total urinary catecholamines. As serum catecholamines are metabolized, several end product metabolites are created, which are excreted in the urine. The primary metabolite is *vanillylmandelic acid* (VMA). Other major metabolites of epinephrine and norepinephrine are metanephrine and normetanephrine. Dopamine's metabolites are 3-methoxy-4-hydroxyphenylacetic acid *(homovanillic acid)* (HVA) and 3,4-dehydroxy-phenylacetic acid ($DOPA_c$).

Purpose of the Test

Urinary catecholamine determinations are usually obtained as a part of the work-up to identify the cause of hypertension and to diagnose pheochromocytoma.

Procedure

A 24-hour urine specimen is collected with an acid preservative added to the container.

Findings

Increase in Catecholamines and Vanillylmandelic Acid

Pheochromocytoma
Neuroblastoma
Ganglioneuroma
Ganglioblastoma

Increase in Homovanillic Acid

Rules out pheochromocytoma
Tumors of the autonomic nervous system

Interfering Factors

- Vary with specific laboratory technique used

CATECHOLAMINE-METABOLITE INTERFERING FACTOR

Epinephrine Norepinephrine Dopamine	Stress Exercise Foods and drugs containing catecholamines High-fluorescent compounds, e.g., tetracycline and quinidine Levodopa Methyldopa
Metanephrine Normetanephrine	Catecholamines and monoamine oxidase (MAO) inhibitors Severe stress
Vanillylmandelic acid	Catecholamines Foods with vanilla Levodopa MAO inhibitors

Nursing Implementation

During the Test

At the start of the test, instruct the patient to void at 8 A.M. and discard this urine. The collection period begins at this time and all urine is collected for 24 hours, including the 8 A.M. specimen on the following morning.

On the requisition slip and specimen label, write the patient's name and the time and date of the start and finish of the test period.

Keep the urine specimen refrigerated or on ice throughout the collection period.

Posttest

Arrange for prompt transport of the cooled specimen to the laboratory.

CORTISOL, PLASMA

(PLASMA)

Background Information

The adrenal cortex produces a group of hormones called glucocorticoids. The primary glucocorticoid is cortisol. Secretion of cortisol is regulated by ACTH, which is secreted by the anterior pituitary gland. When secreted, most of the cortisol in the plasma binds with corticosteroid-binding globulin (CBG). The free cortisol is the biologically active form, whereas the bound hormone acts as a storehouse to replace the free cortisol.

NORMAL VALUES

ADULT

8 A.M.–10 A.M.	5–23 µg/dl *or* SI 138–635 nmol/L
4 P.M.–6 P.M.	3–13 µg/dl *or* SI 83–359 nmol/L

The action of cortisol and the other glucocorticoids are multiple and relate to their plasma concentrations. At normal plasma levels, glucocorticoids, as the name implies, maintains glucose levels by promoting hepatic gluconeogenesis and glycogenolysis, prevents fatigue by making tissues more responsive to glucagon and catecholamines, reduces the secretion of antidiuretic hormone (ADH), increases glomerular filtration rates, and makes the distal tubules of the kidneys more permeable to water reabsorption.

At elevated levels, for example, in times of stress or in pharmacologic doses, the glucocorticoids have an immunosuppressive and antiinflammatory effect. This action assists in control of noninfective inflammatory states and some allergic states.

Cushing syndrome includes excessive secretion of the adrenal cortex hormones resulting from a primary adrenal dysfunction. When a pituitary or hypothalamic disorder causes an increase in the production of glucocorticoids, including cortisol, it is called Cushing disease. The high cortisol levels may be dangerous for the individual, as the inflammatory response is suppressed. The inflammatory response is necessary to destroy invading microorganisms, to wall off infected areas, and to initiate normal wound healing.

Critical Thinking:
A patient in a two-bed room has Cushing syndrome and is awaiting the results of a cortisol level. What medical diagnosis in potential roommates would make them inappropriate for this room assignment?

Purpose of the Test

Plasma cortisol levels are used to diagnose Cushing syndrome, Cushing disease, and primary and secondary adrenal insufficiency. Primary adrenal insufficiency is called Addison disease.

Procedure

Venipuncture is performed to obtain 5 ml of blood in a green-topped tube. If instead of a plasma level, a serum level is desired, 5 ml of blood is collected in a red-topped tube. Varied methods are used to measure cortisol and include RIA, competitive protein-binding assay, fluorimetric assay, and high-performance liquid chromatography.

Findings

Increase	**Decrease**
Stress	Addison disease
Acute illness	Hypophysectomy
Surgery	Postpartum pituitary necrosis

Trauma   Pituitary destruction
Pregnancy
Exogenous estrogen
Anxiety
Starvation
Anorexia nervosa
Alcoholism
Chronic renal failure

Interfering Factors

- Noncompliance with dietary or activity restrictions
- Vary with the laboratory technique used
    With RIA
        Androgens
        Estrogens
        Phenytoin
        Hepatic dysfunction
        Renal failure
    With competitive protein-binding assay
        Prednisolone
        6-Alpha-methylprednisolone
    With fluorimetric assays
        Jaundice
        Renal failure
        Medications
            niacin
            quinacrine
            quinidine
            spironolactone
    With high-performance liquid chromatography
        Prednisone
        Prednisolone

Nursing Implementation

The nurse takes actions similar to those taken in plasma ACTH determinations (see pp. 597–600).

Pretest

Instruct the patient to limit physical activity for 12 hours before the test and to lie down for 30 minutes before the blood is drawn.

DEXAMETHASONE SUPPRESSION TEST

(PLASMA, URINE)

NORMAL VALUES	
Plasma Cortisol:	<5 µg/dl *or* SI <138 nmol/L
Urine 17-Hydroxy-	
corticosteroid (17-OHCS):	<4 ng/24 hours
Urine for Free Cortisol:	<25 µg/24 hours

Background Information

Dexamethasone (Decadron) is a potent glucocorticoid. It will normally suppress ACTH secretion by the pituitary gland via the normal hormonal feedback mechanism. With the suppression of ACTH, the stimulation for cortisol secretion is suppressed in the adrenal cortex, resulting in a decrease in plasma cortisol and urinary corticosteroid levels.

High-dose dexamethasone testing can be helpful in distinguishing Cushing disease (pituitary hypersecretion of ACTH) from adrenal tumors or ectopic secretion of ACTH. With high-dose dexamethasone, pituitary secretion of ACTH can be suppressed, with a resulting decrease in plasma cortisol levels. No change will occur with adrenal tumors or ectopic ACTH production.

Purpose of the Test

The dexamethasone suppression test assesses the hypothalamic-pituitary-adrenal axis. It is usually performed to identify Cushing syndrome. With the dexamethasone test, Cushing disease and ectopic production of ACTH and adrenal tumors can be differentiated.

Procedure

A variety of dexamethasone procedures are possible. Low-dose dexamethasone testing may be carried out overnight or over 2 days. Overnight testing requires the oral administration of 1 mg of dexamethasone at night (10 to 11 P.M.). The next morning, a plasma cortisol level is determined. With the 2-day method, 0.5 mg of dexamethasone is given orally every 6 hours for 2 days. A 24-hour urine specimen is obtained before and after administration (See discussion of 17-OHCS, pp. 659–661) and a plasma cortisol test is performed 6 hours after the last dose of dexamethasone.

High-dose dexamethasone testing begins with a baseline plasma cortisol level being obtained and then 8 mg of dexamethasone being given orally at night, and the next morning another plasma cortisol level is obtained. Another technique requires 2 mg of dexamethasone being given orally every 6 hours for 2 days and a 24-hour urine specimen for 17-OHCS being collected on the second day of administration. A plasma cortisol or free cortisol level is also obtained.

Findings

No Change	Decrease
Cushing syndrome	Cushing disease

Interfering Factors

* Review discussion of 17-OHCS (pp. 659–661), free cortisol, and plasma cortisol (pp. 614–616).

Nursing Implementation

Review discussion of 17-OHCS (pp. 659–661), free cortisol (pp. 621–622), and plasma cortisol (pp. 614–616).

FASTING BLOOD GLUCOSE

(BLOOD, SERUM OR PLASMA)

Synonyms:

FBS, fasting blood sugar

--- **NORMAL VALUES** ---

Children 2 Years to Adult:
  Whole Blood: 60–110 mg/dl *or* SI 3.3–6.1 mmol/L
  Plasma or Serum: 70–120 mg/dl *or* SI 3.9–6.7 mmol/L
Elderly Individuals: 80–150 mg/dl *or* SI 4.4–8.3 mmol/L
Children <2 Years: 60–100 mg/dl *or* SI 3.3–5.6 mmol/L
Infant: 40–90 mg/dl *or* SI 2.2–5.0 mmol/L
Neonate: 30–60 mg/dl *or* SI 1.7–3.3 mmol/L

Background Information

Critical Thinking: The patient's FBS is higher in the morning than in the late afternoon glucose level, which is not a fasting glucose. How can this occur, even though insulin was given?

To meet cellular needs, the body has developed complex mechanisms to take in, use, and store nutrients. A serum glucose level reflects the ability of the body to perform its metabolic tasks. Glucose levels are not static. They vary after eating, so a fasting glucose level is desirable. Many factors influence blood glucose, but it is most frequently used to diagnose and manage diabetes mellitus.

With age, the norms for blood and plasma glucose levels are adjusted by 1 mg/dl per year of life after age 60 years.

One elevated fasting blood glucose level is not considered diagnostic but should be repeated. If a repeated fasting blood glucose level is elevated (>140 mg/dl), it supports the diagnosis of diabetes mellitus.

Purpose of the Test

Fasting blood glucose is evaluated to diagnose and manage patients with diabetes mellitus. The fasting blood glucose level is also obtained as supportive data in many diagnoses, as metabolic factors will influence glucose use and storage. Certain therapies may be evaluated by checking the fasting blood glucose level, for example, hyperalimentation and exogeneous glucocorticoid therapy.

Procedure

After a 12-hour fast, venipuncture is performed to obtain 5 ml of blood in a red-topped tube for a plasma or serum sample or in a green-topped tube for a whole blood sample. Usually serum or plasma sampling is performed because these tests reflect glucose levels in interstitial tissue and are not affected by the hematocrit.

Findings

Increase	Decrease
Acromegaly	Addison disease
Chronic pancreatitis	Advanced liver disease
Cushing syndrome	Alcohol intake, when fasting
Diabetes mellitus	Excessive exogenous insulin
Hyperthyroidism	Islet cell adenoma
Hyperosmolar coma	Leucine sensitivity
Pheochromocytoma	Malnutrition
Stress	

Interfering Factors

- Noncompliance with fasting
- Vigorous exercise
- Stress
- Medications
    Acetaminophen
    Arginine
    Benzodiazepines
    Beta-blockers
    Epinephrine
    Ethacrynic acid

Furosemide
Glucocorticoids
Glucose
Hypoglycemic agents
Insulin
Lithium
MAO inhibitors
Oral contraceptives
Phenothiazines
Phenytoin
Thiazide diuretics

Nursing Implementation

The nurse's actions are similar to those in other venipuncture procedures.

Pretest

Instruct the patient to fast for 12 hours before the blood is drawn.
Explain to the patient who is taking insulin or hypoglycemic agents to withhold the medication until after the blood is drawn.
Observe the patient for clinical manifestations of hypoglycemia.

Posttest

Ensure that the patient receives food and medications that were withheld.
Send blood to the laboratory, as it needs to be centrifuged within 30 minutes for serum and plasma levels.

TABLE 19–2	
COMPLICATIONS OF A FASTING BLOOD SUGAR	
Complication	**Nursing Assessment**
Hypoglycemia	Pallor
	Diaphoresis
	Tachycardia
	Palpitations
	Hunger
	Paresthesia
	Vagueness
	Confusion
	Slurred speech
	Somnolence
	Convulsions
	Coma

Complications

Because a fasting blood glucose determination requires that the patient maintain a nothing by mouth status, hypoglycemia may occur (Table 19–2).

FREE CORTISOL

(URINE)

─────────────── **NORMAL VALUES** ───────────────

0–110 µg/24 hours *or* SI 0–303.6 nmol/24 hours

Background Information

Critical Thinking:
The patient having a free cortisol level done seems very anxious and has a sinus tachycardia, a thickened neck, and bulging eyes. What other assessments and laboratory tests should be done in the interpretation of the free cortisol level?

When secreted by the adrenal cortex, cortisol binds with corticosteroid-binding globulin (CBG) and, to a much lesser degree, albumin. Only a small amount of cortisol circulates unbound or in the free state, which is the biologic active form. Free cortisol is normally excreted in the urine in small amounts.

If there is excessive secretion of cortisol, the CBG binding sites are filled, causing an increase in free cortisol; therefore, the urinary excretion increases. Because of this, an increased secretion of urinary free cortisol is helpful in diagnosing Cushing syndrome. It is not helpful in diagnosing adrenal insufficiency, since it is not sensitive at low levels, and low levels are relatively common in healthy individuals.

CBG is produced by the liver. Liver failure will affect CBG and, therefore, free cortisol levels. CBG is influenced by other factors. CBG levels increase in hyperthyroidism, diabetes, and high-estrogen states such as pregnancy. Genetic disorders may cause an increase or decrease in CBG. Hypothyroidism, protein deficiency, and renal failure may cause a decrease in CBG and influence free cortisol levels.

Procedure

A 24-hour urine specimen is collected and assessed by RIA or competitive protein-binding assay.

Findings

Increase
Cushing syndrome
Adrenal or pituitary tumor
Ectopic ACTH production

Interfering Factors

- Stress
- Physical activity
- Failure to collect all the urine during the 24-hour period
- Failure to store urine on ice or in a refrigerator
- Medications
    Amphetamines
    Morphine sulfate
    Phenothiazines
    Reserpine
    Steroids

Nursing Implementation

Pretest

Instruct the patient to avoid strenuous physical activity.

During the Test

At the start of the test, instruct the patient to void at 8 A.M. and discard this urine. The collection period starts at this time and all urine is collected for 24 hours, including the 8 A.M. specimen of the following morning.

On the requisition slip and specimen label, write the patient's name and the time and date of the start and finish of the test period.

Keep the urine refrigerated or on ice throughout the collection period.

Posttest

Arrange for prompt transport of the cooled specimen to the laboratory.

FREE THYROXINE

(SERUM)

Synonym:

FT_4

━━━━━━━━━━ **NORMAL VALUES** ━━━━━━━━━━

0.9–1.7 mg/dl *or* SI 11.5–21.8 nmol/L

Background Information

The majority of thyroxine (see thyroxine, pp. 669–671) is carried by thyroid-binding globulin, albumin, and prealbumin. It is free thyroxine, which is not bound, that is biologically active and converts to triiodothyronine (T_3) in the peripheral circulation.

The ability to measure free thyroxine has replaced a classic test called protein-bound iodine.

Purpose of the Test

Free thyroxine is used to diagnosis hyper- and hypothyroidism. It is especially helpful when there is abnormal thyroxine-binding globulin levels.

Procedure

Venipuncture is performed to collect 5 ml of blood in a red-topped tube. Laboratory procedures vary in assessing free thyroxine. If RIA is performed, albumin levels and a radionuclide scan within 7 days will affect the results.

Findings

Increase	Decrease
Acute psychiatric disorders	Anorexia nervosa
Hyperthyroidism	Hypothyroidism

Interfering Factors

- Medications
  Carbamazepine
  Exogeneous thyroid therapy
  Heparin
  Phenytoin
  Salicylates

Nursing Implementation

The nurse takes actions similar to those taken in other venipuncture procedures.

FREE TRIIODOTHYRONINE

(SERUM)

Synonym:

FT_3

─────────────── **NORMAL VALUES** ───────────────

0.2–0.52 mg/dl or SI 3–8 nmol/L

Background Information

Triiodothyronine is a hormone secreted by the thyroid gland. Most of the hormone is bound to thyroid-binding globulin. Some triiodothyronine is in the free state, that is, unbound. The unbound or free triiodothyronine is the biologically active form of the hormone.

Purpose of the Test

Free triiodothyronine is used to diagnose hyper- and hypothyroidism.

Procedure

Venipuncture is performed to collect a specimen in a red-topped tube. Laboratory methods to assess free triiodothyronine vary. If RIA is used, albumin levels and a radionuclide scan within 7 days will affect results.

Findings

Increase	Decrease
Hyperthyroidism	Hypothyroidism

Interfering Factors

- Exogenous thyroid therapy

Nursing Implementation

Nursing actions resemble those of other venipuncture procedures.

GLUCAGON, BLOOD

(PLASMA)

―――――――――――――― NORMAL VALUES ――――――――――――――

50–100 pg/ml *or* SI 25 ng/L

Background Information

Glucagon is produced and secreted by the A cells of the islets of Langerhans of the pancreas. Glucagon stimulates the breakdown of stored glycogen and maintains gluconeogenesis. Glucagon is secreted in response to hypoglycemia, helping to meet glucose needs of tissues between the intake of food.

Purpose of the Test

Glucagon levels are assessed in suspected pancreatic tumors, chronic pancreatitis, and familial hyperglucagonemia.

Procedure

Venipuncture is performed to obtain 7 ml of blood in a lavender-topped tube with EDTA. The specimen is placed on ice and sent to the laboratory immediately to be centrifuged.

Findings

Increase	Decrease
Acute pancreatitis	Chronic pancreatitis
Diabetic ketoacidosis	High fatty acid levels
Glucagonoma	Hyperglycemia
Hypoglycemia	Insulinoma
Parasympathetic stimulation	
Pheochromocytoma	
Renal failure	
Stress	
Sympathetic stimulation	

Interfering Factors

- Stress
- Prolonged fasting
- Radioactive scan within 2 days
- Medications
    Catecholamines
    Insulin
    Glucocorticoids

Nursing Implementation

The nurse takes actions similar to those used in other venipuncture procedures.

Pretest

Instruct the patient to fast for 10 to 12 hours before blood is drawn.
Explain to the patient the need to rest for 30 minutes before the test.
Take a medication history and determine if any interfering drugs should be held.
Schedule any radioactive scans after the glucagon determination is obtained.

Place specimen on ice and send to laboratory immediately. (Not all laboratories require the specimen to be placed on ice.)

Posttest

The patient can resume a normal diet and medication regimen.

GLUCOSE, CAPILLARY

(WHOLE BLOOD)

Synonyms:

self-blood glucose monitoring (SBGM), bedside glucose monitoring (BGM)

─────────────── **NORMAL VALUES** ───────────────

60–110 mg/dl *or* SI 3.3–6.1 mmol/L

Background Information

Capillary glucose monitoring has revolutionized the management of patients with insulin-dependent diabetes mellitus (IDDM). Capillary glucose monitoring determines the glucose level of whole blood (which is lower than serum or plasma levels). It evaluates current status, permitting more accurate management and therapy. It has replaced urine glucose testing as the preferred technique to determine insulin replacement requirements in hospitals and in the home.

To perform capillary glucose monitoring, a drop of capillary blood is dropped onto a reagent strip, and the glucose level is determined by the color changes on the strip. The color change can be compared to a color chart or assessed by a glucose meter. Since the visual method is subjective and some diabetics have visual impairment, glucose meters are frequently used. Newer meters are relatively affordable (less than $50). For the diabetic who is blind, there are "talking" meters available, but they are more expensive.

Critical Thinking: As part of the diabetic teaching plan, the nurse instructs the patient on capillary glucose testing. What adaptations to the plan will be necessary if the patient has significant loss of vision?

Non–insulin-dependent diabetics may find the use of capillary glucose monitoring helpful in managing their diabetes. These patients can check their glucose level 2 hours after they eat to see how specific foods affect it and modify their intake by an objective measurement.

For insulin-dependent and non–insulin dependent diabetics, regular capillary glucose testing will produce greater control with more effective long-term treatment. Capillary glucose testing can help the diabetic maintain control during periods of stress, for example, illness, pregnancy, and surgery. Usually, the patient with IDDM will monitor the capillary glucose level before each meal and at bedtime. The patient with non–insulin dependent diabetes (NIDDM) usually monitors the capillary glucose twice a day—before breakfast and 2 hours after dinner.

Nurses need to teach their patients how to monitor capillary glucose, including how to use and care for the glucose meter and reagent strips and how to check the reliability of the meter. This information needs to be reinforced periodically.

Nursing research has also shown the importance of periodic inservice programs for nurses regarding bedside glucose monitors (Amatruda et al., 1989).

Purpose of the Test

Capillary glucose monitoring is carried out to assess and manage patients with diabetes mellitus. It may be used in hospitals to monitor other hyperglycemic patients, such as those on hyperalimentation or high-dose glucocorticoid therapy. Capillary glucose evaluation is *not* used to diagnose diabetes mellitus, but it may indicate a need to perform a glucose tolerance test (Bain et al., 1989).

Procedure

With a lancet, a fingerstick is carried out, and a drop of blood is dropped onto a reagent strip. The intensity of the color change is proportional to the amount of glucose in the blood. The darker the color, the higher the glucose concentration. The color change is assessed visually by comparing it to a color chart or by the blood glucose meter. The meter may read the strip by the process of refractance photometry or by electrochemical technology. Either method will provide a digital readout of the glucose level.

Nursing Implementation

There are many different glucose meters on the market. It is *essential* to follow the manufacturers' guidelines for their use. In addition, there are a number of lancing devices available.

Pretest

QUALITY CONTROL

Glucose meters should be checked daily in hospitals and once a week or when opening a new vial of strips at home with quality control solution containing a known amount of dissolved glucose in water. The meter should also be tested if the meter is dropped or the meter reading does not correlate with clinical assessments.

QUALITY CONTROL

When a fasting blood glucose determination is obtained, a capillary glucose level can also be obtained and the two measures compared. A variance of less than 15% is acceptable.

If the battery in the meter has worn out, recalibrate the meter with the plastic calibration strip provided in the reagent vial according to the manufacturer's guidelines.

Check the code number on the glucose meter and on the reagent strip to ensure that they are the same. Check the expiration date on the reagent strip container and discard outdated strips.

Wear gloves for this procedure, as blood contact is possible.

During the Test

Instruct the patient to wash the hands in warm water and soap. The warm water will help dilate the vessels.

Hospital protocol may require the patient's finger to be wiped with an alcohol swab (this is usually not done in the home). If alcohol is used, it must be allowed to dry out or it will affect the results and increase the painfulness of the procedure.

Have the reagent strip on hand, and puncture the skin. The puncture site should be on the side of the fingertip. The middle of the fingertip is more sensitive to pain, and the side has more capillaries. Instruct the patient to rotate sites.

Milk the fingertip toward the puncture site until a large drop of blood forms.

Let the drop of blood fall on the reagent strip so that the entire pad at the tip is covered with blood. Do not smear the blood or try to add another drop.

Time when to wipe the strip if required according to the manufacturers' guidelines, and when to insert the strip into the meter. Timing is essential for accurate measurement. Some manufacturers require a cotton ball be used to wipe the reagent strip.

Insert the strip into the meter. Read and document the results.

Instruct the patient on how to dispose of the lancet in a heavy plastic container, for example, an empty detergent bottle.

Critical Thinking: On re-admission of a diabetic patient, the nurse has the patient demonstrate the way she does capillary glucose testing at home. The patient makes two errors in technique. How does the nurse correct these mistakes while maintaining the patient's self-esteem and confidence?

Posttest

Administer insulin as ordered.

Instruct the patient to keep an accurate record of the glucose level and insulin replacement. This record should be brought to the physician, diabetic nurse specialist, or clinic on the next visit.

GLUCOSE, URINARY

(URINE)

Synonyms:

───────── **NORMAL VALUES** ─────────

No glucose present

Background Information

As serum glucose levels rise, the renal threshold for glucose will be reached and glucose will "spill out" into the urine. The presence of glycosuria (glucose in the urine) at one time played a major role in regulating the diet and insulin therapy of patients with diabetes mellitus. The urine would be checked four times a day—before each meal and at bedtime—and insulin coverage given depending on how much glucose was spilled.

Today, patients with IDDM and many patients with NIDDM are regulated by self-capillary blood glucose monitoring. Capillary glucose monitoring is superior to urinary glucose testing because it reflects the patient's current glucose status, whereas urine reflects the blood glucose level at the time the urine was formed. Even when the patient performs a "double void," complete emptying of the bladder is questionable and "old" and "fresh" urine will mix. The double void method of obtaining a urine sample requires the patient to void, attempting to empty the bladder. After 30 minutes, the person voids again and uses this urine to check for glucose.

Purpose of the Test

When capillary glucose monitoring is not possible, urinary glucose is measured to determine insulin and dietary requirements of patients with diabetes mellitus.

Procedure

Two methods are commonly used to check for urinary glucose: Copper reduction tests (Clinitest tablets) or the dipstick method. The latter is more frequently used at home.

Findings

Glucosuria may be due to

Diabetes mellitus
Chronic renal failure
Cushing syndrome
Thyroid disorders
Fanconi syndrome
Hyperalimentation
Pregnancy

Interfering Factors

- Failure to use fresh urine
- Urine heavily contaminated with bacteria
- Clinitest tablet or dipstick was exposed to air, light, heat, or moisture
- Medications (partial listing)
  Acetylsalicylic acid
  Chloral hydrate
  Glucocorticoids
  Isoniazid
  Levodopa
  Lithium
  Methyldopa
  Penicillin G
  Probenecid
  Salicylates
  Streptomycin
  Tetramycin
  Thiazide diuretics

Nursing Implementation

Since this test is used for self-monitoring, patient education is an essential part of the nursing role.

Pretest

Critical Thinking: How does the nurse explain to a patient with an enlarged prostate why the "double void" technique for urine testing will not be effective for him?

Instruct the patient on the double void technique.

Explain to the patient the need to collect the specimen in a clean container.

With the Clinitest tablets, heat is created by the chemical action. Warn the patient not to hold the test tube in the hand after dropping the tablet into it.

During the Test

With the Clinitest Tablet

Add to a clean, dry test tube five drops of urine and ten drops of water and then drop a Clinitest tablet into the test tube.

Compare the color change of the urine with the color chart that comes with the tablets.

Record results.

With Dipstick Method (Clinistix, Diastix, Tes-Tape)

The dipstick is dipped in urine. The waiting time is indicated by the manufacturer.

Compare color change with chart provided.
Record results.

Posttest

Clean equipment with soap and water and rinse thoroughly.
Store tablets and dipstick in dry, cool place in their original containers.
Document results on flow sheet.
Adjust insulin dosage as ordered based on the results.

GLYCOSYLATED HEMOGLOBIN ASSAY

(BLOOD)

Synonyms:

glycohemoglobin, GHB, hemoglobin A_1

---------------------- **NORMAL VALUES** ----------------------

GLYCOSYLATED HEMOGLOBIN ASSAY
Normal, healthy person 5.5–8.8% of total hemoglobin *or* SI 0.05–0.08
(fraction of total hemoglobin)
Diabetic under control 7.5–11.4% of total hemoglobin
  Hemoglobin A_{1a} 1.8% of total hemoglobin
  Hemoglobin A_{1b} 0.8% of total hemoglobin
  Hemoglobin A_{1c} 3.5–6% of total hemoglobin

Background Information

Critical Thinking: The hemoglobin A_1 results indicate that the patient's glucose is poorly controlled. When informed, the patient angrily states that he *never* cheated on his diet and *always* took his insulin. How should the nurse respond? Would the response vary if the patient has a history of noncompliance?

Glycosylated hemoglobin refers to hemoglobin that has hooked up with glucose. The major glycosylated hemoglobin is *hemoglobin A_{1c}*, which is approximately 4 to 6% of the total hemoglobin. The other glycosylated hemoglobins are phosphoxylated glucose (A_{1a}) and phosphoxylated fructose (A_{1b}). Usually, a laboratory will report the total glycosylated hemoglobin level (hemoglobin A_1).

The reaction between glucose and hemoglobin is based on the blood glucose concentration. The higher the glucose concentration, the higher percentage of glycosylated hemoglobin. Since the reaction is not reversible, once the glucose adheres to the hemoglobin it remains glycosylated. Since the life span of a red blood cell is normally 120 days, measuring the glycosylated hemoglobin can assist in diabetic control assessment. It is not affected by recent changes in diet or medication, like fasting blood glucose, so the physician can determine diabetic control over a period of weeks or months. Diabetics who are poorly controlled will have a glycosylated hemoglobin value that is more than 12% of the total hemoglobin value.

Purpose of the Test

A glycosylated hemoglobin determination is performed to measure a patient's diabetic control over a period of weeks or months. The maximum period for evaluation of control is the life span of the red blood cells (120 days).

Procedure

Venipuncture is performed to obtain 5 ml of blood in a test tube containing an anticoagulant (lavender-topped tube with EDTA or a green-topped tube with heparin).

Findings

Increase

Poorly controlled diabetes mellitus
Hyperglycemia

Interfering Factors

- Anemia
- Chronic renal failure
- Clotting of specimen
- Fetal-maternal transfusion
- Hemodialysis
- Hemorrhage
- Hemolytic disease
- Phlebotomies
- Thalassemias

Nursing Implementation

The actions of the nurse resemble those used in other venipuncture procedures.

GROWTH HORMONE

(SERUM)

Synonyms:

somatotropin, GH, STH

Background Information

Growth hormone is synthesized and secreted by the anterior pituitary gland under the direction of the hypothalamus. The hypothalamus controls growth

Adult Male:	Undetectable—5 ng/ml *or* SI 0–5 µg/L
Adult Female:	Undetectable—10 ng/ml *or* SI 0–10 µg/L
Child:	Undetectable—16 ng/ml *or* SI 0–16 µg/L

hormone secretion via somatostatin (growth hormone–release-inhibiting hormone) and growth hormone–releasing hormone. The primary function of growth hormone is the promotion of linear growth, which it does by stimulating the production of somatomedin, which is produced by a variety of organs. It is believed that growth hormone also has a direct effect on tissues.

During linear growth and afterward, growth hormone influences protein, carbohydrate, and fat metabolism. It increases protein synthesis, decreases protein catabolism, and activates lipolysis. Excessive growth hormone will decrease carbohydrate use and glucose uptake by the cells.

Critical Thinking: A neighbor's child is the shortest child in his class. His parents ask the nurse if he should be tested. What initial assessments should the nurse make in helping the parents come to a decision?

Since normal basal levels of growth hormone are low, it is sometimes necessary to stimulate the secretion of the hormone to rule out hyposecretion. Various substances can be used in these provocative tests, including arginine, insulin, arginine-insulin, levodopa and, less frequently, vasopressin, glucagon, exercise, or tolbutamide. Careful medical evaluation of the patient is necessary before insulin is used as a provocative agent so that a hypoglycemic crisis can be prevented.

Purpose of the Test

Growth hormone levels are evaluated to diagnose growth disorders and possible pituitary tumors. Abnormal linear growth may be due to several factors: genetics, chronic disease, malnutrition, and so forth. Growth hormone-levels will assist in determining the cause of the growth disorder and thereby influence therapy and prognosis.

Procedure

Serum growth hormone levels are measured by RIA. Five ml of venous blood is drawn into a red-topped tube and is sent to the laboratory.

Findings

Increase	Decrease
Pituitary tumor	Dwarfism
Hypothalamic tumor	Metastatic or anoxic pituitary destruction
Acromegaly	
Gigantism	

Interfering Factors

- Failure to fast for 8 to 12 hours before the test
- Administration of radioactive scan within 7 days
- Medications
    Amphetamines
    Arginine
    Beta-blockers
    Chlorpromazine
    Corticosteroids
    Dopamine
    Glucagon
    Insulin
    L-Dopa
    Methyldopa

Nursing Implementation

Pretest

Instruct the patient to limit activity and not eat or drink for 8 to 12 hours before the specimen is collected.

Obtain a drug history to determine if any interfering medication is being taken.

Inquire if the patient has undergone any recent radioactive scans.

During the Test

The nurse takes actions similar to those of other venipuncture procedures.

Posttest

The patient can resume diet and the medications that were withheld.
Normal activity may be resumed.

GROWTH HORMONE STIMULATION TEST

(SERUM)   *Synonyms:*
arginine test, insulin tolerance test (ITT)

Background Information

Review the preceding section on growth hormone.

━━━━━━━━━━━━━━━━━━━━━━ **NORMAL VALUES** ━━━━━━━━━━━━━━━

With Arginine:	>7 ng/ml *or* SI >7 µg/L
With Insulin (with Serum Glucose of <40 mg/dl):	>20 ng/ml *or* SI >20 µg/L

Purpose of the Test

The growth hormone stimulation test is usually performed to evaluate children and infants with retarded growth. It is also used to support the diagnosis of pituitary tumor.

The insulin tolerance test may be used to distinguish primary versus secondary adrenocorticoid insufficiency by measuring ACTH levels instead of growth hormone levels.

Procedure

Depending on the substance used, there is slight variation in the method used. With arginine, a baseline sample of 5 ml of venous blood is obtained in a red-topped tube. A venous infusion of arginine is then administered. After the arginine infusion is completed (approximately 30 minutes), 30 minutes is allowed to pass. Three venous samples are then obtained at 30-minute intervals. Ion exchange chromatography is used to analyze the blood samples.

If insulin is used, a baseline venous sample is taken, after which 100 U of regular insulin is given intravenously over 2 to 3 minutes. Venous samples are taken at 15, 30, 45, 60, 90, and 120 minutes after the administration of insulin.

Findings

Increase	Decrease
No growth hormone deficiency	Pituitary dwarfism
	Pituitary tumors

Interfering Factors

- Failure to comply with fasting or activity restrictions
- Alcohol
- Medications
    - Amphetamines
    - Beta-blockers
    - Calcium gluconate
    - Estrogen
    - Spironolactone
    - Steroids

Nursing Implementation

Pretest

Critical Thinking: When the nurse questioned an adult patient scheduled for an insulin tolerance test, the patient denied any history of epilepsy or seizure disorders. Later, the nurse discovers that the patient is taking phenytoin (Dilantin). What cultural influences could be responsible for the patient's denial?

Assess patients at risk if a growth hormone stimulation test with insulin is planned. This includes patients with cardiovascular disease, epilepsy, a history of a cerebrovascular accident, or adrenal insufficiency.

Instruct the patient to limit physical activity and not to eat or drink for 12 hours before the test.

Instruct the patient not to drink alcohol for 24 hours before the blood is drawn.

Obtain a medication history to determine if any interfering drug is being taken. Check with prescriber about withholding any interfering medication.

Instruct the patient to lie down quietly for 90 minutes before the blood is drawn.

During the Test

An intravenous catheter (heparin lock) is inserted to prevent multiple venous punctures.

A baseline venous sample is taken.

If arginine is used, an infusion is given over 30 minutes in the arm opposite the heparin lock used for blood sampling. Thirty minutes after the arginine infusion is completed, three additional blood specimens are obtained at 30-minute intervals.

If insulin is used, 100 units of regular insulin is given over 2 to 3 minutes. Blood specimens are drawn at 15, 30, 45, 60, 90, and 120 minutes.

Observe the patient carefully. Stop the test if serious signs of hypoglycemia occur (vertigo, chest pain).

Posttest

The patient can resume medication schedule, diet, and physical activities. Ensure that the patient who received insulin as a stimulant obtains adequate intake.

GROWTH HORMONE SUPPRESSION TEST

(SERUM)

Synonym:

glucose loading test

NORMAL VALUES

Growth hormone levels decrease to undetectable to <3 ng/ml *or* SI <3 µg/L in 30–120 minutes

Background Information

The growth hormone suppression test is performed after high levels of growth hormone are found. Normally, the ingestion of glucose causes a decrease in the secretion of growth hormone. In patients with hypersecretion of growth hormone, however, a significant decrease does not occur.

Purpose of the Test

This test is usually performed to assess an increase in growth hormone levels and to confirm the diagnosis of gigantism in children and acromegaly in adults.

Procedure

A baseline venous blood sample, 5 ml, is drawn into a red-topped tube. The patient ingests a glucose solution. After 1 to 2 hours, another blood sample is drawn. RIA is used to assess the samples.

Findings

Maintenance of High Growth Hormone Levels

Acromegaly
Gigantism

Interfering Factors

* Noncompliance with activity restrictions and fasting
* Radioactive scans within the previous week
* Medications
  Amphetamines
  Arginine
  Beta-blockers
  Chorpromazine
  Dopamine
  Glucagon
  Histamine
  Insulin
  L-Dopa
  Nicotinic acid
  Steroids

Nursing Implementation

Pretest

Instruct the patient about the need to avoid physical activity for 10 to 12 hours before the test and to lie quietly for 30 minutes before the blood is drawn.

Instruct the patient not to eat or drink for 12 hours before the sample is taken.

Obtain a medication history to ensure that an interfering drug has not been taken.

Question the patient or check the patient's chart for any recent radioactive scans.

During the Test

Explain the purpose of two venipunctures.

After the first specimen is obtained in the early morning, instruct the patient to drink the glucose solution *slowly* to minimize nausea.

Ensure that the second specimen is obtained 1 to 2 hours after the ingestion of glucose.

Posttest

The patient resumes normal diet and activity.

2-HOUR POSTPRANDIAL GLUCOSE

(PLASMA)

Synonym:

2-hour postprandial blood sugar

──────────────── **NORMAL VALUES** ────────────────

Fasting Blood Glucose: <140 mg/dl *or* SI <7.78 mmol/L
May be slightly elevated in elderly patients

Background Information

In healthy individuals, the ingestion of food raises the blood glucose level, which is a potent stimulant for insulin release. The insulin level peaks in less than an hour. Normally, within 1½ to 2 hours, the glucose level will return to baseline. It may take slightly longer in older individuals for the value to return to a baseline level. The 2-hour postprandial glucose test evaluates whether the individual has an adequate insulin response to intake. A diabetic is considered in good control if the 2-hour postprandial glucose level is less than 130 mg/dl. In an undiagnosed case, a 2-hour postprandial glucose level greater than 140 mg/dl indicates that an oral glucose tolerance test (OGTT) should be performed because this test has more controlled variables.

Purpose of the Test

The 2-hour postprandial glucose test is performed to support the diagnosis of diabetes mellitus and to evaluate the management of a patient with diabetes mellitus.

Procedure

Two hours after a meal is ingested, venipuncture is performed to obtain 5 ml of blood in a red-topped tube for a plasma or serum glucose level determination.

Findings

A 2-hour postprandial glucose determination greater than 140 mg/dl is consistent with the diagnosis of diabetes mellitus.

Interfering Factors

- Noncompliance with dietary requirements
- Cushing disease or Cushing syndrome
- Infection
- Malabsorption syndrome
- Malnutrition
- Severe stress
- Medications
  Arginine
  Beta-adrenergic blockers
  Epinephrine
  Glucocorticoids
  Glucose administered intravenously
  Hypoglycemic agents
  Insulin
  Lithium
  Phenothiazines
  Phenytoin

Nursing Implementation

Pretest

Instruct the patient to eat normally before the test.

During the Test

The patient ingests a meal containing at least 100 g of carbohydrate. Instruct the patient not to eat or drink for 2 hours after the meal is ingested. Venipuncture is performed to obtain a blood glucose level 2 hours after the meal.

Posttest

The patient resumes a normal diet.

INSULIN, BLOOD

(SERUM OR PLASMA)

NORMAL VALUES

FASTING	**Adult:** 5–25 μU/ml *or* SI 34–172 pmol/L **Newborn:** 3–20 μU/ml *or* SI 21–138 pmol/L **1 Hour After Eating:** 50–130 μU/ml *or* SI 347.3–902.8 pmol/L **Two Hours After Eating:** <30 μU/ml *or* SI <208.4 pmol/L

Background Information

Critical Thinking:
A serum insulin level is planned for a newly diagnosed diabetic. If the insulin level is normal, how does this affect the patient's teaching plan?

Insulin is a protein hormone produced and secreted by the pancreas. It has a short half-life (3 to 5 minutes) and is broken down by the liver and kidneys. Insulin is secreted in response to food intake. It increases in concentration within 10 minutes of eating, peaks in 30 to 45 minutes, and returns to baseline levels within 90 to 120 minutes. Normally, insulin levels increase as blood glucose levels increase.

Without insulin, carbohydrate, protein, and fat metabolism are affected, resulting in hyperglycemia and metabolic acidosis.

Purpose of the Test

Insulin levels are determined to assess for insulin-producing tumors, confirm suspected insulin-resistant states, and as part of the evaluation of glucocorticoid insufficiency.

Procedure

Insulin levels may be assessed by random venous sampling or during a glucose tolerance test. A specimen is obtained by venipuncture and collected in an anticoagulated tube. The specimen is assessed by RIA.

Findings

Increase	Decrease
Acromegaly	IDDM
Cushing syndrome	Hypopituitarism
Hyperinsulinism	
Insulinoma	
Liver disease	
Pancreatic lesions	
Vagal stimulation	

Interfering Factors

- Noncompliance with test protocol
- Insulin antibodies
- Medications
    ACTH
    Catecholamines
    Colchicine
    Diazoxide
    Oral contraceptives
    Phenytoin
    Steroids
    Sulfonylureas
    Thyroid hormones
    Vinblastine

Nursing Implementation

Care varies according to whether a fasting sample is used or the insulin level is being obtained as part of the OGTT (see pp. 647–650 for this test).

Pretest

Take a medication history to determine if any interfering drugs are being taken. Check to determine if these drugs are to be withheld. If the patient is receiving insulin therapy, the insulin is withheld until the test is performed.

Assess the patient's stress level, which may increase endogenous glucocorticoid secretion.

If a fasting insulin sample is to be drawn, instruct the patient not to eat or drink for 7 hours before the blood is drawn.

During the Test

Observe the patient for hyperglycemia if the insulin is withheld and for hypoglycemia because of the fasting state.

If performed with an OGTT, a blood sample for insulin is obtained each time a glucose level specimen is drawn.

Critical Thinking: A newly admitted comatose patient has a finger stick glucose over 900 mg (SI: 49.55 mmol/L). What clinical assessments would make the nurse suspect hyperosmolar coma and a need for a STAT serum ketone level? Would the serum ketone level influence therapy?

QUALITY CONTROL

Send the specimen to the laboratory immediately, as it must be centrifuged within 30 minutes and frozen until the assay can be performed.

Posttest

The patient resumes normal medication schedule and diet therapies.

KETONES, SERUM

(SERUM)

Synonyms:

acetoacetate, acetones

─────── **NORMAL VALUES** ───────

Negative: <1 mg/dl *or* SI <0.1 nmol/L

Background Information

Without adequate insulin, three major ketone bodies accumulate in the blood: acetone, acetoacetate acid, and beta-hydroxybutyric acid.

Purpose of the Test

Serum ketone levels are measured to distinguish between diabetic ketoacidosis and hyperosmolar coma. With diabetic ketoacidosis, incomplete fatty acid metabolism leads to increasing ketones in the blood. Patients with hyperosmolar coma produce minimal or no ketosis in the presence of extremely high levels of serum glucose. The mechanism of maintaining nearly normal ketone levels in hyperosmolar coma is not known. It is theorized that these patients have sufficient insulin to break down fatty acids or are glucagon-resistant.

The severity of the ketosis will influence the therapy for uncontrolled diabetes.

Procedure

Venipuncture is performed to obtain 7 ml of blood in a red-topped tube.

Findings

Increase

Alcoholism
Decreased caloric intake (dieting)
Eclampsia
Isopropanol poisoning
Propranolol poisoning
Starvation
Uncontrolled diabetes mellitus
Gierke disease

Nursing Implementation

The nurse's duties are similar to those performed in other venipuncture procedures.

KETONES, URINARY

(URINE)

Synonyms:

acetoacetate, acetones

―――――――――――――――――――――――― **NORMAL VALUES** ――――――――――

No ketones

Background Information

Without adequate insulin, three major ketone bodies accumulate in the blood and are excreted in the urine. These ketone bodies are acetone, acetoacetic acid, and beta-hydroxybutyric acid. Ketones form as fats and fatty acids are broken down.

There are a variety of commercial products available to test for ketones in the urine. The most popular products are Acetest tablets, Ketostix, and Keto-Diastix. These products measure acetone and acetoacetate acid levels but not beta-hydroxybutyric acid, which may be the dominant ketone in patients with poorly controlled diabetes mellitus.

Urinary ketone testing is usually performed in conjunction with urinary glucose testing. It may be carried out randomly to evaluate a suspected diagnosis of uncontrolled diabetes mellitus or four times a day to regulate insulin coverage.

Purpose of the Test

Urine is tested for ketone bodies to evaluate the patient with diabetes mellitus and to diagnose carbohydrate deprivation. The concentration of urine ketones can be used to adjust insulin requirements in the diabetic and to monitor patients on low-carbohydrate diets.

Procedure

There are a variety of commercial products available for testing ketones in the urine such as the Acetest tablet, Ketostix, and Keto-Diastix. With the Acetest tablet, one drop of urine is dropped on a tablet. With the sticks, the paper strip is dipped in the urine. The color change of the tablet or on the strip is compared to the chart provided by the manufacturer to determine the presence and concentration of ketones.

Findings

Increase

Alcoholic ketoacidosis
Fever
High-fat diets
Hypermetabolic states
Starvation
Uncontrolled diabetes mellitus

Interfering Factors

QUALITY CONTROL
• Using products that have been exposed to light or are outdated
• Bacteria in the urine

Nursing Implementation

Pretest

Instruct the patient about the double void technique.

During the Test

Critical Thinking: When attempting to obtain a urine specimen qid for ketone levels, the patient consistently reports that she has "just voided" and cannot give a specimen. What assessments are needed before the nurse adapts the patient's care plan?

Instruct the patient to void, discard this urine, wait 30 minutes, and void into a clean, dry container.

Check voided urine within 60 minutes.

The method of checking for ketones varies with the product. Follow manufacturer's guidelines.

Posttest

Document the results, usually on a flow chart.

Adjust insulin dosage as ordered based on the results.

LONG-ACTING THYROID STIMULATOR

(SERUM)

Synonym:

LATS

--- **NORMAL VALUES** ---

No long-acting thyroid stimulator

Background Information

Long-acting thyroid stimulator is a globulin that binds to thyroid receptor sites and stimulates thyroid activity. It is present in about half of the patients with Graves disease and may or may not be present in patients with nodular toxic goiter or other thyroid disorders (Zweiman, 1991).

Purpose of the Test

The determination of long-acting thyroid stimulator levels is performed to support the diagnosis of Graves disease.

Procedure

Venipuncture is performed and blood is collected in a heparinized tube. The specimen is assessed by mouse bioassay.

Findings

Increase

Graves disease

Nodular toxic goiter (rare)

Interfering Factors

- Radioactive iodine

Nursing Implementation

The nursing actions are similar to those in other venipuncture procedures.

Pretest

Schedule any test requiring radioactive iodine after blood for long-acting thyroid stimulator levels is drawn.

METYRAPONE TESTING

(SERUM)

Synonym:

metyrapone stimulation test

―――――――――― **NORMAL VALUES** ――――――――――

11-deoxycortisol level >7 µg/dl

Background Information

Critical Thinking: For a patient with no medical or nursing background, how would you explain the purpose of metyrapone testing?

Review the section on plasma ACTH (pp. 597–600). Metyrapone is given to block cortisol synthesis. A decrease in cortisol will normally stimulate ACTH secretion, which, in turn, will increase the secretion of 11-deoxycortisol. If after the metyrapone is given, an increase occurs, ACTH and adrenal function are normal. If an abnormal result occurs, that is, no increase in 11-deoxycortisol, the diagnosis of adrenal insufficiency is established; however, it is not known whether it is primary or secondary adrenal failure.

The *insulin-induced hypoglycemia test* is similar to the metyrapone test. The hypoglycemia causes a stress response normally resulting in the secretion of CRH, which causes an increase in ACTH secretion. This test allows the assessment of the hypothalamic-pituitary axis.

Purpose of the Test

Metyrapone testing is performed to diagnose adrenal insufficiency and to assess pituitary-adrenal reserves.

TABLE 19–3	
COMPLICATIONS OF METYRAPONE TESTING	
Complication	**Nursing Assessment**
Addisonian crisis	Hypotension
	Hyponatremia
	Hyperkalemia
	Muscle weakness
	Shock

Procedure

Metyrapone is given in the evening. The next morning, a venipuncture is performed to obtain 7 to 10 ml of blood in a red- or green-topped tube.

Findings

Adrenal hyperplasia
Adrenal tumor
Ectopic ACTH syndrome

Interfering Factors

- Recent radioisotope therapy or testing
- Medication
    Chlorpromazine

Nursing Implementation

The nursing actions are similar to those carried out in the determination of cortisol levels (see pp. 614–616).

Complications

For a patient with adrenocorticoid insufficiency, the administration of metyrapone, which inhibits cortisol production, may precipitate an addisonian crisis (Table 19–3).

ORAL GLUCOSE TOLERANCE TEST

(PLASMA)   *Synonym:*
          OGTT

──────── **NORMAL VALUES** ────────

Baseline FBS:	70–105 mg/dl *or* SI 3.9–5.8 mmol/L
Thirty Minutes BS:	110–170 mg/dl *or* SI 6.1–9.4 mmol/L
Sixty Minutes BS:	120–170 mg/dl *or* SI 6.7–9.4 mmol/L
Ninety Minutes BS:	100–140 mg/dl *or* SI 5.6–7.8 mmol/L
One Hundred Twenty Minutes BS:	70–120 mg/dl *or* SI 3.9–6.7 mmol/L

Background Information

Fasting blood glucose levels are usually, if repeated, adequate to diagnosis diabetes mellitus if the plasma glucose level is more than 140 mg/dl. However, if the fasting blood glucose level is between 120 and 140 mg/dl and additional clinical indications make diabetes mellitus likely, an OGTT may be performed. Other indications include delivery of an infant weighing more than 9 lb (4.1 kg), frequent vaginal yeast infections, and impotence in males.

The *intravenous glucose tolerance test* (IVGTT) is similar to the OGTT. It is usually ordered when the patient has a problem with gastrointestinal absorption. It is not preferable to the OGTT because it bypasses normal glucose absorption and, therefore, normal changes in gastrointestinal hormones. Patient preparation for the IVGGT is the same as that for the OGTT, except that the glucose load (0.5 gm/kg of ideal body weight) is given intravenously over 2 to 3 minutes. The fasting blood glucose levels after the IVGTT are similar to those after an OGTT, except that the 30-minute ingestion fasting blood glucose level tends to be higher.

Purpose of the Test

The OGTT is performed to confirm the diagnosis of diabetes mellitus.

Procedure

After the ingestion of a glucose load, venous blood samplings for plasma glucose are obtained at the time of ingestion and then at 30, 60, 90, and 120 minutes after the glucose load is given.

Findings

The OGTT confirms the diagnosis of diabetes mellitus if the 2-hour blood glucose level is greater than 200 mg/dl and at least one other blood glucose determination is greater than 200 mg/dl. Blood glucose levels between the diagnostic criteria and normal values are called "impaired glucose tolerance."

Interfering Factors

- Noncompliance with dietary and fasting requirements
- Alcohol ingestion
- Being bedridden
- Cushing syndrome or Cushing disease
- Infection
- Malabsorption syndrome
- Malnutrition
- Pregnancy
- Severe stress
- Medications
  Amphetamines
  Arginine
  Beta-adrenergic blockers
  Diuretics
  Epinephrine
  Glucocorticoids
  Glucose administered intravenously
  Insulin
  Lithium
  Oral contraceptives
  Oral hypoglycemic agents
  Phenothiazines
  Phenytoin
  Salicylates

Nursing Implementation

Pretest

Critical Thinking: In the pretest instruction for OGTT, how is the carbohydrate intake influenced by the patient's culture? How do the American, Chinese, Italian, and Spanish diets differ in carbohydrate content?

Instruct the patient to take in at least 150 to 250 gms of carbohydrates per day for 3 days before the test to optimize insulin secretion.

Instruct the patient not to drink or eat for 8 hours before the test begins. The patient is also instructed to avoid stimulants and not to smoke or perform any unusual activity for 8 hours before the test.

Take a medication history to determine if any interfering drugs are being taken. Check with the prescriber to determine if medications should be withheld. Oral hypoglycemic agents are withheld for 2 weeks before an OGTT is performed.

Question the patient regarding any recent acute illnesses. The OGTT should be delayed for at least 2 weeks after an acute illness.

During the Test

A fasting blood glucose determination is performed (usually in the early morning between 7 A.M. and 9 A.M.).

Critical Thinking: After instructing the patient not to smoke during the OGTT, the nurse smells cigarette smoke in the patient's room and finds the cigarettes in the patient's bedside stand. Does the nurse have the right to remove cigarettes from the patient's room?

Within 5 minutes of obtaining the baseline fasting blood glucose level, the patient drinks 75 g of glucose in 300 ml of water. Children are given 1.5 g of glucose per kilogram of ideal body weight. The glucose solution should be ingested within 5 minutes.

Venipunctures are performed to obtain blood glucose readings at 30, 60, 90, and 120 minutes after the glucose solution is ingested. If a hypoglycemic reaction is suspected, a 3-hour blood specimen is obtained.

Observe the patient for a hyper- or hypoglycemic reaction.

The patient may drink water during the collection period.

Posttest

The patient resumes taking medications that were withheld.
A normal diet and activity level are resumed.

OSMOLALITY, PLASMA

(PLASMA OR SERUM)

Synonyms:

NORMAL VALUES	
Adult:	285–319 mOsm/kg H_2O *or* SI 280–395 mmol/kg
Children:	270–290 mOsm/kg H_2O *or* SI 270–290 mmol/kg

Background Information

Osmolality is a measure of the number of particles dissolved in a solution. In the blood, the osmolality is created by sodium, chloride, bicarbonate, proteins, glucose, and urea dissolved in the plasma. Osmolality will be affected by an increase or decrease in fluid volume or by an increase or decrease in blood particles.

Purpose of the Test

Plasma osmolality is determined to assess the person's fluid status and identify ADH abnormalities.

Procedure

Venipuncture is performed to obtain 7 ml of blood in a heparinized green-topped tube. Osmolality is measured by the freezing point depression of solution using an osmometer or cryoscope or by the vapor pressure or dew point osmometer.

Findings

Increase	Decrease
Alcoholism	Addison disease
Aldosteronism	Fluid overload
Dehydration	Liver failure with ascites
Diabetes insipidus (DI)	Syndrome of inappropriate anti-
High-protein diets	diuretic hormone (SIADH)
Hypercalcemia	
Hyperglycemia	
Hypernatremia	
Hyperkalemia	

Interfering Factors

- Hemolysis of specimen
- Medications
  Diuretics
  Mineralocorticoids

Nursing Implementation

The nursing actions are similar to those of other venipuncture procedures.

OSMOLALITY, URINE

(URINE)

Synonyms:

NORMAL VALUES

With normal diet and fluid intake:
500–800 mOsm/kg H_2O or SI 500–800 mmol/kg
Range: 50–1400 mOsm/kg H_2O or SI 50–1400 mmol/kg

Background Information

Osmolality is a measure of the number of particles that are dissolved in a solution. Thus, urine osmolality varies based on the person's fluid status and the metabolic waste products being excreted. If the patient is overhydrated, the urinary osmolality decreases as output increases. If the person is dehydrated, the urine osmolality increases as the output decreases. Urine osmolality is based on the concentration ability of the kidneys and the serum levels of sodium, chloride, bicarbonate, proteins, glucose, and urea.

Purpose of the Test

Urine osmolality is determined to assess the ability of the kidneys to concentrate or dilute urine and to identify ADH abnormalities.

Procedure

Ten ml of urine is collected in a sterile container and is sent to the laboratory.

Findings

Increase	Decrease
Addison disease	Aldosteronism
Azotemia	DI
Cirrhosis of the liver	Glomerulonephritis
Dehydration	Hypocalcemia
Diabetes mellitus	Hyponatremia
Diarrhea	Overhydration
Hyperglycemia	Sickle cell anemia
Hypernatremia	
SIADH	

Interfering Factors

- Noncompliance with the nothing-by-mouth status
- Glucosuria
- Recent scans requiring radiopaque dyes
- Medications
    Antibiotics
    Diuretics
    Volume expanders

Nursing Implementation

Pretest

Instruct the patient not to eat or drink overnight before the urine is collected.

During the Test

Obtain 10 ml of urine in a sterile container.

Posttest

Send to the laboratory immediately.

PARATHYROID HORMONE

(SERUM)

Synonyms:
parathormone, PTH

NORMAL VALUES

(Interpreted in relation to serum calcium levels)
Intact parathyroid hormone: 210–310 pg/ml *or* SI 210–310 ng/L
N-terminal fraction: 230–630 pg/ml *or* SI 230–630 ng/L
C-terminal fraction: 410–1760 pg/ml *or* SI 410–1760 ng/L

Background Information

Parathyroid hormone is produced and secreted by the parathyroid glands. Its role in the body is the regulation of calcium. Its secretion is based on a negative feedback mechanism with calcium (Fig. 19–3).

Parathyroid hormone affects calcium levels by stimulating osteoclast activity in the bone and inhibiting osteoblast activity. This causes bone reabsorption, which shifts calcium and phosphate out of the bone into the blood. Parathyroid hormone also causes increased reabsorption of calcium at the kidney's distal tubules and decreased reabsorption of phosphate at the proximal tubules. The result of parathyroid hormone's activity is an increase in calcium in the blood with a decrease in plasma phosphate levels.

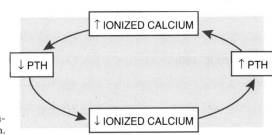

FIGURE 19–3. Regulation of parathyroid hormone (PTH) secretion.

Purpose of the Test

A parathyroid hormone determination is performed to diagnose suspected parathyroid disorders. It may be performed to differentiate between clinical diagnoses that result in calcium and phosphate abnormalities.

Procedure

Parathyroid hormone is measured by RIA, which can measure biologically active intact parathyroid hormone. This fraction represents only a small portion of the total parathyroid hormone. Alternatively, RIA can measure C-terminal or N-terminal portions of the hormone. Two venous samples, 3 ml each in red-topped tubes, are needed.

Findings

Increase	Decrease
Hyperparathyroidism	Hypoparathyroidism
	Lung, kidney, pancreatic, or ovarian cancer

Interfering Factors

- Noncompliance with fasting requirements
- Elevated lipid levels

Nursing Implementation

The actions of the nurse are similar to those carried out in other venipuncture procedures.

Pretest

Instruct the patient not to eat or drink for 12 hours before the test.

Posttest

The patient may resume a normal diet.

RENIN, PLASMA

(PLASMA)

Synonym:
plasma renin activity, PRA

NORMAL VALUES

Recumbent Position:	12–79 mU/L *or* SI 12–79 mU/L
Upright Position:	13–114 mU/L *or* SI 13–114 mU/L

Background Information

Renin is a proteolytic enzyme produced and secreted by the juxtaglomerular cells of the kidneys. Renin is secreted whenever there is a reduction of blood pressure to the kidneys. Renin in the circulation acts on angiotensinogen to form angiotensin I, which is converted to angiotensin II—a powerful vasoconstrictor and stimulant for aldosterone secretion. This action is called the renin-angiotensin-aldosterone system or axis (see Fig. 19–2).

Because renin is a powerful vasoconstrictor, its role in hypertension has been studied. Most patients with hypertension have normal renin levels. Some hypertensive patients with excessive fluid retention have low renin levels, and other hypertensive patients have high renin levels.

It has been difficult to correlate renin levels with clinical states, as renin levels vary between individuals and because laboratory techniques vary in the measurement of these levels. In addition, many factors will influence secretion rates of renin, including dietary ingestion of sodium. For this reason, some clinicians will correlate renin levels with the sodium content of the patient's diet. The sodium content of the diet is measured by a 24-hour urine sodium level.

Another method to evaluate renin is to perform a *sodium-depleted renin test*, during which a diuretic (usually furosemide) is given.

Purpose of the Test

Plasma renin levels are determined as part of hypertension screening and to diagnose primary aldosteronism.

Procedure

Procedures vary. A random renin test simply requires a venipuncture to obtain 10 ml of blood in a lavender-topped tube containing EDTA. The specimen is placed on ice and immediately sent to the laboratory. If the renin level is to be correlated with sodium intake, a 24-hour urine specimen is required.

If a renin determination from a renal vein is planned, it is carried out under fluoroscopy; a catheter is inserted into the renal vein via the femoral vein. The specimen is assayed by RIA.

Findings

Increase	Decrease
Hypertension	Fluid retention with high-sodium diet
Cirrhosis	Primary aldosteronism
Hypovolemia	Excessive licorice intake
Hypokalemia	Hypertension with fluid retention
Addison disease	Cushing syndrome
Chronic renal failure	

Interfering Factors

- Noncompliance with dietary and medication restrictions
- Improper positioning during test
- Medications
    - Antihypertensives
    - Clonidine
    - Diuretics
    - Estrogen
    - Minoxidil
    - Nitroprusside
    - Propranolol
    - Reserpine
    - Vasodilators

Nursing Implementation

The actions of the nurse vary depending on the technique used.

Pretest

Critical Thinking: A random renin level is ordered for a young child. The physician orders it done after the patient has been in the upright position for 2 hours. How can a busy nurse ensure this positioning?

Instruct the patient on the technique

If a random sampling is ordered, instruct the patient to maintain a prone position or an upright position for 2 hours before the test. The position is based on physician preference.

If a renal vein level is ordered, explain the need to go to the radiology department for fluoroscopy. Explain equipment, groin preparation, and local anesthesia.

If a sodium depletion renin test is ordered, assess the patient's cardiovascular status before a diuretic is given. Instruct the patient to maintain a low-sodium diet for 3 days before the test.

Check with the prescriber regarding withholding interfering medications, for example, hypertensives, vasodilators, diuretics, or oral contraceptives, before the test.

TABLE 19–4
COMPLICATIONS OF ADRENAL VEIN RENIN LEVELS

Complication	Nursing Assessment
Bleeding	Observe puncture site and under patient for blood
	Restlessness
	Tachycardia
	Decreased urinary output
	Hypotension
Hematoma	Observe site for swelling
	Check distal pulses
	Check extremity for color and temperature

Posttest

If the femoral approach to the renal vein is used, assess the site for hematoma and bleeding.

Complications

The only complications expected with renin evaluation are those associated with femoral vein access: bleeding and hematoma formation (Table 19–4).

RESIN TRIIODOTHYRONINE UPTAKE

(SERUM)

Synonyms:

T_3 resin uptake test, RT_3U, T_3 uptake ratio

NORMAL VALUES	
	25–35% *or* SI 0.25–0.35
Free thyroxine index	1.3–4.2
Free triiodothyronine index	24–67

Background Information

The triiodothyronine resin uptake is determined to estimate the *free triiodothyronine index* and the *free thyroxine index* (see pp. 622–624 for discussion of free triiodothyronine and free thyroxine). In many institutions, the assay of free thyroid hormones have replaced the free triiodothyronine and thyroxine index because the indexes are estimates of the free hormone levels.

The resin triiodothyronine uptake assesses the capacity of the blood proteins to bind with thyroid hormones. It does not measure the hormones themselves.

Purpose of the Test

The triiodothyronine resin uptake test is performed to diagnose hyper- and hypothyroidism.

Procedure

Venipuncture is performed to obtain a serum specimen to which radioactive triiodothyronine is added. Radioactive triiodothyronine is used instead of thyroxine because more triiodothyronine is bound to the resin, as it has a lower affinity to endogenous protein-binding sites. After the resin is mixed with the radioactive triiodothyronine in serum, it is removed and the amount of radioactivity absorbed is measured.

The measurement of the free thyroxine and free triiodothyronine index is obtained by multiplying the resin uptake and the total thyroid hormone concentration. The indexes are not direct measurements of the free thyroid hormones, but estimates. However, the indexes do correlate with true free thyroid levels.

Findings

Increase	Decrease
Hyperthyroidism	Hypothyroidism

Interfering Factors

- Renal failure
- Malnutrition
- Metastatic disease
- Liver dysfunction
- Critical illness
- Medications
  ACTH
  Androgens
  Barbiturates
  Chlorpromazine
  Estrogen
  Furosemide
  Glucocorticoids
  Heroin
  Lithium
  Methadone
  Phenylbutazone

Propylthiouracil
Thyroid replacement

Nursing Implementation

The nurse takes actions similar to those taken in other venipuncture procedures.

17-HYDROXYCORTICOSTEROIDS

(URINE)

Synonym:

17-OHCS

--- **NORMAL VALUES** ---

Adult Male:	4.5–12 mg/24 hours *or* SI 12.4–33.1 µmol/24 hours
Adult Female:	2.5–10 mg/24 hours *or* SI 6.9–27.6 µmol/24 hours
Children:	
8–12 Years:	<4.5 mg/24 hours *or* SI <12.4 µmol/24 hours
<8 Years:	<1.5 mg/24 hours *or* SI <4.14 µmol/24 hours

Background Information

17-OHCS are urinary steroids (cortisol and cortisone metabolites) used to assess adrenal function. An increase in 17-OHCS in the urine reflects an increase in plasma cortisol. With the direct measurement of plasma cortisol and free cortisol, the frequency of 17-OHCS determinations has significantly decreased.

When assessing 17-OHCS values, it is necessary to consider the patient's body type. Obese or muscular individuals will have higher 17-OHCS levels than will those with normal body types because of an increase in cortisol metabolism. To adjust to body type, some clinicians correlate the 17-OHCS to the creatinine clearance (norm: 2 to 6.5 mg/g of urinary creatinine).

Purpose of the Test

17-OHCS levels are obtained to assess adrenal function.

Procedure

A 24-hour urine specimen is obtained. The urine is assessed by colorimetric reaction.

Findings

	Increase	Decrease
	Adrenal cancer	Addison disease
	Cushing syndrome	Hypothyroidism
	Extreme stress	Starvation
	Hyperthyroidism	Liver failure
	Pituitary tumor	Renal failure
		Pregnancy

Interfering Factors

- Failure to collect all the urine during the 24-hour collection period
- Failure to keep specimen on ice or refrigerated
- Medications
    Chloral hydrate
    Chlorpromazine
    Colchicine
    Erythromycin
    Estrogens
    Oral contraceptives
    Paraldehyde
    Quinidine
    Quinine
    Reserpine
    Spironolactone

Nursing Implementation

Pretest

Take the patient's medication history to assess for interfering factors.

Explain collection procedure to the patient, especially the need to collect *all* the urine for 24 hours.

Instruct the patient to avoid excessive physical activity during the testing period.

Critical Thinking: After collecting a 24-hour urine specimen for a 17-OHCS, the nurse tells the aide to bring it to the laboratory. Two hours later, the nurse finds the specimen on the radiator in the patient's room. What should the nurse do? How can this be prevented in the future?

During the Test

At the start of the test, instruct the patient to void at 8 A.M. and discard this urine. The collection period begins at this time and all the urine is collected for 24 hours, including the 8 A.M. specimen of the following morning.

On the requisition slip and specimen label, write the patient's name and the time and date of the start and finish of the test period.

Keep the urine and collection container refrigerated or on ice during the collection period.

Posttest

Arrange for prompt transport of the cooled specimen to the laboratory.

17-KETOGENIC STEROIDS

(URINE)

Synonym:

17-KGS

NORMAL VALUES

Adult Male:	4–14 mg/24 hours *or* SI 13–49 µmol/24 hours
Adult Female:	2–12 mg/24 hours *or* SI 7–42 µmol/24 hours
Children:	
11–14 Years:	2–9 mg/24 hours *or* SI 7–31 µmol/24 hours
<11 Years:	0.1–4 mg/24 hours *or* SI 0.3–14 µmol/24 hours

Background Information

17-Ketogenic steroids (17-KGS) include the metabolites of cortisol and other steroids. 17-KGS determination is not performed often because direct measurement of plasma cortisol and free cortisol has become more common.

Purpose of the Test

Determination of 17-KGS levels is performed to assess adrenal function and support the diagnosis of Cushing syndrome or Addison disease.

Procedure

A 24-hour urine specimen is collected. The urine is assessed colorimetrically.

Findings

Increase	**Decrease**
Adrenal cancer	Addison disease
Adenoma	Cretinism
Adrenogenital syndrome	Hypopituitarism
Cushing syndrome	
Extreme stress	

Interfering Factors

- Failure to collect all the urine during the 24-hour collection period
- Failure to keep specimen cool during the collection period
- Physical exercise
- Physical or emotional stress, or both
- Medications
  Estrogens
  Hydralazine
  Penicillin
  Phenothiazines
  Quinine
  Reserpine
  Steroids
  Thiazides

Nursing Implementation

Pretest

Critical Thinking: A 17-KGS is ordered for an outpatient. Develop a teaching plan to ensure a proper collection of the specimen. What nursing assessment would indicate the patient's inability to perform this function?

Take the patient's medication history to assess for interfering factors.

Explain to the patient the need to collect *all* the urine for 24 hours.

Instruct the patient to avoid excessive physical activity during the collection period.

During the Test

At the start of the test, instruct the patient to void at 8 A.M. and discard this urine. The collection period begins at this time and all the urine is collected for 24 hours, including the 8 A.M. specimen of the following morning.

On the requisition slip and specimen label, write the patient's name and the time and date of the start and finish of the test period.

Keep the urine and collection container refrigerated or on ice throughout the test period.

Arrange for prompt transport of the cooled specimen to the laboratory.

17-KETOSTEROIDS, URINARY

(URINE)

Synonym:
17-KS

Background Information

Urinary 17-ketosteroids measure the metabolites of androgens. Determination of 17-ketosteroids is rarely carried out because (1) plasma levels of the

---
NORMAL VALUES

Adult Male:	10–25 mg/24 hours *or* SI 35–87 μmol/24 hours
Adult Female:	6–14 mg/24 hours *or* SI 21–49 μmol/24 hours
Children:	
10–14 Years:	1–6 mg/24 hours *or* SI 2–21 μmol/24 hours
<10 Years:	<3 mg/24 hours *or* SI <10 μmol/24 hours

androgens are available, (2) it requires a 24-hour urine specimen, and (3) multiple drugs interfere with an accurate measurement.

Purpose of the Test

Determination of 17-ketosteroids is performed to assess adrenal and gonadal function.

Procedure

A 24-hour urine specimen is collected and assessed by colorimetric analysis.

Findings

Increase	**Decrease**
Adrenal carcinoma	Addison disease
Adenoma	Cretinism
Cushing syndrome	Hypopituitarism
Extreme stress	

Interfering Factors

- Failure to collect all the urine in the 24-hour period
- Failure to keep urine on ice or refrigerated during collection period
- Hematuria
- Contrast dyes
- Increased exercise
- Stress
- Medications
    ACTH
    Estrogens
    Glucocorticoids
    Hydralazine
    Morphine

Oral contraceptives
Penicillin
Phenothiazines
Quinine
Reserpine
Thiazides

Nursing Implementation

Pretest

Instruct the patient to avoid excessive physical activity and stressful situations.

Take a medication history to determine if interfering drugs are being taken.

Explain to the patient the need to obtain *all* the urine during the collection time.

During the Test

At the start of the test, instruct the patient to void at 8 A.M. and discard this urine. The collection period starts at this time and all urine is collected for 24 hours, including the 8 A.M. specimen of the following morning.

On the requisition slip and specimen label, write the patient's name and the time and date of the start and finish of the collection period.

Keep the urine and collection container refrigerated or on ice throughout the collection period.

Posttest

Arrange for prompt transport of the cooled specimen to the laboratory.

THYROGLOBULIN AUTOANTIBODIES

(SERUM)

Synonym:

antithyroid antibodies

NORMAL VALUES

Titer less than 1:100 by immunofluorescence; negative by hemagglutination method

Background Information

Some thyroid disorders may be autoimmune in origin. To evaluate this potential cause, antithyroid antibodies are measured. One of these antibodies is thyroglobulin autoantibody. The thyroglobulin antibodies act on the antigen thyroglobulin, the storage form of thyroid hormones. Although the presence of these antibodies helps confirm the diagnosis of autoimmune disease, their absence does not rule out the potential diagnosis.

Purpose of the Test

Thyroglobulin antibodies are evaluated to detect autoimmune-based thyroid disease.

Procedure

Venipuncture is performed to obtain 7 ml of blood in a red-topped tube. The specimen is assessed by immunofluorescence or hemagglutination technique.

Findings

Increase

Graves disease
Hashimoto thyroiditis
Hyperthyroidism
Hypothyroidism
Nontoxic nodular goiter
Pernicious anemia
Rheumatoid arthritis
Systemic lupus erythematosus
Thyroid cancer

Interfering Factor

- Oral contraceptives

Nursing Implementation

The nursing actions are similar to those of other venipuncture techniques.

THYROID MICROSOMAL AUTOANTIBODIES

(SERUM)

Synonym:
antithyroid antibodies

─────────────────── **NORMAL VALUES** ───────────────────

> Titer less than 1:100 by immunofluorescence method; negative by hemagglutination method

Background Information

Antithyroid antibodies are present in autoimmune diseases of the thyroid gland. Thyroid microsomal antibodies act against the lipoprotein microsomal antigen found in the thyroid gland. Evaluation of the antibody formation provides help in diagnosing autoimmune-based disorders of the thyroid gland. Although the presence of the antibody helps confirm the cause of the disorder, its absence does not usually rule out the potential cause.

Purpose, Procedure, Findings, and Nursing Implementation

The purpose of the thyroid microsomal autoantibody test, the procedure, the findings, and the nursing implementation are as for the thyroglobulin autoantibodies.

THYROTROPIN

(SERUM)

Synonyms:

thyroid-stimulating hormone, TSH

─────────────────── **NORMAL VALUES** ───────────────────

Adult:	0.4–8.9 U/ml *or* SI 0.4–8.9 mU/L
Newborn, Whole Blood:	<20 U/ml *or* SI <20 mU/L

Background Information

Thyrotropin is secreted by the anterior pituitary gland via a negative feedback mechanism (see Fig. 19–4). Thyrotropin causes the thyroid gland to increase its production and secretion of thyroid hormones.

Because of thyrotropin's regulatory mechanism with the thyroid hormones, its level will be affected by primary thyroid abnormalities. If the patient has hyperthyroidism, thyrotropin will be suppressed. If the patient has primary hypothyroidism, thyrotropin secretion will become markedly elevated. This elevation may create a compensatory euthyroid state. Exogenous thyroid hormones will also suppress thyrotropin secretion.

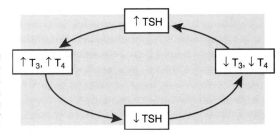

FIGURE 19–4. Thyroid hormone regulation. Thyroid hormone production and secretion is based on a negative feedback mechanism with thyroid-stimulating hormone (TSH) secreted by the anterior pituitary gland.

Purpose of the Test

Thyrotropin levels are obtained to (1) diagnose hypothyroidism, (2) distinguish between primary and secondary hypothyroidism, and (3) monitor patient response to thyroid replacement therapy.

Procedure

Venipuncture is performed to obtain 7 ml of blood in a red-topped tube. If the test is required on a newborn, a heelstick is performed and the blood is collected on filter paper.

Findings

Increase	Decrease
Addison disease	Hyperthyroidism
Goiter (some forms)	Overdose of exogenous thyroid replacement
Hyperpituitarism	Secondary hypothyroidism
Pituitary adenoma	Tertiary hypothyroidism
Primary hypothyroidism	Thyroiditis
Thyroid cancer	

Interfering Factors

- Radioisotope administration within 1 week
- Extreme stress
- Medications
    - Aspirin
    - Corticosteroids
    - Dopamine
    - Heparin
    - Lithium
    - Potassium iodide
    - Thyroid replacement therapy

Nursing Implementation

Nursing actions resemble those of other venipuncture procedures.

Pretest

Assess for and report any clinical states that would increase the patient's endogenous glucocorticoid levels.

Check with prescriber regarding withholding medications that may interfere with test results.

THYROTROPIN-RELEASING HORMONE TEST

(SERUM)

Synonyms:

TRH test, TSH-releasing hormone, TSH stimulation test

─────────────── **NORMAL VALUES** ───────────────

After TRH is given, TSH increases:
Males: 14–24 µU/ml *or* SI 14–24 mU/L
Females: 16–26 µU/ml *or* SI 16–26 mU/L

Background Information

Thyrotropin-releasing hormone (TRH) is produced and secreted by the hypothalamus. It acts as moderator of the thyroid hormone–thyrotropin negative feedback mechanism. In response to synthetic TRH being given intravenously, the anterior pituitary gland will normally increase its secretion of thyrotropin within 5 minutes. The thyrotropin levels peak in 20 to 30 minutes and will return to baseline within 2 to 4 hours (Howanitz, 1991).

Purpose of the Test

TRH determinations are rarely performed today because the thyrotropin (TSH) test is usually adequate to support the diagnoses. TRH testing is performed when clinical manifestations of thyroid dysfunction are evident, but other tests are not clear.

Procedure

TRH determinations may be performed in a number of ways with the dose and route of the TRH varying. The most common method is the bolus intravenous administration of 200 to 500 μg of synthetic TRH after blood is drawn for a baseline thyrotropin level. After 30 minutes (and sometimes again after 60 minutes), when the thyrotropin response is normally peaking, a second specimen is drawn for a thyrotropin determination.

Findings

Increase	Decrease
Normal response	Cushing syndrome
Hypothyroidism	Depression
	Hyperthyroidism
	Multinodular goiter
	Pituitary lesions
	Renal failure

Interfering Factors

- Corticosteroids
- Levodopa
- Salicylates (high-dose)

Nursing Implementation

The nursing implementation for this test is similar to those for thyrotropin testing (see pp. 666–668).

Pretest

Explain to the patient the need for multiple venipuncture procedures.

THYROXINE, SERUM

(SERUM)

Synonym:

T_4

NORMAL VALUES	
Adult:	5–12 μg/dl *or* SI 64.4–154.4 nmol/L
Children:	
10–20 Years:	4.2–11.8 μg/dl *or* SI 54.1–151.9 nmol/L
1–10 Years:	6.4–15 μg/dl *or* SI 82.4–193.1 nmol/L
2–10 Months:	7.8–16.5 μg/dl *or* SI 100.4–212.4 nmol/L
Newborn:	6.4–23.2 μg/dl *or* SI 82.4–298.6 nmol/L

Background Information

The thyroid gland produces and secretes the hormones thyroxine and triiodothyronine. This gland takes up iodide from the extracellular fluid and uses the iodide to produce thyroglobulin, the precursor of all thyroid hormones. The thyroglobulin is stored in the thyroid gland until thyroxine and triiodothyronine are processed before secretion from the gland. Secretion of triiodothyronine and thyroxine is primarily regulated by a negative feedback mechanism with thyrotropin. Thyrotropin is secreted by the anterior pituitary gland (Fig. 19–4).

Once secreted by the thyroid gland, triiodothyronine and thyroxine are bound primarily to thyroid-binding globulin and to a lesser degree to albumin and prealbumin. The small amount of the hormones not bound to protein is called free thyroxine and free triiodothyronine. It is the free hormones that are biologically active. The bound hormones are released from the protein as the hormones are needed. In the peripheral circulation, thyroxine will lose one of its iodide molecules and become triiodothyronine, the more potent of the thyroid hormones.

Because the majority of the thyroid hormones are bound to protein, the evaluation of thyroid hormone levels should include the person's protein levels. If the patient has decreased proteins to carry the hormone, a greater amount of the hormone will be in the free state or active form. RIA measures both bound and unbound thyroxine.

When needed, thyroxine converts to triiodothyronine to bind with its target cells. Its action is to increase the basal metabolic rate; therefore, its effect is widespread. By increasing the basal metabolic rate, thyroid hormones increase oxygen consumption and produces heat. Triiodothyronine and thyroxine are needed for conversion of carotene to vitamin A in the liver, are essential for normal growth and development, stimulate secretion of growth hormone, and increase the affinity of beta-adrenergic receptors to catecholamines.

Purpose of the Test

Thyroxine levels are obtained to evaluate thyroid function, confirm the diagnosis of hyper- or hypothyroidism, and evaluate therapy for hyper- or hypothyroidism.

Procedure

Venipuncture is performed to obtain 5 ml of blood in a red-topped tube. RIA is used to assess the hormone level.

If a thyroxine determination is ordered on a newborn, umbilical cord blood may be used *or* a heelstick can be performed. With the heelstick method, special filter paper is used to blot the blood, and the filter paper is sent to the laboratory in a container that protects against light.

Findings

Increase	**Decrease**
Hyperthyroidism	Hypothyroidism

Interfering Factors

- Liver disorders, which affect blood protein levels
- Protein-wasting diseases such as chronic renal failure
- Medications
    Androgens
    Aspirin
    Chlorpropamide
    Chlorpromazine
    Estrogen
    Heparin
    Iodides
    Thyroid replacement medications
    Lithium
    Methadone
    Phenothiazines
    Phenytoin
    Reserpine
    Steroids
    Sulfonamides
    Sulfonylureas
    Tolbutamide

Critical Thinking: After a heelstick is performed on an infant to obtain a thyroxine level, the mother begins to sob uncontrollably. How can the nurse best help the mother? What nursing diagnosis should be validated by nursing assessments?

Nursing Implementation

Nursing actions are similar to those used in other venipuncture procedures.

During the Test

If a heelstick is performed, the heel is first cleansed with antiseptic and the skin is pierced with a sterile lancet. Completely saturate the circles on the filter paper.

Since pregnancy will normally cause an increase in thyroxine levels, indicate on the requisition slip if the patient is pregnant.

Posttest

Send filter paper to the laboratory in a container that protects against light.

THYROXINE-BINDING GLOBULIN

(SERUM)

Synonym:

TBG

────────────── **NORMAL VALUES** ──────────────

16–34 µg/ml *or* SI 16–34 mg/L

Background Information

Thyroxine-binding globulin (TBG) is the primary protein carrier of thyroxine and triiodothyronine. The thyroid hormones bound to TBG provide a store house of the hormones, which are released from the protein as needed. Since TBG carries approximately 70% of the total amount of thyroid hormones in the circulation, TBG levels significantly affect total hormone concentrations. In addition to increased or decreased levels of TBG affecting hormone levels, there may be factors that affect the binding capacity of triiodothyronine and thyroxine to TBG. These factors may interfere with test results (see further on).

Purpose of the Test

TBG is evaluated when clinical manifestations of thyroid dysfunction and thyroid hormone levels do not correlate.

Procedure

Venipuncture is performed to collect 7 ml of blood in a red-topped tube. TBG levels are assessed by RIA or electrophoresis.

Findings

Increase	Decrease
Congenital abnormality	Androgens
Estrogen therapy	Cirrhosis of the liver
Hepatitis, acute	Congenital abnormality
Hypothyroidism	Glucocorticoids
Pregnancy	Hyperthyroidism
	Recent surgery
	Renal failure
	Starvation

Interfering Factors

- Heparin
- Phenylbutazone
- Phenytoin
- Salicylates

Nursing Implementation

The nurse takes actions similar to those taken in other venipuncture procedures.

Pretest

Obtain a medication history to determine if any drug is being taken that affects normal thyroid binding.

TOLBUTAMIDE STIMULATION TEST

(SERUM)

Synonyms:

━━━━━━━━━━━━━━━━━━━━━━━━━━ **NORMAL VALUES** ━━━━━━━━━━━━

Serum Insulin Level:	<195 µU/ml *or* SI 1354 pmol/L

Background Information

Tolbutamide (Orinase) is an oral hypoglycemic agent. Its duration of action is short, being rapidly inactivated by the liver. For this reason, tolbutamide is used in stimulation tests to evaluate exaggerated and prolonged insulin secretion. This condition may occur with insulinoma, which is an insulin-secreting tumor of the pancreatic islets of Langerhans. It presents with spontaneous fasting hypoglycemia.

The goal in giving tolbutamide is to create a hypoglycemic state and see the insulin response to the induced hypoglycemia. If the insulin secretion stays at high levels and is prolonged, the test result is positive.

Purpose of the Test

The tolbutamide stimulation test is performed to identify insulin-producing tumors of the pancreas.

Procedure

The tolbutamide stimulation test is performed by administering 1 g of tolbutamide intravenously over a 2-minute period. Serum insulin levels are obtained every 5 minutes for 15 minutes.

Findings

If the insulin level is maintained or prolonged, the test confirms the diagnosis of insulinoma.

Interfering Factors

- Liver disorders
- Renal failure
- Medications
    Chloramphenicol
    Dicumarol
    MAO inhibitors
    Phenylbutazone
    Salicylates
    Sulfonamides

Nursing Implementation

See section on serum insulin, pp. 640–642.

Pretest

Explain to the patient the need for several venipuncture procedures.

During the Test

Observe the patient for a reaction to tolbutamide, which is most commonly a skin rash.

Posttest

Observe the patient for prolonged hypoglycemia, especially in elderly individuals.

Complications

Prolonged hypoglycemia may occur with the administration of tolbutamide (Table 19–5).

TABLE 19–5
COMPLICATIONS OF TOLBUTAMIDE STIMULATION TEST

Complication	Nursing Assessment
Hypoglycemia	Anxiety
	Diaphoresis
	Hunger
	Palpitations
	Tachycardia
	Tremulousness
	Vagueness
	Ataxia
	Convulsions
	Coma

TRIIODOTHYRONINE

(SERUM)

Synonym:

T_3

NORMAL VALUES

Adult:	40–204 ng/dl *or* SI 0.6–3.1 nmol/L
Children:	
10–20 Years:	80–213 ng/dl *or* SI 1.2–3.3 nmol/L
1–10 Years:	105–269 ng/dl *or* SI 1.6–4.1 nmol/L
1–12 Months:	105–245 ng/dl *or* SI 1.6–3.7 nmol/L
Newborn:	100–740 ng/dl *or* SI 1.5–11.4 nmol/L

Background Information

See the discussion of thyroxine (pp. 669–671).

Purpose of the Test

Triiodothyronine levels are obtained as part of the diagnostic process to determine hyper- or hypothyroidism and to diagnose triiodothyronine toxicosis.

Procedure

Venipuncture is performed to obtain 3 ml of blood in a red-topped tube.

Findings

Increase	Decrease
Hyperthyroidism	Hypothyroidism
Pregnancy	Liver disease
Toxic adenoma of the thyroid gland	Recent surgery
Toxic nodular goiter	Renal disease

Interfering Factors

- Significant increase or decrease in thyroxine-binding globulins
- Medications
  - Estrogen
  - Heparin
  - Iodides
  - Triiodothyronine replacement therapy
  - Lithium
  - Methadone
  - Methimazole
  - Methylthiouracil
  - Phenylbutazone
  - Phenytoin
  - Progestins
  - Propranolol
  - Propylthiouracil
  - Reserpine
  - Salicylates
  - Steroids
  - Sulfonamides

Nursing Implementation

Nursing actions are similar to those for other venipuncture procedures.

VASOPRESSIN, PLASMA

(SERUM)

Synonyms:

ADH, antidiuretic hormone

NORMAL VALUES

If serum osmolality >290 mOsm/kg: 2–12 pg/ml *or* SI 1.85–11.1 pmol/L
If serum osmolality <290 mOsm/kg: <2 pg/ml *or* SI <1.85 pmol/L

Background Information

Vasopressin (ADH) is produced by the hypothalamus and stored in the posterior pituitary gland. Its major function in the body is to act on the cells in the collecting ducts of the kidney, making them more permeable to water. The result is an increased reabsorption of water. This action is independent of electrolyte levels, and electrolytes are *not* reabsorbed with the water. The purpose of this action is to maintain normal plasma osmolality. ADH also has a vasopressor effect. It causes arteriole smooth muscles to constrict, thus elevating the blood pressure.

ADH is released from the posterior pituitary gland in response to several stimuli. The major stimulus is an increase in plasma osmolality. Whenever the osmoreceptors in the anterior hypothalamus sense even minor changes in plasma osmolality, neural stimulation of the pituitary gland will result in an increased secretion of ADH, which will result in an increased reabsorption of water at the renal collecting ducts. With the increase in water in the extracellular fluid, blood tonicity will decrease and urine osmolality will increase. As the increase in water results in decreased blood osmolality, the osmoreceptors will cease the neural stimulation necessary for ADH secretion (Fig. 19–5).

Another stimulant for ADH release is the extracellular fluid volume. A drop in blood volume is sensed by stretcher receptors primarily in the vena cava and right atrium. By way of the brain stem, these receptors tell the hypothalamus to stimulate the release of ADH from the posterior pituitary gland. The resultant increase in fluid volume from water retention results in a decrease in stretcher receptor stimulation. In addition, as arterial blood pressure drops, pressor receptors found in the aorta and coronary sinuses will stimulate the release of ADH to increase extracellular fluid volume and thus the person's blood pressure.

ADH secretion may be increased by drugs (e.g., nicotine, opiates, barbiturates, chlorpropamide) and severe pain, stress, and hyperthermia. Decreased sensitivity of the kidneys to ADH occurs with the intake of lithium carbonate and demeclocycline.

FIGURE 19–5. Vasopressin (ADH) regulation. ADH is secreted by the posterior pituitary gland primarily in response to an increase in plasma osmolality.

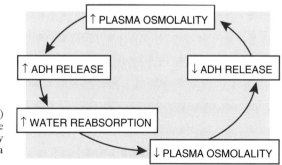

Purpose of the Test

A serum ADH determination is obtained to diagnose DI and SIADH.

Procedure

Venipuncture is performed to obtain 5 ml of blood in a red-topped tube.

Findings

Increase	Decrease
SIADH	DI

Interfering Factors

- Noncompliance with diet, activity, and medication restrictions
- Pain
- Stress
- Mechanical ventilation
- Alcohol
- Medications
  Anesthetics
  Carbamazepine
  Chlorothiazide
  Cyclophosphamide
  Estrogen
  Oxytocin
  Vincristine

Nursing Implementation

Pretest

Instruct the patient not to eat or drink for 12 hours before the test.
Instruct the patient not to drink alcohol for 24 hours before the test.
Instruct the patient to limit physical activity for 12 hours before the test. The patient should lie down and rest for 30 minutes before the blood is drawn.
Obtain a medication history to determine if any interfering drugs are being taken. Check with the prescriber to determine if these drugs are to be withheld or continued.
Assess the patient for pain and stress, which may interfere with results.

During the Test

Venipuncture is performed.

Posttest

Instruct the patient to resume normal activity and diet. Administer prescribed medications that were withheld for the test.

VITAMIN D, ACTIVATED

(SERUM OR PLASMA)

Synonym:
1,25-dihydroxycholecalciferol

―――――――――――――― **NORMAL VALUES** ――――――

25–45 pg/ml *or* SI 60–108 nmo/L

Background Information

Activated vitamin D is produced from vitamin D by the liver and kidneys. Vitamin D is derived from the action of ultraviolet light on a group of provitamins in the skin. Vitamin D is also derived from vitamin D–enriched foods. The vitamin D is first converted in the liver to 25,hydroxycholecalciferol and then to 1,25-dehydroxycholecalciferol in the kidney. Activated vitamin D elevates plasma calcium and phosphate levels by increasing intestinal absorption of calcium and phosphate and increasing the release of calcium from bone into blood.

Purpose of the Test

Activated vitamin D levels are assessed to evaluate causes of hypocalcemia. It is usually obtained with parathyroid hormone levels.

Procedure

A fasting venous specimen is needed. If a serum level is ordered, 5 ml of blood is collected in a red-topped tube. If a plasma level is desired, 5 ml of blood is collected in a green-topped tube.

Findings

Increase	Decrease
Hyperparathyroidism	Anticonvulsants
Overdose of vitamin D	Hepatic failure

Sarcoidosis	Hypoparathyroidism
	Isoniazid
	Malabsorption syndrome
	Osteomalacia
	Pseudohypoparathyroidism
	Renal failure

Interfering Factors

- Phosphorus deficiency
- Prolonged lack of exposure to sunlight

Nursing Implementation

The nurse performs actions similar to those in other venipuncture procedures.

Pretest

Instruct the patient not to eat or drink for 8 hours before the test.

WATER DEPRIVATION TEST

(URINE)

Synonyms:

dehydration test, concentration test

--- **NORMAL VALUES** ---

Specific Gravity:	1.025–1.032
Osmolality:	>800 mOsm/kg *or* SI >800 mmol/kg

Background Information

Normally, as fluid intake is withheld, blood osmolality increases and urine output decreases, whereas urinary osmolality increases. The increase in serum osmolality causes an increase in ADH secretion. In patients with DI, there is not a normal response to increased plasma osmolality; instead little or no increase in ADH occurs, resulting in little or no change in urinary output or osmolality.

DI may be caused by a defect in production, release, or utilization of ADH. If DI is due to a problem in production (hypothalamic) or release (pituitary) of ADH, it is called neurogenic or central DI. If DI is caused by a failure of the kidney to respond to ADH, it is called nephrogenic DI. The water deprivation test supports the diagnosis of DI.

As part of the water deprivation test, a *vasopressin stimulation test* or *vasopressin test* may be performed to distinguish between neurogenic and nephrogenic DI. This distinction is important in determining appropriate treatment plans.

Purpose of the Test

The water deprivation test is performed to diagnose DI and to assess the kidney's ability to concentrate urine based on extracellular fluid load.

Procedure

During the test, the patient is deprived of fluid intake, and periodic urine specimens are obtained for osmolality and specific gravity determinations. The urine is collected in separate clean containers and placed on ice or refrigerated. Strict urinary output measurements are maintained.

If a vasopressin stimulation test is included, hypertonic saline or nicotine is given to stimulate ADH release. If complete neurogenic DI is present, no change is noted on urinary output or osmolality. If partial neurogenic DI is present, only minor changes occur. If desired, a vasopressin test may be performed. After vasopressin is given, no change will occur in urinary output or osmolality if nephrogenic DI is present. With central DI, the urine osmolality will increase and urinary output will decrease.

Findings

If there is no change in urine osmolality, the diagnosis is DI.

Interfering Factors

- Noncompliance with fluid restrictions
- Inability to complete test because of hypovolemia
- Glucosuria
- Administration of radiopaque dyes within 7 days

Nursing Implementation

Pretest

Assess patient's hemodynamic status. If vasopressin test is planned, check for a history of coronary artery disease, as vasopressin may cause coronary artery spasm.

Obtain baseline serum and urine specimens for osmolality determinations.

Baseline weight is obtained before the evening meal on the day before testing.

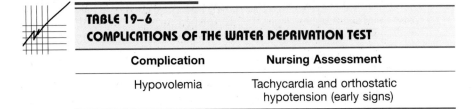

TABLE 19–6 COMPLICATIONS OF THE WATER DEPRIVATION TEST	
Complication	**Nursing Assessment**
Hypovolemia	Tachycardia and orthostatic hypotension (early signs)

During the Test

Assess the patient for hypovolemia (tachycardia, orthostatic hypotension).
Observe the patient to ensure compliance with the nothing by mouth status.
Obtain a urine specimen every 2 hours. Label each specimen with the time and the amount obtained. Document urinary output.
Weigh patient every 2 to 4 hours. Maintain the patient on the nothing-by-mouth status until 2 to 5% of the patient's weight is lost (takes approximately 6 to 12 hours).
After 2 to 5% of body weight is lost and urinary output continues with urinary osmolality plateauing, an ADH stimulation test may be performed by administering hypertonic saline (3% sodium chloride) or nicotine as ordered.
Continue to collect urine specimens for amount and osmolality.
If a vasopressin test is to be performed, check the patient's blood pressure and document; notify the physician if the patient is hypertensive. Aqueous vasopressin is given subcutaneously or intravenously. Collect the urine specimen for the amount and osmolality 1 hour after vasopressin administration. Another method is to give long-acting vasopressin in oil intramuscularly the night before the test. Urine is collected in the morning three times at hourly intervals. This method cannot be performed in conjunction with the water deprivation test.

Critical Thinking: When a water deprivation test is being done, how would a nurse assess for psychogenic polydipsia? If psychogenic polydipsia is suspected, what should the nurse do?

Complications

Hypovolemia may occur with the water deprivation test (Table 19–6). Patients with DI will continue to put urine out even though they have no intake. If a vasopressin test is performed, the administration of vasopressin may produce the complications of high blood pressure or coronary artery spasms, or both (Table 19–7).

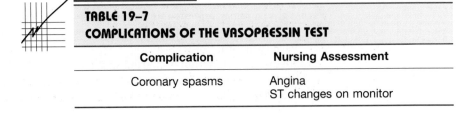

TABLE 19–7 COMPLICATIONS OF THE VASOPRESSIN TEST	
Complication	**Nursing Assessment**
Coronary spasms	Angina ST changes on monitor

WATER-LOADING TEST

(PLASMA AND URINE)

Synonyms:

NORMAL VALUES

Urinary output increases and plasma and urine osmolality decrease.

Background Information

Review the discussion of plasma ADH (pp. 676–679). Normally, with an increase in fluid intake, urinary output will increase to maintain a normal plasma osmolality. As the urine volume increases, its osmolality decreases. However, patients with SIADH will not respond to increasing fluid intake.

Purpose of the Test

The water-loading test is performed to diagnose SIADH.

Procedure

With the water-loading test, the patient orally ingests a water load of 20 to 25 ml/Kg body weight. Hourly serum and urine osmolality and urine outputs are recorded for 4 hours.

Findings

Little or no change in urinary output or plasma and urine osmolality readings supports the diagnosis of SIADH.

Interfering Factors

- Patient is unable to drink required volume of fluid
- Medications
    Demeclocycline
    Diuretics
    Lithium carbonate

Nursing Implementation

Pretest

Assess the patient for hyponatremia.

TABLE 19–8	
COMPLICATIONS OF THE WATER-LOADING TEST	
Complication	**Nursing Assessment**
Water intoxication	Hyponatremia
	Lethargy
	Confusion
	Stupor
	Muscular twitching
	Convulsions
	Coma

Obtain a cardiac history on the patient, the results of which may require that the test be cancelled.

Weigh the patient.

During the Test

Instruct the patient to drink the required fluid.

Obtain hourly output measurements and send blood and urine to the laboratory for osmolality determination. On the requisition slip, indicate the hour of the specimen, with zero hour being the time the patient ingested the fluid. See discussion of plasma and urine osmolality for the nursing procedures associated with the collection of these samples.

Observe the patient for water intoxication.

Posttest

Weigh the patient.

Complications

When patients with SIADH undergo the water-loading test, their output is not increased. The increased fluid load in the extracellular fluid can cause a dilutional hyponatremia (Table 19–8).

Critical Thinking: An elderly female patient is having a waterloading test. How can the nurse ensure that the fluid intake is adequate?

DIAGNOSTIC PROCEDURES

COMPUTED TOMOGRAPHY OF THE ADRENAL GLANDS

(IMAGING)

Synonym:

CT scan of the adrenal glands

──────────────── NORMAL VALUES ────────────────

Negative; no tumor or enlargement

Background Information

A CT scan of the abdomen is performed to visualize the adrenal glands. Its purpose is to identify adrenal tumors (adrenal carcinomas and adenomas) and to differentiate tumors from hyperplasia. CT scanning has almost completely replaced adrenal arteriography.

An adrenal CT scan is performed using iodocholesterol iodine-131 as the contrast agent.

Nursing Implementation

Pretest

Check for allergy to iodine.

(Review Chapter 12 for discussion of CT scanning and the other nursing responsibilities for this procedure.)

COMPUTED TOMOGRAPHY OF THE PANCREAS

(IMAGING)

Synonym:

CT scan of the pancreas

──────────────── NORMAL VALUES ────────────────

Negative; no tumor or inflammation

Background Information

CT scanning of the pancreas is performed to diagnose tumors (benign or malignant) and pancreatitis (acute or chronic) and to localize abscesses. The scan may be carried out with or without contrast medium, usually depending on whether the person is allergic to the dye.

(Review Chapter 12 for a discussion of CT scanning and the nursing responsibilities for this diagnostic procedure.)

PANCREATIC ULTRASONOGRAPHY

(ULTRASOUND)

Synonym:

pancreatic sonogram

―――――――――――――――― **NORMAL VALUES** ――――――――――――

Normal size and morphologic features

Background Information

The pancreas is both an exocrine and an endocrine organ. The exocrine function consists of the production and excretion of digestive enzymes required for the absorption of ingested food. The endocrine function consists of the production and secretion of hormones necessary for cellular nutrition.

A pancreatic sonogram assesses the size, shape, and positioning of the organ. Inflammation of the pancreas as well as calculi, cysts, pseudocysts, and tumors can be identified by ultrasound.

Purpose of the Test

An ultrasound of the pancreas is performed to support the diagnosis and progression of pancreatitis and to identify tumors, cysts, and pseudocysts. Ultrasound may be used as a guide for fine needle biopsy of the pancreas.

Procedure

See Chapter 8 on ultrasound.

Findings

Abscess
Acute or chronic pancreatitis
Cancer
Cyst
Pseudocyst

Interfering Factors

• Barium or gas in the bowel
• Dehydration

- Noncompliance with fasting
- Obesity

Nursing Implementation

Review Chapter 8.

Pretest

Instruct the patient not to eat or drink for 12 hours before the test.
Schedule any barium studies *after* the sonogram.
Explain to the patient the need to distend the stomach to visualize the entire pancreas.

During the Test

Encourage the patient to drink the prescribed fluid (500 to 1000 ml of juice).
Place the patient in the supine position. The patient is usually repositioned during the procedure to a sitting position.

Posttest

The patient resumes a normal diet.

PITUITARY MAGNETIC RESONANCE IMAGING

(IMAGING)

Synonyms:
none

────────────── **NORMAL VALUES** ──────────────

Normal pituitary size and configuration

Background Information

MRI has significantly affected endocrine diagnoses because of its ability to identify small lesions of the pituitary gland. In most cases, it has eliminated the need for angiography in patients with suspected aneurysms or vascular malformations. With MRI, the pituitary stalk and gland as well as the optic chiasm and the intercavernous portion of the carotid artery are visualized.

Purpose of the Test

MRI of the pituitary gland is performed to identify suspected hypothalamic-pituitary tumors and vascular abnormalities, including aneurysms, infarctions, and malformations.

Procedure

MRI of the pituitary gland is usually performed once without contrast dye and then with a contrast agent. Usually, gadolinium DPTA is given intravenously as the contrast medium.

Findings

Critical Thinking: A patient with claustrophobia requires an MRI. What assessments can the nurse make and what measures can she take to support the patient through the procedure?

Adenomas
Aneurysm
Arachnoid cysts
Craniopharyngiomas
Hemochromatosis
Germinomas
Gliomas
Vascular malformations

Interfering Factors

• Claustrophobia

Nursing Implementation

See Chapter 12 for the nursing responsibilities associated with this diagnostic procedure.

RADIOACTIVE IODINE UPTAKE

(IMAGING)

Synonym:
RAIU

──────────────── **NORMAL VALUES** ────────────────

After 6 hours: 3–13%
After 24 hours: 8–29%

Background Information

Radioactive iodine uptake can be a helpful index of thyroid function because the thyroid gland takes up from the extracellular fluid only the amount of iodide it needs for the synthesis of the thyroid hormones. The iodide not used is excreted in the urine. The thyroid gland does not distinguish between radioactive and nonradioactive iodine.

The thyroid uptake of radioactive iodine will be influenced by dietary iodine, which will be taken up at the same time as the radioisotope. Generally, the greater the amount of thyroid hormone produced, the greater the need for iodide and the higher the radioactive iodine uptake. Usually, radioactive iodine uptake increases with hyperthyroidism and decreases with hypothyroidism.

Purpose of the Test

The radioactive iodine uptake test assesses thyroid function to confirm the diagnosis of hyper- or hypothyroidism.

Procedure

Sodium iodide-123 is given to the patient orally. After 6 hours and again after 24 hours a gamma scintillation counter is used to measure the radioactivity over the thyroid gland.

Findings

Increase	Decrease
Hashimoto thyroiditis	Excessive iodide intake
Hyperthyroidism	Hypothyroidism
Hypoalbuminemia	Thyrotoxicosis due to
Iodine-deficient goiter	Ectopic thyroid metastasis
Lithium ingestion	Spontaneously resolving hyperthyroidism
	Subacute thyroiditis
	Thyrotoxicosis factitia

Interfering Factors

- Dietary intake of iodized foods (salt, bread, and so on)
- Iodine-deficient diet
- Previous radiographic studies with iodine-based dye
- Severe diarrhea
- Renal failure
- Noncompliance with dietary restrictions
- Medications
  Anticoagulants

Antihistamines
Antithyroid medications
Corticosteroids
Lithium
Multivitamins
Penicillin
Phenothiazides
Phenylbutazone
Salicylates
Thyroid hormones

Nursing Implementation

Pretest

Instruct the patient not to eat or drink for 12 hours before the test.
Obtain a medication history to determine if any interfering drugs were taken.
Schedule any x-ray studies requiring dyes after the radioactive iodine uptake study.
Describe the scanning equipment to the patient. The probe is placed over the anterior portion of the neck. Emphasize that no discomfort is involved but that the patient must lie absolutely still while the scan is performed.
Ensure that a signed consent form has been obtained.
Tell the patient that the oral radioactive iodine must be ingested. It has little or no taste. It comes in capsule or liquid form.
Explain to the patient the need for two scans, since the uptake of the radioactive iodine is usually maximized at 24 hours, but some thyroid conditions may cause the peak uptake to occur earlier.

During the Test

Two hours after ingestion of the radioactive iodine, a light meal may be consumed.
Transport the patient to the nuclear medicine laboratory when scheduled.

Critical Thinking: When handling the patient's bedpan after a radioactive iodine uptake, how can the nurse explain to the patient the need for gloves without making the patient feel fearful or isolated?

Posttest

The patient resumes a normal diet.
Observe for allergic response to the dye.
Wear gloves for 24 hours after the test when handling the patient's bedpan or urinal. Wash hands with soap and water after removing gloves.
Instruct the patient to wash hands with soap and water after voiding for 24 hours.

RADIONUCLIDE THYROID SCANNING

Synonyms:

──────────── **NORMAL VALUES** ────────────

Normal anatomic position and size

Background Information

To produce its hormones, the thyroid gland must extract iodide from the extracellular fluid. Once it has taken up enough iodide to meet its needs, the iodide left in the extracellular fluid is excreted in the urine. The thyroid gland cannot distinguish between dietary iodine and radioactive iodide. Thus, it will take up the radioactive iodide, which can be scanned by a gamma camera. The functioning of the thyroid gland can be evaluated by the amount of radioactive iodide it takes up. In thyrotoxic states, more iodide is needed and the uptake is increased, whereas in hypothyroid states, less than normal amounts of iodide are needed, and thus less is taken up by the thyroid gland.

Findings

Increased Uptake	**Decreased Uptake**
Hyperthyroidism	Hypothyroidism
	Cretinism

In addition to an increase or decrease in uptake by the thyroid gland, scanning may also identify "hot" or "cold" spots. Cold nodules are areas of the gland that do not take up or take up less radioactive iodine. Hot nodules are areas that take up more radioactive iodine than does the surrounding tissue. Cold spots may indicate cancer, whereas hot spots are usually not malignant. An echogram (sonogram) may be obtained to distinguish if the cold spot is a solid or semicystic lesion or a pure cyst. Pure cysts are rarely cancerous.

Interfering Factors

- Ingestion of foods and medications containing iodine
- Recent studies using iodine-based dyes

Nursing Implementation

Pretest

Inquire if the patient is allergic to iodine or seafood.
Ask women if they are pregnant or breast-feeding.

Ask if any x-ray studies requiring contrast media have been performed within the past 2 months.

Instruct the patient to avoid iodized salt or iodinated salt substitutes and seafood for a week before the test.

Instruct the patient not to eat or drink for 12 hours before the test.

Check with the prescriber to determine if interfering medications are to be withheld.

Ensure that an informed consent form is signed.

Warn the patient that when the intravenous radioactive iodine is given, he or she may feel warm, flushed, and nauseous. Deep breathing may relieve the nausea.

During the Test

Transport the patient to the nuclear medicine laboratory.

Iodine-123 is given orally and intravenously.

Posttest

Iodine-123 is excreted in the urine within 24 hours. The patient resumes a normal diet.

THYROID BIOPSY

(PATHOLOGY)

Synonyms:

───────────────────────── **NORMAL VALUES** ─────────────────

Normal cells

Background Information

A thyroid biopsy is usually performed by fine needle aspiration (FNA). FNA has replaced surgical removal as a diagnostic technique because it avoids surgical risk and is less traumatic for the patient.

Purpose of the Test

A biopsy is performed to differentiate the cause of thyroid nodules or lumps. Thyroid nodules are more common in women and occur at any age. Thyroid cancer is rare; most nodules are benign. The biopsy will identify malignant thyroid nodules, follicular neoplasms, and benign lesions.

Procedure

FNA is usually carried out in the operating room to maintain sterile technique. It usually requires a local anesthetic only, which permits it to be performed on an outpatient basis. A 23- or 25-gauge biopsy needle is used to aspirate tissue from the nodule. The tissue is assessed by cytologic examination.

Findings

Benign thyroid nodules
Cancer of the thyroid gland
Follicular neoplasm (cancerous or benign)

Interfering Factors

• Noncompliance with dietary restrictions
• Failure to place specimen in preservative immediately after aspiration
• Inadequate amount of tissue obtained

Nursing Implementation

Pretest

Assess the patient's level of anxiety, as fear of cancer may be significant or may interfere with the patient's ability to understand explanations.
Instruct the patient not to eat or drink for 12 hours before the test.
Prepare the patient for the operating room according to hospital protocol.
Ensure that a signed informed consent form has been obtained.
Administer preprocedure medication as prescribed.

During the Test

The patient is positioned on the back with a small pillow under the shoulders.
Usually, a local anesthetic is given. General anesthesia may be required in some cases.
Encourage the patient not to move or swallow as the local anesthetic is being given.
Support the patient, who will feel pressure as the procedure is performed.

Posttest

Reassure the patient that tenderness at the biopsy site is normal.
Position the patient in a semi-Fowler position with a small pillow under the head to remove stress from the site.

TABLE 19–9	
COMPLICATIONS OF THYROID BIOPSY	
Complication	**Nursing Assessment**
Bleeding	Overt bleeding
	With hematoma
	Swelling
	Stridor
	Dyspnea
Edema	Swelling
	Stridor
	Dyspnea
Infection	Malaise
	Fever
	Tenderness
	Redness

Instruct the patient to support the head when changing position. Keep site clean and dry.

Complications

Complications of a thyroid biopsy are rare. Most patients complain only of some tenderness, but the nurse should observe for bleeding, edema, and infection (Table 19–9).

REFERENCES

Amatruda, J., Vallone, B., Schuster, T., et al. (1989). Importance of periodic reeducation of hospital-based nurses in capillary blood glucose monitoring and an evaluation of the usefulness of reflectance meters. *The Diabetes Educator, 15*, 435–439.

American Diabetes Association. (1990). Consensus statement: Self-monitoring of blood glucose. *Clinical Practice Recommendation: Supplement to Diabetes Care, 13*, 41–46.

Bain, O., Brown, K., Sacher R., et al. (1989). A hospital-wide blind control program for bedside glucose meters. *Archives of Pathology and Laboratory Medicine, 13*, 1370–1375.

Burke, C.W. (1992). The pituitary megatest: Outdated? *Clinical Endocrinology, 36*, 133–134.

Buthcher, G.P., Zambon, M., Moss, S., et al. (1993). Addisonian crisis presenting with normal short tetracosactrin stimulation test. In *Yearbook of endocrinology.* St. Louis: CV Mosby.

Chernecky, C.C., Krech, R. L., & Berger, B.J. (1993). *Laboratory tests and diagnostic procedures.* Philadelphia: W.B. Saunders.

Daniels, D.L., Mark, L., & Haughton, V.M. (1990). Diagnostic imaging of the sellar region. In *Principles and practice of endocrinology and metabolism* (pp. 196–203). Philadelphia: J.B. Lippincott.

Fitzgerald, P. A. (1994). Endocrine disorders. In *Current Medical Diagnosis and Treatment* (pp. 912–976). Norwalk, CT: Lange Medical.

Greenspan, F.S., & Rapoport, B. (1991). Thyroid gland. In F.S. Greenspan & J.D. Baxter (Eds.), *Basic and Clinical Endocrinology* (3rd ed.). Norwalk, CT: Appleton & Lange.

Hambling, C., Jung, R.T., Gunn, A., et al. (1992). Re-evaluation of the captopril test for the diagnosis of primary hyperaldosteronism. A.B. Grossman (Ed.), *Clinical Endocrinology* (pp. 495–503). Cambridge, Blackwell Scientific.

Harding, K. (1993). A comparison of four glucose monitors in a hospital medical surgical setting. *Clinical Nurse Specialist, 7*, 13–18.

Hardy, K., Mead, B., & Gill, G. (1993). Adrenal apoplexy after coronary artery by-pass surgery leading to addisonian crisis. In *Yearbook of endocrinology*. St. Louis: C.V. Mosby.

Howanitz, J.H., Howanitz, P.J., & Henry, J.B. (1991). Evaluation of endocrine function. In *Clinical diagnosis and management by laboratory methods*. Philadelphia: W.B. Saunders.

Johnson, M.R., Hoare, R.D., Cox, T., et al. (1992). The evaluation of patients with suspected pituitary microadenoma: Computer tomography compared to magnetic resonance imaging. *Clinical Endocrinology, 36*, 335–338.

Jurney, T.H., et al. (1987). Spectrum of serum cortisol response to ACTH in ICU patients. *Chest, 92*, 292–305.

Karam, J. H., Salber, P.R., & Forsham, P.H. Pancreatic hormones and diabetes mellitus. (1991). In F.S. Greenspan and J.D. Baxter (Eds.), *Basic and clinical endocrinology* (3rd ed.). Norwalk, CT: Appleton & Lange.

Loriaux, D.L. (1990). Tests of adrenocorticortical function. In K.L. Becker (Ed.), *Principles and practice of endocrinology and metabolism* (pp. 591–595). Philadelphia: J.B. Lippincott.

Marston, R.A. (1992). Primary adrenocortical failure masked by exogenous steroid administration. *Clinical Endocrinology, 36*, 519–520.

Moseley, I. (1992). Computed tomography and magnetic resonance imaging of pituitary microadenoma. *Clinical Endocrinology, 36*, 333.

Pavord, S. R., et al. (1992). A retrospective audit of the combined pituitary function test, using the insulin stress test, TRH and GRH in a district laboratory. *Clinical Endocrinology, 36*, 135–136.

Pitzinger, R. (1992). Diabetes aids and products for people with visual or physical impairment. *The Diabetes Educator, 18*, 121–138.

Philippon, G., Koutras, D. A., Piperingos, G., et al. (1992). The effect of iodine on serum thyroid hormone levels in normal persons, in hyperthyroid patients and in hypothyroid patients on thyroxine replacement. *Clinical Endocrinology, 36*, 573–578.

Resner, C. (1990). Adrenal disorders. *Critical Care Nursing Quarterly, 13*, 67–73.

Smallridge, R.C. (1990). Evaluation of thyroid function: Blood test. In E.L. Becker (Ed.), *Principles and practice of endocrinology and metabolism* (pp. 278–284). Philadelphia: J.B. Lippincott.

Walker, E. A. (1993). Quality assurance for blood glucose monitoring: The balance of feasibility and standards. *Nursing Clinics of North America, 28*, 61–70.

Wall, S.D. (1994). Imaging. In *Current medical diagnosis and treatment*. Norwalk, CT: Appleton & Lange.

Weir, G.C., & O'Hare, J.A. (1990). Evaluation of metabolic control in diabetes. In *Principles and practice of endocrinology and metabolism*. Philadelphia: J.B. Lippincott.

Wilson, J.D. Assessment of endocrine function. In *Harrison's principles of internal medicine* (13th ed., pp. 1889–1891). New York: McGraw-Hill.

Zweiman, B., & Lisak, R.P. (1991). Autoantibodies: Autoimmunity and immune complexes. In J.B. Henry (Ed.), *Clinical diagnosis and management by laboratory methods* (18th ed., pp. 885–911). Philadelphia: W.B. Saunders.

CHAPTER 20

Renal and Urinary Tract Function

The kidneys perform the processes of regulation, excretion, and hormonal production. Under normal anatomic and physiologic conditions, the kidneys help maintain body tone, fluid volume, acid-base balance, and the chemical balance of extracellular fluids.

The ureters, bladder, and urethra are the other components of the urologic system that guide the flow of urine in excretory functions. The prostate gland surrounds part of the bladder neck and urethra in the male. Alterations in the anatomy or physiology of these parts can result in urinary obstruction.

The laboratory tests presented in this chapter evaluate renal function based on changes in blood chemistry test results and urine analyses. Blood test results can also indicate the presence of prostate cancer markers. There are additional laboratory tests that are appropriate for the evaluation of renal function and other functions throughout the body. These multisystem laboratory tests are presented in Chapter 5.

The diagnostic procedures presented in this chapter are used to identify abnormalities of structure and function of the renal and urologic system. The tests evaluate sources of obstruction, abnormalities in renal blood flow, and changes in the cells. The structural abnormalities can also alter renal function, as measured by the blood and urine laboratory tests.

CALCIUM, SERUM

(SERUM)

Synonyms:

Ca, total serum calcium

696

LABORATORY TESTS

NORMAL VALUES

Adult:	8.2–10.2 mg/dl *or* SI 2.05–2.54 mmol/L
Infant–1 Month:	7–11.5 mg/dl *or* SI 1.75–2.87 mmol/L
Child, 1 Month–1 Year:	8.6–11.2 mg/dl *or* SI 2.15–2.79 mmol/L

Background Information

Calcium is one of the essential mineral elements of the body. Almost all of it is concentrated in bone. The remainder is present in the cells or extracellular fluids, including the serum, in which about half the total calcium is in a free or ionized state and is physiologically active. A little less than half of the total calcium is bonded to albumin and other plasma proteins.

In the serum and other extracellular fluids, the normal level of calcium is maintained in homeostatic balance by the actions of the small intestine, bones, and kidneys. For the regulation of calcium, these target organs are governed by the interplay of parathyroid hormone, calcitonin hormone, and vitamin D_1, an active form of vitamin D.

Parathyroid hormone prevents hypocalcemia by increasing the amount of calcium in the extracellular fluids. It does this by (1) acting on bones to increase bone resorption, (2) acting on the kidneys to increase the resorption of calcium, and (3) acting on the kidneys to convert vitamin D to the active form of vitamin D_1, which acts on the small intestine to absorb a greater amount of dietary calcium.

Calcitonin, a hormone manufactured by the thyroid gland, works in a manner opposite that of parathyroid hormone and vitamin D_1. Calcitonin prevents hypercalcemia by lowering the amount of calcium in the extracellular fluids. Its action is to decrease or limit the resorption of calcium by the bones and kidneys.

Calcium is needed for the process of bone formation and is an essential element in bone structure. It is also needed for many other physiologic functions, including coagulation of the blood, excitation of cardiac and skeletal muscle, maintenance of muscle tone, conduction of neuromuscular impulses, and

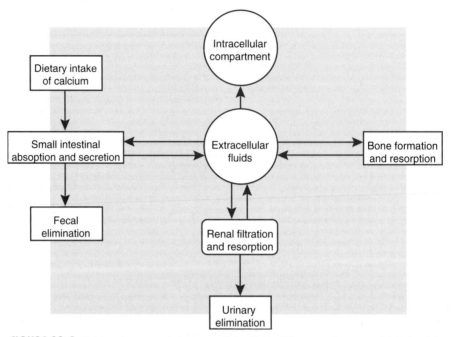

FIGURE 20–1. Calcium homeostasis in extracellular fluids. The normal serum calcium level is regulated by a complex interaction of intestinal, bone, and renal functions. Excess amounts of calcium are excreted in feces or urine.

synthesis and regulation of the endocrine and exocrine glands. On the cellular level, calcium preserves the integrity and permeability of the cell membrane, particularly for sodium and potassium exchange.

In normal physiology, calcium is obtained from dietary sources. About 20% of the daily intake is absorbed in the duodenum of the small intestine (Bourke and Delaney, 1993). As the absorbed calcium enters the blood, it is used in cells and bone formation or it remains in the extracellular fluid. The glomeruli of the kidneys filter out the calcium from the blood. Most of it is then resorbed by the renal tubules and reenters the circulation and extracellular fluid. The excess dietary calcium is excreted in feces. The excess calcium in the extracellular fluid and serum is excreted by the kidneys, and a small amount is excreted in sweat (Fig. 20–1).

In the individual, the endocrine-regulating mechanisms maintain a steady serum calcium level with little variation. There is a higher normal value in infants and children than in adults and a lower normal value in older adult men and pregnant women. Daily, the normal level fluctuates in a diurnal rhythm, with a lower serum calcium level in the later afternoon. The reference values vary among laboratories because of different methods of analysis. To ensure accuracy in laboratory testing, the specimen is always drawn in the early morning to minimize the diurnal variation. An abnormally elevated value is routinely validated by repeating the test two additional times.

HYPERCALCEMIA. An elevated level of calcium in the blood is called hypercalcemia. It alters the function of most body organs and can result in coma. A potential life-threatening serum elevation is 14 mg/dl or greater (SI, 3.49 mmol/L). Hyperparathyroidism and malignancy are the most common causes of hypercalcemia. In hyperparathyroidism, an excess of parathyroid hormone increases the resorption of calcium from the bones and renal tubules. Malignancy and multiple myeloma increase the level of total serum proteins. The calcium level increases as the calcium bonds to the excess protein concentration.

HYPOCALCEMIA. A decreased level of calcium in the serum is called hypocalcemia. It causes neuromuscular hyperactivity, depression or psychosis, laryngeal stridor, tetany, convulsions, hypotension, and decreased myocardial contractility. A severe decrease is equal to or less than 6 mg/dl (SI, 1.5 mmol/L). Total serum calcium is lowered in conditions that decrease plasma proteins, impair intestinal absorption, alter renal filtration and resorption functions, or decrease the amount of parathyroid hormone.

Critical Thinking: Your East Indian patient has a serum calcium level of 7 mg/dl (SI: 1.75 mmol/L). She states that she never drinks milk because it gives her gas. Considering her cultural food tastes, how can she supplement her dietary intake of calcium with alternative foods?

Purpose of the Test

The serum calcium level is measured to assist in the diagnosis of acid-base imbalance, coagulation disorders, pathologic bone disorders, endocrine disorders, cardiac arrhythmia, and muscle disorders.

Procedure

Adult: A red-topped tube is used to collect 7 to 10 ml of venous blood.
Infant: A capillary pipette is used to collect capillary blood via the heelstick method.

QUALITY CONTROL

The tourniquet is applied briefly. Venipuncture technique must be smooth, with a flow of blood that fills the vacuum tube readily. If there is venous stasis and pooling or excessive hemolysis, the serum calcium level will be falsely elevated.

Findings

ELEVATED VALUES

Hyperparathyroidism
Metastatic cancer
Multiple myeloma
Vitamin D intoxication
Milk-alkali syndrome
Overuse of calcium antacids
Paget disease
Idiopathic hypercalcemia of infancy

Polycythemia vera
Pheochromocytoma
Sarcoidosis
Adrenal insufficiency
Thyrotoxicosis
Bacteremia
Dehydration

DECREASED VALUES

Hypoparathyroidism   Acute pancreatitis
Vitamin D deficiency   Anterior pituitary hypofunction
Chronic renal failure   Alcoholism
Renal tubular disease   Hypoalbuminemia
Cirrhosis of the liver   Massive blood transfusions
Malnutrition   Prolonged intravenous fluid therapy
Neonatal prematurity

Interfering Factors

- Upright position or prolonged activity before the test
- Venous stasis or hemolysis during the blood collection procedure
- Prolonged storage of the blood specimen

Nursing Implementation

Pretest

Instruct the patient to fast from food for 8 hours and arrange to have the blood drawn in the early morning (Jacobs et al., 1990).

Some medications (i.e., thiazides and other diuretics, lithium, and calcium salts) cause a rise in the serum value and may be withheld during the period in which the patient ingests nothing by mouth, as prescribed.

Posttest

Arrange for prompt transport of the specimen to the laboratory.

QUALITY CONTROL

The blood specimen may require refrigeration in the laboratory, but the analysis must be performed on a fresh sample. Prolonged storage or a delay in performing the analysis results in a false elevation of the calcium value.

CALCIUM, URINE

(URINE)

Synonyms:

calcium, 24-hour urine

Background Information

Calcium is maintained in homeostatic balance in the blood by the functions of the intestine, bones, and kidneys (Fig. 20–1). This balance is regulated by the

─────────────── **NORMAL VALUES** ───────────────

Adult (Normal calcium intake):	100–300 mg/day *or* SI 2.5–7.5 mmol/day
Adult (Low calcium intake):	50–100 mg/day *or* SI 1.25–3.75 mmol/day
Adult (Calcium-free diet):	5–40 mg/day *or* SI 0.13–1 mmol/day
Infant and Child:	<6 mg/kg/day *or* SI <0.15 mmol/kg/day

interplay of parathyroid hormone, calcitonin, and vitamin D_1, the active form of vitamin D. The daily intake of calcium in food provides a continual renewal of the supply of calcium that is available for the body. In daily excretion of excess supply, the glomeruli of the kidneys filter calcium out of the blood and the renal tubules resorb the amount needed to maintain a normal serum value. Excess calcium is removed from the body in urine, feces, and sweat.

Parathyroid hormone prevents hypocalcemia by increasing the resorption of calcium by the bones and the renal tubules. When the renal tubules resorb calcium, there is less calcium present in the urine. Calcitonin works in the opposite way. It prevents hypercalcemia by decreasing the resorption of calcium by the bones and renal tubules. When the renal tubules resorb less calcium, there is more calcium present in the urine. Vitamin D_1 acts on the mucosa of the small intestine to allow the absorption of dietary calcium.

The normal excretion of urinary calcium varies with dietary intake. The average calcium intake for adults is 600 to 800 mg/day (SI, 15–20 mmol/day). Patients who follow a calcium-restricted diet or who consume less than an average amount of daily calcium have a lower normal value of calcium in the urine.

HYPERCALCIURIA. An excessive calcium level in the urine is called hypercalciuria. It is identified as a calcium value in the urine of more than 350 mg/day (SI, 8.75 mmol/day). The excess urinary calcium can result from increased intestinal absorption, increased bone resorption, or impaired renal tubular resorption. Increased intestinal absorption can result from low serum phosphorus levels, excessive loss of phosphorus from the kidneys, or excessive vitamin D intake. Increased bone resorption means that excess calcium is released from bone. The excess calcium enters the serum and ultimately is released in the urine. This can occur with immobility; bone diseases, including malignancy; and endocrine disorders including hyperparathyroidism, thyrotoxicosis, and Cushing disease.

Excess calcium in the urine can cause the formation of urinary calculi. The most common calcium stones are composed of calcium oxalate, and a few are composed of calcium phosphate.

HYPOCALCIURIA. A diminished amount of calcium in the urine is called hypocalciuria. It can result from a deficiency of parathyroid hormone, vitamin D disorders, renal diseases that limit glomerular filtration or cause loss of serum proteins, bone diseases that increase the skeletal uptake of calcium, and digestive disorders that inhibit the intestinal absorption of calcium.

Purpose of the Test

The urinary calcium level is used to evaluate bone disease, parathyroid disorders, nephrolithiasis, calcium metabolism, and idiopathic hypercalciuria.

Procedure

Urine is collected for 24 hours and stored in a clean plastic container or a special glass container that is acid-washed prior to use.

Findings

ELEVATED VALUES

Hyperparathyroidism	Vitamin D toxicity
Malignancy of bone	Renal tubular acidosis
Sarcoma	Nephrolithiasis
Multiple myeloma	Thyrotoxicosis
Paget disease	Sarcoidosis
Osteoporosis	Schistosomiasis
Skeletal immobility	Degenerative liver disease
Cushing disease	Diabetes mellitus

DECREASED VALUES

Hypoparathyroidism	Hypothyroidism
Pseudohypoparathyroidism	Celiac disease
Nephrosis	Steatorrhea
Acute nephritis	Hypocalciuric hypercalcemia
Renal osteodystrophy	Vitamin D–resistant rickets
	Vitamin D deficiency

Interfering Factors

• Failure to collect all urine in the 24-hour collection period.

Nursing Implementation

Pretest

If the test is used to evaluate nephrolithiasis, instruct the patient to eat the usual diet for 3 days before the test. If the patient is already receiving a calcium-restricted diet as part of the calcium stone prevention treatment, instruct the patient to maintain the dietary restriction before and during the test period.

When thiazide diuretics are used to prevent formation of calcium stones, instruct the patient to continue the medication before and during the test. Thiazides are effective in lowering the urine calcium levels, and the benefits of the medication can be evaluated.

Instruct the patient to void at 8 A.M. and discard the specimen.

For 24 hours thereafter, all urine is collected and placed in the large collection container. The 8 A.M. specimen of the following day is included in the collection period.

Posttest

No special nursing implementation is needed.

CALCULUS ANALYSIS

(QUALITATIVE CHEMI-
CAL ANALYSIS)

Synonyms:

kidney stone analysis, renal calculus analysis, nephrolithiasis analysis

——————————————————— NORMAL VALUES ———————————————————

There are no kidney stones present in the urine.

Background Information

A renal calculus is commonly called a stone. It forms in the renal pelvis; descends through the ureter, bladder, and urethra; and exits from the body in the urine. Calculi are of various sizes, textures, colors, and chemical compositions.

CALCIUM STONES. The most common type of renal calculi are calcium stones. They are caused by excess calcium in the urine. These calculi consist of calcium phosphate or calcium oxalate, or a combination of the two chemical salts. These dark-colored stones are usually hard and have a rough surface. The underlying causes of calcium stone formation are thought to be increased intestinal absorption of dietary calcium, poor renal tubular resorption of calcium, a loss of calcium from bone, or any combination of these factors. Calcium homeostasis is regulated by parathyroid hormone. Hyperparathyroidism also causes increased turnover of bone and excess calcium in the blood and urine (Henry, 1991).

STRUVITE STONES. This type of stone is sometimes called an "infection stone" because of its association with chronic urinary tract infection. Although it is not known whether the stone causes the infection to occur or the infection causes the stone to form, the bacteria that are associated with this calculus are *Proteus,*

Pseudomonas, Klebsiella, and *Staphylococcus aureus* (Frank and Resnick, 1989). This pale stone is usually large and soft. The stone is also called a staghorn calculus because of its characteristic shape as it forms within the renal pelvis. The chemical composition consists of magnesium ammonium phosphate and carbonate apatite. It is sometimes called a phosphate stone based on its chemical composition.

URIC ACID STONES. These stones consist of uric acid and urate crystals. They are yellow-brown and moderately hard. They form in the presence of excess uric acid and concentrated acidic urine. Underlying causes include primary gout, dehydration, and some medications, including thiazide diuretics and salicylates.

CYSTINE STONES. These stones occur infrequently. They are dark yellow-brown and greasy. Their formation is caused by an autosomal recessive inborn error in metabolism that impairs the absorption of amino acids. Because of this deficit in metabolism, cystine and other amino acids are excreted in urine. The precipitate forms both crystals and stones.

Critical Thinking:
The patient, an office worker, has not passed his urinary calculus. As you prepare him for discharge, make suggestions about how to strain his urine samples at home and during the work hours.

Purpose of the Test

The analysis of urinary calculus is used in the work-up for nephrolithiasis. It determines the chemical composition of the stone and provides data regarding the metabolic factors that result in stone formation.

Procedure

All urine is strained by the use of a gauze strainer or a fine mesh sieve. Any stones that are recovered are placed in a glass bottle or plastic container and sent to the laboratory for qualitative analysis.

Findings

ABNORMAL VALUES

Urolithiasis	Hypercalciuria
Hyperparathyroidism	Gout
Primary cystinuria	Dehydration
Urinary tract infection	Infection

Nursing Implementation

Pretest

Teach the patient to use a clean container to collect the urine every time he or she voids. The first voided specimen of the morning is particularly important because the stone may pass during the night.

Each collected specimen is to be poured through the strainer or sieve. The gauze or mesh is examined to see if a stone is present. Teach the patient to look carefully because it can be as small as the head of a pin.

If a stone is recovered, it is placed in a clean, lidded container. Label the container with the patient's name, other identifying data, and the date, time, and source of the stone.

Posttest

Send the stone to the laboratory in the labeled container. If the stone is enmeshed in the gauze, place both the stone and gauze in the container. Specify on the requisition form that the source of the stone is urinary and include the date and time that the stone was passed.

QUALITY CONTROL

Do not wrap or place the stone on adhesive tape to secure it. The adhesive interferes with the infrared spectroscopy examination that is used to analyze the stone.

CREATININE CLEARANCE, 24-HOUR URINE

(URINE)

Synonyms:

Ccre, Ccr, urine creatinine

━━━━━━━━━━━━━━ **NORMAL VALUES** ━━━━━━━━━━━━━━

MEAN CREATININE CLEARANCE	
Adult Male:	1–2 g/day *or* SI 8.8–17.7 mmol/day
	90–139 ml/minute/1.73 m^2 *or* SI 0.87–1.34 mL/second/m^2
Adult Female:	0.8–1.8 g/day *or* SI 7.1–15.9 mmol/day
	80–125 ml/minute/1.73 m^2 *or* SI 0.77–1.2 mL/second/m^2
Child:	70–140 ml/minute/1.73 m^2 *or* SI 1.17–2.33 mL/second/m^2

Background Information

Creatinine is an amino acid waste product that is derived from muscle creatinine, a product of protein metabolism. It is distributed throughout body fluids and is excreted by the kidneys. In the process of urinary elimination, creatinine is freely filtered by the glomeruli, usually without resorption by the tubules. Additional creatinine is secreted by the proximal renal tubules. The total amount of creatinine excreted in urine is called creatinine clearance.

In the course of renal failure, there is diminished glomerular filtration. Once the glomerular filtration rate is reduced by half, the renal tubules compensate by an increase in their secretion of creatinine. As chronic renal failure or uremia becomes severe, there is an eventual reduction in the excretion of creatinine by both the glomeruli and the tubules (Finn, 1990), but there is also an additional nonrenal source of elimination of creatinine. Although it is not fully proved, the nonrenal excretion is probably via the gastrointestinal tract (Duarte and Preuss, 1993).

The amount of urinary creatinine is increased significantly by muscle necrosis and muscle atrophy because of protein catabolism. It is decreased significantly in acute and advanced chronic renal failure because of the kidneys' inability to filter and secrete this waste product.

The urinary creatinine clearance test is usually accompanied by a serum creatinine test. The blood test may be performed at the midpoint in urinary collection or at the start and completion of the urine collection, depending on laboratory protocol. A complete discussion of the serum creatinine is found in Chapter 5.

Purpose of the Test

The urine creatinine clearance test is performed to help assess renal function and creatinine excretion. It is also used to monitor the progress of renal disease.

Procedure

The test usually requires urine collection for 24 hours, but collection periods of 4 or 12 hours are sometimes prescribed.

Findings

ELEVATED VALUES

Muscular dystrophy
Paralysis
Hyperthyroidism
Leukemia

Polymyositis
Muscular inflammatory disease
Anemia

DECREASED VALUES

Glomerulonephritis
Acute tubular necrosis
Shock
Renal malignancy
Bilateral ureteral obstruction

Congestive heart failure
Advanced pyelonephritis
Polycystic kidney disease
Dehydration
Nephrosclerosis

Interfering Factors

- Excessive exercise in the test period
- Failure to collect all the urine

- Failure to time the test accurately
- Warming of the urine specimen
- High protein intake prior to the test

Nursing Implementation

Pretest

Instruct the patient to avoid excessive intake of meat on the day before the test.

Instruct the patient to collect all urine for the 24-hour period of the test, storing the container in the refrigerator or on ice.

Encourage adequate hydration before and during the test, omitting coffee and tea during the test.

During the Test

At 8 A.M., instruct the patient to void and discard the urine. The test begins at this time and all subsequent urine specimens are collected for 24 hours, including the 8 A.M. specimen of the next morning.

Advise the patient to avoid vigorous exercise during the test period.

Ensure that the patient's name and the time and date of the start and finish of the test are written on the label and requisition slip.

Posttest

Arrange for prompt transportation of the refrigerated specimen to the laboratory.

ELECTROLYTES, 24-HOUR URINE

(URINE)

Synonyms:

sodium, urine; chloride, urine; potassium, urine

Background Information

Electrolytes are ions that are present in body fluids. Potassium is the major intracellular cation. Sodium, chloride, and bicarbonate are the major anions in extracellular fluid. The concentrations of these electrolytes are important determinants of osmolarity, pH, and hydration in both intracellular and extracellular fluid. The concentrations of intracellular and extracellular electrolytes also regulate membrane potentials and the functions of nerve, heart, and muscle tissue.

In normal physiology, the daily intake of foods includes a renewing supply of sodium, chloride, and potassium. These electrolytes are absorbed in the intestine

━━━━━━━━━━━━━━━ **NORMAL VALUES** ━━━━━━━━━━━━━━━

SODIUM

Adult: 40–220 mEq/24 hours *or* SI 40–220 mmol/24 hours

Child (6–10 Years): Male: 41–115 mEq/24 hours *or* SI 41–115 mmol/24 hours
Female: 20–69 mEq/24 hours *or* SI 20–69 mmol/24 hours

Child (10–14 Years): Male: 63–117 mEq/24 hours *or* SI 63–117 mmol/24 hours
Female: 48–168 mEq/24 hours *or* SI 48–168 mmol/24 hours

CHLORIDE

Adult: 110–250 mEq/24 hours *or* SI 110–250 mmol/24 hours

Adult (>60 Years): 95–195 mEq/24 hours *or* SI 95–195 mmol/24 hours

Child (<6 Years): 15–40 mEq/24 hours *or* SI 15–40 mmol/24 hours

Child (6–10 Years): Male: 36–110 mEq/24 hours *or* SI 36–110 mmol/24 hours
Female: 18–74 mEq/24 hours *or* SI 18–74 mmol/24 hours

Child (10–14 Years): Male: 64–176 mEq/24 hours *or* SI 64–176 mmol/24 hours
Female: 36–173 mEq/24 hours *or* SI 36–173 mmol/24 hours

Infant: 2–10 mEq/24 hours *or* SI 2–10 mmol/24 hours

POTASSIUM

Adult: 25–125 mEq/24 hours *or* SI 25–125 mmol/24 hours

Child (6–10 Years): Male: 17–54 mEq/24 hours *or* SI 17–54 mmol/24 hours
Female: 8–37 mEq/24 hours *or* SI 8–37 mmol/24 hours

Child (10–14 Years): Male: 22–57 mEq/24 hours *or* SI 22–57 mmol/24 hours
Female: 18–58 mEq/24 hours *or* SI 18–58 mmol/24 hours

Infant: 4.1–5.3 mEq/24 hours *or* SI 4.1–5.3 mmol/24 hours

and maintained in a steady concentration in the intracellular and extracellular fluid. The glomeruli filter the electrolytes from the blood, and the renal tubules resorb most of them for recirculation and redistribution as needed. Electrolyte excesses are not resorbed and are excreted in the urine.

The normal urinary excretion of electrolytes is dependent on the amount of intake, the serum level, and the state of hydration of the body. The equilibrium of water and electrolytes is controlled by renal, adrenal, posterior pituitary, and hypothalamic functions.

SODIUM AND CHLORIDE. In patients with endocrine deficiency, an excess amount of diuretic medication, or renal disease that affects the renal tubules, the kidneys cannot conserve the sodium and chloride through renal tubular resorption. Thus, the urinary electrolyte levels rise as the electrolytes are lost from the body.

Nonrenal causes of low levels of sodium and chloride in the urine include intestinal problems that affect the digestion or absorption of the electrolytes or losses of these electrolytes via other mechanisms of excretion. Additionally, problems that cause water retention dilute the concentration of the electrolytes in the body fluids. The kidneys respond by greater resorption and conservation of the sodium and chloride, and there is a lower amount of excretion of these electrolytes in the urine. Aldosterone and other adrenocorticoid hormones promote the resorption of sodium and chloride, with less loss of electrolytes in the urine.

When renal conditions cause low levels of sodium and chloride in the urine, conditions that cause prerenal azotemia or acute oliguria prevent glomerular filtration of blood. Depending on the severity of the condition, fewer electrolytes are removed from the blood, and urinary excretion of electrolytes is minimal.

POTASSIUM. A nonrenal condition that results in excess potassium in the urine includes excessive potassium intake in food or medication. Excess aldosterone or adrenocortical hyperfunction both promote potassium excretion in the urine. Catabolism and lysis of cells cause the release of potassium into the extracellular fluid and ultimately into the urine. Renal conditions that cause excess potassium in the urine include metabolic acidosis and renal tubular disease that prevents resorption of the potassium.

Nonrenal causes of decreased urinary potassium include conditions that either prevent intestinal absorption of this electrolyte or cause a loss of the electrolyte via another route. When the serum level is low, the kidneys will compensate and resorb more potassium, allowing less to be lost in the urine. Additionally, adrenocortical hypofunction and a deficiency of aldosterone promotes potassium resorption by the renal tubules, with less potassium to be excreted in the urine.

Renal causes of low levels of potassium in the urine are due to acute or advanced chronic renal disease. When there is diminished renal circulation and diminished glomerular filtration, there is less production of urine and less elimination of the excess serum potassium.

Purpose of the Test

Urine electrolytes are used to help monitor renal function, fluid and electrolyte balance, and acid-base balance.

Procedure

A 24-hour urine specimen is collected in a large, clean urine collection container. Alternative methods include a 12-hour urine collection or a single random urine sample for electrolyte testing. If a 24-hour urine test for protein or creatinine clearance is also ordered, these tests can be performed simultaneously with the urine electrolyte test, using the same specimen.

Findings

ELEVATED VALUES

Sodium and Chloride	Potassium
Increased sodium chloride intake	Increased potassium intake
Adrenal failure	Cushing syndrome
Addison disease	Aldosteronism
Nephritis (salt-wasting)	Renal tubular disease
Renal tubular acidosis	Metabolic acidosis
Syndrome of inappropriate antidiuretic hormone	Adrenocorticotropic hormone or cortisone treatment
Alkalosis	Salicylate poisoning
Diuretic therapy	
Acute or chronic renal failure	

DECREASED VALUES

Sodium and Chloride	Potassium
Decreased sodium chloride intake	Addison disease
Cushing syndrome	Acute glomerulonephritis
Cirrhosis (with ascites)	Pyelonephritis
Congestive heart failure	Nephrosclerosis
Nephrotic syndrome	Malabsorption syndrome
Prerenal azotemia	Metabolic alkalosis
Vomiting, diarrhea	
Intestinal fistula	
Severe burns	
Excessive sweating	
Metabolic acidosis	

Interfering Factors

- Blood in the urine
- Warming of the specimen

Nursing Implementation

Pretest

Obtain a urine collection container from the laboratory for the collection of all urine in the 24-hour test period.

During the Test

Instruct the patient to void at 8 A.M. and discard the specimen. The test begins immediately thereafter, and all urine is collected for the next 24 hours, including the 8 A.M. specimen of the next morning.

Keep the urine in the refrigerator or on ice throughout the collection period.

Ensure that the patient's name and the date and time of the start and finish of the test are written on the label and the requisition slip.

Posttest

Arrange for prompt transport of the chilled specimen to the laboratory.

ERYTHROPOIETIN

(SERUM)

Synonym:
EP

─────────────── **NORMAL VALUES** ───────────────

5–36 µU/ml *or* SI 5–35 IU/L

Background Information

Erythropoietin is a hormone manufactured primarily by the kidney. Its action is to regulate erythropoiesis, meaning that it stimulates or promotes the proliferation, differentiation, and maturation of erythrocyte precursor cells of the bone marrow. In normal kidneys, the stimulus to produce erythropoietin is hypoxia and decreased renal oxygenation.

In the anemia of renal disease, the erythropoietin level is low. In cases of end-stage renal disease or after bilateral nephrectomy, the ability to produce erythropoietin is greatly reduced, and erythropoiesis by the bone marrow is limited.

In chronic iron deficiency anemia and other types of anemia and after a moderate blood loss, the erythropoietin level is elevated as the kidneys respond to the need for more red blood cells and oxygen. The erythropoietin level rises dramatically in pregnancy and with erythropoietin-producing tumors.

Purpose of the Test

Measurement of erythropoietin is performed to investigate some anemias and the anemia of end-stage renal disease. It also may be used to differentiate between primary and secondary polycythemia vera or to detect the recurrence of an erythropoietin-producing tumor.

Procedure

A red-topped tube is used to collect 7 ml of venous blood.

Findings

ELEVATED VALUES

Anemias
Secondary polycythemia (pulmonary fibrosis, chronic obstructive pulmonary disease)
Erythropoietin-producing tumor (cerebellar hemangioblastoma, renal tumor, hepatoma, pheochromocytoma)
Polycystic kidney disease
Early renal transplant rejection

DECREASED VALUES

End-stage renal failure
Primary polycythemia (polycythemia vera)

Interfering Factors

• Pregnancy

Nursing Implementation

No specific patient instruction or intervention is needed.

MAGNESIUM, SERUM

(SERUM)

Synonym:
Mg^+

Background Information

Magnesium is one of the major intracellular cations of the body. Almost all magnesium is stored in soft tissue, muscle, and bone, with only 1% of the total

═══════════════════ **NORMAL VALUES** ═══════════════════

Adult	1.3–2.1 mEq/L *or* SI 0.65–1.05 mmol/L
Child	
12–20 Years	1.56 ± 0.21 mEq/L *or* SI 0.78 ± 0.11 mmol/L
6–12 Years	1.56 ± 0.18 mEq/L *or* SI 0.78 ± 0.09 mmol/L
5 Months–6 Years	1.65 ± 0.23 mEq/L *or* SI 0.83 ± 0.12 mmol/L
Infant	
Newborn–4 Days	1.2–1.8 mEq/L *or* SI 0.6–0.9 mmol/L

magnesium present in the serum and extracellular fluid. Because so little of the magnesium is in the serum, total body magnesium is difficult to measure accurately. Often, a low serum level of magnesium is followed up by a 24-hour urine measurement to provide additional data (Quamme, 1993).

Serum magnesium is maintained in homeostatic balance by the functions of gastrointestinal absorption and excretion and renal resorption and excretion. As seen in Figure 20–2, magnesium is obtained from food. The magnesium is absorbed in the small intestine and enters the blood and extracellular fluid. From there, the largest amount of magnesium is stored in bone. An equivalent amount is stored in the soft tissue and bones, and a small amount is stored in the erythrocytes. In the kidneys, the glomeruli filter the magnesium, and the renal tubules are responsible for resorption. Excess magnesium is removed from the body in feces and urine.

HYPOMAGNESEMIA. A low level of magnesium in the blood is called hypomagnesemia. In a normal physiologic response to a low serum level of magnesium, the metabolites of vitamin D and the action of parathyroid hormone respond by increasing the amount of intestinal absorption of magnesium. Additionally, parathyroid hormone causes the renal tubules to resorb a greater amount of magnesium, with less to be excreted in the urine. Renal tubular resorption exerts the most powerful effect on the conservation of magnesium and the restoration of the homeostatic balance. If these responses are inadequate, hypomagnesemia results. The deficiency of magnesium is usually associated with deficiencies of calcium and potassium.

Hypomagnesemia causes neuromuscular changes that include weakness, tremors, tetany, convulsions, and cardiac arrhythmias. If the serum value falls to less than 1.2 mEq/dl (SI, 0.5 mmol/L), these symptoms will appear, and the deficit is considered to be severe. In the patient who has had a recent myocardial infarction, the danger is even greater. In these patients, a serum value of less than 2 mEq/dl (SI, 0.82 mmol/L) can trigger a ventricular arrhythmia. Hypomagnesemia is considered to be more serious than hypermagnesemia.

HYPERMAGNESEMIA. This is an elevation of the serum value of magnesium in the blood. In a normal physiologic response to a rising level of magnesium in the blood, the intestines respond by absorbing less of the dietary sources of

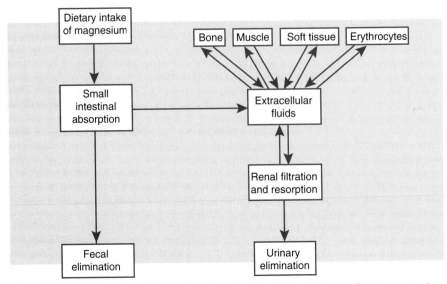

FIGURE 20–2. Homeostasis of magnesium in extracellular fluids. The normal serum magnesium level is regulated by intestinal and renal function. Most of the body's magnesium is stored in bones, muscle, and soft tissues.

Critical Thinking:
The patient is receiving magnesium sulfate infusion therapy. If there is excessive replacement and hypermagnesemia, what ECG changes would occur?

magnesium and eliminating the excess magnesium in feces. More powerfully, the renal tubules resorb less magnesium, and a greater amount of magnesium is excreted in the urine. If these physiologic responses are inadequate, hypermagnesemia results.

Most cases of hypermagnesemia are caused by advanced renal failure, with a decreased glomerular filtration rate and a resultant rise in the serum value of magnesium. The effects of hypermagnesemia include a slowing of cardiac conduction as well as heart block, hypotension, muscle flaccidity, loss of deep tendon reflexes, and muscle paralysis. The toxic effects will appear when the serum value rises to greater than 4.9 mg/dl (SI, 2 mmol/L). At values greater than 14.6 mg/dl (SI, >6 mmol/L), respiratory paralysis, general anesthesia, and cardiac arrest will occur.

Purpose of the Test

The measurement of serum magnesium helps to evaluate electrolyte disorders, hypocalcemia, hypokalemia, and acid-base imbalance. It is also used to monitor patients who have a cardiac disorder because the low magnesium levels are dangerous. The test is also performed to monitor the pregnant patient with severe toxemia during the intravenous administration of magnesium sulfate.

Procedure

A red-topped tube is used to obtain 7 to 10 ml of venous blood.

QUALITY CONTROL

The tourniquet should be applied for no longer than 1 minute to avoid venous stasis. Venipuncture technique must be smooth, with a blood flow that fills the vacuum tube readily. If there is stasis or if the blood has excessive turbulence because of flawed venipuncture technique, the hemolysis of erythrocytes will cause a false elevation of the results.

Findings

ELEVATED VALUES
Advanced renal failure
Addison disease
Administration of multiple magnesium sulfate enemas
Excessive ingestion of magnesium-containing antacids
Magnesium sulfate infusion therapy

DECREASED VALUES
Early renal disease
Chronic glomerulonephritis
Chronic alcoholism
Hypercalcemia
Pancreatitis
Hemodialysis therapy
Pregnancy
Prolonged hyperalimentation
Diabetic ketoacidosis (during treatment)

Inadequate dietary intake
Malabsorption
Prolonged nasogastric drainage
Severe burns
Hypoparathyroidism
Hyperaldosteronism
Cisplatin therapy
Prolonged intravenous therapy

Interfering Factors

- Venous stasis
- Hemolysis

Nursing Implementation

Pretest

Instruct the patient to fast from food and fluids for 8 hours before the test.

Posttest

Send the specimen to the laboratory, without delay.

QUALITY CONTROL
To avoid the clumping of erythrocytes and invalid test results, the blood must be centrifuged quickly. The serum must then be refrigerated until it is analyzed.

MAGNESIUM, 24-HOUR URINE

(URINE)

Synonym:

Mg^+

―――――――――――― **NORMAL VALUES** ――――――――――――

7.3–12.2 mg/dl *or* SI 3–5 mmol/day

Background Information

The magnesium cation is derived from the intake of food. Most of the magnesium cation is stored in soft and hard tissues and a small amount is maintained in homeostatic balance in the serum and extracellular fluid. The excess dietary intake is not absorbed and is eliminated in feces. The kidneys maintain major control of the serum level by conserving magnesium in tubular resorption processes or eliminating the excess in the urine (Fig. 20–2).

In normal physiologic function, an excess of serum magnesium causes the renal tubules to resorb less, resulting in a greater amount of magnesium in the urine. A low level of serum magnesium causes the renal tubules to resorb more magnesium, resulting in less of the cation in the urine.

In pathophysiologic processes, an excess of magnesium in the urine can be caused by damage to the renal tubules, with a failure to resorb the magnesium. As a result of the renal loss, the serum value can become low. A low level of magnesium in the urine can be caused by advanced renal failure with an inability of the glomeruli to filter out the magnesium from the blood. If the magnesium does not enter the nephrons, it does not appear in the urine. There are also other diverse causes of excess or reduced magnesium in the urine.

The physiology of magnesium is not fully understood, and its measurement by laboratory analysis is not standardized. There is little of this cation present in the serum because so much of it is stored in the soft tissue, muscle, and bone. When the serum value is abnormal, the urine is usually tested to obtain additional data. One of the problems of urine testing is that there is little agreement regarding the normal range of urine values. Because the normal values vary among laboratories and geographic regions, the reference value of a particular laboratory may vary from the value listed in this text.

Purpose of the Test

This test is used to determine the amount of magnesium present in the urine, particularly when there is a low serum magnesium value. It is also used to help evaluate the effect of kidney disease.

Procedure

A 24-hour specimen is collected in a large plastic, acid-washed container.

Findings

ELEVATED VALUES

Chronic renal disease
Chronic alcoholism
Ingestion of excess magnesium
Diuretic therapy

Addison disease
Bartter syndrome
Cisplatin therapy

DECREASED VALUES

Advanced kidney failure
Diabetic acidosis
Pancreatitis
Primary aldosteronism

Acute or chronic diarrhea
Starvation
Dehydration
Malabsorption

Interfering Factors

- Contact of urine with metal
- Loss of part of the urine specimen
- Failure to refrigerate the specimen

Nursing Implementation

Pretest

Instruct the patient to use the special laboratory container to collect the urine. If a bedpan or urinal is used for voiding, it must be made of plastic, not metal.

To begin the test, instruct the patient to void and discard the 8 A.M. specimen. For the next 24 hours, all urine is saved, including the 8 A.M. specimen of the next morning.

Instruct the patient to refrigerate the specimen container throughout the test period.

Posttest

Label the bottle with the patient's name and the time and date of the start and completion of the test.

Arrange for prompt transport of the chilled specimen to the laboratory.

PHENYLALANINE, BLOOD

(BLOOD)

Synonyms:

Phe, PKU test, phenylalanine screening test, Guthrie screening test

---

NORMAL VALUES

GUTHRIE TEST
<2 mg/day/L *or* SI 121 µmol/L
FLUOROMETRY METHOD
Normal Newborn: 1.2–3.4 mg/dl *or* SI 73–206 µmol/L
Premature Newborn: 2–7.5 mg/dl *or* SI 121–454 µmol/L
Adult: 0.8–1.8 mg/dl *or* SI 48–109 µmol/L

Background Information

Critical Thinking:
After drinking chocolate milk at school, a 7-year-old child with PKU has a slightly elevated blood phenylalanine level. This is not the first time that she has eaten prohibited foods. How can the nurse help the child follow her diet?

In normal amino acid metabolism, the enzyme phenylhydroxylase is needed to convert phenylalanine to tyrosine. When this enzyme or its cofactor BH_4 is absent, the level of phenylalanine and phenylpyruvic acid, a phenylalanine metabolite, rises in the blood and urine.

Phenylketonuria (PKU) is an inherited disorder of amino acid metabolism that is characterized by elevated levels of phenylalanine and phenylpyruvic acid. Unless there is early detection and proper dietary intervention, the elevated blood level of phenylalanine will cause central nervous system damage and mental retardation. The possible panic range of the Guthrie test is 4 mg/dl or higher (SI, 242 µmol/L). Within 10 days of birth, a newborn with undetected and untreated hyperphenylalaninemia may have a serum level of 15 to 30 mg/dl (SI, 907–1815 µmol/L).

The phenylalanine level is not elevated at birth because there has been no dietary intake of protein. In the infant who has a defect in amino acid metabolism, the serum level begins to rise within 24 hours after starting to feed with milk or formula. The ideal time to screen the blood for phenylalanine is 48 to 72 hours after birth or 2 days after the newborn begins to feed.

State laws require PKU testing of all newborns within a specified period. If the blood phenylalanine test is performed in the first 24 hours of life, the test should be repeated after feeding has begun. The repeat test would greatly reduce the chance of a false-negative result.

The blood phenylalanine test is a screening tool that only identifies hyperphenylalaninemia. Further testing is needed to verify the cause of the elevated blood level. If there is an elevated result, the test is repeated in 24 hours to ensure accuracy.

Premature or low-birth-weight infants have higher serum values than do full-term, infants of normal weight. This "false-positive" serum elevation is caused by immaturity of the liver. Antibiotics also interfere with the Guthrie method of analysis and cause a "false-positive" result.

Purpose of the Test

The blood phenylalanine test is performed to detect PKU and other causes of hyperphenylalaninemia. It is also used to monitor patients who have PKU and are being maintained on a phenylalanine-restricted diet.

Procedure

A heelstick puncture is used to obtain a few drops of blood. The blood sample is collected by capillary tube or PKU card or filter paper. The circles are filled by blotting the blood onto the paper.

QUALITY CONTROL

With the filter paper or card, only one side of the paper is blotted to fill the circles. The paper should not be turned over to soak the other side. Cord blood cannot be used for this test.

Findings

ELEVATED VALUES

PKU   Severe burns
Hyperphenylalaninemia   Liver disease
Sepsis   Galactosemia

Interfering Factors

- Little to no ingestion of milk
- Insufficient quantity of blood
- Antibiotics

Nursing Implementation

Pretest

Ensure that the laboratory requisition slip includes the name, date, time of the test, date of birth, and time of the first milk feeding. Note the administration of antibiotics or blood transfusion.

Posttest

Arrange for prompt transport of the specimen to the laboratory.

PHENYLALANINE, URINE

(URINE)

Synonym:
PKU urine test

NORMAL VALUES

FERRIC CHLORIDE METHOD
Green color is positive for phenylpyruvic acid.
PHENASTIX METHOD (URINE REAGENT DIP STRIP)
Persistent blue-gray to green-gray color is positive for phenylpyruvic acid.

Background Information

In normal amino acid metabolism, phenylalanine is converted to tyrosine. The enzyme phenylalanine hydroxylase and other cofactors must be present for this conversion to take place. Normal renal function provides for glomerular filtration of the amino acids, with tubular resorption of the filtrate.

When the enzyme or its cofactors are absent, and there is an intake of protein as the source of amino acids, the levels of phenylalanine and phenylpyruvic acid (the phenylalanine metabolite) rise in the blood. The increase of amino acids in the plasma concentration results in an increase in glomerular filtration, but the renal tubules cannot resorb all the excess. Thus, the overflow of phenylalanine and phenylpyruvic acid is excreted in the urine.

PKU is one type of aminoaciduria. It is an inherited disorder of amino acid metabolism caused by the absence of phenylalanine hydroxylase. If the condition remains undetected or uncontrolled by dietary therapy, damage to the central nervous system and mental retardation will occur.

Phenylpyruvic acid is not present in the urine at birth because there must first be an intake of protein from breast milk or infant formula. If the amino acid metabolism is impaired, there will be a rapid rise of phenylalanine in the blood. This can be detected readily by the serum phenylalanine test, which is the primary screening test for PKU.

In hyperphenylalanemia, the presence of phenylpyruvic acid is not detectable in the urine for 2 to 6 weeks after birth. Once the serum level of phenylpyruvic acid rises to 10 to 20 ng/dl, the metabolite appears in the urine. Because of the time delay, the phenylalanine urine test is not used as an initial screening test for PKU.

Purpose of the Test

The urine phenylalanine test is used to assist in the detection of hyperphenylalanemia, including PKU. The test is also used to monitor the effect of dietary treatment for patients who have a defect in amino acid metabolism.

Procedure

A freshly voided specimen of urine is collected in a plastic urine collection container.

Findings

ABNORMAL VALUES
PKU
Non-PKU hyperphenylalanemia

Interfering Factors

- Inadequate labeling
- Improper collection procedure
- Diluted urine

Nursing Implementation

Pretest

For testing infants and small children, teach the mother to apply the urine collection bag and transfer the urine to a collection container.

Posttest

Ensure that the time and date of voiding are written on the label and requisition slip.
Arrange for the transport of the urine to the laboratory within 1 hour.

PHOSPHORUS

(SERUM)

Synonyms:
P, inorganic phosphate, $PO_4^=$

Background Information

Phosphorus is a mineral element that is present in bone cells and extracellular fluid, including serum. The dietary intake of phosphorus is partially absorbed by

━━━━━━━━━━ **NORMAL VALUES** ━━━━━━━━━━

SERUM PHOSPHORUS (P)

Adult (12–60 Years):	2.7–4.5 mg/dl *or* SI 0.87–1.45 mmol/L
(>60 Years):	2.3–3.7 mg/dl *or* SI 0.74–1.2 mmol/L
Child (2–12 Years):	4.5–5.5 mg/dl *or* SI 1.45–1.78 mmol/L
(10 Days–2 Years):	4.5–6.7 mg/dl *or* SI 1.45–2.16 mmol/L
Infant (0–10 Days):	4.5–9 mg/dl *or* SI 1.45–2.91 mmol/L
Premature Infant (1 Week):	5.4–10.9 mg/dl *or* SI 1.74–3.52 mmol/L
Cord Blood:	3.7–8.1 mg/dl *or* SI 0.85–1.5 mmol/L
PLASMA PHOSPHATE (PO₄⁼):	
Adult:	8.2–14.5 mg/dl *or* SI 0.85–1.5 mmol/L

the small intestine and provides the renewing source of the mineral. The homeostatic balance of the mineral in the extracellular fluid is maintained by the actions of parathyroid hormone, calcitonin, and vitamin D. Excess phosphorus is excreted in the feces and urine.

There is an inverse relationship between the serum levels of phosphorus and calcium. If the serum level of either mineral falls, the serum level of the other mineral rises.

The homeostatic regulation of serum phosphorus is based on the body's ability to detect alterations in the level of serum phosphorus and adjust accordingly. In hypophosphatemia, the kidneys possess the most rapid and best ability to raise the serum level by an increase of tubular resorption and a reduction of the urinary excretion of the mineral. The small intestine also responds by absorbing more phosphorus.

In the extracellular fluid, most phosphorus is present in the form of free phosphate ions, and the small remainder is bound to plasma proteins. Most of the body content of phosphorus is not in the plasma, however, but is stored in bone as a component of the bone matrix. The mineral is stored and used as part of new bone formation. As bone resorption or bone turnover occurs, the phosphorus is rereleased into the extracellular fluid.

Serum phosphorus concentrations have a diurnal rhythm. The level is highest in the morning and lowest in the evening. The normal values also vary over a life span, with the highest serum values occurring in infants and children and the lowest values occurring in elderly individuals.

HYPERPHOSPHATEMIA. This is defined as a fasting serum phosphorus level greater than 4.7 mg/dl (SI, >1.5 mmol/L) in the adult. Severe hyperphosphatemia causes hypocalcemia, with hypotension and tetany from the calcium depletion. The most common cause of the hyperphosphatemia is a decreased glomerular filtration rate from acute or chronic renal failure. The renal failure is usually in an advanced stage, with a loss of about 75% of glomerular filtration, before the serum phosphorus level rises (Bourke & Yanagawa, 1993). Other sources of hyperphosphatemia include conditions that cause increased tubular resorption in the kidneys and diseases that cause increased bone turnover, releasing more phosphorus into the extracellular fluids.

HYPOPHOSPHATEMIA. This condition is of serious consequence because it can affect neuromuscular, neuropsychiatric, skeletal, gastrointestinal, and cardiopulmonary function. Symptoms of organ dysfunction appear when the serum value falls to less than the critical level of 1 mg/dl (SI, 0.32 mmol/L).

Purpose of the Test

Serum phosphorus helps diagnose kidney disorders and acid-base imbalance. It is also used to detect disorders of calcium, bone, or endocrine origin.

Procedure

A red-topped tube is used to collect 7 to 10 ml of venous blood. For infants and small children, a heelstick puncture and capillary tube are used to collect a blood sample.

QUALITY CONTROL

Venipuncture technique must be smooth, with a blood flow that fills the vacuum tube readily. If the blood has excessive turbulence because of flawed technique, the hemolysis of the erythrocytes will alter the results.

Findings

ELEVATED VALUES

Renal failure
Hypovolemia
Dehydration
Milk alkali syndrome
Acromegaly
Osteolytic metastatic bone
   cancer
Sarcoidosis

Cirrhosis of the liver
Pulmonary embolism
Diabetes, ketoacidosis
Vitamin D toxicity
Respiratory acidosis
Lactic acidosis
Postanesthesia hyperthermia
Hypoparathyroidism

DECREASED VALUES

Osteomalacia
Osteoblastic bone cancer
Acute gout
Vitamin D deficiency
Renal tubular disease
Severe malabsorption
Starvation
Respiratory alkalosis

Acute respiratory infection
Prolonged intravenous glucose
   therapy
Prolonged nasogastric drainage
Hyperparathyroidism
Serum calcium elevation
Vomiting, diarrhea
Sepsis

Interfering Factors

- Hemolysis
- Carbohydrate-rich meals
- Recent phosphate enema

Nursing Implementation

Pretest

Schedule the test for early morning.

Instruct the patient to discontinue all food and fluids for 8 hours before the test.

QUALITY CONTROL

It is best to obtain a fasting specimen because carbohydrate intake and recent food intake tend to decrease the serum phosphate level. Early morning hours are used to obtain the blood to avoid the diurnal fluctuations.

Do not administer a phosphate enema just prior to the test because some of the phosphate is absorbed by the colonic mucosa.

Posttest

Arrange for prompt transport of the specimen.

QUALITY CONTROL

A delay in centrifuge of the specimen results in a false rise of the serum value.

PROSTATE-SPECIFIC ANTIGEN

(SERUM)

Synonym:

PSA

─── **NORMAL VALUES** ───

Male (15 Years and Older):
0.81 ± 0.89 ng/ml *or* SI 0.81 ± 0.89 µg/L

TABLE 20–1
ABNORMAL VALUES OF PROSTATE-SPECIFIC ANTIGEN

Condition	Laboratory Values
Male with benign prostate hypertrophy	10.2 ± 8.97 ng/ml *or* SI 10.2 ± 8.97 µg/L
Prostate cancer	
Stage A	9.39 ± 8.09 ng/ml *or* SI 9.39 ± 8.09 µg/L
Stage B	17.45 ± 16.83 ng/ml *or* SI 17.45 ± 16.83 µg/L
Stage C	55.14 ± 51.65 ng/ml *or* SI 55.14 ± 51.65 µg/L
Stage D	118.92 ± 50 ng/ml *or* SI 118.92 ± 50 µg/L

Background Information

Prostate-specific antigen is a tumor marker for adenocarcinoma of the prostate gland. This antigen is an enzyme that is manufactured exclusively by the prostate gland, establishing its specificity and usefulness in detecting abnormal prostatic tissue growth. Prostate-specific antigen is produced by the epithelial cells of the gland in normal, benign hypertrophy and malignant prostate conditions, but the amount of the enzyme varies with each type of condition (Table 20–1).

BENEFITS. The best use of the prostate-specific antigen test is to monitor patients after treatment for adenocarcinoma of the prostate gland. The test is highly predictive of residual or recurrent disease after treatment by radical prostatectomy, radiation therapy, or antiandrogen treatment. Following treatment, the patient is monitored by the prostate-specific antigen test for a number of years. It will detect renewed malignant growth in localized or distant metastatic sites long before the recurrence can be detected by all other diagnostic methods (Saito, 1993).

In 1994, the Food and Drug Administration approved the use of prostate-specific antigen as a screening tool for prostate cancer when the prostate-specific antigen test is used together with the digital rectal examination. In combination, the abnormal results are valid indicators for a biopsy of the prostatic tissue. About 50% of the patients who are positive for both the prostate-specific antigen and digital rectal examination will actually have prostate cancer (*New York Times*, 1994).

LIMITATIONS. Even though this is the first and only organ-specific tumor marker and it is a valuable test in specific situations, the test has some problems of reliability and specificity. By itself, prostate-specific antigen cannot be used as a cancer screening tool for the healthy male population because it is not specific enough to consistently distinguish between benign and malignant conditions.

The recent Food and Drug Administration decision regarding the prostate-specific antigen–digital rectal examination as an approved screening tool raises concerns about the cost of testing (and follow-up biopsy) when the test, even in combination, still has a high false-positive rate.

The prostate-specific antigen test lacks specificity to distinguish between benign prostatic hypertrophy and an early stage of prostatic malignancy (Oester-ling, 1991). As seen in Table 20–1, the elevated value for benign prostatic hypertrophy may be in the same range as the value for stage A of the malignant growth.

Prostate-specific antigen cannot be used by itself to stage the malignancy. As seen in Table 20–1, the abnormal values often rise proportionately with the severity or extent of the malignancy. This correlation, however, is not always consistent or reliable, particularly in the early stages of the malignancy. The prostate-specific antigen test is used together with digital examination, other tumor marker tests, and radionuclide bone scanning to stage the prostatic adenocarcinoma (Chybowski, 1991).

Purpose of the Test

As a tumor marker for adenocarcinoma of the prostate gland, the test is used most effectively to monitor the postsurgical patient who has had a radical prostatectomy. It is used to evaluate for recurrence or residual tumor and helps identify the need for additional treatment. In combination with the digital rectal examination, it is recommended as a screening tool for all men over the age of 50 years and for men over the age of 40 years who have additional risk factors, including African-American men and men who have a positive family history of prostate cancer.

Procedure

A red-topped tube is used to collect 7 to 10 ml of venous blood.

Findings

ELEVATED VALUES
Adenocarcinoma of the prostate
Benign prostatic hypertrophy
Prostatitis
Urinary retention
Prostatic infarct

Interfering Factors

• Recent urethral instrumentation

Nursing Implementation

Pretest

Schedule the test at least 2 weeks after any urethral instrumentation procedure such as a transurethral resection, prostatic biopsy, or cystoscopy because these procedures will cause a release of the prostate-specific antigen (Oesterling, 1991).

Since a fasting specimen is preferred (Jacobs et al., 1990), instruct the patient to discontinue food intake for 8 hours before the test.

Posttest

Arrange for prompt transport of the specimen to the laboratory.

QUALITY CONTROL

Once the blood is centrifuged and the serum extracted, the serum is stable at room temperature for 24 hours. Thereafter, it must be stored at −20° C or less.

PROSTATIC ACID PHOSPHATASE

(SERUM, VAGINAL SECRETIONS)

Synonyms:

PAP, acid phosphatase

NORMAL VALUES

SERUM	
4-Nitrophenyl Phosphate Method	
at 37° C (Male):	0.13–0.63 U/L
Tartrate Resistance Fraction (Male):	0.2–3.5 U/L *or* SI 2.2–10.5 U/L
Thymolphthalein Monophosphate	
Method at 37° C:	<1.9 U/L
VAGINAL SECRETIONS:	<2 U/L

Background Information

Acid phosphatase is an enzyme that is present in high concentrations in the prostate gland and its secretions. In the serum, its value is elevated in association with metastatic cancer of the prostate, but it is more likely to remain in a normal range during the early stage of the disease. The normal value varies with the method of analysis used.

There are other acid phosphatase isoenzymes present in body tissues, including platelets, erythrocytes, liver, spleen, and bone marrow. These tissue sources can also release small amounts of prostatic acid phosphatase into the serum and cause a false elevation of the serum value (Oesterling, 1991).

SERUM. For many years, prostatic acid phosphatase was used as a tumor marker to diagnose and help stage adenocarcinoma of the prostate gland, but there were problems of accuracy and reliability (Saito, 1993). In addition to nonprostate sources of the enzyme, the values may be elevated because of a bone or metabolic disorder. Today, the prostate-specific antigen test has surpassed the prostatic acid phosphatase test in the diagnosis and evaluation of carcinoma of the prostate gland. The prostatic acid phosphatase test is still used with the prostate-specific antigen test in the evaluation and staging of metastatic prostate cancer. The tartrate-resistant method of analysis remains an important diagnostic test for hairy cell leukemia.

VAGINAL SECRETIONS. Prostatic acid phosphatase is present in prostatic secretions and therefore in semen. In cases of alleged rape, the vaginal secretions are tested for acid phosphatase as part of the forensic laboratory testing. Following coitus, the acid phosphatase level of the vaginal secretions rises from a normal low level to a value greater than 50 U/L (Henry, 1991).

Purpose of the Test

Acid phosphatase is used to assist with the staging of metastatic adenocarcinoma of the prostate gland. After treatment for the malignancy, it assists in the evaluation for recurrence of the disease.

Procedure

A red- or purple-topped tube with ethylenediaminetetraacetic acid or acid phosphatase anticoagulant is used to collect 7 ml of venous blood.

QUALITY CONTROL

Venipuncture technique must be smooth, with a blood flow that fills the vacuum tube readily. If the blood has excessive turbulence because of flawed venipuncture technique, the hemolysis of the erythrocytes will alter the results.

Findings

ELEVATED VALUES

Metastatic cancer of the prostate
Gaucher disease
Niemann-Pick disease
Benign prostatic hypertrophy
Metastatic cancer of bone

Hairy cell leukemia
Hemolytic diseases
Advanced Paget disease
Prostatitis
Prostatic infarct

Interfering Factors

• Hemolysis

- Warming of the specimen
- Failure to maintain a nothing-by-mouth status
- Lipemia

Nursing Implementation

Pretest

To avoid a false-positive elevation, schedule this test several days after any diagnostic test that manipulates the prostate gland (transurethral resection, bladder catheterization, digital examination).

Instruct the patient to discontinue all food and fluids for 8 hours before the test because lipemia interferes with the laboratory analysis.

Posttest

Arrange for prompt transport of the specimen to the laboratory.

QUALITY CONTROL

The blood must be centrifuged promptly and the serum tested or put on ice for rapid cooling. If the specimen is warmed, within 1 hour the serum value will be lowered falsely.

PROTEIN ELECTROPHORESIS, 24-HOUR URINE

(URINE)

Synonym:

urine protein electrophoresis

───────────────── **NORMAL VALUES** ─────────────────

40–150 ng/24 hours *or* SI 40–150 mg/24 hours
No monoclonal gammopathy (M protein) noted

Background Information

Normally, there is a small amount of protein in the urine. About one third of it is albumin and the remainder consists of plasma proteins, including many small globulins.

When excessive protein appears in the urine, the causes can be broadly categorized as glomerular disorders, tubular disorders, or overflow proteinuria. In the first two categories, the problems are related to renal damage. The third category is characterized by excessive protein produced by nonrenal disease. The proteins are filtered by the glomeruli, but the large amount prevents the tubules from effective resorption. Thus, there is an "overflow" of protein into the urine.

Protein electrophoresis is a laboratory method used to identify the predominant proteins in the urine. In abnormal glomerular permeability, albumin, alpha$_1$-proteins, and transferrin are predominant. In tubular proteinemia, alpha$_2$- and beta$_2$-microglobins are predominant.

The Bence-Jones protein is one of the proteins of overflow proteinuria. Its presence in the urine is associated with multiple myeloma, macroglobulinemia, and malignant lymphoma. Protein electrophoresis analyzes for the presence of monoclonal gammopathy (M protein). On the electrophoresis pattern, the M protein is demonstrated by a sharp spike in the globulin region.

Purpose of the Test

Protein electrophoresis of the urine is used to identify the different types of protein loss in the urine and to evaluate patients with known or suspected multiple myeloma.

Procedure

A single voided specimen of urine is placed in a clean urine container.

Findings

ABNORMAL VALUES

Glomerular-Pattern Proteinuria
Glomerular diseases
Nephrotic syndrome
Overflow-Pattern Proteinuria
Multiple myeloma
Macroglobulinemia of Waldenström
Lymphoma
Amyloidosis
Tubular-Pattern Proteinuria
Falconi syndrome
Cystinosis
Wilson disease
Pyelonephritis
Renal transplant rejection

Interfering Factors

• Hematuria

Nursing Implementation

Pretest

Instruct the patient to collect a routine urine specimen.
Instruct female patients to collect the urine at a time when there is no menstrual flow.

Posttest

Refrigerate the urine until it is transported to the laboratory.

URIC ACID

(URINE)

Synonyms:

NORMAL VALUES

Average Diet (Adult):	250–750 mg/24 hours *or* SI 1.48–4.43 mmol/24 hours
Low Purine Diet (Male):	<420 mg/24 hours *or* SI <2.83 mmol/24 hours
Low Purine Diet (Female):	<400 mg/24 hours *or* SI <2.36 mmol/24 hours
High Purine Diet (Adult):	<1000 mg/24 hours *or* SI <5.9 mmol/24 hours

---

Background Information

As an end product of protein metabolism, uric acid and urate crystals are excreted by the kidneys and bowel. Hyperuricosuria, a high level of uric acid in the urine, may be caused by excess secretion or excess production of uric acid.

URIC ACID EXCRETION. The excretion of uric acid is influenced by a number of normal variables. A high intake of purine foods results in a high level of uric acid excretion in the urine. Normal urine has a saturated level of uric acid, with urate crystals in the sediment of the urine. If the urine is acidic and concentrated, uric acid becomes insoluble and produces greater quantities of urate crystals. Abundant crystals form a thick sludge that can block renal tubules or cause uric acid stone formation.

URIC ACID PRODUCTION. Some pathologic conditions cause increased uric acid production and ultimately excess uric acid excretion. These conditions include metabolic abnormalities such as gout and glycogen storage diseases. Intestinal changes such as ileostomy or other intestinal diversions cause the urine to become acidic. The acidity increases the urinary precipitation of urate crystals.

When leukemia is treated with cytotoxic drugs or when malignant tumors are irradiated, there is tumor necrosis and a metabolic breakdown of nucleoprotein. The massive amount of uric acid and urate crystal production can cause an acute or dangerous elevation of the urine uric acid level. The urate crystals can block the renal tubules and ureters, resulting in renal failure.

If there is mild to severe renal failure or other kidney disease that inhibits renal function, the urinary excretion of uric acid will be low, even though there is normal to excessive uric acid production and a high serum uric acid level.

Purpose of the Test

Urinary uric acid measures the urinary excretion of uric acid in patients with renal calculi or those at risk for the development of a calculus. The test is also used to assess the effect of enzyme deficiency or metabolic abnormality that results in the overproduction of uric acid.

Procedure

A 24-hour urine collection is used to measure the amount of daily uric acid that is excreted.

Findings

ELEVATED VALUES

Uric acid nephrolithiasis	Viral hepatitis
Gout	Glycogen storage disease
Leukemia, chronic myeloid	Lesch-Nyhan syndrome
Acute leukemia of childhood	Radiation therapy
Lymphatic leukemia	Crohn disease
Lymphosarcoma	Ulcerative colitis
Wilson disease	Ileostomy
Cystinosis	Surgical jejunoileal bypass
Sickle cell anemia	Polycythemia vera
Tumor lysis syndrome	

DECREASED VALUES

Chronic glomerulonephritis	Collagen disease
Diabetic glomerulosclerosis	Lead toxicity
Folic acid deficiency	Xanthinuria

Interfering Factors

• Failure to collect all urine during the test period

- Failure to store the specimen properly
- High or low purine diet
- Many medications (including aspirin, antiinflammatory drugs, diuretics, vitamin C, and x-ray contrast medium)

Nursing Implementation

Pretest

Instruct the patient to collect all urine of the test period and store it in a large container. Some laboratories require the specimen to be refrigerated or stored on ice during the test period. Other laboratories do not require refrigeration, but the specimen container has sodium hydroxide added to maintain alkalinity of the urine. This prevents precipitation of urate crystals in an acid medium.

During the Test

Critical Thinking:
The patient's 24-hour urine collection is underway when you notice that there is no written documentation about the time that the test started. How can you resolve this problem?

Discard the 8 A.M. specimen and then start the test. All urine is collected for 24 hours, including the 8 A.M. specimen of the following morning.
Ensure that the label and requisition slip contain the patient's name and the time and date of the start and finish of the test.

Posttest

List all medications taken by the patient on the requisition slip.
Arrange for transport of the specimen to the laboratory.

URINE PROTEIN, 24-HOUR

(URINE)

Synonyms:

───────────────── **NORMAL VALUES** ─────────────────

40–150 mg/24 hours *or* SI 40–150 mg/24 hours

Background Information

Protein is minimally present in the urine of individuals with normal renal function. The urinary proteins consist of albumin and many small globulins. In normal renal anatomy and physiology, the albumin molecules are quite large and most cannot be filtered through the glomerular membrane. The smaller globulins are filtered by the glomeruli, but most are resorbed by the proximal tubules. Additional glycoproteins are secreted by cells in the distal tubules and the ascending loop of Henle. These minimal losses of protein into the urine are considered to be normal protein losses.

Urinary protein levels can increase after strenuous exercise, with salt depletion, or during a period of dehydration or febrile illness. These events cause a higher level of proteinuria but are not considered to be indications of renal or urinary tract disease.

When proteinuria is detected by urinalysis, it is an indicator of renal disease. As a follow-up study, the 24-hour specimen measures the amount of protein in the urine. Repeat tests may be performed to determine if the problem is intermittent or persistent. Additional tests of renal function, urine sediment, and urine culture are also performed to assess for renal disease or urinary tract infection (Henry, 1991).

Purpose of the Test

The urine protein test is used to help confirm the presence of renal disease.

Procedure

A 24-hour urine specimen is collected in a large, clear glass or plastic container.

Findings

ELEVATED VALUES

Glomerulonephritis	Renal transplant rejection
Tubular necrosis	Chronic pyelonephritis
Nephrotic syndrome	Diabetic glomerulosclerosis
Renal failure	Urinary tract infection
Toxemia of pregnancy	Multiple myeloma
Congestive heart failure	Malignant hypertension

Interfering Factors

- Contamination of the specimen with mucus, vaginal or prostatic secretions, or white cells
- Dilute urine from excessive fluid intake
- Failure to collect all urine
- Warming of the specimen

Nursing Implementation

Pretest

Instruct the patient to collect all urine for a 24-hour period. The specimen must be refrigerated or kept on ice throughout the test period.

Advise the patient to drink a regular amount of fluids during the test period.

QUALITY CONTROL

Excessive fluid intake will dilute the urine and give a false-negative value.

During the Test

Have the patient void at 8 A.M. and discard the urine.

The test period starts at this time and all urine is collected for 24 hours, including the 8 A.M. specimen of the following morning.

Ensure that the patient's name and the time and date of the start and finish of the test are written on the label and requisition slip.

Posttest

Keep the specimen refrigerated until it is transported to the laboratory.

DIAGNOSTIC PROCEDURES

ANGIOGRAPHY, RENAL

(RADIOGRAPHY)

Synonyms:

The arterial circulation to the kidneys and within the kidneys is visualized by using an iodinated contrast medium and radiography. The contrast material is administered via a femoral or brachial artery. An arterial catheter is passed through the aorta and into the right and left renal arteries. As the dye is injected via the catheter, timed, rapid x-ray films are taken to visualize the arterial circulation and tissue perfusion.

Arterial circulatory impairment includes aneurysm, arteriosclerosis, renal artery stenosis, and renal artery infarction. Abnormalities of renal tissue include chronic pyelonephritis, renal abscess, tumor, cyst, pseudotumor, and hematoma.

A complete discussion of angiography is presented in Chapter 11.

BIOPSY, PROSTATE

(TISSUE BIOPSY)

Synonyms:

core biopsy of the prostate gland, fine needle aspiration biopsy of the prostate gland

──────── **NORMAL VALUES** ────────

Normal prostate tissue with no evidence of tumor or infection

Background Information

Prostate cancer usually consists of multiple tumors that originate in the peripheral area of the prostate gland. The majority of these cases are adeno-carcinomas.

A biopsy of the prostate gland is indicated when there is a palpable nodule; alteration in size, shape, or texture of prostate tissue; abnormal findings on ultrasound of the prostate, or elevated blood levels of the tumor markers prostatic acid phosphatase or prostate-specific antigen.

The microscopic study of the biopsy tissue confirms the diagnosis. If it is malignant, the tissue sample provides the identification of the tumor type, including the tumor grading and local staging of the cancer. The data identify the biologic behavior of the tumor and help determine the best method of treatment (Yazdi, 1991).

There are a number of methods that can be used to obtain the biopsy sample. An open biopsy means that the peritoneal area is incised and a wedge of prostate tissue is removed surgically. The tissue sample may also be obtained during a transurethral resection procedure. Each of these methods requires general or spinal anesthesia.

Needle aspiration biopsy is performed via a transrectal or perineal approach. Ultrasound may be used during the procedure to guide the placement of the needle and confirm the presence of the needle in the tumor tissue (Fig. 20–3). A core biopsy procedure uses a larger needle (14 to 18 gauge) that may be attached to an automated core biopsy gun. The core biopsy needle has a higher accuracy rate in establishing the diagnosis. A fine needle aspiration biopsy uses a narrow, flexible prostatic aspiration needle (23 gauge). One advantage of the fine needle is the ability to biopsy small nodules (Narayan et al., 1991).

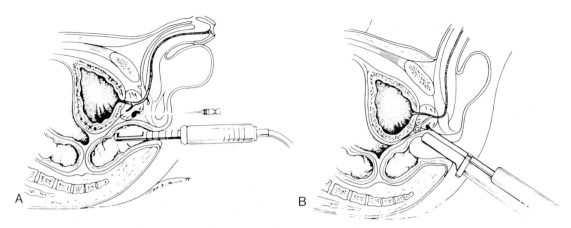

FIGURE 20-3. Ultrasound-guided prostate biopsy. *A,* Transperineal approach. *B,* Transrectal approach. (Reproduced with permission from Muldoon, L., & Resnick, M.I. [1989]. Results of ultrasonography of the prostate. *Urologic Clinics of North America, 16,* 699.)

A needle biopsy can result in tumor tracking or tumor seeding. This means that as a result of the needle being inserted into the tumor, the malignant cells can grow into the needle track or extend into surrounding prostate tissue (Bastacky et al., 1991).

Purpose of the Test

A prostate biopsy is used to determine the cause of an enlarged prostate gland and to diagnose prostate cancer.

Procedure

Using aseptic technique and local anesthesia to the perineum, a needle is inserted into the prostate tumor. Suction or a syringe is used to aspirate several samples of the tissue.

Findings

ABNORMAL VALUES

Cancer of the prostate gland
Benign prostatic hypertrophy
Lymphoma
Prostatitis

Interfering Factors

- Failure to maintain a nothing-by-mouth-status
- Acute prostatitis

Nursing Implementation

Pretest

Instruct the patient regarding the procedure and obtain written consent from the patient or person legally designated to make the patient's health care decisions.

Inform the patient to take a disposable phosphate (Fleet) enema on the night before or in the early morning. No food or fluids are permitted for 12 hours before the test in preparation for possible anesthesia (Narayan et al., 1991).

Assist the patient in removing all clothes and putting on a hospital gown.

Have the patient void to empty the bladder.

Place the patient in the lithotomy position.

During the Test

For the transperineal approach, assist with the preparation of the local anesthetic. It will be injected by the physician into the perineal area between the scrotum and the rectum.

Provide comfort and reassurance to the patient who is anxious and afraid. Momentary pain is felt as the anesthetic is injected. Additionally, there is worry about the possible diagnosis.

Place the biopsy specimen in a sterile container with a preservative such as formalin or Zenker's fluid. In some cases, cultures or tissue slides are prepared immediately. Label all specimens with the patient's name and the tissue source.

Send the specimens to the laboratory without delay.

Apply an adhesive bandage to the perineal biopsy site. No dressing is used for the transrectal approach.

Posttest

Take vital signs and record the results. If general anesthesia was used or if the patient is unstable, continue monitoring the vital signs at regular intervals.

Assess for pain and offer pain medication as needed.

Observe the biopsy site for signs of bleeding into the dressing or into local tissue.

Assess for difficulty in voiding or hematuria.

Instruct the patient to take the prescribed antibiotic for 2 days to prevent infection.

Complications

Biopsy of the prostate is considered a safe procedure, with an overall complication rate of 2% (Bastacky et al., 1991). The most common complication

TABLE 20–2
COMPLICATIONS OF BIOPSY OF THE PROSTATE

Complication	Nursing Assessment
Sepsis	Redness
	Localized swelling
	Fever
	Pain
	Purulence
Bladder or urethral puncture	Hematuria
	Frequency
	Urinary retention
Bleeding	Ecchymosis
	Hematoma
	Swelling
	Pain
	Hematuria

of this procedure is infection, particularly in patients who had unknown prostatitis or a history of rheumatoid disorder (Yazdi, 1991). It is also possible for the biopsy needle to penetrate the bladder or prostatic urethra or for bleeding to occur.

The complications of prostate biopsy are presented in Table 20–2.

BIOPSY, RENAL

(TISSUE BIOPSY)

Synonyms:

kidney biopsy, fine needle aspiration biopsy of the kidney

─────────────── **NORMAL VALUES** ───────────────

Normal renal tissue is present, with no indication of inflammation, fibrosis, necrosis, or tumor cells.

Background Information

Biopsy of the kidney provides specific information regarding the pathophysiologic changes in the tissue. The need for biopsy is determined on an individualized case basis. Other laboratory tests and noninvasive procedures are performed first to obtain as much diagnostic information as possible. The broad categories of pathophysiologic conditions that require renal biopsy include acute renal failure, renal tumor, renal transplant rejection, transplant failure, asymptomatic hematuria, proteinuria of unknown origin, or questions regarding drug toxicity and untoward reaction to medication.

In acute renal failure, the pathologic changes have many possible causes, with variation among patients as to the location and severity of the change. The type of renal failure is categorized by the location of the pathologic change, including *prerenal failure* caused by reduced circulation to the kidneys, *postrenal failure* caused by obstruction to the flow of urine, and *intrarenal (parenchymal) failure* caused by damage to the glomeruli, tubules, or interstitial tissue (Jennette & Falk, 1990). Renal biopsy is used to investigate intrarenal failure.

Needle biopsy is also performed to diagnose renal cancer. It is used when computed tomography (CT) or magnetic resonance imaging (MRI) findings are inconclusive, to investigate metastatic disease or recurrence of cancer, and to diagnose the type of renal tumor in the patient who is a poor surgical risk. With fine needle aspiration biopsy, there is a small risk that the tumor will disseminate along the needle track, but research demonstrates that this complication does not affect the 5-year survival rate (Yazdi, 1991).

In renal transplant patients, the donor kidney can show signs of transplant rejection. Without biopsy, early accurate diagnosis of rejection is difficult because of other possible causes of renal dysfunction that produce the same symptoms. Fine needle aspiration biopsy is minimally invasive and can be used repeatedly on the same patient (Simpson et al., 1991).

Critical Thinking:
The 15-year-old student with end-stage renal disease has a nursing diagnosis of *Ineffective individual coping related to loss of health.* Develop some expected outcomes for change that can start to be implemented during the hospitalization.

Purpose of the Test

Renal biopsy is used to determine the exact pathologic state and diagnosis of the renal disorder, monitor the progression of the renal disease, evaluate the response to treatment, and assess for rejection of the renal transplant.

Procedure

After administration of local anesthesia, a biopsy needle is inserted percutaneously or through a small incision in the lower back. While the needle is advanced into the kidney, ultrasound or x-ray films are used to guide the exact placement and location. A syringe is used to aspirate a small core of tissue from the renal cortex. The total time needed to obtain the specimen is about 15 minutes. In the laboratory, the tissue is prepared and examined by light, immunofluorescent, and electron microscopy (Moore and Carome, 1993).

Findings

ABNORMAL VALUES
Acute or chronic glomerulonephritis
Goodpasture syndrome
Amyloid infiltration of the kidney
Systemic lupus erythematosus

Renal transplant rejection or failure
Renal cell carcinoma
Wilms tumor

Interfering Factors

- Failure to maintain a nothing-by-mouth status
- Coagulation disorder
- Urinary tract infection
- Nonfunction of one kidney

Nursing Implementation

Pretest

Inform the patient about the procedure and obtain a written consent from the patient or person legally responsible for the patient's health care decisions.

Ensure that all screening tests are completed and that the results are posted in the patient's chart. Coagulation studies, including prothrombin time, activated partial thromboplastin time, platelet levels, and hematocrit, are performed to verify clotting ability. Urinalysis identifies the presence of any infection. An intravenous pyelogram or renal scan demonstrates renal function in both kidneys.

Take baseline vital signs and record the results.

During the Test

Cleanse the skin of the lower back with antiseptic.

Provide reassurance to the patient to help alleviate anxiety.

When the needle is to be inserted, instruct the patient to take a deep breath and hold it. Assist the patient in remaining still. There may be brief pain, but it is mild.

After the needle is removed, apply pressure to the puncture site for 20 minutes to help promote clotting.

Apply a sterile dressing and adhesive bandage to the puncture site.

Place the biopsy specimen in a sterile container with normal saline.

Ensure that the container is labeled with the patient's name and the tissue source of the specimen.

Arrange for immediate transport of the specimen to the laboratory.

QUALITY CONTROL

On arrival at the laboratory, the specimen must be fresh and moist to ensure accurate analysis.

Posttest

Take the vital signs every 15 minutes for 1 hour, every 30 minutes for the next hour, and at regular intervals thereafter.

At frequent intervals, observe the dressing and surrounding tissue for signs of bleeding.

For 8 hours, monitor each voided specimen for hematuria. Initially, a small amount of blood may be present, but it should disappear within the 8-hour period. In some institutions, the protocol is to collect every urine specimen separately, with a notation of the time and date of voiding written on the container. Over time, there should be progressively less blood, and the urine should return to its normal color.

Encourage the patient to drink extra fluids to help promote urination.

Eight hours after the test, ensure that a specimen for hemoglobin and hematocrit determinations is drawn. When bleeding is excessive, different time intervals and repeat testing may be necessary.

Instruct the patient to lie flat for 12 to 24 hours. A sandbag in the flank area may be used to help promote compression of the tissue. After this period of immobility, bed rest or limited activity is maintained for 24 hours to prevent the onset of fresh bleeding.

Instruct the patient to avoid physical exertion, heavy lifting, and trauma to the lower back for several days.

Complications

Although renal biopsy is considered safe, with a low complication rate, there are some risks to the procedure. Major complications occur in 0.75 to 1.4% of patients. These complications include perirenal hemorrhage, pneumothorax, and infection. The minor complication of microscopic hematuria occurs in 6.5% of patients (Espinel, 1993). A summary of the complications of renal biopsy appears in Table 20–3.

COMPUTED TOMOGRAPHY, KIDNEY

(TOMOGRAPHY)

Synonyms:
CT, CAT, CT scan

CT of the kidney produces many axial slices for imaging renal tissue. Tumors, cysts, and other lesions are clearly demonstrated. The scan can also be used to detect or evaluate calculi, obstruction, congenital abnormalities, infections, and polycystic disease. An iodine-based contrast medium is used to provide a sharp, clear image (Moss et al., 1992).

A complete discussion of CT is presented in Chapter 12.

TABLE 20–3
COMPLICATIONS OF RENAL BIOPSY

Complication	Nursing Assessment
Bleeding	Hematuria (microscopic or gross)
	Dizziness, weakness
	Pallor
	Falling hematocrit value
	Falling hemoglobin value
	Tachycardia
	Hypotension
	Pain (dorsal, flank, or shoulder)
Infection	Fever
	Burning on urination
	Urinary frequency
Pneumothorax	Dyspnea
	Cyanosis
	Hypotension
	Restlessness, apprehension

CYSTOSCOPY

(ENDOSCOPY)

Synonyms:

———————————————— **NORMAL VALUES** ————————————————

No anatomic or structural abnormalities are present.

Background Information

Cystoscopy provides direct visualization of the urinary bladder. When the urethra also is examined, the procedure is called cystourethroscopy.

The examination is performed with a cystoscope—a thin, lighted tube with a telescopic lens. The procedure may be performed in the urologist's office or in the operating room with local, spinal, or general anesthesia. Following the diagnostic component, treatment may include dilation of stricture, cauterization of bleeding spots, removal of superficial tissue, implantation of radium seeds, and placement of a ureteral stent or catheter.

Cystoscopy is used to investigate the cause of painless hematuria, particularly when cancer of the epithelial lining is suspected. It also is part of the investigation into the cause of urinary incontinence or retention. The examiner is able to visualize the location, extent, and exact nature of the problem.

Purpose of the Test

Cystoscopy is used to diagnose and evaluate structural and functional changes of the urinary bladder.

Procedure

Under local anesthesia, the cystoscope is inserted through the urethra into the urinary bladder. Once the bladder is filled with saline for irrigation, all aspects of the bladder walls are examined. Biopsy samples for tissue examination and cell washings for cytologic analysis may be carried out. Urine samples may be collected from the bladder or from each ureter. The procedure takes 30 to 45 minutes.

Findings

ABNORMAL VALUES

Cancer of the bladder
Diverticulum of the bladder
Bladder stones
Congenital anomaly
Cancer of the prostate
    gland

Polyps
Bladder fistula
Bladder neck stricture
Benign prostatic hypertrophy

Interfering Factors

- Failure to maintain a nothing-by-mouth-status
- Acute infection of the bladder, urethra, or prostate gland

Nursing Implementation

Pretest

Inform the patient about the procedure and obtain a written consent from the patient or person legally designated to make health care decisions for the patient.

When bowel emptying is part of the protocol, instruct the patient to administer an enema the night before or the morning of the test.

For general or spinal anesthesia preparation, instruct the patient to fast from food and fluid for 8 hours before the procedure. For local anesthesia, fasting from food is required, but clear liquids on the morning of the test are permitted.

Take baseline vital signs and record the results.

Preoperative sedatives or antispasmodics may be prescribed.

During the Test

Provide reassurance to the patient who is awake during the procedure. The instillation of the local anesthetic into the urethra is mildly painful until the tissue becomes numb. When the bladder is filled with saline, discomfort and the urge to void are normal sensations.

Assist with the collection of specimens.

- The biopsy tissue is placed in a sterile glass container with formalin preservative.
- For the cytologic study, 50 to 75 ml of bladder irrigation fluid is placed in a sterile jar with 50% alcohol as a preservative. Identify the source of the fluid as bladder washings (Yazdi, 1991).

Assist with the collection of urine specimens and mark their source (bladder, right ureter, left ureter).

Posttest

Take vital signs and record the results. For patients who have undergone general anesthesia, continue monitoring the vital signs every 15 to 30 minutes until the patient is stable.

Assess for pain or bladder spasms and medicate as needed.

Encourage extra oral fluids to promote adequate hydration and the voiding of urine.

Instruct the patient to void within 8 hours after the test.

Reassure the patient that it is normal to have a burning sensation on voiding and to see a small amount of blood or pink-tinged urine. These problems should disappear after the third voiding.

At home, warm tub baths can help alleviate the discomfort or pain of bladder spasms. Instruct the patient to avoid alcohol for 48 hours because of its irritant effect on the bladder mucosa.

To prevent infection, instruct the patient to take the prescribed antibiotic for 1 to 3 days.

TABLE 20–4
COMPLICATIONS OF CYSTOSCOPY

Complication	Nursing Assessment
Bleeding	Persistent, painless hematuria Bright red urine Passage of blood clots
Urinary obstruction	Inability to urinate within 8 hours despite a full bladder and desire to void
Infection	Flank or abdominal pain Chills Fever Pyuria

Complications

The more common complications of cystoscopy are persistent bleeding, infection, and urinary retention. Because the patient usually goes home soon after the test, a review of abnormal problems should be provided and the patient advised to notify the urologist when these problems occur. The complications of cystoscopy are presented in Table 20–4.

INTRAVENOUS PYELOGRAM

(RADIOGRAPHY)

Synonyms:

IVP, excretory urogram, EUG, intravenous urography, IVU, IUG

─────── **NORMAL VALUES** ───────

There are no anatomic or physiologic abnormalities noted in the kidneys, ureters, or bladder.

Background Information

The intravenous pyelogram is a basic urologic procedure that uses contrast medium and radiography to visualize the anatomy and function of the urinary tract. The intravenous contrast material is filtered from the blood by the kidneys. The x-ray films demonstrate the contrast medium entering the renal pelvis of each kidney and then flowing through the ureters and into the bladder (Fig. 20–4).

When there is a time delay before the injected contrast medium reaches the renal pelvis, the delay is an indication of prerenal vascular obstruction or poor renal function. The x-ray films also demonstrate abnormalities of position, shape, size, or structure of the organs of the urinary tract. There is clear detail and precise location of a stricture, dilation, calculus, obstruction, tumor, or filling defect.

The role of the intravenous pyelogram is under some debate because of newer, more effective alternatives (Little et al., 1989). Alternatives include CT, ultrasound, and digital subtraction angiography. The contrast medium used in an intravenous pyelogram can be toxic to the kidney or can cause an allergic type of reaction that can be severe. Although studies indicate that the risks are few and not always serious, the intravenous pyelogram is not used as often as it once was.

Purpose of the Test

The intravenous pyelogram is used to evaluate the structure and function of the kidneys, ureters, and bladder. It assesses the cause of nontraumatic hematuria,

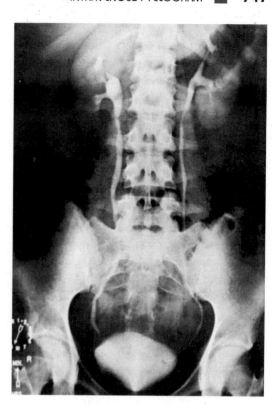

FIGURE 20–4. Intravenous pyelogram (IVP). The calyces of the kidneys, ureters, and bladder appear white because of the use of contrast medium. (Reproduced with permission from Thompson, M.A. [1994]. *Principles of imaging science and protection* [vol. 2, Slide 291A]. Philadelphia: W.B. Saunders.)

locates the precise site of obstruction, and investigates the cause of flank pain or renal colic.

Procedure

A scout film is taken to provide baseline information. After an intravenous injection of contrast material, timed radiographs are taken of the urinary tract. Films at 1 minute visualize the kidneys; at 3 to 5 minutes, the renal collecting system is visualized; at 10 minutes, the ureters are seen; and at 20 to 30 minutes filling of the bladder is seen. A postvoiding film demonstrates the ability of the bladder to empty. The test requires 1 to 1½ hours to complete.

Findings

ABNORMAL VALUES

Hydronephrosis
Hydroureter
Tumor
Renal tuberculosis
Congenital anomalies

Renal or ureteral calculi
Polycystic kidney disease
Pyelonephritis
Absent kidney
Nonfunctioning kidney

Interfering Factors

- Renal failure
- Feces, gas, or barium in the colon
- Recent gallbladder series
- Failure to maintain a nothing-by-mouth status

Nursing Implementation

Pretest

Ask the patient about any history of allergy to shellfish or iodine or a previous reaction to an x-ray study that used contrast medium.

Schedule the intravenous pyelogram before any barium test or gallbladder series that also used iodinated contrast material.

Explain the procedure to the patient and obtain a written consent from the patient or person legally designated to make health care decisions for the patient.

Instruct the patient regarding the pretest bowel cleansing procedure that removes gas and fecal matter. This includes taking the prescribed laxative or cathartic the night before the test and an enema or suppository on the morning of the test.

Instruct the patient to discontinue food intake for 8 hours before the test. Fluids are permitted.

QUALITY CONTROL

Patients who are dehydrated are at high risk for the development of renal failure as a result of the toxic effect of the contrast medium on the kidney tissues. Adequate hydration before and after the test is essential (Little et al., 1989).

Ensure that recent blood urea nitrogen and creatinine test results are posted in the chart. These tests help identify patients who are at risk and help determine a safe dose of contrast medium.

Record baseline vital signs.

During the Test

Assist the patient as the contrast medium is administered. It is common for the patient to experience a brief burning sensation or a metallic taste, or both. Up to 50% of patients will experience nausea or vomiting (Little et al., 1989).

Posttest

Take the vital signs and record the results.

TABLE 20–5
COMPLICATIONS OF INTRAVENOUS PYELOGRAPHY

Complication	Nursing Assessment
Vasovagal response	Flushing
	Hypotension
	Bradycardia
Allergic-type reaction	Hives, rash
	Urticaria
	Flushing
	Hypotension
	Tachycardia
	Dyspnea
	Stridor
	Laryngospasm
Nephrotoxicity	Elevated blood urea nitrogen level
	Elevated creatinine
	Oliguria

Continue the intravenous fluid replacement and encourage the patient to take oral fluids.

Complications

During the test, a small number of patients have a vasovagal response to the contrast material. Atropine is kept on hand to overcome this side effect. An allergic or anaphylactic response can occur immediately or hours later. This response varies from a rash and hives to acute respiratory distress. A mild reaction is treated with antihistamines or steroids. A severe reaction is treated with intravenous epinephrine and oxygen, with additional measures taken as needed. An emergency cart is maintained in the radiology suite at all times.

Impaired renal function can occur from 1 to 4 days after the study is completed. Most times it is a transitory problem and the kidneys return to their baseline level of function. Patients with a combination of diabetes and preexisting renal insufficiency are vulnerable to this complication (Cronan, 1991). A summary of the complications of intravenous pyelography is presented in Table 20–5.

MAGNETIC RESONANCE IMAGING, URINARY TRACT

(TOMOGRAPHY)

Synonym:

MRI

The role of MRI in urinary tract disorders is in evolution. Uses continue to be developed and findings validated, but it is not yet proved that MRI is better than CT or ultrasound in the imaging of the urinary system (Little et al., 1989).

It is not used to evaluate most urinary lesions but may be used when alternative tests fail to produce a clear image (Newhouse, 1991).

MRI produces a sharp image of the kidneys and can distinguish the renal cortex from the renal medulla. The vascular system can be imaged without the use of contrast material, and the staging of renal cell carcinoma is effective. Bladder tumors and their malignant extension into perivesicular fat or lymph nodes are shown clearly. The MRI can distinguish benign from malignant growth in the prostate and it can detect cancer invasion into seminal vesicles and pelvic lymph nodes.

A complete discussion of MRI is presented in Chapter 12.

PLAIN X-RAY FILM, RENAL TRACT

(RADIOGRAPHY)

Synonyms:

KUB; kidney, ureter, bladder

The plain x-ray film of the renal tract is a basic radiologic film that demonstrates the size, shape, and position of the organs of the renal tract. It can identify enlargement of the kidneys, as in hydronephrosis or tumor growth, and shrinkage of the kidney from chronic pyelonephritis or renal ischemia. Visible calcifications include calculi of the kidney, ureter, or bladder; renal tuberculosis; renal tubular acidosis; and calcifications in the bladder wall and ureters from the *Schistosoma* parasite.

A complete discussion of radiography is presented in Chapter 9.

RENAL SCAN

(RADIONUCLIDE IMAGING)

Synonyms:

The renal scan uses radionuclides to investigate renal failure and evaluate the function of the renal vascular system, the kidneys, and the ureters. The renal scan assesses the kidneys or renal transplant for adequacy of renal blood flow, tissue perfusion, glomerular filtration, tubular excretion, and ureteral function.

The scan can demonstrate the prerenal disorders of renal artery stenosis or occlusion. Within the kidney, renal perfusion, glomerular filtration rates, and tubular transport rates can be semiquantified. Intrarenal disorders identified by the renal scan include acute tubular necrosis, glomerulonephritis, vasculitis, and acute interstitial nephritis. The scan also demonstrates postrenal problems including obstruction of the ureter or ureters or ureterovesicular reflux.

A complete discussion of nuclear diagnostic tests is presented in Chapter 10.

RETROGRADE PYELOGRAPHY

(RADIOGRAPHY)

Synonyms:

The retrograde pyelogram provides radiographic visualization of the bladder, ureters, and renal pelvis following the retrograde instillation of sterile contrast medium into the renal collecting system. Generally, this procedure is used during or after cystoscopy or to evaluate the placement of a ureteral stent or catheter.

In the past, the procedure was used to diagnose postrenal obstruction. It was also an alternative imaging procedure when intravenous pyelography was not possible or when the intravenous pyelogram results were not clear. Today, because of improvements in the contrast medium used in intravenous pyelography and the use of ultrasound, retrograde pyelography is used much less frequently. Retrograde pyelography carries the risk of severe urinary tract infection and sepsis.

ULTRASOUND, RENAL

(ULTRASOUND)

Synonyms:

Renal ultrasound clearly defines the kidneys—their size, shape, position, collecting systems, and surrounding tissues. Renal masses greater than 2 cm are readily detected. Renal cysts are the most common finding (Little et al., 1989). The procedure also identifies the location and severity of obstruction with resulting hydronephrosis (Cronan, 1991). In addition to its diagnostic uses, renal ultrasound may be used as a guide for needle placement in renal biopsy, drainage of a renal abscess, or for placement of a nephrostomy tube.

A complete discussion of ultrasound is presented in Chapter 8.

ULTRASOUND, TRANSRECTAL

(ULTRASOUND)

Synonyms:

Transrectal ultrasound is a procedure that positions the ultrasound instrument and its high-frequency transducer in the rectum. The sound wave echoes are converted into images of the prostate gland. One use of ultrasound is to differentiate malignant from benign prostatic disease.

The malignant prostate gland is often enlarged and deformed. An irregular echo is a characteristic finding. Benign hyperplasia of the prostate gland shows an enlarged gland that is semilunar or circular. The wall of the capsule is thickened, and a regular echo is the characteristic finding (Watanabe, 1989).

Other uses of transrectal ultrasound include monitoring the size of the gland, staging prostate cancer, evaluating treatment, evaluating urodynamics, and providing visualization of the prostate gland during a prostate biopsy procedure (Lee et al., 1989) (Fig. 20–3).

A complete discussion of ultrasound is presented in Chapter 8.

UROFLOWMETRY

(MANOMETRY)

Synonyms:

NORMAL VALUES

GENDER	AGE RANGE	URINE VOLUME	FLOW RATE
Male	66–80 years	≥ 200 ml	9 ml/second
Female	66–80 years	≥ 200 ml	10 ml/second
Male	46–65 years	≥ 200 ml	12 ml/second
Female	45–65 years	≥ 200 ml	15 ml/second
Male	14–45 years	≥ 200 ml	21 ml/second
Female	14–45 years	≥ 200 ml	18 ml/second
Male	8–13 years	≥ 100 ml	12 ml/second
Female	8–13 years	≥ 100 ml	15 ml/second
Male	4–7 years	≥ 100 ml	10 ml/second
Female	4–7 years	≥ 100 ml	10 ml/second

Background Information

The broad category of urodynamic studies consists of several tests that evaluate voiding and lower urinary tract function. Uroflowmetry is the initial test that is performed to assess bladder and sphincter function. Generally, patients who need this test have incontinence or retention of urine.

Urinary incontinence is the involuntary leakage of urine through the urethral meatus. When incontinence is defined by its symptomatology, the problem is called urge incontinence, stress incontinence, or total incontinence. When the incontinence is defined by its cause, the problem is one of bladder storage, bladder emptying, or urinary sphincter dysfunction (Snyder and Lipsitz, 1991). In urinary retention or obstruction, the classification is one of bladder or urethral dysfunction.

Determination of the urinary flow rate is a noninvasive procedure that provides measurable baseline data about the patient's ability to void. The data measure the volume of urine voided, the pattern of micturition, and the time and rate of voiding. The patient's data are compared with normal micturition patterns and numeric values of the flow rate. When the patient's values are higher than normal, there is a problem of incontinence. When the patient's values are lower than normal, there is a problem of impaired urinary flow (O'Donnell, 1991).

In any person, the urinary flow rate varies with the volume of urine that is voided. The patient's results are compared with normal values based on the volume voided. The flow rate of any individual also varies from one voiding episode to another. The uroflowmetry test is repeated several times to obtain comprehensive data. Additionally, normal voiding rates vary between males and females and among different age groups across the life span. The interpretation of the patient's values is age- and gender-specific.

Purpose of the Test

Uroflowmetry is used to help evaluate lower urinary tract dysfunction.

Procedure

The patient urinates into a toilet that is equipped with a funnel and uroflowmeter. As voiding activates the uroflowmeter and its transducer, electronic data are received, transmitted, analyzed, and recorded. Specific variations in the procedure are based on manufacturers' variations in the equipment and laboratory protocol. The total time for completion of the test is 10 to 15 minutes.

Findings

ELEVATED VALUES
Conditions that cause reduced urethral resistance
Incontinence (stress, urge, or total)

DECREASED VALUES
Urethral or bladder neck obstruction
Poor muscular contraction of the bladder

Interfering Factors

- Body movement during voiding
- Toilet tissue in the apparatus
- Straining during urination

Nursing Implementation

Pretest

Instruct the patient to drink fluids and refrain from voiding for several hours before the test.

Ensure the patient's privacy for the test. The bathroom contains a toilet with the uroflowmeter installed in it.

Instruct the patient to void into the urometer funnel without straining or body movement. No toilet tissue is to be discarded into the funnel or collection container (Benner, 1990).

Posttest

No specific patient instruction or intervention is needed.

REFERENCES

Bastacky, S.S., et al. (1991). Needle biopsy associated with tumor tracking of adenocarcinoma of the prostate. *Journal of Urology, 145,* 1003–1007.

Benner, J. (1990). How I help the patient through urodynamic studies. *Urologic Nursing, 10,* 24–25.

Bourke, E., & Delaney, V. (1993). Assessment of hypocalcemia and hypercalcemia. *Clinics in Laboratory Medicine, 13,* 151–181.

Bourke, E., & Yanagawa, N. (1993). Assessment of hyperphosphatemia and hypophosphatemia. *Clinics in Laboratory Medicine, 13,* 183–207.

Chybowski, F. M. (1991). Predicting radionuclide bone scan findings in patients with newly diagnosed untreated prostate cancer: Prostate specific antigen is superior to all other clinical parameters. *Journal of Urology, 145,* 313–318.

Cronan, J.J. (1991). Contemporary concepts in imaging urinary tract obstruction. *Radiology Clinics of North America, 29,* 527–542.

Duarte, C.G., & Preuss, H.G. (1993). Assessment of renal function—Glomerular and tubular. *Clinics in Laboratory Medicine, 13,* 33–52.

Espinel, C.H. (1993). Diagnosis of acute and chronic renal failure. *Clinics in Laboratory Medicine, 13,* 89–102.

F.D.A. approves prostate blood test. (1994). *New York Times,* August 31, 1994, Section C, 9.

Finn, W.F. (1990). Diagnosis and management of acute tubular necrosis. *Medical Clinics of North America, 74,* 873–891.

Frank, S.H. & Resnick, M.I. (1989). Urolithiasis in primary care. *Primary Care, 16,* 967–979.

Henry, J.B. (Ed.). (1991). *Clinical diagnosis and management by laboratory methods* (18th ed.). Philadelphia: W.B. Saunders.

Jacobs, D.S., et al. (Eds.). (1990). *Laboratory test handbook* (2nd ed.). Baltimore: Williams & Wilkins.

Jennette, J.C., & Falk, R.J. (1990). Diagnosis and management of glomerulonephritis and vasculitis. *Medical Clinics of North America, 74,* 893–906.

Lee, F., et al. (1989). Diagnosis of prostate cancer by transrectal ultrasound. *Urologic Clinics of North America, 16,* 663–673.

Little, D.N., Thompson, M.E., & Thompson, D.E. (1989). The diagnostic evaluation: History, physical examination, urinalysis, and imaging. *Primary Care, 16,* 857–871.

Moore, J., & Carome, M.A. (1993). Proteinuria. *Clinics in Laboratory Medicine, 13,* 21–31.

Moss, A.A., Gamsu, G., & Genant, H.K. (Eds.). (1992). *Computed tomography of the body with magnetic resonance imaging* (2nd ed., vol. 2: Abdomen and pelvis). Philadelphia: W.B. Saunders.

Muldoon L., & Resnick, M.I. (1989). Results of ultrasonography of the prostate. *Urologic Clinics of North America, 16,* 693–702.

Narayan, P., et al. (1991). Core biopsy instrument in the diagnosis of prostate cancer: Superior accuracy to fine needle aspiration. *Journal of Urology, 145,* 795–797.

Newhouse, J.H. (1991). Clinical use of urinary tract magnetic resonance imaging. *Radiologic Clinics of North America, 29,* 455–474.

O'Donnell, P.D. (1991). Pitfalls of urodynamic testing. *Urologic Clinics of North America, 18,* 257–267.

Oesterling, J.E. (1991). Prostate specific antigen: A critical assessment of the most useful tumor marker for adenocarcinoma of the prostate. *Journal of Urology, 145,* 907–923.

Quamme, G.A. (1993). Laboratory evaluation of magnesium status: Renal function and free intracellular magnesium concentration. *Clinics in Laboratory Medicine, 13,* 209–223.

Saito, Y. (1993). Laboratory assessment of prostate status. *Clinics in Laboratory Medicine, 13,* 279–286.

Simpson, M.A., Madras, P.N., & Monaco, A. (1991). Immunologic heterogeneity among potential transplant recipients. *Clinics in Laboratory Medicine, 11,* 733–762.

Snyder, J.A., & Lipsitz, D.U. (1991). Evaluation of female urinary incontinence. *Urologic Clinics of North America, 18,* 197–209.

Teitz, N.W. (Ed.). (1990). *Clinical guide to laboratory tests* (2nd ed.). Philadelphia: W.B. Saunders.

Watanabe, H. (1989). History and applications of transrectal sonography of the prostate. *Urological Clinics of North America, 16,* 617–623.

Yazdi, H.M. (1991). Genitourinary cytology. *Clinics in Laboratory Medicine, 11,* 369–401.

CHAPTER 21

Reproductive Function

This chapter addresses the tests that are related to reproduction and childbearing. The span of diagnostic tests is extensive. Some are measurements of sexual maturation and others are assessments that are performed before conception, during pregnancy, during labor, or after delivery. Also included are diagnostic tests and procedures that investigate infertility, genetic alteration, hormonal imbalance, the effects of aging, and malignancy of the reproductive organs.

Patients who undergo tests that are related to reproduction represent the entire spectrum of the human life span. Because of new prenatal technology in diagnostic testing and treatment, the concept of life span has expanded to include the embryo and fetus.

The development of new diagnostic technologies and the expanded understanding of genetics have increased our knowledge and ability to identify causes of prenatal risk. Laboratory tests that are performed on cord blood provide direct diagnostic data about the fetus itself. This allows intervention and treatment at a much earlier stage of gestation than was possible in the past.

A number of the diagnostic tests and procedures include genetic analysis of the parents and family. The analyses may be performed before or after conception. The blood of the developing fetus also may be examined to detect an inherited or acquired genetic abnormality that could adversely affect growth and development. The results of genetic testing provide knowledge, but they do not always provide certainty about the eventual outcome and health status of the offspring.

Knowledge about the future can be a blessing for the prospective parents, but it can also create a painful burden or a serious dilemma for them. Prenatal diagnostic technology promotes outcomes based on "choice rather than chance." The diagnostic knowledge forces the prospective parents to make conscious, rational decisions and influences the path of life for the fetus (Satish, 1992).

The rapid advances in diagnostic testing also create ethical and legal dilemmas. Some of the advances are powerful enough to create eventual changes within society itself. In nursing, these advances also create changes in professional practice. There is an ongoing need for the nurse's knowledge to grow regarding the new diagnostic technologies. The nurse must also understand the implications of the findings for the patient.

During the period of diagnostic testing, the patient can experience anxiety. The fears are often related to the possible results of the tests and may also be related to the risk of the tests, such as potential harm to the pregnancy or fetus.

The patient may express feelings of depression, irritability, invasion of privacy, personal inadequacy, or even failure. The tests are often expensive and multiple, causing varying degrees of financial strain.

The interaction between the nurse and the patient can help alleviate the stress, correct misconceptions, and provide empathetic support as the patient makes decisions about treatment, the continuation or termination of the pregnancy, or the future health care needs of the child.

LABORATORY TESTS

ANDROSTENEDIONE

(SERUM)

Synonyms:

Background Information

Androstenedione is an androgen precursor hormone that converts to testosterone in the male and to estrogens in the female. It is synthesized by the adrenal cortex in males and females and is also synthesized in the ovaries of females. In normal physiology, the level of the hormone rises sharply after

━━━━━━━━━━━━━━━━ **NORMAL VALUES** ━━━━━━━━━━━━━━━━

ADULT	
Male:	75–205 ng/dl *or* SI 2.6–7.2 nmol/L
Female:	85–275 ng/dl *or* SI 3–9.6 nmol/L
CHILD	
10–17 Years:	8–240 ng/dl *or* SI 0.3–8.4 nmol/L
1–10 Years:	8–50 ng/dl *or* SI 0.3–8.4 nmol/L
1–12 Months:	6–68 ng/dl *or* SI 0.2–2.4 nmol/L
Newborn:	20–290 ng/dl *or* SI 0.7–10.1 nmol/L

puberty and peaks in the young adult. After menopause, the level decreases abruptly in women. The hormone has a diurnal pattern and peaks in the blood level about 7 A.M., with the lowest blood level at 4 P.M. each day.

The hirsute female experiences excessive growth of body hair, similar to the hair distribution of the male. An elevated level of androstenedione may be the cause of the virilization. The possible panic value of the hormone is an elevated level of more than 1000 ng/dl (SI, >34.9 nmol/L). This extreme level suggests a diagnosis of a virilizing tumor.

Purpose of the Test

This test may be used to evaluate androgen production in the hirsute female. It also may be used to identify the cause of gonadal impairment, menstrual irregularity, and premature sexual development.

Procedure

A red-topped tube is used to collect 7 ml of venous blood.

Findings

ELEVATED VALUES

Cushing syndrome
Congenital adrenal hyperplasia
Adrenal tumor
Ovarian tumor
Polycystic ovaries
Gynecomastia (in the male)
Ovarian hyperplasia

Stein-Leventhal syndrome
Endometriosis
Premature sexual development
  in the child
Osteoporosis
Hirsutism
Testicular tumor

DECREASED VALUES

Sickle cell anemia
Ovarian failure
Adrenal failure

Interfering Factors

- Menstruation
- Recent radioactive isotope scan

Nursing Implementation

Pretest

For the menstruating female, schedule the test at least 1 week before or 1 week after menstruation. For all patients, schedule this test before a nuclear scan because the radioisotopes of the scan would interfere with the method of laboratory analysis.

Instruct the patient that it is preferable to fast from food and fluids for 8 hours before the test (Jacobs, 1990). The blood should be drawn early in the morning (7 A.M.) because of the diurnal rhythm of the hormone.

Posttest

Place the specimen on ice and arrange for prompt transport. The laboratory analysis should be performed within 1 hour. If there is a delay, the serum is frozen until it can be analyzed.

CANCER ANTIGEN 125

(SERUM, BODY FLUIDS)

Synonym:
CA 125

──────────── NORMAL VALUES ────────────

<35 U/mL *or* SI <35 kU/L

Background Information

Cancer antigen 125 is a tumor marker for ovarian cancer. The serum antigen is produced by the genes of malignant cells and normal endometrial and uterine tissue. The antigen has a minimal presence in the blood and body fluids unless there is destruction of these tissues and release of the antigen from the cells. The antigen can be detected by laboratory radioimmunoassay methodology.

There are a variety of different malignant and benign disorders that cause a rise in cancer antigen 125. The level rises in the first trimester of pregnancy, during menstruation, and in some nonmalignant disorders. It also rises in gynecologic malignancy and in metastatic disease of a nongynecologic origin. In addition, the test does not always detect early stage ovarian cancer. Because of these variables, cancer antigen 125 cannot be used as a screening test for ovarian cancer (Jacobs et al., 1990).

Despite the problems with sensitivity and reliability that prevent its use for screening, cancer antigen 125 is valuable in selected situations. In the patient with a pelvic mass, a serum value >65 U/ml (SI, >65 kU/L) correlates well with pelvic malignancy. Additionally, a persistently rising value may be associated with advancing malignancy, particularly advanced ovarian cancer. Conversely, in the patient with known ovarian cancer, a decline in the cancer antigen 125 value indicates a good response to treatment.

In cases of suspected malignancy in the abdominal or pleural cavity, the body fluid obtained during paracentesis or thoracentesis may be analyzed for cancer antigen 125. The malignant cells of cancers of the pancreas and lung release this antigen into the fluid of the body cavity.

Critical Thinking:
The CA 125 level is elevated in a patient with a known history of ovarian cancer. The patient is aware of her diagnosis and the significance of this test result. What are potential ways of providing support for her during this difficult time?

Purpose of the Test

The serum cancer antigen 125 level is used to monitor the progress of disease in patients with ovarian cancer after the surgical removal of the tumor. The analysis of body fluids for cancer antigen 125 helps diagnose malignancy of an organ in the body cavity.

Procedure

Serum: A red-topped tube with a serum separator is used to collect 7 ml of venous blood.

Body Fluid: During the aspiration procedure, some of the body fluid is collected in three sterile tubes (red, green, and lavender tops). Because a series of tests will be performed on the specimens, there must be sufficient fluid available. Two of the tubes contain anticoagulant to prevent clotting by fibrinogen.

Findings

ELEVATED VALUES
Ovarian cancer
Adenocarcinoma of the cervix, endometrium, or fallopian tubes
Adenocarcinoma of the lung, colon, pancreas, or breast
Acute pelvic inflammatory disease
Pregnancy
Endometriosis
Menstruation
Ovarian-tubal abscess

Interfering Factors

• Inadequate specimen identification
• Recent radioactive isotope scan

Nursing Implementation

Pretest

Schedule this test before or at least 7 days after any radioimmunoassay scan. The radioisotopes of the scan would interfere with the radioimmunoassay method of analysis.

If this test is to be performed on a body fluid sample obtained by thoracentesis or paracentesis, follow the nursing care procedures described in Chapters 13 and 18 of this text.

For the patient with a history of cancer, provide empathetic support. Her anxiety level is likely to be high because of the implications of a potentially elevated test result.

Posttest

Before leaving the patient's bedside or the treatment table, ensure that the specimen tubes are correctly identified. When the specimen is a body fluid, ensure that the source of the fluid (thoracentesis or paracentesis fluid) is written on the requisition slip.

Arrange for prompt transport of the specimen to the laboratory.

QUALITY CONTROL

The serum must be separated from the cells quickly. It is frozen until it can be analyzed.

When the patient with a known history of cancer of the ovary has a rising or elevated level of cancer antigen 125, there is a high probability that the cause is progression or recurrence of the malignancy. Before new treatment is instituted, additional diagnostic testing (including surgery or biopsy, or both) to examine abnormal tissue is indicated (Jacobs, 1990). Provide additional emotional support to help the patient cope during the stress of additional testing and in the decision-making that is part of the overall treatment plan.

ESTRADIOL, SERUM

(SERUM)

Synonym:

E_2

Background Information

The ovaries, testes, and placenta are capable of the biosynthesis of all steroids, including the sex hormones. Estradiol is the most potent of the estrogen

ADULT
PREMENOPAUSAL FEMALE: 30–400 pg/ml *or* SI 110–1468 pmol/L
POSTMENOPAUSAL FEMALE: 0–30 pg/ml *or* SI 0–110 pmol/L
MALE: 10–50 pg/ml *or* SI 37–184 pmol/L

Critical Thinking:
Your female patient has started her infertility work-up. She expresses feelings of sadness because of the inability to conceive. What other assessment findings would validate a nursing diagnosis of self-esteem disturbance?

hormones. Estradiol is secreted by the ovaries in the female, and it is produced by the testes in the male. The estradiol level is sharply decreased or absent in postmenopausal women.

Purpose of the Test

The measurement of serum estradiol aids in the analysis and evaluation of female infertility, menstrual irregularity, amenorrhea, or sexual precocity in the child. In the male, this test may be used to help evaluate a feminizing condition.

Procedure

A red-topped tube is used to collect 7 ml of venous blood.

Findings

ELEVATED VALUES

Polycystic ovary	Adrenal tumor
Ovarian neoplasm or tumor	Gynecomastia
Hepatic cirrhosis	Hyperthyroidism

DECREASED VALUES

Anorexia nervosa	Amenorrhea
Ovarian dysfunction	Ovarian hypofunction

Interfering Factors

• Recent radioactive isotope scan

Nursing Implementation

Pretest

Schedule this test before or at least 7 days after radioimmunoassay scan. The radioisotopes of the scan would interfere with the radioimmunoassay method of analysis.

Posttest

To assist in the correct interpretation of the results, include the patient's age, phase of menstrual cycle, and the time that the test specimen was obtained.

Arrange for prompt transport of the blood to the laboratory.

QUALITY CONTROL

The serum must be extracted from the blood sample and frozen within 1 hour.

ESTRIOL, PREGNANCY

(SERUM, URINE)

Synonyms:

E_3; total serum estriol, pregnancy; total urine estriol, pregnancy

NORMAL VALUES

SERUM (TEITZ, 1990)	
Weeks of Gestation	
28–30 Weeks:	38–140 ng/ml *or* SI 132–486 nmol/L
32–34 Weeks:	35–260 ng/ml *or* SI 121–902 nmol/L
36–38 Weeks:	48–570 ng/ml *or* SI 167–1978 nmol/L
40 Weeks:	95–460 ng/ml *or* SI 330–1596 nmol/L
URINE (TEITZ, 1990)	
Weeks of Gestation	
28–30 Weeks:	5–18 mg/24 hours *or* SI 17–62 µmol/L
32–34 Weeks:	2–26 mg/24 hours *or* SI 24–90 µmol/L
36–38 Weeks:	10–36 mg/24 hours *or* SI 35–125 µmol/L
40 Weeks:	13–42 mg/24 hours *or* SI 45–146 µmol/L

Background Information

During pregnancy, estriol is the predominant estrogen present in the serum and urine. Because this hormone is synthesized by the placenta, the serum and urine values are considered a measure of the integrity and well-being of the fetal-placental-maternal unit. Because the normal serum values vary greatly according to the test methodology used, the nurse uses the reference values provided by the laboratory that performed the test.

Because serum levels rise progressively during a normal pregnancy, the number of weeks of gestation is a necessary consideration in the interpretation of the test result. The serum level of estriol also fluctuates in a diurnal rhythm, with the highest value occurring at midday. To increase the reliability of the test results, each test specimen is drawn at the same time of day. Because of the fluctuations in values, no single test specimen is used for interpretation. Instead, a series of test values are used to calculate the average test result.

When the serial test results are declining or are at a lower than normal level, the fetus is considered to be in danger. Immediate further investigation of the status of fetal health is indicated. This is particularly true in the high-risk pregnancy. The possible panic range for urinary estriol levels is less than 4 or 40% less than the average result. The average urinary result is calculated from the results of the three prior test results (Jacobs, 1990). Because there are alternative tests and technologic procedures that are better able to visualize the fetus or monitor for fetal distress, this test may not be used in most facilities.

Purpose of the Test

In the later stages of pregnancy, the results of the serial estriol tests are used to evaluate fetal well-being and placental function, especially in the high-risk pregnancy.

Procedure

Serum: A red- or green-topped tube is used to obtain 5 to 7 ml of venous blood from the pregnant female.

Urine: A special laboratory container is used to collect a 24-hour specimen.

Findings

DECREASED VALUES

Diabetes mellitus
Postmaturity
Preeclampsia
Erythroblastosis fetalis
Hemoglobinopathy

Fetal growth retardation
Fetal encephalopathy
Fetal adrenal aplasia
Intrauterine death

Interfering Factors

- Recent radioisotope scan.
- Improper urine collection procedure.
- Failure to collect all the urine of the test period.
- Failure to refrigerate the urine specimen.
- Improper labeling.

Nursing Implementation

Pretest

Urine Collection

Provide both written and verbal instructions regarding the collection of the urine. These instructions must include the specific times for the collection period.

During the Test

The first voided specimen of the morning is discarded and the urine collection period begins at 8 A.M.

The patient places all urine for 24 hours into the container. This includes the first voided specimen of the next morning.

Keep the specimen and container on ice or refrigerated during the collection period. This prevents deterioration of the urine.

During the collection period, all urine is added to the container. If any urine spills or if a specimen is discarded accidentally, the test is invalidated. The stored specimen is discarded and a new collection period is started on the following day.

Posttest

Serum and Urine

Label the urine container (not the lid) with the patient's name and other appropriate identifying data. Include the time and date of the start and completion of the urine collection period.

Include the weeks of gestation on the requisition slip of each test.

Arrange for prompt delivery of the specimen to the laboratory.

QUALITY CONTROL

For the serum specimen, the cells must be separated from the serum, and the serum is frozen immediately. The urine specimen must be refrigerated continuously until the urine is analyzed.

ESTROGEN-PROGESTERONE RECEPTOR ASSAY

(TISSUE BIOPSY)

Synonym:

ER-PgR

Background Information

The biopsy specimen of malignant breast tissue is tested to identify the presence of estrogen receptor sites and progesterone receptor sites. Although the

─────────── **NORMAL VALUES** ───────────

Negative:	<3 fmol/mg cytosol protein *or* SI <3 nmol/kg cytosol protein
Borderline:	3–10 fmol/mg cytosol protein *or* SI 3–10 nmol/kg cytosol protein
Positive:	>10 fmol/mg cytosol protein *or* SI >10 nmol/kg cytosol protein

Critical Thinking: The postmastectomy patient learns that her estrogen-progesterone assay result is positive. Which nursing interventions can help the patient as she considers the treatment option of hormonal therapy with tamoxifen?

name of the assay is written as a single entity, the tests are actually two different assays. One is for estrogen and the other is for progesterone. Generally, both tests are performed on the tissue sample to provide the most information regarding the potential effectiveness of hormonal therapy on the malignant tumor.

When the results of the estrogen receptor assay or of both the estrogen and the progesterone assays are positive, the tumor is likely to respond to androgen therapy or tamoxifen as a supplemental or palliative method of treatment. In each test, a value greater than 100 fmol/mg cytosol protein (SI, >100 nmol/kg cytosol protein) is considered strongly positive and has the best potential for an effective treatment result. The laboratory term "fmol/mg cytosol protein" or its SI equivalent is the measurement of the binding capacity of the protein that is present at the receptor sites. The test results are usually available 1 week after the biopsy is performed.

Purpose of the Test

The assay is used to identify primary or metastatic tumors of the breast that would respond favorably to hormonal therapy.

Procedure

A biopsy specimen of abnormal breast tissue is obtained and placed in a jar or waxed cardboard container. This jar or container is placed immediately in a larger container with ice.

Findings

POSITIVE VALUES

Breast cancer that may respond to hormonal therapy

Interfering Factors

- Use of a fixative on the tissue specimen
- Delay in transport of the specimen
- Inadequate tissue specimen

Nursing Implementation

Pretest

The pretest preparation of the patient is presented in the section on breast biopsy later in this chapter.

If the patient receives hormonal therapy for contraception, menopausal therapy, or antiestrogen therapy, these hormones should be discontinued before the breast biopsy is performed.

On the requisition slip, identify the source and site of the tissue (left or right breast).

During the Test

Ensure that the tissue is not fixed with a preservative and place the container on ice.

Deliver the specimen to the pathologist present in the operating suite or have the specimen sent to the laboratory. The specimen is sent as soon as it is obtained, without waiting for closure of the incision or completion of the biopsy procedure.

QUALITY CONTROL

The specimen must be prepared for frozen section within 15 to 30 minutes to prevent deterioration of the proteins at the receptor sites.

Posttest

The posttest nursing care consists of postoperative care for the patient with a breast biopsy.

ESTROGENS, 24-HOUR URINE

(URINE)

Synonym:

total urinary estrogens

Background Information

The ovaries, placenta, testes, and adrenal gland are capable of the biosynthesis of all steroids, including the sex hormones. The liver and many other organs metabolize and conjugate estrogen. Ultimately, the conjugated forms of estrogen are excreted in the urine or feces. Estradiol, estrone, and estriol are three estrogen hormones measured in the total urinary estrogen test. The amount and composition of the estrogens varies between the sexes and among age groups, based on differences of physiologic function.

=========== **NORMAL VALUES** ===========

Postmenopausal Female:	<20 µg/24 hours *or* SI 69 µmol/24 hours
Premenopausal Female:	15–80 µg/24 hours *or* SI 52–277 µmol/24 hours
Male:	15–40 µg/24 hours *or* SI 52–139 µmol/24 hours
Child:	<10 µg/24 hours *or* SI <35 µmol/24 hours

In the nonpregnant female, estradiol is the most potent estrogen, and it is secreted from the follicular fluid of the ovaries. Most estrone is produced by conversion of the adrenal steroidal hormone, but some is secreted from the ovaries or is converted from estriol. The amount of estrogen fluctuates during the menstrual cycle. The highest level occurs during the ovulation cycle. In pregnancy, estriol is produced by the fetal-placental unit.

The postmenopausal woman produces a lower amount of total estrogen because of the decreased estrogen secretion from the ovaries. The primary source of this woman's estrogen is the conversion of adrenal hormone to estrone. The testes of the male also produce some estrogen in the form of estradiol and some estrone.

Purpose of the Test

The measurement of urinary estrogen is used to evaluate ovarian function, predict ovulation, determine the cause of amenorrhea, evaluate excess or decreased estrogen conditions, or help diagnose a testicular tumor.

Procedure

A special plastic collection bottle with a boric acid preservative is used to collect all urine for a 24-hour period.

Findings

ELEVATED VALUES

Male	**Nonpregnant Female**
Testicular tumor	Ovarian tumor
	Adrenocortical tumor
	Adrenocortical hyperplasia

DECREASED VALUES

Ovarian dysfunction	Pituitary gland hypofunction
Ovarian insufficiency	Adrenal gland hypofunction
Menopause	Anorexia nervosa

Interfering Factors

- Improper storage of the specimen
- Incomplete collection of the urine

Nursing Implementation

Pretest

Provide both written and verbal instructions regarding the collection of urine. These instructions must include the specific times for the collection period.

During the Test

The first voided specimen of the morning is discarded and the urine collection period begins at 8 A.M.

All urine for a 24-hour period is placed in the container. This includes the first voided specimen of the next morning.

Maintain the specimen and container on ice or refrigerated during the collection period. This prevents deterioration.

During the time period, all urine is added to the collection container. If any urine spills or if a specimen is discarded accidentally, the test is invalidated.

Posttest

Label the urine container (not the lid) with the patient's name and other appropriate identifying data. Include the time and date of the start and completion of the urine collection period.

For the pregnant woman, include the weeks of gestation on the requisition slip. For all patients, include the patient's gender and age on the requisition slip.

Arrange for prompt delivery of the specimen to the laboratory.

QUALITY CONTROL

The urine specimen must be refrigerated continuously until the urine is analyzed.

FOLLICLE-STIMULATING HORMONE

(SERUM, URINE)

Synonyms:

FSH, follitropin

━━━━━━━━━━━━━━━━━━ **NORMAL VALUES** ━━━━━━━━━━━━━━━━━━

SERUM
Adult Male: 1–7 mU/ml *or* SI 1–7 U/L
Adult Female:
   Follicular phase: 1–9 mU/ml *or* SI 1–9 U/L
   Midcycle peak: 6–26 mU/ml *or* SI 6–26 U/L
   Luteal phase: 1–9 mU/ml *or* 1–9 U/L
   Postmenopausal
     phase: 30–118 mU/ml *or* SI 30–118 U/L
Child 6 Months–
10 Years: <1–3 mU/ml *or* SI <1–3 U/L
URINE
Adult Male: 4–18 U/24 hours *or* SI 4–18 U/24 hours
Female:
   Follicular phase: 3–12 U/24 hours *or* SI 3–12 U/24 hours
   Midcycle peak: 8–60 U/24 hours *or* SI 8–60 U/24 hours
Child 1–8 Years:
   Male: 0.5–4.5 U/24 hours *or* SI 0.5–4.5 U/24 hours
   Female: 0.5–4 U/24 hours *or* SI 0.5–4 U/24 hours
Child 13–14 Years:
   Male: 2–12 U/24 hours *or* SI 2–12 U/24 hours
   Female: 1–10 U/24 hours *or* SI 1–10 U/24 hours

Background Information

Follicle-stimulating hormone (FSH), like luteinizing hormone, is a gonadotropin manufactured by the anterior pituitary gland. This hormone is regulated by the hypothalamic gonadotropin-releasing hormone and by the serum levels of progesterone and estrogen in the female or by testosterone in the male (O'Brien, 1989). The target organs of FSH are the ovaries and testes. Often, the determination of the FSH level is carried out at the same time as the luteinizing hormone (LH) level because of the common source of tissue synthesis and action on target organs (Smith, 1992).

In the ovulating female, the FSH level is somewhat high in the preovulatory phase. Just prior to midcycle, it surges to a peak level. Thereafter, there is a sharp decline and maintenance of the lower level of FSH during the luteal phase. In both the male and female, as the FSH and LH levels suddenly rise, their combined function is to stimulate the granulosa cells of the ovaries or the Leydig cells of the testes. This assists with the maturation of the oocyte and spermatozoa.

The flow of FSH is described as pulsatile or intermittent throughout the day and night. For the female patient, some laboratories require three separate blood samples at 15- to 30-minute intervals. This provides control for the problem of episodic secretion. For the adult male, the secretion of FSH is somewhat episodic but not as much as in the female. In the young child, the FSH level is low and rises gradually with the onset of puberty. By midpuberty, the FSH level is equivalent to that of the adult.

Urinary collection may be used because the 24-hour collection period is not affected by the pulsatile, episodic variations that can alter the results of the blood test.

Purpose of the Test

The measurement of FSH is used to differentiate between primary and secondary gonadal failure of pituitary or hypothalamic origin. It is used to help diagnose gonadal dysfunction or failure, including delayed sexual maturation, menstrual disturbance, or amenorrhea. It is also used to evaluate infertility in the female and testicular dysfunction in the male.

The urinary values are most useful for children with precocious puberty. The urine study is also used to identify the time of ovulation when in vitro fertilization is planned.

Procedure

Serum: A red- or green-topped tube is used to collect 5 to 7 ml of venous blood.

QUALITY CONTROL

Venipuncture technique must be smooth, with a blood flow that fills the vacuum tube readily. If the blood has excessive turbulence because of flawed venipuncture technique, the hemolysis of the erythrocytes will alter the test results.

Urine: A large plastic urine container is used to collect all urine for 24 hours. Some laboratories recommend boric acid preservative and others do not.

Findings

Critical Thinking:
The rise in the FSH level confirms the onset of menopause in a 50-year-old patient. What manifestations of self-esteem disturbance can occur? How can the nurse help her?

ELEVATED VALUES
Primary testicular failure
Klinefelter syndrome
Idiopathic precocious puberty
Central nervous system lesion

Ovarian agenesis
Castration
Menopause
Orchitis

DECREASED VALUES
Polycystic disease of the ovary
Anterior pituitary hypofunction
Hypothalamic disorder
Congenital adrenal hypoplasia

Pregnancy
Anorexia nervosa
Adrenal tumor
Sickle cell disease

Interfering Factors

- Recent radioactive isotope scan
- Incomplete urine collection
- Inadequate preservation of the urine
- Hemolysis

Nursing Implementation

Pretest

Schedule this test before nuclear scan examination because the radioactive isotopes of the scan would interfere with the radioimmunoassay examination used in this test.

Urine Collection

Provide both written and verbal instructions regarding the collection of the urine. These instructions must include the specific times of the collection period.

During the Test

The first voided specimen of the morning is discarded, and the urine collection period begins at 8 A.M.

All urine is collected for 24 hours and placed in the container. This includes the first voided specimen of the next morning.

Maintain the specimen and container on ice or refrigerated during the collection period. This prevents deterioration.

All urine is added to the collection container during the 24 hours. If any urine spills or if a specimen is discarded accidentally, the test is invalidated.

Posttest

On the urine requisition slip, write the time and date of the start and completion of the test.

For both tests, write the date of the last menstrual period on the requisition slip.

For both the blood and urine tests, the specimen must be delivered to the laboratory without delay. The urine must be kept chilled or refrigerated. In the laboratory, FSH is stable for 4 hours at a cool temperature. Thereafter, the urine must be frozen until the analysis is performed. The blood is centrifuged to separate the serum from the cells. The serum is then frozen until the analysis is performed.

HUMAN CHORIONIC GONADOTROPIN, SERUM

(SERUM)

Synonym:

hCG

NORMAL VALUES

QUALITATIVE MEASUREMENT	Negative
QUANTITATIVE MEASUREMENT	
Male and Nonpregnant Female:	<5 mU/ml *or* SI <5 UL
Pregnant Female:	
1 week gestation:	5–50 mU/ml *or* SI 5050 UL
4 weeks gestation:	1000–30,000 mU/ml *or* SI 1000–30,000 UL
6–8 weeks gestation:	12,000–270,000 mU/ml *or* SI 12,000–270,000 UL
12 weeks gestation:	15,000–270,000 mU/ml *or* SI 15,000–270,000 UL

Background Information

Human chorionic gonadotropin (hCG) is a hormone normally produced by the developing placenta. In abnormal conditions, it is also produced by some germ cell malignancies and malignancy of other organs. This glycoprotein hormone consists of two subunits called alpha- and beta-hCG. The serum assay usually measures the beta subunit (Teitz, 1990).

The measurement of the beta subunit detects a normal pregnancy within 6 to 10 days after the fertilized egg is implanted. During the early part of a normal pregnancy, the amount of hCG shows a dramatic rise in the blood. The level generally peaks in the 7th to 10th week of gestation. Very high values suggest a multiple pregnancy. In ectopic pregnancy, however, the secretion of hCG is much lower and does not progress in the same pattern.

Benign or malignant trophoblastic disease is usually associated with an hCG level greater than 100,000 mU/ml (SI, >100,000 UL). The trophoblastic abnormalities include hydatiform mole, invasive mole, and choriocarcinoma. After surgical removal of a hydatiform mole, the serum level recedes and returns to normal within 8 to 12 weeks. Once the serum level is normal for several consecutive weeks, the patient is considered free of disease. The serum levels continue to be monitored monthly for 1 year.

Malignant trophoblastic diseases include an invasive mole or choriocarcinoma with or without metastases. These conditions are also monitored by beta-hCG levels. After the surgical removal of the hydatiform mole, a persistently elevated level of hCG or a return to an elevated level is an indication for additional diagnostic tests. Radiation therapy or chemotherapy may be needed.

Purpose of the Test

The serum measurement of hCG is used to detect an early pregnancy, help confirm the diagnosis of a trophoblastic disorder, and monitor the patient after the surgical removal of the tumor. In these postsurgical cases, the follow-up tests help evaluate the need for additional treatment.

Procedure

A red-topped tube is used to obtain 7 ml of venous blood.

QUALITY CONTROL

Venipuncture technique must be smooth, with a blood flow that fills the vacuum tube readily. If the blood has excessive turbulence because of flawed venipuncture technique, the hemolysis of the erythrocytes will alter the test results.

Findings

ELEVATED VALUES

Pregnancy
Islet cell neoplasm of the pancreas
Ovarian-testicular teratoma

Hydatidiform mole
Choriocarcinoma
Cancer of the lung, stomach, liver
  or colon

DECREASED VALUES

Ectopic pregnancy

Threatened abortion

Interfering Factors

- Recent radioactive isotope scan
- Hemolysis

Nursing Implementation

Pretest

It is preferable to schedule this test before or at least 7 days after a nuclear scan.

QUALITY CONTROL

Some laboratories use a radioimmunoassay method of analysis. If this method is used, the radioisotopes of the scan would interfere with the analysis and results.

Posttest

On the requisition slip, include the date of the patient's last menstrual period. This information is used to help determine whether the results are within normal limits.

Arrange for prompt transport of the specimen to the laboratory.

QUALITY CONTROL

Once the cells have been separated out, the serum can be maintained for 24 hours at a temperature of 2 to 8° C. If there is additional delay, the serum must be frozen.

HUMAN CHORIONIC GONADOTROPIN, URINE

(URINE)

Synonyms:

pregnancy test; beta subunit, human chorionic gonadotropin, urine; hCG

──────────────── NORMAL VALUES ────────────────

Male, Nonpregnant Female:	Negative
Pregnant Female:	Normal, positive

Background Information

Almost immediately after the fertilized ovum is implanted, hCG production and secretion begins. During the early phase of the pregnancy, the serum hCG rises rapidly and reaches a peak about 60 to 80 days after the last menstrual period. Thereafter, it tapers off a bit but is sustained at an elevated level throughout the pregnancy.

The urinary level of this hormone is also elevated in the same pattern as the serum level. Once the pregnancy is completed or terminated, the urinary value converts to negative within 2 weeks.

In addition to pregnancy, there are some malignancies that produce hCG. The serum and urine levels are elevated in these conditions.

Purpose of the Test

This urine test confirms pregnancy within 6 days of conception. If a teratogenic medication or treatment such as X-ray, chemotherapy, or radiotherapy must be given to a young, sexually active female, the test can screen for an unknown pregnancy before treatment begins.

Procedure

A clean plastic container is used to collect a first-voided morning specimen of urine.

Findings

Critical Thinking: In the third month of pregnancy, the patient's urinary hCG value declines sharply. Until the viability of the fetus can be determined, how can the nurse provide support to the patient?

POSITIVE VALUES

Pregnancy

Lung, colon, pancreatic, or stomach cancer

Melanoma

Choriocarcinoma

Ovarian tumor

Testicular tumor

Multiple myeloma

NEGATIVE VALUES

Threatened abortion

Ectopic pregnancy

Interfering Factors

- Hematuria
- Bacteriuria
- Proteinuria
- Detergent or soap in the specimen container

Nursing Implementation

Pretest

Instruct the patient to collect a single specimen of urine in the laboratory collection container. The urine should be from the first-voided morning specimen, collected on arising from sleep. This urine sample is more concentrated and would produce the most accurate result.

Posttest

Ensure that the container has a lid in place and that there is a label with correct identification on the container.

Arrange for prompt delivery of the urine to the laboratory.

QUALITY CONTROL

The urine is stable for 4 hours at room temperature. If there is a delay before analysis is performed, the laboratory can refrigerate the urine at 4° C for up to 3 days.

LUTEINIZING HORMONE

(SERUM, URINE)   *Synonyms:*

LH, lutropin

NORMAL VALUES

SERUM	
Adult Male:	1–8 mU/ml *or* SI 1–8 U/L
Adult Female:	
Follicular phase:	1–12 mU/ml *or* SI 1–12 U/L
Midcycle peak:	16–104 mU/ml *or* SI 16–104 U/L
Luteal phase:	1–12 mU/ml *or* SI 1–12 U/L
Postmenopausal:	16–66 mU/ml *or* SI 16–66 U/L
Child (6 Months–10 Years):	1–5 mU/ml *or* SI 1–5 U/L
URINE	
Adult Male:	9–23 U/24 hours
Adult Female:	4–30 U/24 hours
Male Child (1–10 Years):	<1–5.6 U/24 hours
Female Child (1–10 Years):	1.4–4.9 U/24 hours

Background Information

Luteinizing hormone is a gonadotropin synthesized and secreted by the anterior pituitary gland. The regulation of the flow of the hormone is carried out by hypothalamic gonadotropic-releasing hormone. Hypothalamic and pituitary control is influenced by the feedback of the serum levels of estrogen and progesterone in the female and testosterone in the male. The target organs of LH are the ovaries of the female and the testes of the male (O'Brien, 1989).

In the course of the menstrual cycle, the serum level of LH is low in the follicular phase. It surges to a peak at midcycle and then sharply decreases to a low level during the luteal phase. The LH preovulatory stimulus initiates ovarian activity, including progesterone production and the maturation of the oocyte. All these activities must occur before a mature oocyte is released in ovulation.

In the male, LH secretion is more episodic, with smaller surges throughout each day. LH is needed for the maturation of spermatozoa.

In the early years of childhood, the serum level of LH remains low. The LH concentration increases during puberty, and by the end of puberty it is equivalent to that of the adult.

The urine measurement of LH is used to detect the day of the LH surge in the preovulatory phase of the menstrual cycle. The test provides data on LH production without the variables of diurnal fluctuation.

The LH test is often performed with the FSH test. These hormones have similar structure and secretion patterns, and they are both manufactured by cells of the anterior pituitary gland.

Purpose of the Test

The measurement of LH is used to help diagnose gonadal dysfunction or failure, including delayed sexual development, amenorrhea, and menstrual irregularity. It also is used as part of infertility evaluation in the female and testicular dysfunction in the male (Smith, 1992).

Procedure

Serum: A red-topped or green-topped tube is used to collect 5 to 7 ml of venous blood.

Urine: A large bottle is used to collect urine for 24 hours. Some laboratories require the addition of boric, acetic, or hydrochloric acid. Other laboratories require no preservative in the bottle.

Findings

ELEVATED VALUES

Primary gonadal dysfunction
Post menopause
Castration

Polycystic ovary syndrome
Pituitary adenoma
Ovarian failure

DECREASED VALUES

Pituitary or hypothalamic syndrome
Malnutrition
Isolated gonadotropic deficiencies
Delayed puberty

Severe stress
Anorexia nervosa
Congenital adrenal hyperplasia
Adrenal tumor

Interfering Factors

• Recent radioactive isotope scan

Nursing Implementation

Pretest

Schedule this test before or at least 7 days after a nuclear scan.

QUALITY CONTROL

The measurement of LH is carried out by radioimmunoassay. The radioisotopes of the scan would interfere with the analysis and results.

Urine Collection

Provide both written and verbal instructions regarding collection of urine. These instructions must include the specific times for the collection period.

During the Test

The first-voided specimen of the morning is discarded and the urine collection period begins at 8 A.M.

All urine collected in the 24-hour period is placed in the container. This includes the first-voided specimen of the next morning.

Keep the specimen and container on ice or refrigerated during the collection period. This prevents its deterioration.

All urine collected during this period is added to the collection container. If any urine spills or if a specimen is discarded accidentally, the test is invalidated.

Posttest

On the urine requisition slip, write the time and date of the start and completion of the test.

For both tests, write the date of the last menstrual period on the requisition slip.

For both the blood and urine tests, the specimen must be delivered to the laboratory without delay. The urine must be kept chilled or refrigerated. In the laboratory, the urine must be frozen until the analysis is performed. The blood is centrifuged to separate the serum from the cells. The serum is then frozen or refrigerated until the analysis is performed.

PROGESTERONE

(SERUM)

Synonym:

P_4

Background Information

The androgenic sex hormone progesterone is synthesized in various body tissues. In the male and nonmenstruating female, the source is the adrenal gland and the conversion of pregnenolone and pregnenolone sulfate. In the menstruating female, it is produced by the ovaries. During pregnancy, progesterone is synthesized in great quantity by the placenta, and the serum level rises progressively throughout the term of the pregnancy.

In the menstruating female, the corpus luteum of the ovary produces a small but steady supply during the preovulatory or follicular phase of the menstrual

―――――――――――― **NORMAL VALUES** ――――――――――――

Adult Male:	13–97 ng/dl *or* SI 0.4–3.1 nmol/L
Menstruating Female:	
Follicular phase:	15–70 ng/dl *or* SI 0.5–2.2 nmol/L
Luteal phase:	200–2500 ng/dl *or* SI 6.4–79.5 nmol/L
Pregnant Female:	
7–13 weeks gestation:	1025–4400 ng/dl *or* SI 32.6–139.9 nmol/L
30–42 weeks gestation:	6500–22,900 ng/dl *or* SI 206.7–728.2 nmol/L

Critical Thinking: In the female, what are the possible psychologic effects of habitual abortion?

cycle. After ovulation, the progesterone level rises over a 4 to 5-day period in the luteal phase of the menstrual cycle. The serum level reaches and maintains its peak for about 1 week and then falls rapidly before the start of menstruation.

Progesterone functions to help prepare the endometrium of the uterus for the implantation of the fertilized ovum. To determine the day of ovulation, serial blood samples are obtained during the menstrual cycle.

Purpose of the Test

Serum progesterone levels are used to determine ovulation and to assess the function of the corpus luteum, particularly in cases of habitual abortion or infertility.

Procedure

A red-topped tube is used to obtain 7 ml of venous blood.

Findings

ELEVATED VALUES
Congenital adrenal hyperplasia
Molar pregnancy
Ovarian tumor

DECREASED VALUES
Threatened abortion
Short luteal phase syndrome

Interfering Factors

• Recent radioactive isotope scan

Nursing Implementation

Pretest

Schedule this test before or at least 7 days after a nuclear scan.

QUALITY CONTROL

The measurement of progesterone is performed by the radioim-munoassay method of analysis. The radioisotopes of the scan would interfere with the analysis and results.

When a series of blood tests throughout the menstrual cycle are required, make sure that the patient understands the testing plan and schedule of test dates.

Posttest

On the requisition slip, write the pertinent data, including the patient's sex, date of the patient's last menstrual period, and the trimester of pregnancy. These data are used to help determine whether the results are within normal limits. Arrange for prompt transport of the specimen to the laboratory.

QUALITY CONTROL

Once the cells have been separated out, the serum must be refrigerated or frozen.

PROLACTIN

(SERUM)

Synonyms:

PRL, lactogenic hormone, lactogen

─────────── **NORMAL VALUES** ───────────

Adult:	0–20 ng/ml *or* SI 0–20 µg/L
Pregnancy:	
First trimester:	<84 ng/ml *or* SI <84 µg/L
Second trimester:	18–306 ng/ml *or* SI 18–306 µg/L
Third trimester:	34–306 ng/ml *or* SI 34–306 µg/L
Lactating Mother:	<40 ng/ml *or* SI <40 µg/L
Child (12 weeks):	
Male:	5–15 ng/ml *or* SI 5–15 µg/L
Female:	5–25 ng/ml *or* SI 5–25 µg/L
Newborn:	<300 ng/ml *or* SI <300 µg/L

Background Information

Prolactin is a hormone produced by the anterior pituitary gland that is needed for lactation. Its production and release into the blood is controlled by the inhibiting and releasing factors of the hypothalamus and a number of other internal and external variables.

It has a diurnal rhythm; the serum level rises during sleep and is at its highest level several hours after waking. It rises progressively during pregnancy, and after delivery it returns to a baseline value in the woman who does not breastfeed. The hormone is usually mildly elevated in the breast-feeding mother. The hormone prolactin is at an elevated level in the fetus and neonate but declines to a normal level a few weeks after birth. Serum levels also can rise after stress, exercise, and during the venipuncture procedure.

The serum prolactin level can be less than normal because of damage to the pituitary gland. The low level would prevent lactation in the postpartum mother. In the male or female with excess flow of this hormone, the cause can be a problem in the hypothalamus, pituitary gland, or adrenal gland. The elevated level affects gonadal function and can cause galactorrhea (inappropriate lactation), anovulation, hirsutism, or infertility. A prolactin-secreting tumor causes a dramatic rise in the serum.

Purpose of the Test

The measurement of serum prolactin is used to evaluate oligorrhea, amenorrhea, or galactorrhea. It may assist in the diagnosis of pituitary gland or hypothalamic dysfunction.

Procedure

A chilled, red-topped tube is used to collect 7 ml of venous blood 3 to 4 hours after arising from sleep.

QUALITY CONTROL

Venipuncture technique must be smooth, with a blood flow that fills the vacuum tube readily. If the blood has excessive turbulence because of flawed venipuncture technique, the hemolysis of the erythrocytes will alter the test results.

Findings

ELEVATED VALUES

Hypothalamus-pituitary disease (sarcoidosis, metastatic cancer)
Hypothyroidism
Renal failure
Cirrhosis of the liver

Prolactin-secreting pituitary tumor
Acromegaly
Anorexia nervosa
Adrenal insufficiency

DECREASED VALUES
Pituitary infarction or necrosis

Interfering Factors

- Alcohol intake
- Failure to fast in the pretest period
- Recent radioactive isotope scan
- Warming of the specimen
- Hemolysis
- Sleep disturbance

Nursing Implementation

Pretest

Schedule this test before or at least 7 days after a nuclear scan.

QUALITY CONTROL

The measurement of progesterone is carried out by radioimmunoassay. The radioisotopes of the scan would interfere with the analysis and the results.

Instruct the patient to abstain from alcohol in the 24 hours before the blood is drawn and to fast from food for 8 hours before the test.

Schedule the blood to be drawn between 8 A.M. and 10 A.M. or 3 to 4 hours after arising from sleep. This helps to control for the diurnal fluctuations.

Posttest

Ensure that the blood is placed on ice immediately.
Arrange for prompt transport of the specimen to the laboratory.

QUALITY CONTROL

The cells must be separated from the serum by refrigerated centrifuge. The serum can be maintained for 24 hours at a temperature of 4° C. If there is additional delay before analysis, the serum must be frozen.

SEMEN ANALYSIS

(EJACULATE)

Synonyms:

sperm analysis, sperm count, seminal cytology

━━━━━━━━━━━━━━━━━━━ **NORMAL VALUES** ━━━━━━━━━━━━━━━━━━━

PHYSICAL ANALYSIS
Appearance: Opalescent gray-white color
Volume: 2–5 ml
Coagulation-Liquefaction: Coagulates rapidly; forms water droplets in 10–60 minutes
pH: 7.2–7.8
CHEMICAL ANALYSIS
  Acid phosphatase: >200 U per ejaculate
  Citric acid: >52 µmol per ejaculate
  Fructose: >13 µmol per ejaculate
  Zinc: >2.4 µmol per ejaculate
MICROSCOPIC ANALYSIS
  Motility: >50% sperm with moderate to rapid linear (forward) motion
  Concentration: $20–250 \times 10^6$ spermatozoa per ml of ejaculate
  Morphology: >50% of spermatozoa that have normal structure and shape
  Viability: >50% of spermatozoa are alive
  Leukocytes: $<1 \times 10^6$/ml of ejaculate

Background Information

Semen consists of secretions from the testes, epididymis, seminal vesicles, and prostate gland. The spermatozoa are produced in the testes and released into the semen. The semen serves as the transport medium for the mature spermatozoa.

In infertility, the analysis of the semen is usually the first test to be performed on the male. Infertility may result from a decreased amount of sperm, or oligospermia. Sterility results from nonviable sperm, or azoospermia. The semen specimen is examined for physical and chemical characteristics and then for microscopic visualization of the sperm and a leukocyte count. Because the concentrations of sperm can vary significantly, two to three samples are examined in a 2 to 3-month period.

PHYSICAL ANALYSIS. The semen is a liquid having a characteristic grayish white, opalescent color. Abnormal color changes can include red, often caused by blood, or yellow, as associated with certain drugs. Clear semen is often due to a low sperm count. The semen is usually somewhat viscous. It usually coagulates after ejaculation but then liquefies in about 30 minutes. The failure to liquefy after 60 minutes is abnormal. A greater than normal volume is associated with infertility (O'Brien, 1989).

CHEMICAL ANALYSIS. The pH of fresh semen is in the range of 7.2 to 7.8. A lower than normal pH is associated with a problem in the epididymis, vas

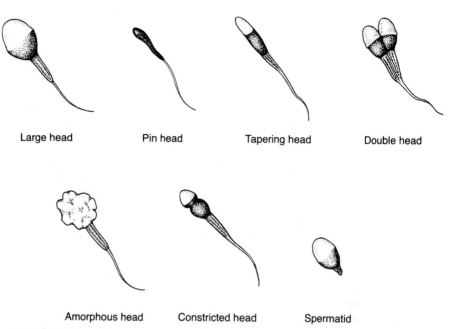

Large head   Pin head   Tapering head   Double head

Amorphous head   Constricted head   Spermatid

FIGURE 21-1. Abnormal sperm morphologic features. (With permission from Brunzel, N.A. [1994]. *Fundamentals of urine and body fluid analysis.* Philadelphia: W.B. Saunders.)

deferens, or seminal vesicles. A higher than normal pH is associated with infection. Seminal fluid fructose is a common clinical test in the analysis of semen. A normal value verifies the secretory ability of the seminal vesicles and the integrity of the ejaculatory ducts and vas deferens. A low fructose level is associated with a low sperm count. The levels of zinc, citric acid, and acid phosphatase are measures of the secretory ability of the prostate gland.

MICROSCOPIC EXAMINATION. The mobility of the sperm is an important characteristic because mobile sperm are able to reach the ovum. Both speed and linear (forward) progression are evaluated. The concentration is a measure of the quantity of sperm. Sperm counts of less than 20 million per ml or greater than 250 million per ml are abnormal and are associated with infertility. Sperm morphologic features or the measurement of the head, midpiece, and tail are part of the analysis for defects. Some of the common abnormal morphologic conditions are presented in Figure 21-1. When greater than 50% of the sperm have a normal structure, the sperm morphologic state is called normal.

The semen is also examined microscopically for viable sperm. In a fresh normal specimen, at least 50% of the sperm are alive. The ejaculate is examined for cells, particulate matter, and debris. When there are more than 1 million leukocytes present, the results indicate inflammation that probably originates in the prostate gland or seminal vesicles.

Under the microscope, immature sperm may be present in great numbers and are indicative of infertility. The sperm may also agglutinate, or clump together.

Critical Thinking: When an infertility work-up is indicated, cultural or religious conflicts can occur. For the Orthodox Jew, the Roman Catholic, and the Arab American, what are some of the beliefs and values that create conflict for the patient or spouse? How can medical and nursing practice be modified to accommodate cultural differences?

This occurs in the presence of IgG or IgA antibodies, and the clumping is associated with infertility. Either the male or female may produce the antibodies, but once there is agglutination, the sperm cannot reach the ovum (Brunzel, 1994).

The semen specimen is a potential biohazard that may contain an infectious organism, such as the human immunodeficiency virus, hepatitis virus, or herpesvirus. To prevent accidental transmission, universal precautions must be used when handling the semen specimen.

Purpose of the Test

Semen analysis is used to investigate infertility in the male. It is also used to evaluate the effectiveness of vasectomy. In special situations, it may be part of medicolegal testing, such as in cases of alleged rape or sexual abuse.

Procedure

A special wide-mouthed, clean plastic or glass container is used to collect ejaculate, which is usually produced by masturbation. Two to three specimens are usually required. They are collected at least 7 days apart and within a 3-month period.

QUALITY CONTROL

Some plastic containers are toxic to spermatozoa. The container should be provided by the laboratory.

If the patient cannot produce the sperm by masturbation, special, nonspermicidal condoms can be provided by the laboratory (Smith, 1992). Regular condoms are not acceptable because of the lubricant and the spermicidal preparation that is on or in them.

Findings

ABNORMAL VALUES

Testicular failure
Obstruction of the ejaculatory ducts
Genital infection
Cryptorchidism

Hyperpyrexia
Prostatic dysfunction
Postvasectomy azoospermia

Interfering Factors

- Exposure of the ejaculate to intense sunlight or chilling temperatures
- Delay in the analysis of the specimen
- Use of lubricant or over-the-counter condom
- Incomplete collection of the ejaculate

Nursing Implementation

Pretest

Instruct the patient regarding the method of specimen collection. The instructions are given verbally in a professional and sensitive manner. A written copy of the instructions is also given to the patient. These instructions include the following:
- Use the sterile container that is provided by the laboratory.
- Collect the specimen by masturbation. If this is not possible or acceptable, a special condom provided by the laboratory can be used. Coitus interruptus is also acceptable, but the amount of ejaculate will be less.
- Instruct the patient to practice sexual abstinence for at least 2 days but not more than 7 days before the specimen is collected.

Provide a clean, comfortable room for the patient. It should be in or near the laboratory because of the short time before liquefaction occurs. If these arrangements are not possible, the specimen can be obtained at home. Special transport instructions are provided regarding avoidance of sunlight, cooling, spillage, and delay in delivery of the specimen to the laboratory.

During the Test

To protect the spermatozoa from cold shock, the collection container should be at room temperature or warmed before the ejaculate is produced. The container can be warmed under the patient's arm or next to his body (Brunzel, 1994).

The complete ejaculate must be placed in the specimen container.

Posttest

Ensure that the container and the requisition slip are labeled, including the patient's name, date, and time of specimen collection. The period of sexual abstinence is included in the documentation.

Ensure that the specimen is delivered to the laboratory within 1 hour. The specimen must be analyzed within 3 hours.

To protect the specimen from deterioration during transport, instruct the patient to:
- Place the lid securely on the container.
- Protect the specimen from chilling and sunlight by placing it next to the body, in an inside coat pocket, or under the arm.

QUALITY CONTROL

The specimen must not be exposed to chilling or sunlight because these negative conditions would reduce the motility of the sperm.

TESTOSTERONE, TOTAL, FREE

(SERUM)

Synonyms:

─────────────── **NORMAL VALUES** ───────────────

TOTAL TESTOSTERONE	
Adult Male:	300–1000 ng/dl *or* SI 10.4–34.7 nmol/L
Adult Female:	20–75 ng/dl *or* SI 0.69–2.6 nmol/L
Child (1–10 Years):	<3–10 ng/dl *or* SI <0.1–0.35 nmol/L
FREE TESTOSTERONE	
Adult Male:	52–280 pg/ml *or* SI 180.4–971.6 pmol/L
Adult Female:	1.6–6.3 pg/ml *or* SI 5.6–21.9 pmol/L
Child (1–10 Years):	0.15–0.66 pg/ml *or* SI 0.5–2.1 pmol/L

Background Information

Total testosterone consists of the measurement of testosterone that is free, loosely bound to albumin, and strongly bound to sex hormone–binding globulin. Free testosterone is the amount of the total hormone that is unbound in the serum. Because free testosterone is the active form of the hormone, it is the more significant test (O'Brien, 1989).

In the male, almost all the testosterone is synthesized by the testes. In the female, small amounts are synthesized by the ovaries and adrenal glands, and additional amounts are converted from androstenedione. Testosterone is the dominant androgen and in the male is responsible for spermatogenesis (O'Brien, 1989). Androgens affect many other organs and tissues, resulting in increased total body mass and hirsutism—the distribution of body hair. When hirsutism is excessive, it is due to excessive testosterone or its hormonal precursor, androstenedione.

Purpose of the Test

The measurement of serum testosterone is used to diagnose precocious sexual development in the boy who is less than 10 years old. It helps diagnose deficient activity of the testes or ovaries. It is part of the testing that determines the cause of male infertility or sexual dysfunction. In the female, it helps determine the cause of hirsutism or virilization.

Procedure

A red-topped tube is used to collect 7 ml of venous blood.

Findings

ELEVATED VALUES

Ovarian tumor

Hyperthyroidism

Testicular tumor

Central nervous system
lesion

Adrenal tumor

Congenital adrenal hyperplasia

Idiopathic precocious puberty

DECREASED VALUES

Cirrhosis of the liver

Hypopituitarism

Severe obesity

Malnutrition

Cryptorchidism

Excessive alcohol intake

Estrogen therapy

Renal failure

Down syndrome

Interfering Factors

• Recent radioactive isotope scan

Nursing Implementation

Pretest

Schedule this test before or at least 7 days after a nuclear scan.

QUALITY CONTROL

The measurement of testosterone is carried out by radioimmu-noassay. The radioisotopes of the scan would interfere with the analysis and the results.

Posttest

Arrange for prompt transport of the specimen to the laboratory.

QUALITY CONTROL

Once the cells have been separated out, the serum must be refrigerated. It will be stable for 2 days. Thereafter it must be frozen at –20° C until the analysis is performed.

URINARY PREGNANETRIOL

(URINE)

Synonyms:

───────────────── **NORMAL VALUES** ─────────────────

Adult:	<2 mg/day *or* <5.9 µmol/day
Child:	
(0–6 Years):	<0.2 mg/day *or* SI <0.6 µmol/day
(7–16 Years):	<0.3–1.1 mg/day *or* SI <0.9–3.3 µmol/day

Background Information

17-Hydroxyprogesterone is a substrate needed to produce cortisol, an adrenocortical steroid. Pregnanetriol is a metabolite of 17-hydroxyprogesterone. When there is normal adrenal function, minute amounts of pregnanetriol are present in the urine. If there is adrenal insufficiency that prevents or limits the synthesis of cortisol, there is an increase in adrenocorticotropic hormone production, increased release of adrenal androgens, and increased release of 17-hydroxyprogesterone into the serum. The increase of serum 17-hydroxyprogesterone causes an increase in pregnanetriol in the urine.

The increase in adrenal androgens results in virilization of the female. The infant female may show masculinization of the external genitals at birth, and female secondary sex characteristics can fail to develop in the older female child. The increase in adrenal androgens can cause precocious development in the male child.

Purpose of the Test

The measurement of this urinary metabolite helps confirm the diagnosis of adrenal hyperplasia. It also is used to monitor cortisol replacement.

Procedure

A large, clean collection bottle is used to collect urine for 24 hours.

QUALITY CONTROL

Some laboratories require a boric acid preservative to be added to the container. To preserve the urine, the specimen is refrigerated or cooled throughout the collection period.

Findings

ELEVATED VALUES

Congenital adrenal hyperplasia
Insufficient cortisol replacement
21-Hydroxylase deficiency

Ovarian tumor
Adrenal tumor
Stein-Leventhal syndrome

Interfering Factors

- Muscular exercise
- Warming of the specimen
- Failure to collect the entire specimen

Nursing Implementation

Pretest

Instruct the patient or the parent of the small child that there can be no physical exertion before or during the test period. This is because physical activity increases the urinary metabolic output and causes a falsely elevated test result.

Provide both written and verbal instructions regarding the collection of urine. These instructions must include the specific times for the collection period.

For the infant or small child, the pediatric collection bag is to be taped to the clean perineal area. A diaper is applied over the bag to help maintain its position and to prevent removal of the bag by the child.

During the Test

The first voided specimen of the morning is discarded and the urine collection period begins at 8 A.M.

All urine is collected for 24 hours and placed in the container. This includes the first voided specimen of the next morning.

Maintain the specimen and container on ice or keep refrigerated during the collection period. This prevents deterioration.

DIAGNOSTIC PROCEDURES

During the period of collection, all urine is added to the collection container. If any urine spills or if a specimen is discarded accidentally, the test is invalidated.

Posttest

On the urine requisition slip, write the time and date of the start and completion of the test.

The specimen must be delivered to the laboratory without delay. The urine must be kept chilled or refrigerated. In the laboratory, the urine can be frozen until the analysis is performed.

AMNIOCENTESIS

(AMNIOTIC FLUID)

Synonyms:

Background Information

Amniotic fluid is the fluid that surrounds the fetus in the uterus. During pregnancy, it provides the medium for water, electrolyte, and other solute exchange with the fetus. The fetus swallows the amniotic fluid for hydration and urinates into the fluid to eliminate metabolic wastes. Throughout the pregnancy, the amniotic fluid bathes the fetal lungs. The amniotic fluid is also in continuous exchange with maternal plasma, so there is a complete cleansing and change of the fluid every 2 to 3 hours.

Amniocentesis is used to obtain an amniotic fluid sample. As seen in Table 21–1, there are several reasons to perform amniocentesis. The biochemical and cytologic analyses provide the data regarding the fetus and the pregnancy. When the purpose of the amniocentesis is to screen for fetal abnormality, it is performed early in the second trimester. By that time, there are fetal cell samples available for chromosomal study and there is sufficient amniotic fluid available to obtain the fluid and cell samples. When the amniocentesis is guided by high-resolution ultrasound, it may be performed as early as 12 to 14 weeks' gestation. If the procedure is performed by the 15th to 17th week of gestation, there is still sufficient time to provide the appropriate counseling and discuss treatment alternatives. The mother or parents can consider the option of abortion when the fetus is abnormal.

When the purpose of the amniocentesis is to evaluate a problem pregnancy or to identify a change in the health status of the fetus, the procedure is performed in the late part of the second trimester or during the third trimester. In high-risk pregnancy, it may be advisable to terminate the pregnancy early because of severe maternal illness or a maternal condition that adversely affects the fetus. In either

━━━━━━━━━━━ **NORMAL VALUES** ━━━━━━━━━━━

AMNIOTIC FLUID ANALYSIS

Chromosomes Analysis:	normal karyotype
Alpha$_1$-fetoprotein:	0.5–3 MoM (multiple of median value)
Acetylcholinesterase:	negative
Rh incompatibility:	
Freda classification:	negative or 1+
Optical density at 450 nm (delta 450):	0–0.2
Bilirubin:	0.01–0.03 mg/dl *or* SI 0.02-0.06 µmol/L
Creatinine:	
36 weeks of gestation:	1.6–1.8 mg/dl *or* SI 141–159 µmol/L
37–38 weeks of gestation:	>2 mg/dl *or* SI >177 µmol/L
Lecithin/sphingomyelin Ratio:	>2
Phosphatidylglycerol:	Present
Pulmonary Surfactant:	Positive Foam Stability Index: >0.48
Meconium:	Absent

situation, the status of fetal health and fetal maturity are considerations that influence the decision-making and timing of the delivery.

AMNIOTIC FLUID ANALYSIS. Normal amniotic fluid is colorless to pale yellow. When the fluid is a darker yellow or amber, the cause is excessive bilirubin and biliverdin. A dark green color is caused by meconium. Blood colors the fluid pink to red. There should be no blood in the specimen. If there is, it may come from a maternal vein, the placenta, the fetus, or the cord. One possibility is that it is caused by the insertion of the needle during the procedure.

CHROMOSOMAL ANALYSIS. Chromosomal abnormalities are detected in the analysis of fetal cells that are harvested from cell cultures. Trisomy 21 and other trisomy conditions caused by the translocation of genes have the highest incidence in women older than 35 years of age. Chromosome analysis can also detect neural tube defects that include anencephaly, myelomeningocele, and spinal bifida. The analysis can also detect genetic abnormalities that cause more than 80 different types of inborn errors of metabolism. They include disorders of lipid, carbohydrate, glycoprotein, mucopolysaccharide, amino acid, and organic acid metabolism. The use of gene probe technology can also identify other genetic disorders, including cystic fibrosis, muscular dystrophy, sickle cell anemia, and hemophilia.

When a genetic abnormality is encountered, the parents need comprehensive information about the health status of the fetus. They need to make an informed decision about the pregnancy, and the choices are painful. The alternatives

Critical Thinking: When a genetic abnormality of the fetus is identified, what are the ethical and religious dimensions of the decision to abort or continue the pregnancy? Does the severity of the defect influence the decision?

TABLE 21–1
AMNIOCENTESIS: TIMING, PURPOSES, AND POTENTIAL FINDINGS

Gestation	Indications	Potential Abnormalities
15–17 weeks	Maternal age >35 years	Trisomy 21 (Down syndrome) Neural tube defect (spinal bifida, anencephaly)
	Sex determination of the fetus	Sex-linked recessive disorders (hemophilia, Duchenne muscular dystrophy)
	Family history of chromosomal abnormality	
	Family history of metabolic disorder	Inborn errors of metabolism (Tay-Sachs disease, Gaucher disease, Niemann-Pick disease; galactosuria, maple syrup disease, homocystinuria)
	Family history of hemoglobinopathy	Hemoglobin disease (thalassemia, sickle cell anemia)
20–42 weeks	Management of a problem pregnancy	Maternal heart disease, diabetes, endocrine disorder; analysis of amniotic fluid for fetal thyroid hormone, glucose, estriol, L/S ratio
	Assessment of fetal distress	Rh incompatibility, infection, fetal pulmonary immaturity

L/S = lecithin/sphingomyelin.

include termination of the pregnancy or completion of the pregnancy with preparation for the special health care needs of the newborn. Genetic counseling precedes the amniocentesis and is also provided when a genetic abnormality is encountered.

ALPHA₁-FETOPROTEIN. Alpha$_1$-fetoprotein is a glycoprotein that is made in the yolk sac, fetal intestinal tract, and liver. It is present in the fetal serum and the amniotic fluid. The amount increases steadily during fetal growth, with a maximal level at about 12 weeks' gestation. Thereafter, the concentration decreases as a greater proportion of amniotic fluid is produced (Sundaram et al., 1992).

Amniotic fluid alpha$_1$-fetoprotein is used to detect neural defects, such as spina bifida or anencephaly, and nonneural defects, such as congenital nephrosis or atresia in the upper gastrointestinal tract.

ACETYLCHOLINESTERASE. This enzyme is present in high concentrations in cerebrospinal fluid. It is not present in the amniotic fluid with a normal fetus, but if there is a neural tube defect, such as anencephaly or spina bifida (open or closed), the cerebrospinal fluid leaks into the amniotic fluid. If the fetus has a ventral wall defect such as an omphalocele, acetylcholinesterase also leaks into the amniotic fluid and the test result is positive (Sundaram et al., 1992).

Rh INCOMPATIBILITY. Amniocentesis can usually detect Rh incompatibility after 30 weeks' gestation. The analysis is based on the amount of free bilirubin in the fluid. Higher values indicate the degree of hemolysis that is occurring in the fetus. The possible panic range of the delta 450 spectral analysis is 0.3 to 0.7. On the Freda scale, a value of 3+ indicates severe fetal distress. Higher values indicate impending fetal death.

BILIRUBIN. Unconjugated bilirubin is produced by the fetus during normal erythrocyte destruction. The amount of bilirubin is minimal and is removed by the placenta and maternal circulation. With hemolytic disease, however, there is a continual and excessive destruction of the fetal erythrocytes. The amount of unconjugated bilirubin rises dramatically in the amniotic fluid in direct correlation with the severity of the disease.

The most common cause of hemolytic disease of the newborn is incompatibility of the maternal antibodies with the fetal erythrocyte antigen. The problem is usually due to the mix of the Rh-negative antibodies of the mother with the Rh_oD antigen of the fetus, but other Rh antibodies can also cause hemolysis of fetal erythrocytes. In measuring the bilirubin level, the possible panic value is more than 0.47 mg/dl (SI, 8 μmol/L). It is an indication of fetal distress.

CREATININE. Creatinine levels are a measure of renal function and renal maturity of the fetus. They are also a measure of fetal lung maturity because the development of the lungs is dependent on the normal development of the kidneys. The possible panic range is a creatinine level of less than 1.6 mg/dl (SI, <141 μmol/L). This lower than normal value implies that the fetus is immature or premature. If it is delivered at this stage of development, the fetus is likely to experience respiratory distress syndrome.

LECITHIN/SPHINGOMYELIN RATIO. The lecithin/sphingomyelin (L/S) ratio is a major indicator of fetal pulmonary maturity. Lecithin is the major compound of pulmonary surfactant, the phospholipid substance needed for alveolar function. Sphingomyelin is produced in cell membranes, but its function is unknown. In the early stages of gestation, these two substances are produced in approximately equivalent amounts (a ratio of 1:1 or 1).

As the fetus matures beyond 34 to 36 weeks of gestation, the concentration of lecithin increases and the sphingomyelin remains stable. Thus, a ratio of greater than 2 means that there is about twice as much lecithin as sphingomyelin. The L/S ratio of greater than 2 indicates fetal lung maturity. In a normal pregnancy, this value usually occurs at about the 36th week of gestation and thereafter. A ratio of less than 1.5 to 2 is the indicator of fetal lung immaturity, with the increased likelihood that the fetus would experience respiratory distress syndrome. In diabetic mothers, an L/S ratio of greater than 3.5 is the normal value for fetal lung maturity. This higher value is due to increased surfactant production in the fetus of the diabetic mother.

PHOSPHATIDYGLYCEROL. This is a lipid component of pulmonary surfactant that normally appears in the amniotic fluid after the 35th week of gestation. It is an indicator of fetal pulmonary maturity. Once it appears, there is little risk that the fetus will experience respiratory distress syndrome. Generally this test is used with the L/S ratio to assess fetal lung maturity. Phosphatidylglycerol is also useful as a criterion for delivery in the high-risk pregnancy that is complicated by diabetes mellitus, type I.

PULMONARY SURFACTANT. The lungs are one of the late-maturing organs of the fetus. Surfactant is a lipid and protein substance produced by the mature epithelial cells of the alveoli. Surfactant enables the walls of the alveoli to expand and contract in the function of respiration. Since amniotic fluid bathes the lungs of the fetus, a certain amount of surfactant produced appears in the fluid. The amount of surfactant is one of the predictors of fetal maturity and viability.

Pulmonary surfactant is measured by the "shake test," also known as the foam stability index (FSI). In the laboratory, amniotic fluid samples are mixed with different amounts of ethanol in test tubes. The tubes are shaken to produce foam and bubbles that indicate that surfactant is present. The FSI represents the highest concentration of the mixture that produces a foam that does not dissolve. FSI values greater than 0.48 indicate fetal pulmonary maturity (Brunzel, 1994).

MECONIUM. Meconium staining is caused by the release of mucus-like fetal intestinal secretions into the amniotic fluid. It is an abnormal sign that indicates fetal distress and the need for immediate delivery of the fetus.

Purpose of the Test

Amniocentesis is used to detect genetic or chromosomal abnormalities in the fetus. It is also used to assess fetal maturity or fetal distress in the management of a problem pregnancy.

Procedure

Ultrasound is used to locate the position of the fetus, placenta, and the pool of amniotic fluid, and it guides the insertion of the needle. Using sterile technique, several syringes and a long needle are used to aspirate 10 to 20 ml of amniotic fluid from the uterus (Fig. 21–2). The fluid is placed in sterile brown plastic containers for transport to the laboratory.

QUALITY CONTROL

Glass containers cannot be used because cells adhere to the surface of the glass. An amber-colored container is used to protect the solution and bilirubin from the sunlight. If such a container is not available, a clear container can be used. It is covered immediately with aluminum foil to prevent oxidation from sunlight.

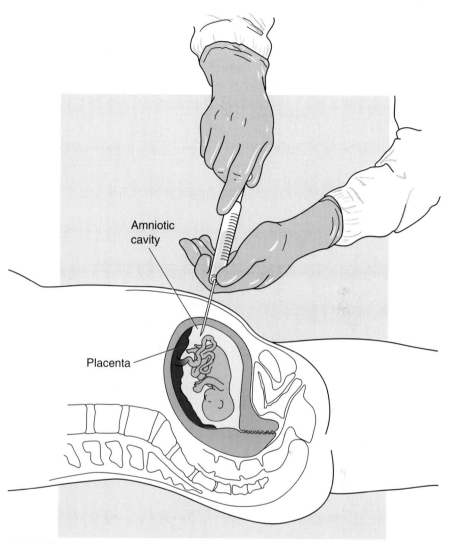

FIGURE 21–2. Amniocentesis. Once the needle is inserted through the skin and uterine wall, a sample of amniotic fluid is aspirated with a syringe.

Findings

ELEVATED VALUES

Alpha$_1$-Fetoprotein

Neural Tube Defects
Anencephaly
Spina bifida
Myelocele
Hydrocephaly

Nonneural Tube Defects
Congenital nephrosis
Esophageal atresia
Duodenal atresia

Acetylcholinesterase
Neural tube defect
Fetal thyroid disease

Rh Incompatibility
Fetal hemolysis of erythrocytes
(erythroblastosis fetalis)

Bilirubin
Rh incompatibility

L/S Ratio
Maternal diabetes

Pulmonary Surfactant
Maternal diabetes
Intrauterine growth retardation
Toxemia
Hypertension
Malnutrition

Placenta previa
Premature rupture of membranes
Hemoglobinopathy
Drug addiction

Meconium
Fetal distress

DECREASED VALUES

Bilirubin
Fetal immaturity

Creatinine
Fetal immaturity

L/S Ratio
Fetal pulmonary immaturity

Phosphatidylglycerol
Fetal pulmonary immaturity

Pulmonary Surfactant
Polyhydramnios
Liver disease
Renal disease
Advanced maternal age

Hypothyroidism
Anemia
Syphilis
Toxoplasmosis

Interfering Factors

- Exposure of specimen to sunlight
- Contamination of specimen (blood, meconium)
- Recent radioactive isotope scan
- Position of the placenta
- Delay in delivery of specimen to laboratory

Nursing Implementation

Pretest

After the patient receives a complete explanation of the amniocentesis procedure from the physician, obtain written consent from the patient or person who is legally responsible for her care.

Provide instructions regarding pretest preparation. These instructions vary, depending on the gestation of the pregnancy.

- For a pregnancy that is less than 20 weeks of gestation, instruct the woman to drink extra fluids 1 hour before the test and not to urinate until the test is completed. A full bladder raises the uterus up and out of the pelvis so that the uterine contents can be visualized.

- For a pregnancy that is greater than 20 weeks of gestation, there are no requirements for fluid intake. Instruct the woman to void before the procedure begins. With the larger size of the uterus, an empty bladder is less likely to be punctured during the procedure.

Assist the patient in removing her clothes, putting on a hospital gown, and lying supine on the examining table.

Obtain and record vital signs, including the blood pressure, temperature, pulse, respirations, and fetal heart rate. This establishes the baseline values that are needed for comparison in the posttest period.

Provide emotional support for the patient. Anxiety about the procedure and the status of the fetus' health are common concerns.

During the Test

Position the patient with her hands behind her head to help prevent contamination of the sterile field.

After ultrasound has located the fetus' position, the placenta, and the pool of amniotic fluid, wash the abdomen with povidone-iodine solution and drape the sterile field.

Comfort the patient during the administration of the local anesthetic in the intended area of the abdomen. Some stinging may be felt during the injection.

After the fluid sample is withdrawn, assist with its placement in the specimen containers.

Once the needle is withdrawn, place a small adhesive bandage over the site of the needle puncture.

Posttest

Monitor and record the blood pressure, pulse, respirations, and fetal heart rate every 15 minutes for 30 to 60 minutes. They should remain within normal limits and be comparable to the pretest data.

Ensure that the specimen is correctly labeled. The requisition slip should state the source of the fluid and the period of gestation of the pregnancy. Arrange for prompt transport of the specimen to the laboratory.

Critical Thinking: Does the fetus have the right to safe and effective health care? What are the issues related to the fetus's right to life, the parent's right to know the health status of the fetus, and the risks associated with complication from amniocentesis?

QUALITY CONTROL

In the laboratory, the specimen used for cellular analysis is kept at room temperature. The specimen used for biochemical analysis is centrifuged and refrigerated or placed on ice. Phospholipid is metabolized when kept uncentrifuged at room temperature. This specimen is also kept in a dark place to prevent photooxidation of the bilirubin.

If the patient feels faintness, nausea, or cramps, place her on her right side to relieve the uterine pressure.

TABLE 21–2
COMPLICATIONS OF AMNIOCENTESIS

Complication	Nursing Assessment
Premature labor	Leakage of fluid from the vagina Severe, persistent uterine cramping Uterine contractions
Bleeding	Blood in the amniotic fluid (port wine–colored fluid) Fetal lethargy or hyperactivity
Infection	Chills, fever Purulent drainage at the puncture site Uterine cramping Fetal lethargy

At the time of discharge, instruct the patient to rest at home until the cramping subsides. Light activity can then resume.

Provide the patient with written instructions to notify the physician immediately about any symptoms of itching, fever, leakage of fluid, severe abdominal pain, or unusual (increased or decreased) fetal activity.

Complications

There is a 0.5% incidence of complications from amniocentesis (Satish, 1992). The complications include spontaneous rupture of the membranes, premature labor, spontaneous abortion, stillbirth, bleeding from a traumatic tap, and infection.

The nursing assessment of complications of amniocentesis is presented in Table 21–2.

BIOPSY, BREAST

(TISSUE BIOPSY)

Synonyms:

─────── **NORMAL VALUES** ───────

No malignant cells are seen.

Background Information

A suspicious palpable or nonpalpable lesion of the breast requires a biopsy to determine the cause and differentiate between benign and malignant tissue. A mammogram is often performed before the biopsy to visualize the size and location of the growth. There are several methods that can be used to obtain the tissue specimen.

SURGICAL BIOPSY. This procedure is performed with local or general anesthesia. A surgical incision is made over the area of abnormal tissue. In an *excisional biopsy*, the cyst, fibroadenoma, or calcified area is removed. With larger tumors, a wedge of tissue is removed from the mass. Sutures or surgical clips are used to close the incision. There are disadvantages to the incisional biopsy procedure. Many nonpalpable lesions are benign. The external scar may be disfiguring, and the internal scarring impairs visualization in future mammography examinations. Because of bleeding or slippage of the localizing wire, the abnormal tissue may not be removed. In this case, the biopsy must be repeated.

NEEDLE ASPIRATION BIOPSY. This procedure is performed by inserting a hollow needle into the lump or cyst. Aspiration removes the fluid of the cyst or a sample of tissue from a solid tumor. Needle aspiration has advantages that include the ability to drain or collapse a benign cyst, remove a small lesion by aspiration, and obtain a tissue sample without disfigurement. The disadvantage is that without direct visualization, it is difficult to locate the abnormal tissue with pinpoint accuracy.

STEREOTACTIC NEEDLE ASPIRATION BIOPSY. This is a relatively new procedure in the United States. Automated mammography and computers provide a three-dimensional view for precise localization of the abnormal tissue. Based on imaging, computer control, and the alignment of needle holders and guides, the needle is inserted and guided to the precise location and depth of the lesion. The radiologist can then inject blue dye or insert a wire hook to identify the location for the surgeon. Alternatively, the radiologist can perform a needle aspiration biopsy to obtain the tissue sample. The patient may find this procedure difficult to tolerate because she must remain motionless for 20 to 60 minutes as the coordinates are determined (Doogan, 1991).

The advantages of this method are the removal of the biopsy tissue without a scar and pinpoint accuracy in the exact location of the abnormal tissue. The disadvantage is that there is a 1 to 30% chance of a false-negative test result (Peart, 1992). One of the causes of this problem is insufficient aspiration of cellular material because the needle is too narrow. As this technique gains greater use, the accuracy rate should improve.

The woman who must undergo breast biopsy experiences deep anxiety and stress regardless of the technique used. The anxiety begins at the time the lump is discovered before there is knowledge about the biopsy result. The fears are focused on a possible malignancy, fear of the unknown, concerns about family health, and fear of pain from the biopsy procedure (MacFarlane and Sony, 1992).

Purpose of the Test

The biopsy distinguishes benign from malignant breast disease.

Procedure

Fluid or tissue is removed from the breast lesion. The fluid aspiration sample will be used to make slides for microscopic analysis. The tissue slides will be examined by frozen section and permanent slides. An estrogen-progesterone assay may be performed.

Findings

ABNORMAL VALUES

Fibroadenoma	Fat necrosis
Carcinoma	Abscess
Duct papilloma	Mastitis
Fibroplasia	Lipoma
Calcification	Cystosarcoma
Granular cell tumor	

Interfering Factors

- Inadequate tissue sample

Nursing Implementation

Pretest

After the patient has been informed of the procedure and the need for it, obtain a written consent from the patient or person legally responsible for the patient's health care decisions.

If surgical biopsy and general anesthesia are planned, instruct the patient to fast from food and liquids for 8 hours before the surgery.

Assist the patient in removing all clothes and putting on a hospital gown.

Assess and record the vital signs, including temperature, blood pressure, pulse, and respirations.

Provide emotional support through the personalization of care. Assist the patient in reducing her stress by listening, providing explanations, or using diversions, as indicated (MacFarlane and Sony, 1992).

For needle aspiration or incisional biopsy, place the patient in a supine position. For stereotactic needle biopsy, the patient sits erect in a chair with the breast compressed between the module and the compression plate.

During the Test

Clean the breast tissue with povidone-iodine.

With the surgical or fine needle biopsy approach, apply the sterile drapes over the correct breast.

Assist with the preparation of the local anesthetic.

Once the tissue is obtained, place the specimen in a sterile, dry, labeled container. Place the container on ice and arrange for immediate transport of the specimen to the laboratory. The specimen may also be given directly to the pathologist or technician who is waiting in the room.

When microscopic slides are prepared, the aspirated material is used to prepare two to four slides. The smears are fixed immediately with 95% alcohol or a spray-on cytologic fixative. The slides are then transported to the laboratory within minutes (Hajdu and Gaston, 1991).

Apply a dry, sterile dressing to the incision or puncture site.

Posttest

Take vital signs and record the results. When a general anesthetic is used, monitor the vital signs every 15 to 30 minutes until the patient is reactive, alert, and stable.

To help cope with postoperative depression or anxiety, encourage the patient to return to normal activity as soon as possible. After a surgical procedure, however, vigorous exercise must be avoided for 2 weeks.

To relieve surgical pain, instruct the patient to use warm, moist compresses or a heating pad and to wear a supportive bra.

Instruct the patient to shower or bathe as usual, using unscented soap for the needle puncture site. Cleansing of the surgical incision is prescribed by the surgeon. The surgical dressing is changed once a day.

Advise the patient to inform the surgeon of inflammation, infection, or excessive pain in the incision.

Complications

The complications of incisional biopsy are cellulitis and hematoma. The needle aspiration methods can produce bruising, particularly when there are multiple needle insertions and aspirations during the procedure. The nursing assessment of complications of breast biopsy is presented in Table 21–3.

COLPOSCOPY

(ENDOSCOPY)

Synonyms:
none

──────────── **NORMAL VALUES** ────────────

No abnormalities of the vagina or cervix are noted.

TABLE 21-3
COMPLICATIONS OF BREAST BIOPSY

Complication	Nursing Assessment
Cellulitis, infection	Fever
	Headache
	Malaise
	Pain in the breast
	Redness
	Swelling
Hematoma	Swelling in the breast
	Pain
	Ecchymosis
	Leakage of blood from the incision

Background Information

The colposcope is a microscope with a bright light that is inserted into the vagina. In the examination of the vagina and cervix, it provides 10 to 40 times the magnification of the surface epithelium and underlying connective tissue. The goal is to identify precursor changes in cervical tissue before the changes advance from benign or atypical cells to cervical cancer. The location of the changes is often at or near the squamocolumnar junction (Ramzy and Mody, 1991).

The colposcopy procedure examines for cellular and vascular changes in the surface epithelium of the cervix and vagina. Endocervical curettage is used to scrape the tissue and obtain cell samples of the endocervical canal, and a biopsy forceps is used to nip small samples of tissue from the cervix. After a biopsy, bleeding is controlled with an application of silver nitrate, pressure, or sutures.

Significantly abnormal tissue that may be invasive carcinoma appears as a large lesion, one that is dull gray-white, or has dilated blood vessels that are visible. A low-grade lesion that has tiny red dots or a mosaic pattern from the connection of capillaries is also suspicious. The colposcopy examination takes 10 to 15 minutes to perform.

Purpose of the Test

Colposcopy is performed to further evaluate an abnormal Papanicolaou smear, to monitor for precancerous abnormalities, or to evaluate a lesion of the vagina or cervix.

Procedure

A colposcope is inserted into the vagina to provide magnification and illumination of vaginal and cervical tissue. A tissue biopsy may also be performed.

Findings

ABNORMAL VALUES

Atrophic cellular changes	Cervical intraepithelial neoplasia (CIN)
Condyloma	Infection, inflammation
Cervical erosion	Invasive carcinoma
Papilloma	

Interfering Factors

- Vaginal creams
- Menstruation

Nursing Implementation

Pretest

Schedule the procedure in the early part of the menstrual cycle, preferably between days 8 and 12. In this period, the cervical mucus is clear and thin and allows maximum visibility (Ferris, 1992).

Instruct the patient to refrain from the application of any creams or vaginal medications because they obscure the view of the cervix.

After the patient has been informed about the procedure, obtain written consent from the patient or person legally responsible for the patient's health care decisions.

Assist the patient in removing all clothes and putting on a hospital gown.

During the Test

Place the patient in the lithotomy position with the legs supported in stirrups.

During the insertion of the colposcope, instruct the patient to breathe through the mouth to help relax the muscles.

Once the glass slides are prepared with cell scrapings, apply the fixative to prevent drying of the cells. If biopsy specimens are taken, place the tissue on hard brown paper or on a nonstick gauze (Telfa). Each sample is placed in a separate specimen jar that contains fixative.

Posttest

Ensure that all specimens are labeled appropriately and that the requisition slip identifies the source of the tissue.

Arrange for prompt transport of the specimen to the laboratory.

When a cervical biopsy is performed, instruct the patient to refrain from sexual intercourse and avoid the insertion of anything into the vagina until the lesion is healed. Arrange for a follow-up appointment to evaluate the healing process.

COMPUTED TOMOGRAPHY, PELVIS

(TOMOGRAPHY)

In the evaluation of the female pelvis, computed tomography (CT) with intravenous contrast material produces clear, cross-sectional images of the pelvic tissues and organs. The pelvic CT scan is often used to determine the extent of malignancy or the source of infection. For these purposes, the scan usually includes the abdomen and the pelvis so that nearby organs, structures, and blood vessels are visualized. Oral and rectal barium contrast material may be administered to opacify the bowel loops. If a pelvic tumor or abscess is located, the CT scan is used to guide the placement of a needle in a percutaneous aspiration biopsy or in a percutaneous needle drainage of the purulence.

The scout view of the CT scan may be used to perform CT pelvimetry on the pregnant woman, particularly when the fetus is in a breech position. When compared with radiography, the CT measurements are more accurate and there is less radiation exposure for the mother and the fetus (Friedman and Rosenfield, 1992).

More extensive discussion of the CT scan is presented in Chapter 12.

CORDOCENTESIS

(FETAL BLOOD)

Synonyms:

percutaneous umbilical cord sampling, PUBS

─────────── **NORMAL VALUES** ───────────

FETAL BLOOD ANALYSIS	
Chromosomal Analysis:	Normal karyotpye
Hematologic Evaluation:	Within normal limits for gestational age
Biochemistry Analysis:	Within normal limits for gestational age
IgG Antibodies:	Within normal limits
IgM Antibodies:	Within normal limits
Coagulation Factors:	Factors II, V, VIII, and IX are present

Background Information

Cordocentesis is a newer and accepted method of obtaining a fetal blood specimen during pregnancy through venipuncture of an umbilical vein. Since this procedure has a lower rate of complication, cordocentesis has begun to replace fetoscopy. The cordocentesis procedure can be performed in the second or third trimester, but for the purpose of genetic studies, the procedure is performed around the 15th week of gestation (Satish, 1992). The direct sampling of the fetal blood provides more rapid test results than does amniocentesis and a more definitive diagnosis than is obtained by testing amniotic fluid or maternal blood. The normal values of fetal cord blood vary, based on the gestational age of the fetus.

Critical Thinking: Will the identification of a chromosomal abnormality and the right to abortion ultimately result in the procreation of "perfect children only"?

FETAL BLOOD ANALYSIS

Prenatal Chromosomal Analysis. This procedure is performed on fetal lymphocytes obtained in the blood sample. The karyotype results are available in 2 to 3 days. The karyotype consists of the characteristics of the chromosomes—their number, form, size, structure, and grouping in the cell nucleus—with identification of chromosomal abnormality in the fetus (Wax and Blakemore, 1992).

The documentation of serious or severe chromosomal abnormality causes great emotional distress for the parents. Genetic counseling is an essential component of care and helps the parents make an informed choice about the continuation of the pregnancy. In obstetric management, the alternatives include continuation or termination of the pregnancy. If the pregnancy is continued, plans are made for intensive antepartal monitoring, possible cesarian section for fetal distress during labor, and plans for the special postdelivery needs of the newborn.

Congenital Infection. Such infection occurs when infection in the pregnant woman crosses the placental barrier and infects the fetus. Some of these infections are teratogenic and have a devastating effect on the health and development of the fetus. The fetal blood analysis for infection includes measurement of fetal antibodies, white blood cells, eosinophils, liver enzymes, and platelets. Viral culture of the fetal blood and the amniotic fluid may be performed to identify the infectious organism (McGowan and Hodinka, 1992).

Since fetal antibodies do not develop until the 22nd week of gestation, fetal cord blood samples cannot verify the infection before this time. Because of the legal limits of pregnancy termination, there is little time left to perform the cordocentesis, verify the fetal infection, and inform the parents. If the woman decides to terminate the pregnancy, the abortion procedure must be scheduled quickly.

Thrombocytopenia. This is a low platelet count, which can result in fetal intracranial bleeding during pregnancy, labor, or the neonatal period. In most cases, the mother has immune thrombocytopenia and passively transmits the maternal antiplatelet antibodies to the fetus. If the fetus is affected, the treatment depends on the cause of the disorder and the severity of the platelet deficit. Several cordocentesis procedures may be performed to monitor the problem, and the fetus can receive a platelet transfusion by cordocentesis.

Red Cell Isoimmunization. This occurs when the fetus has Rh-positive red blood cell antigens and the mother has Rh-negative erythrocytes. The maternal antibodies are transmitted to the fetus and result in fetal hemolysis of erythrocytes. If the erythrocyte incompatibility is not prevented or controlled, the fetus experiences a hemolytic anemia called erythroblastosis fetalis or Rh disease.

If the maternal serum antibody titer is greater than 1:64, the fetal risk increases and cordocentesis is indicated. The fetal cord blood is tested for blood type, the presence of Rh antigens, hematocrit, and reticulocyte count. The treatment is individualized, but repeated cordocentesis is used to monitor the problem and administer a fetal intravascular transfusion in utero as needed.

Purpose of the Test

Cordocentesis is used to obtain fetal blood for the identification of chromosomal abnormality, detection of fetal infection, and assessment for fetal anemia or other hematologic abnormality. It is also used to monitor fetal growth and development and the state of fetal health during the gestational period.

Procedure

Guided by ultrasound, a sterile 20- to 22-gauge spinal needle is inserted through the woman's abdomen and uterus. The needle is then advanced into the umbilical cord until it is placed in one of the umbilical veins (Fig. 21–3). Once the needle placement is verified, a syringe is used to aspirate 0.5 to 3 ml of venous blood. The blood is then transferred to microtubes for the specific laboratory analyses.

Findings

ABNORMAL VALUES

Chromosomal Disorder
Trisomy
Fragile X syndrome
Sex chromosome mosaicism
Dysmorphic syndromes
Inborn errors of metabolism

Coagulopathy
Hemophilia A
Hemophilia B
von Willebrand disease

Hemolytic Anemia
Rh disease
Minor antigen disorders

Immunodeficiency
Severe combined immunodeficiency
    disorder

Infection
Toxoplasmosis
Rubella
Varicella
Cytomegalovirus
Human parvovirus B19

Erythrocyte Disorders
Sickle cell anemia
Thalassemias
Spherocytosis
Enzyme deficiency G-6-PD

Platelet Disorder
Thrombocytopenia

Miscellaneous
Familial hypercholesterolemia
Adrenoleukodystrophy

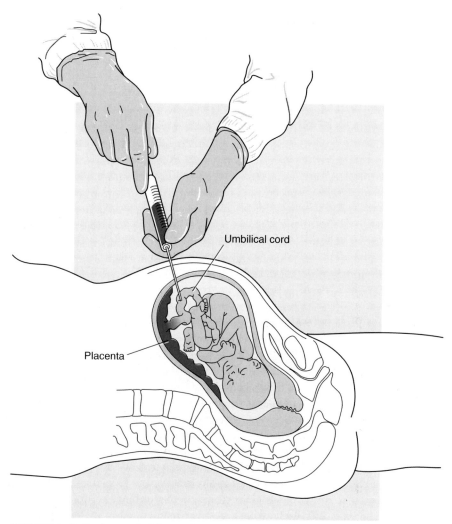

FIGURE 21–3. Cordocentesis. The needle is advanced through the skin and into the uterus. Once the needle punctures the umbilical cord and one of the uterine veins, cord blood is aspirated by syringe.

Chronic granulomatous disease   Hyperphenylalaninemia
Wiscott-Aldrich syndrome
Ataxia telangiectasia
Homozygous C3 deficiency
Chediak-Higashi syndrome

Interfering Factors

- Maternal obesity
- Uncooperative behavior

- Severe polyhydramnios
- Unfavorable fetal position
- Specimen contamination (amniotic fluid or blood)

Nursing Implementation

Pretest

Once the woman has been informed of the procedure by her physician and has agreed to have the cordocentesis, obtain her written consent.

Assist the patient in removing all clothes and putting on a hospital gown.

Place the patient in a lateral position on the examining table.

Assess and record the mother's vital signs and the fetal heart rate.

Provide emotional support. The patient's anxiety level is often high because of concern for the safety of the fetus, fear of the procedure, or anxiety about the potential of abnormal test results.

During the Test

Thoroughly cleanse the woman's abdomen with the appropriate povidone-iodine or surgical soap solution and then place the surgical drape.

Assist with the preparation of the local anesthetic.

Reassure the patient when the injection causes a slight stinging sensation in the injection site on the abdomen.

Begin the frequent assessment and recording of the fetal heart rate. The fetal cardiac contractions can be counted during the imaging of the fetus on the ultrasound monitor.

Prepare any additional medications, as prescribed. If the fetus moves excessively, the mother may receive intravenous sedation to limit fetal movement. As an alternative, the fetus may receive an intravenous sedative or muscle relaxant via the umbilical vein (Wax and Blakemore, 1992).

Once the blood is obtained, assist with depositing it in the microtubes. Ensure that all blood samples and requisition forms are properly labeled. The data include the mother's name and age and the gestation of the pregnancy. Each requisition slip clearly identifies the specimen as fetal blood (cord blood) obtained by cordocentesis.

Posttest

Once the needle is removed, begin the monitoring of the fetal heart rate and also assess and record the mother's vital signs.

In the recovery area, begin the external fetal monitoring of the fetal heart rate and uterine contractions. It is common for the mother to have mild uterine cramping for a short while. The fetal monitoring is discontinued when the fetal heart rate remains stable in a normal range and the uterine contractions cease.

At regular intervals, observe the abdomen for signs of bleeding. The small sterile dressing that covers the puncture site should remain dry and intact. Administer the prophylactic antibiotics, as prescribed.

In preparation for discharge, instruct the patient to rest for the remainder of the day. She should take her temperature at least two times per day. Fever greater than 100° F should be reported to her physician without delay. The patient is instructed to return to the physician for a follow-up evaluation and to learn of the test results.

Complications

Although the cordocentesis procedure is a potential risk for the fetus, the overall complication rate of 1% or less is low (Wax and Blakemore, 1992). Bleeding is the most common occurrence. Many patients have minimal bleeding that ceases a few minutes after the needle is removed. If the bleeding from the cord is prolonged, the fetus may become anemic.

The more serious complications can have severe consequences. Fetal death can occur as a result of cordocentesis. If there is prolonged fetal bradycardia or excessive bleeding, an emergency cesarian section may be performed. With rupture of the membranes or ongoing preterm labor, the fetus may be delivered prematurely.

A summary of the complications of cordocentesis is presented in Table 21–4.

FETAL MONITORING, EXTERNAL

(ELECTRIC MONITORING)

Synonym:

external EFM

NORMAL VALUES	
Baseline Fetal Heart Rate:	120–160 beats per minute
Variability:	±5–25 beats per minute

Background Information

The fetal heart rate is a reliable indicator of fetal well-being. It is also an indirect measurement of placental function. Placental blood flow provides oxygen to the fetal central nervous system and the reflexes that control fetal heart rate. The baseline fetal heart rate varies with the gestational age of the fetus. The normal rate is higher in the early months of gestation. It drops proportionately with advancing gestation, as the maturing fetal CNS exerts greater control over the fetal heart rate (Eganhouse and Burnside, 1992).

TABLE 21–4
COMPLICATIONS OF CORDOCENTESIS

Complication	Nursing Assessment
Fetal bradycardia	Fetal heart rate <120 beats per minute Fetal lethargy

Infection, fetal or maternal	*Maternal:*
	  Fever of 100° F or higher
	  Chills
	  Uterine cramping
	  Possible redness, swelling, or purulence at the puncture site
	Fetal:
	  Lethargy

Premature labor	Continual uterine contractions recorded on the fetal monitor Sensations of uterine cramping, pain, or rhythmic contraction and relaxation of the uterus Vaginal leakage of amniotic fluid
Bleeding, fetus, cord	Blood in the amniotic fluid Fetal lethargy Fetal hyperactivity Continued staining or wetness of the dressing; pink drainage

External monitoring is used to assess the fetus, particularly when there is a complication in the pregnancy. The fetal heart rate is monitored by a cardiotachometer, which amplifies the sounds and records the results on a graph. Simultaneously, a tokodynamometer measures and graphically records the pressure of uterine contractions (Fig. 21–4).

Measurements

The normal baseline *fetal heart rate* is 120 to 160 beats per minute, with a variability of ±5 to 25 beats per minute. The fetal heart rate can change in response to uterine contractions, or the change in rate can be unrelated to contractions. In addition, the fluctuations of the fetal heart rate are assessed in terms of amplitude, lag time, and recovery time. The *amplitude* is the difference of beats per minute between the baseline value and the maximum or minimum number of beats. The *lag time* is the difference between the peak of uterine contractions and the lowest point of deceleration. The *recovery time* is the difference between the end of the contraction and the return of the fetal heart rate to the baseline value.

ANTEPARTAL MONITORING. The *nonstress test* assesses the fetal heart rate in response to fetal movement. The test monitors the fetal heart rate for 40 minutes during fetal rest or sleep as well as during fetal activity or movement. The fetal heart rate should increase in response to fetal movement. The normal nonstress

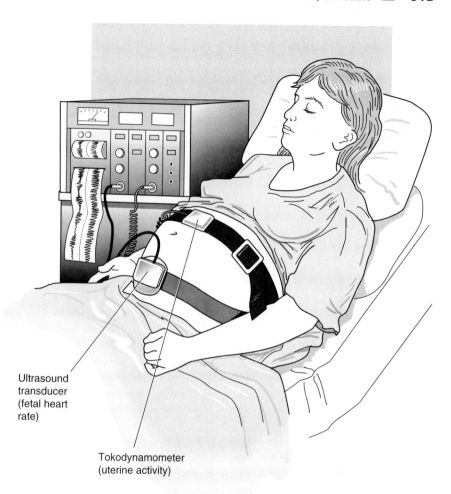

Ultrasound
transducer
(fetal heart
rate)

Tokodynamometer
(uterine activity)

FIGURE 21–4. External fetal monitoring. The heart rate of the fetus is evaluated, particularly in response to uterine activity or contractions.

test is also a good predictor of the health status of the fetus and a positive outcome of the pregnancy (Paine et al., 1992).

The *contraction stress test* identifies the fetus that already has diminished oxygenation to the CNS. The contraction is a source of stress because there is decreased uterine and placental blood flow during the contraction. When contractions occur, the healthy fetus sustains a normal baseline heart rate, with no decelerations. The fetus with compromised health or already diminished blood flow responds to the contractions with late decelerations.

To obtain adequate data for the contraction stress test, the monitoring must evaluate the fetal response to at least three contractions in a 10-minute period. The contractions may occur naturally or they may be stimulated. The stimulation can be carried out by having the patient rub one of her nipples to stimulate prolactin release and contractions or it can be carried out by administering an intravenous dose of oxytocin.

INTRAPARTUM MONITORING. External electronic fetal monitoring during labor provides a graphic recording of the fetal heart rate during contractions. Continual monitoring is not recommended for the patient who is at low risk and has had a normal pregnancy and normal labor. It is, however, highly informative in the moderate- to high-risk pregnancy or in cases of suspected or known problems with the fetus and its state of health.

Purpose of the Test

External fetal monitoring assesses fetal health and the fetal heart rate in nonstress situations during pregnancy or in stress situations that are provoked or occur during the contractions of labor.

Procedure

Using conductive gel on the skin, the cardiotachometer is placed on the woman's abdomen at the location at which the fetal heart tone is loudest. The tokodynamometer is placed over the fundus of the uterus to record the pressure of the contractions. Each transducer is attached with an abdominal belt or secured with an adhesive strip. The transducer is also connected by cable to the fetal monitor. After the recorder is set and adjusted, the recording of simultaneous linear graphic recordings occurs.

Findings

ABNORMAL VALUES

Fetal Problems	**Maternal Problems**
Bradycardia	Fever
Arrhythmia	Tachycardia
CNS depression	Hypertension
Hypoxia	Hypotension
Acidosis	Excess dosage of narcotics, sedatives, or tranquilizers
Infection	Uteroplacental insufficiency
Malposition	Hyperthyroidism
Temporary compression of the head during contractions	
Transitory umbilical cord compression	

Interfering Factors

- Maternal obesity
- Excessive movement of the fetus or mother
- Polyhydramnios

Nursing Implementation

Pretest

When monitoring is performed in the antepartum period, instruct the mother to eat a full meal before the test. This increases fetal activity. When the monitoring is performed during labor, the mother must remain without food and fluids.

Assist the mother in removing all clothes and putting on a hospital gown.

Position her in a semi-Fowler or left lateral position with the abdomen exposed.

As the equipment is prepared and applied, explain the purpose and show how the procedure benefits the mother and fetus. The woman should be reassured that the equipment cannot harm her or the fetus and that it does not interrupt the progress of labor.

During the Test

Critical Thinking: During labor, what are the possible reactions of the mother to the recordings of the fetal monitor? In response, how would you assist her?

Once the monitoring begins, instruct the mother to avoid body movement for the first few minutes until the baseline recording is completed. Thereafter, she may move to change her position. During labor, she may move out of bed within the distance allowed by the monitoring cables to which she is attached.

Record any special events on the graph paper, including a change of the patient's position, administration of medications, or procedures.

At intervals, check the positioning of the belts and transducers. They may fall off or slip out of position with the woman's activity.

Continuously evaluate the graphic recordings for abnormal results. When the fetal heart rate indicates persistent fetal distress, cesarian section may be an urgent necessity.

Posttest

Once the monitoring is completed, remove the belts and transducers. Cleanse the skin to remove the conductive gel.

When the woman has diabetes mellitus, hypertension, a pregnancy of more than 42 weeks' gestation, or preterm labor, or there is fetal growth retardation, the test is repeated on a weekly basis. Arrange the next appointment date.

FETAL MONITORING, INTERNAL

(ELECTRONIC
MONITORING)

Synonyms:

internal EFM, direct fetal monitoring

—————————————————— **NORMAL VALUES** ——————————————————

Baseline Fetal Heart Rate:	120–160 beats per minute
Variability:	±5–25 beats per minute

Background Information

Internal electronic fetal monitoring provides an accurate recording of the fetal heart rate and uterine contractions during labor. It is an invasive procedure that poses some risk to the mother and fetus, but the benefit is a more accurate assessment and monitoring of the fetus during labor. It is used in the high-risk pregnancy or when the fetal health is at risk or already compromised.

The fetal heart rate is monitored by a fetal electrode that is applied to the presenting part, often the scalp (Fig. 21–5). The electrode is connected by a wire to a metal plate on the mother's thigh. A cord goes from the plate to the monitor for a fetal heart rate graphic recording. The strength of the uterine contractions are monitored by an intrauterine pressure catheter. Within the tip of the catheter, the transducer or computer chip measures the pressures of the uterus during contraction and relaxation. The catheter is also connected by cable to the fetal monitor. The uterine pressure tracing is recorded simultaneously with the fetal heart rate.

To implant each monitor in the uterine cavity, the membranes must be ruptured. If they are still intact, amniotomy is performed. During implantation of the electrode, care is taken to avoid its placement in the eye, fontanelle, face, or genitals of the fetus.

Purpose of the Test

Internal fetal monitoring is used to assess the heart rate of the fetus who is at risk for uteroplacental insufficiency or fetal compromise. It is also used to monitor the strength of uterine contractions—particularly when oxytocin has been administered, when uterine dystocia is suspected, or when there is a trial of labor after a previous delivery by cesarian section.

Procedure

An electrode is inserted through a guide in the vagina and is implanted under the skin of the fetus. The monitoring device is connected to a metal plate on the mother's thigh and then to the fetal cardiac monitor. The internal pressure catheter is passed through the guide and advanced into the uterine cavity until its tip is located between the fetal head and the uterine cervix. This monitoring device is connected by a cord to a pressure reading device and then by cable to the monitor.

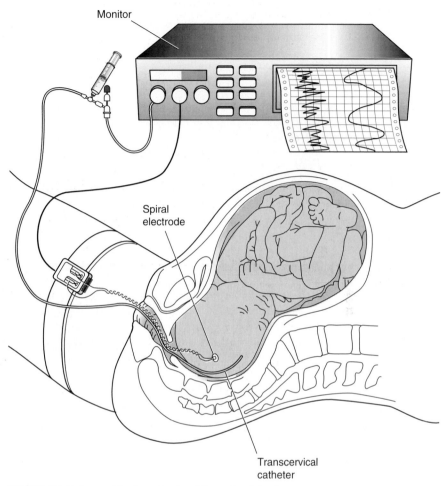

Monitor

Spiral
electrode

Transcervical
catheter

FIGURE 21–5. Internal fetal monitoring. The scalp of the fetus is punctured by the implantation of the electrode. After delivery, the nurse assesses the puncture site for signs of bleeding, hematoma, tissue injury, and potential infection.

Findings

ABNORMAL VALUES

Fetus	Mother
Bradycardia	Infection, fever
Malposition	Hypotension
Hypoxia	Tachycardia
Arrhythmia	Anemia
Congenital anomalies (cardiac or cerebral)	Hyperthyroidism
Growth retardation	Overmedication with a CNS depressant
	Uterine dystocia

Interfering Factors

- Maternal obesity
- Excessive maternal or fetal activity
- Closed cervix
- Presenting part not fully descended or engaged

Nursing Implementation

Pretest

Once the woman receives a complete explanation of the procedure, obtain a written consent.

Assist the woman into the lithotomy position with her legs in stirrups.

During the Procedure

Assist the nurse-midwife or physician with the equipment needed for a sterile vaginal examination and placement of the monitors.

Apply conductive gel to the leg plate and use the strap to secure the plate to the mother's thigh. The uterine catheter is taped to the thigh. Connect the wires and cables correctly.

Turn on the recording device, run a test pattern, and begin the continuous monitoring. Observe for abnormal patterns.

If it helps the mother and her support person to relax, provide simple explanations about the variations in the recordings. Some individuals, however, are made more anxious by knowing every detail. Continue to provide encouragement to the mother as she progresses through labor.

On the paper recording strip, write the patient's name, identification number, weeks of gestation, and the time and date that the monitoring began. Whenever there is a change in maternal or fetal activity, addition of medication, or change of equipment, record the data on the electronic fetal monitor strip.

In the patient's chart, record the woman's vital signs, time of the initiation of internal fetal monitoring, and any special procedures such as amniotomy that were performed.

Posttest

Once the electrode and catheter are removed and the infant is delivered, inspect the skin and puncture site for signs of laceration or infection. Record the results.

Apply an antiseptic or antibiotic solution to the site of skin puncture.

FETAL SCALP BLOOD SAMPLING

(ENDOSCOPY, CAPIL-
LARY BLOOD)

Synonyms:

NORMAL VALUES

Fetal pH: 7.25–7.35

Background Information

Critical Thinking: During labor, there was some meconium staining and the fetal scalp blood had a pH reading of 7.1. In the nursery, which nursing assessments of this newborn should take priority?

During labor, fetal distress and fetal hypoxia are indicated by a number of assessment findings. The fetal monitor may demonstrate late or variable deceleration, a change in heart rate (either bradycardia or tachycardia), or a loss of beat-to-beat variability. In addition, there may be some meconium staining of the amniotic fluid.

The pH of the capillary blood is similar to that of the arterial blood. The pH of fetal capillary blood is a direct assessment for fetal acidosis. In cases of fetal hypoxia, the pH of the fetal blood falls to less than normal levels. A borderline result is indicated by a pH of 7.2 to 7.25. When this slight decline occurs, additional blood specimens are obtained in 15 to 30 minutes. Acidosis is defined as a fetal pH of 7.2 or less, usually demonstrated in two consecutive blood samples. The acidosis confirms that the fetus is hypoxic and health is compromised. Immediate delivery by forceps or cesarian section is indicated.

To obtain the capillary blood sample, there must be access to the scalp or skin of the fetus. The mother must be in active labor, with the membranes ruptured, the cervix partially dilated, and the presenting part engaged. To obtain pertinent and timely data, the blood must be analyzed within 10 to 15 minutes.

Purpose of the Test

Fetal scalp blood sampling is carried out to determine the fetal capillary pH and to identify or confirm fetal acidosis.

Procedure

Under sterile conditions, an endoscope with a light is inserted through the vagina and up to the fetal scalp or presenting part (Fig. 21–6). After the fetal skin is cleansed, a scalpel blade is passed through the endoscope and is used to nick the fetal scalp or skin. Three long heparinized microtubes are used to collect the capillary blood specimen. Once the bleeding ceases, the endoscope is removed.

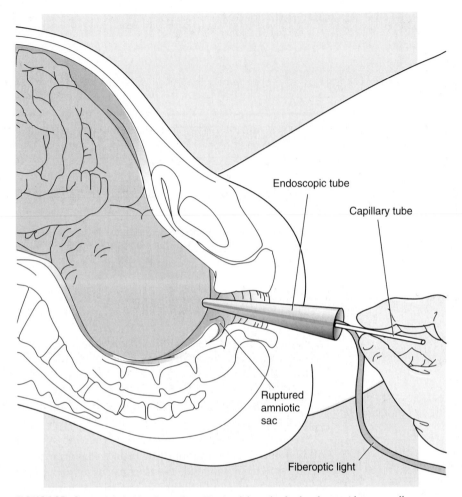

FIGURE 21–6. Fetal scalp blood sampling. During labor, the fetal scalp provides an excellent source of capillary blood, particularly useful for measuring pH. Once the infant is delivered, the nurse assesses the scalp for signs of bleeding, hematoma, tissue injury, and potential infection.

Findings

DECREASED VALUES

Fetal hypoxia
Fetal acidosis
Acute fetal distress

Interfering Factors

• Intact membranes
• Undilated cervix

- Acute and ominous conditions that require immediate delivery (placenta previa, abruptio placentae)

Nursing Implementation

Pretest

Once the need for the test is explained to the mother, obtain her written consent to test the fetal blood.

Although there is urgency in the situation, provide appropriate support to the mother and her partner. Their anxiety level will be high.

Place the mother in the lithotomy or lateral position.

Notify the laboratory if the fetal blood sample requires immediate analysis.

During the Test

Control the endoscopy light and pass the needed equipment to the individual obtaining the sample.

If the cervix is dilated manually, reassure the mother that it is normal to feel uterine cramping.

On receipt of the blood tubes, seal them with clay or wax. Place the tubes on ice to minimize cellular respiration and alteration of the pH.

Label all specimens. Write the identification data, time, date, and source of the blood on the requisition slip. Send the blood to the laboratory immediately.

Posttest

Assist the mother to a lateral position.

As the mother and her partner await the test results, encourage them to support each other.

Document the procedure in the patient's chart.

If labor continues, assess the vaginal fluid for signs of additional blood that could come from the fetal puncture site. Continued fetal bleeding puts the fetus at greater risk.

After delivery, assess the puncture site and document its size and location. Cleanse the skin with an antiseptic and apply antibiotic ointment.

HYSTEROSALPINGOGRAPHY

(RADIOGRAPHY)

Synonym:

hysterosalpingogram

—————————————— **NORMAL VALUES** ——————————————

> There is normal flow of dye through the uterus and fallopian tubes.

Background Information

As part of the infertility work-up in the female, the hysterosalpingogram is performed to identify anatomic abnormality of the uterus or occlusion of the fallopian tubes. The lumen of each of these structures is visualized. The tubes can be blocked because of external compression from an abdominal or pelvic abnormality or there can be internal blockage from scarring. The uterus may have an anatomic abnormality such as that caused by incomplete development of the uterus or congenital abnormality due to intrauterine exposure to diethystibestrol. Uterine abnormality causes about 15% of recurrent spontaneous miscarriages (Smith, 1992).

In normal anatomy, once the radiopaque dye is instilled into the uterine cavity, the effects of gravity and positional changes promote the flow of dye through the fallopian tubes and into the abdominal cavity. If the contrast material does not enter the abdominal cavity, one or both tubes are blocked. The test requires 30 to 45 minutes to complete.

Purpose of the Test

Hysterosalpingography is used to assess the patency of the fallopian tubes as part of infertility studies of the female. It also can identify abnormal development of the uterus and the presence of a uterine fistula.

Procedure

Radiopaque contrast medium is instilled through a catheter into the uterus. The patient's positional changes and a tilting of the table promote gravity flow of the contrast material. Fluoroscopic and x-ray films provide visualization of the interior surfaces of the uterus and fallopian tubes. This procedure may be performed during laparoscopy, with direct visualization of the contrast medium as it enters the abdominal cavity.

Findings

ABNORMAL VALUES

Partial or complete obstruction
  of the fallopian tubes
Uterine fistula
Foreign body (i.e., intrauterine
  device)

Adhesions
Fibroid tumor of the uterus
Uterine malformation

Interfering Factors

- Menstruation
- Pregnancy
- Active uterine bleeding
- Pelvic inflammatory disease
- Allergy to the contrast medium

Nursing Implementation

Pretest

Schedule this test during the early part of the menstrual cycle, before ovulation occurs. This prevents interference with ovulation, irradiation of the oocyte, or the possibility of an early phase of pregnancy.

Ensure that the patient has no current vaginal bleeding or gynecologic infection. When these conditions exist, the contrast material could be absorbed into the vasculature, or its flow could introduce microorganisms into the fallopian tubes.

Identify any patient with a history of allergy to iodine or shellfish or a reaction to a previous x-ray study that used iodinated contrast medium. If there is a positive allergic history, plans are made to premedicate the patient with steroids or an antihistamine, or both.

Once the patient is informed of the procedure, obtain written consent.

In the pretest preparation, instruct the patient to take the prescribed laxative on the night before the test. On the morning of the procedure, she administers cleansing enemas until the returns are clear (Snopek, 1992).

Assist the patient in removing all clothes and putting on a hospital gown. Instruct the patient to void to empty the bladder. This prevents displacement of the uterus and fallopian tubes by an enlarged bladder.

Take the patient's vital signs and record the results.

During the Test

Place the patient in the lithotomy position.

Provide reassurance as the vaginal speculum is inserted, the cervix is cleansed with povidone-iodine, and the cannula is inserted. As the contrast material is instilled, the patient may experience temporary sensations of nausea, dizziness, bradycardia, or uterine cramping.

Between radiographic images, help the patient change position so that the contrast medium flows through the fallopian tubes.

Posttest

Take and record the patient's vital signs.

If an oily contrast material is used, instruct the patient to return in 24 hours for a delayed x-ray of the abdomen. This is carried out to ensure that the contrast medium has entered the peritoneal cavity and is not trapped by an obstruction in the fallopian tubes (Snopek, 1992).

Instruct the patient to gradually return to pretest activity levels.

Complications

An allergic reaction to the contrast medium can cause hives, urticaria, or hypotension.

LAPAROSCOPY

(ENDOSCOPY)

Synonym:

peritoneoscopy

NORMAL VALUES

No abnormalities of the ovaries, fallopian tubes, uterus, or peritoneal cavity are noted.

Background Information

The laparoscope is a fiberoptic telescope that is used to visualize the peritoneal cavity, ovaries, uterus, and fallopian tubes. If a determination of tubal patency is to be included, hysterosalpingography is performed. Additional surgical procedures such as tissue biopsy or tubal ligation may be part of the procedure.

Under general or local anesthesia, the peritoneal cavity is inflated with 2 to 3 L of carbon dioxide. The gas distends the abdomen wall so that the instruments can be inserted safely. The laparoscope is inserted through a small incision just below the umbilicus. If surgical procedure is to be performed, a second incision is made in the lower abdomen for insertion of the additional instruments. To prevent trauma or injury, an indwelling catheter is used to keep the urinary bladder deflated.

Purpose of the Test

Laparoscopy is used to investigate the cause of pelvic pain, detect endometriosis or an ectopic pregnancy, identify a pelvic mass, or determine if cancer is present or has metastasized.

Procedure

A laparoscope is used to visualize the size and shape of the uterus, ovaries, and fallopian tubes. The peritoneal cavity and peritoneum are observed for signs of infection, abscess, or adhesions. Biopsy of abnormal tissue may be performed.

Findings

ABNORMAL VALUES

Ovarian cyst	Endometriosis
Ectopic pregnancy	Uterine fibroid tumors
Pelvic abscess	Pelvic inflammatory disease
Adhesions	Abnormality of the fallopian tubes
Malignancy	

Interfering Factors

- Failure to maintain a nothing-by-mouth status
- Obesity
- Adhesions
- Advanced abdominal wall malignancy

Nursing Implementation

Pretest

Instruct the patient to discontinue all food and fluids for 8 hours before the procedure is performed.

After the patient has been informed about the procedure, obtain written consent from the patient or person legally responsible for the patient's health care decisions. Ensure that all preoperative laboratory work is completed and that the results are posted in the chart.

Assist the patient in removing all clothes and putting on a hospital gown.

Assess and record the vital signs, including the temperature, blood pressure, pulse, and respirations.

Place the patient in the lithotomy position, with the legs supported in stirrups.

During the Test

Insert the indwelling catheter into the bladder and connect it to the urinary collection system.

To help alleviate anxiety, provide reassurance or distraction, as indicated.

If a biopsy specimen is obtained, place the tissue in a glass container with preservative. Identify the tissue source on the requisition slip.

Posttest

Monitor the vital signs every 30 minutes for 4 hours or until stable.

Ensure that the small dressing or dressings remain dry and intact.

Once the catheter is removed, monitor for voiding and urinary output.

TABLE 21–5
COMPLICATIONS OF LAPAROSCOPY

Complication	Nursing Assessment
Hemorrhage	Hypotension
	Tachycardia
	Dizziness
	Grossly bloody drainage from the incision
Infection	Fever
	Malaise
	Diaphoresis
	Tachycardia
	Abdominal pain

Once the patient is alert, encourage ambulation and the oral intake of fluids. Carbonated beverages are avoided for 24 to 36 hours because the excess carbon dioxide in the abdomen and the intake of carbonated beverage can cause vomiting.

Provide pain medication as needed. Advise the patient that some pain in the abdomen and shoulder is to be expected for 24 to 36 hours. The cause is the carbon dioxide gas, which will gradually be absorbed and exhaled from the lungs.

Instruct the patient to restrict physical activity for a few days until the incisions are healed. The patient must notify the physician of increasing abdominal pain, fever, or abnormal drainage.

Complications

Laparoscopy can cause bleeding from the puncture of a blood vessel, infection from external contamination, or the accidental puncture of the intestine. Although these events can occur, they are quite rare. The complications of laparoscopy are presented in Table 21–5.

MAMMOGRAPHY

(RADIOGRAPHY)

Synonym:

mammogram

Background Information

Mammography is used as a screening tool for breast cancer in asymptomatic women because it can identify tumors less than 5 mm in diameter (Bassett and Butler, 1991). This small size is not palpable on physical examination. In the

─────────────────── **NORMAL VALUES** ───────────────────

The breast tissue is within normal limits.

patient with an irregular area of tissue or a palpable growth, this x-ray method is used to obtain additional data about the abnormality.

The normal breast tissue of the younger woman consists of fibroglandular tissue that is dense. After childbearing and in older age, the glandular tissue atrophies and is replaced with fatty tissue. Because fatty tissue is radiolucent, lesions or masses are visible on mammography films.

Malignancy of the breast appears as a dense mass with irregular margins or spiricules. The malignancy may also appear as numerous tiny clusters of calcification. The calcification can be caused by the secretion of calcium from tumor cells or tissue necrosis, or it can be caused by benign fibrocystic disease (Bassett and Butler, 1991). Additional abnormalities that appear on mammography and may indicate malignancy include a newly developed area of density and asymmetry of the breast. Benign growths are also visible, for example, fibroadenoma, cysts, and lymph glands. On mammography, these growths appear more rounded and have well-defined margins.

Purpose of the Test

Mammography is used to screen for breast cancer, and it investigates a symptomatic change in the breast tissue. It helps differentiate between benign and malignant diseases of the breast.

Procedure

X-ray films of each breast are taken from different angles (Fig. 21–7).

Findings

ABNORMAL VALUES

Benign cyst	Microcalcifications
Fibroadenoma	Malignancy of the breast

Interfering Factors

- Jewelry and clothing
- Scar tissue from previous surgery
- Body powders, creams, deodorants

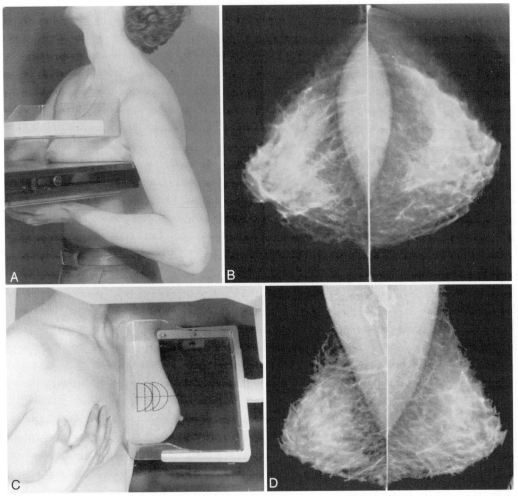

FIGURE 21–7. Mammography positioning and corresponding radiographic views. *A*, Positioning for craniocaudal view. *B*, Radiographs depicting properly positioned craniocaudal views. *C*, Positioning for mediolateral oblique view. *D*, Radiographs depicting properly positioned mediolateral oblique views. (Reproduced with permission from Prue, L.K. [1994]. *Atlas of mammographic positioning* [pp. 16, 17, 23, 24]. Philadelphia: W.B. Saunders.)

Nursing Implementation

Pretest

Instruct the patient to omit the use of body creams, powders, and deodorants on the day of the test. The metallic elements in these products interfere with visualization of the tissues.

Instruct the patient to remove all jewelry and clothing above the waist. The hospital gown is put on with the opening to the front.

During the Test

Critical Thinking: During a health teaching class at the senior center, the nurse discovers that only a few women have had a recent mammogram. Identify possible reasons for their omission of this health care screening test. How would you intervene?

Although the nurse does not perform the mammogram, he or she may be asked to describe the procedure.

The patient is positioned by seating her in front of the machine, with the breast placed on the platform over the x-ray cassette. The compressor is applied to the top of the tissue. The breast is squeezed between the two surfaces to hold the tissue firmly in place. The sensation is one of compression, but it is not painful. Each breast is radiographed separately.

Posttest

No special posttest nursing measures are needed.

PAPANICOLAOU SMEAR

(CYTOLOGIC STUDY)

Synonyms:

Pap smear, cervicovaginal cytology, cervical smear

NORMAL VALUES

BETHESDA SYSTEM CLASSIFICATION
Normal; within normal limits

Background Information

The Papanicolaou smear is an inexpensive screening test to detect premalignant and malignant lesions of the cervix, vagina, and endometrium. In the past, the Papanicolaou smear test results were classified as class I (normal) through class V (invasive cancer). Today, the Bethesda system is the accepted standard for reporting the cervical cytologic results.

The report informs about the adequacy of the specimen and the descriptive findings regarding infection or abnormal cell changes (Table 21–6). Cervical intraepithelial neoplasm (CIN) is measured on a continuum of severity (I, II, III) and documents cervical dysplasia, a precancerous state. Squamous intraepithelial lesions (SIL) are graded from low grade to high grade. The low-grade squamous intraepithelial lesion consists of mild dysplasia–CIN I. A high-grade squamous intraepithelial lesion ranges from moderate dysplasia (CIN II) to severe dysplasia (CIN III), carcinoma in situ. Invasive carcinoma or adenocarcinoma may also be diagnosed.

Abnormal Papanicolaou smear results, the patient's history of relevant risk factors, and the findings of the pelvic examination are the basis for an individualized treatment plan. This may include treatment for infection, repeat

TABLE 21–6
REPORTING SYSTEMS FOR SQUAMOUS CELL NEOPLASIAS OF THE CERVIX

Papanicolaou	World Health Organization	CIN System	Bethesda System
Class I (normal)	Normal	Normal	Normal
Class II (atypical)	Atypical		Other
			Infection (except HPV)
			Reactive and reparative
Class III (suggestive for cancer)	Dysplasia, mild	CIN 1	Low-grade SIL
Class IV (strongly suggestive for cancer)	Moderate to severe, CIS	CIN 2	High-grade SIL
		CIN 3	
Class V (conclusive for cancer)	Invasive squamous cell cancer	Invasive squamous cell cancer	Invasive squamous cell cancer

From Copeland, L.J. (1993). *Textbook of gynecology*. Philadelphia: W.B. Saunders, modified from American Medical Association, Council on Scientific Affairs. Quality assurance in cervical cytology: The Papanicolaou smear. *JAMA*, 1989; 262:1672. Copyright 1989, American Medical Association.

Papanicolaou smear testing at specific intervals, or colposcopy with possible biopsy.

When results of the Papanicolaou smear are abnormal, some women experience fear of cancer, the potential loss of sexual or reproductive function, or the follow-up test procedures. The anxiety may be expressed verbally, somatically (as with loss of sleep or weight gain), emotionally with crying, anger, or irritation. Coping with the abnormal results is a process that appears to have different phases. The needs vary among individuals and at different intervals during the testing process (Lauver and Rubin, 1991).

Purpose of the Test

The Papanicolaou smear is used to detect inflammation, premalignant changes, and malignancy or infection of the vagina and cervix. It is also used to evaluate the response of the cervix to chemotherapy or radiotherapy in the treatment of cancer.

Procedure

Using a vaginal speculum to enhance visibility, secretions and cells from the cervix and vagina are collected. The fluid and tissue scrapings are placed on glass slides and sprayed with or immersed in a fixative.

QUALITY CONTROL

The speculum is not lubricated before insertion because the lubricant would interfere with the microscopic viewing of the slides. The fixative must be applied promptly to prevent drying of the cells.

Findings

ABNORMAL VALUES
Cervical dysplasia or cervical intraepithelial neoplasia
Genital infection (viral, fungal, parasitic)
Cervicovaginal endometriosis
Condyloma
Human papillomavirus
Lymphogranuloma venereum
Carcinoma in situ
Adenocarcinoma

Interfering Factors

- Menstruation
- Recent douching
- Vaginal infection or medication

- Recent sexual intercourse
- Drying of the specimen
- Inadequate specimen

Nursing Implementation

Pretest

Schedule the test when the patient is not menstruating.

Instruct the patient to refrain from sexual intercourse, douching, and vaginal medication for 48 hours before the test. Sexual intercourse can cause inflammation of the tissue. Douching can remove surface cells before the test sample is obtained. Medication obscures the microscopic examination of the cells. If vaginal infection is present, it will be treated and the Papanicolaou test postponed for 2 to 4 weeks (Lucci and Berman, 1992).

Prior to the examination, instruct the patient to void.

During the Test

Help the patient to lie on the table in the lithotomy position with the legs supported by stirrups. The elderly patient may need extra assistance in positioning because of stiffness and arthritis pain (Blesch and Prohaska, 1991).

After the tissue and fluid samples are obtained, apply the fixative by spraying or immersing in solution. Identify each slide with the patient's name.

Posttest

Help the patient get down from the table.

On the requisition slip, write the patient's name, age, date of last menstrual period, and the source of the specimen. The pertinent clinical data are also included, such as history of an abnormal Papanicolaou smear, carcinoma, radiation, chemotherapy, abnormal vaginal bleeding, exposure to diethylstibestrol, a visible lesion, or recent pregnancy.

When the woman is informed of abnormal Papanicolaou test results, she often requires additional information about the meaning of the results and the follow-up measures. Recognize the patient's anxiety or confusion and intervene appropriately to help with the emotional stress. Additional information and repetition of the instructions may be needed (Lauver and Rubin, 1991).

ULTRASOUND, PELVIS

(ULTRASOUND)

Gynecologic ultrasound can be performed transabdominally to scan multiple planes of the abdomen and pelvis. In a transvaginal approach, the ultrasound

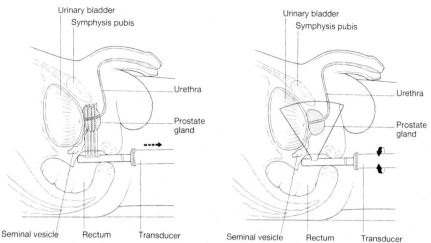

FIGURE 21–8. Ultrasound of the male pelvis. *Left,* Transverse plane—rectal approach. *Right,* Sagittal plane—rectal approach. (Reproduced with permission from Tempkin, B.B. [1993]. *Ultrasound scanning: Principles and protocols* [p. 197]. Philadelphia: W.B. Saunders.)

performs the scans in the coronal plane. In a comprehensive examination of the female, both approaches are used (Wade, 1993). Male pelvic ultrasonography usually uses an endorectal approach to examine the pelvic organs and structures (Fig. 21–8).

ULTRASOUND IN PREGNANCY. In conditions related to pregnancy, ultrasound identifies an early ectopic pregnancy, a multiple pregnancy, fetal abnormality, and assessment of fetal growth. It is also used to guide aspiration procedures such as amniocentesis, cordocentesis, and the aspiration of multiple oocytes for in vitro fertilization.

FEMALE PELVIC ULTRASOUND. In the diagnosis of gynecologic problems, ultrasound is used to identify an ovarian malignancy at an early stage. In the case of abnormal uterine bleeding, it will identify submucous leiomyomas and evaluate the thickness of the uterine wall. Pelvic ultrasound often precedes any invasive gynecologic diagnostic test such as dilation and curretage.

MALE PELVIC ULTRASOUND. Ultrasonography in the male is used to assess the texture, size, and condition of the prostate gland, prostatic urethra, seminal vesicles, and vas deferens. It is also used to guide the placement of the needle during biopsy of the prostate gland.

A complete discussion of ultrasound is presented in Chapter 8.

REFERENCES

Bassett, L.W., & Butler, D.L. (1991). Mammography and early breast cancer. *American Family Physician, 43,* 547–557.

Blesch, K.S., & Prohaska, T.R. (1991). Cervical cancer screening in older women: Issues and interventions. *Cancer Nursing, 14,* 141–147.

Brunzel, N.A. (1994). *Fundamentals of urine and body fluid analysis.* Philadelphia: W.B. Saunders.

Daddario, J.B. (1992). Fetal surveillance in the intensive care unit: Understanding fetal monitoring. *Critical Care Clinics of North America, 4,* 711–719.

Davis, J.M. (1991). Pap tests needed for women of all ages. *Postgraduate Medicine, 89,* 27, 30.

Doogan, R.A. (1991). The role of mammography in the early detection of breast cancer. *Nurse Practitioner Forum, 2,* 217–224.

Dubin, S.B. (1992). Assessment of fetal lung maturity by laboratory methods. *Clinics in Laboratory Medicine, 18,* 603–620.

Eganhouse, D.J. (1991). Electronic fetal monitoring: Education and quality assurance. *Journal of Obstetrical, Gynecologic and Neonatal Nursing, 20,* 16–22.

Eganhouse, D.J., & Burnside, S.M. (1992). Nursing assessment and responsibilities in monitoring the preterm pregnancy. *Journal of Obstetrical, Gynecologic and Neonatal Nursing 21,* 355–363.

Ferris, D.G. (1992). Colposcopy for early detection of cervical cancer. *Emergency Medicine, 24,* 115–118, 121.

Friedman, W.N., & Rosenfield, A.T. (1992). Computed tomography in obstetrics and gynecology. *Journal of Reproductive Medicine, 37,* 3–18.

Hajdu, S.I., & Gaston, J.P. (1991). Aspiration cytology of the breast. *Clinics in Laboratory Medicine, 11,* 357–368.

Henry, J.B. (Ed.) (1991). *Clinical diagnosis and management by laboratory methods* (18th ed.). Philadelphia: W.B. Saunders.

Jacobs, D.S., et al. (Eds.). (1990). *Laboratory Test Handbook* (2nd ed.). Baltimore: Williams & Wilkins.

Lauver, D., & Rubin, M. (1991). Women's concerns about abnormal Papanicolaou test results. *Journal of Obstetrical, Gynecologic and Neonatal Nursing, 20,* 154–159.

Lucci, J.A., & Berman, M.L. (1992). Improving the accuracy of the Pap smear. *Emergency Medicine, 24,* 87–92, 95–96, 98.

MacFarlane, M.E., & Sony, S.D. (1992). Women, breast lump discovery, and associated stress. *Health Care for Women International, 13,* 23–32.

McGowan K.L., & Hodinka, R.L. (1992). Laboratory diagnosis of fetal infections. *Clinics in Laboratory Medicine, 12,* 523–552.

Murphy-Black, T. (1991). Fetal monitoring in labor [RCM supplement]. *Nursing Times, 87,* 58–59.

Nugent, L.S., et al. (1992). The colposcopy experience: What do women know? *Journal of Advanced Nursing, 17,* 514–520.

O'Brien, J.M. (1989). Male factor infertility. *Primary Care, 16,* 1057–1068.

Paine, L.L., et al. (1992). A comparison of the auscultated acceleration test and the nonstress test as predictors of perinatal outcomes. *Nursing Research, 41,* 87–91.

Peart, O. (1992). Stereostatic localization pinpoints breast lesions. *Radiologic Technology, 63,* 234–239.

Ramzy, I., & Mody, D.R. (1991). Gynecologic cytology. *Clinics in Laboratory Medicine, 11,* 271–292.

Satish, J. (1992). Prenatal genetics in laboratory medicine. *Clinics in Laboratory Medicine, 12,* 493–502.

Smith, S. (1992). Use of the laboratory in infertility and recurrent spontaneous miscarriage. *Clinics in Laboratory Medicine, 12,* 393–410.

Snopek, A.M. (1992). *Fundamentals of special radiographic procedures* (3rd ed.). Philadelphia: W.B. Saunders.

Sundaram, S.G., et al. (1992). Alpha-fetoprotein and screening markers of congenital disease. *Clinics of Laboratory Medicine, 18,* 481–492.

Teitz, N.W. (Ed.). (1990). *Clinical Guide to Laboratory Tests* (2nd ed.). Philadelphia: W.B. Saunders.

Wade, N. (1993). Gynecologic applications of real-time ultrasound. *Applied Radiology, 22,* 15–19.

Wax, J.R., & Blakemore, K.J. (1992). What can be learned from cordocentesis? *Clinics in Laboratory Medicine, 18,* 503–521.

Neurologic function

Neurologic laboratory tests and diagnostic procedures include both general and highly specific measures that provide data about the nervous system. The tests focus on the assessment of the skull, brain, spinal cord, central and peripheral nerves, and the extracranial and intracranial circulation. The tests are used to confirm the presence and location of a lesion and to provide data about the cause of the problem. The tests are also used to gauge the progression of the disease or the patient's response to treatment.

Many of these tests provoke anxiety in the patient and the patient's family because of fear of pain, the potential for a severe complication as a result of the procedure, and the threatening nature of the potential neurologic diagnosis.

Often, the patient who must have a neurologic diagnostic procedure already has abnormal assessment findings that result from disease or trauma. For example, he or she may be in a coma, mentally confused, paralyzed, or in severe pain. The patient's pretest condition and limitations are incorporated into the plan of care for each diagnostic test or procedure. The nurse's assistance provides accurate pretest preparation, patient safety, measures to meet emotional, physical, and cognitive needs, with accurate assessment before, during, and after each test.

LABORATORY TESTS

CEREBROSPINAL FLUID ANALYSIS AND LUMBAR PUNCTURE

(CEREBROSPINAL FLUID)

Synonyms:

CSF analysis, spinal tap, LP

―――――――――― **NORMAL VALUES** ――――――――――

CEREBROSPINAL FLUID ANALYSIS

Pressure:	90–180 mm H_2O (lateral recumbent position)
Appearance:	clear, colorless
Microscopic Examination	
Leukocyte Count:	
Adult:	0–5 cells per µl *or* SI 0–5 × 10^6/L
Child (5–18 years):	0–10 cells per µl *or* SI 0–10 × 10^6/L
Neonate–1 year:	0–30 cells per µl *or* SI 0–30 × 10^6/L
Differential Count:	
Adult:	
Lymphocytes:	40–80%
Monocytes:	15–45%
Neutrophils:	0–6%
Neonate:	
Lymphocytes:	5–35%
Monocytes:	50–90%
Neutrophils:	0–8%
Chemistry Analysis	
Lactate:	10–22 mg/dl *or* SI 1.1–2.4 mmol/L
Glucose:	50–80 mg/dl *or* SI 2.75–4.4 mmol/L
Total Protein:	15–45 mg/dl *or* SI 150–450 mg/L
Albumin:	10–30 mg/dl *or* SI 100–300 mg/L
IgG:	1–4 mg/dl *or* SI 10–40 mg/L
Protein Electrophoresis (% of Total Protein):	
Prealbumin:	2–7%
Albumin:	56–76%
Alpha$_1$-globulin:	2–7%
Alpha$_2$-globulin:	4–12%
Beta globulin:	8–18%
Gamma globulin:	3–12%
Myelin–Basic Protein:	0–5 µg/L

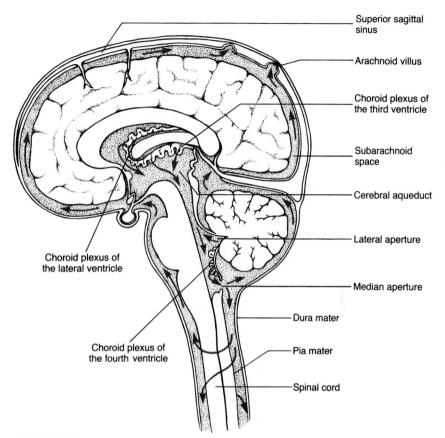

FIGURE 22–1. Circulation of the cerebrospinal fluid. A schematic representation of the brain and spinal cord, including the circulation of the cerebrospinal fluid. (Reproduced with permission from Brunzel, N. [1994]. *Fundamentals of urine and body fluid analysis* [p. 366]. Philadelphia: W.B. Saunders.)

Background Information

About 70% of the cerebrospinal fluid is produced in the ventricles of the brain, with the remainder coming from the interstitial spaces of the cells of the brain and spinal cord. There is continuous production-secretion and reabsorption so that the volume of the cerebrospinal fluid remains relatively constant. The total volume of cerebrospinal fluid for the adult ranges from 90 to 150 ml, and the total volume for the neonate is 10 to 60 ml. The fluid circulates throughout the subarachnoid space and continuously bathes the brain and spinal cord (Fig. 22–1).

The fluid protects and supports the central nervous system and provides the medium for the exchange of nutrients and metabolic wastes. Although the chemical composition of the cerebrospinal fluid includes measurable electrolytes, ions, enzymes, and carbon dioxide, the significance of these values is not clearly understood (Brunzel, 1994). The chemistry values of protein, glucose, and lactate help in the diagnoses of neurologic disease as does the presence of cells and microorganisms.

Lumbar Puncture

Lumbar puncture is used to obtain the sample of cerebrospinal fluid for analysis. This procedure involves the insertion of a sterile spinal needle between the lumbar vertebrae into the subarachnoid space. Because the spinal cord ends at L1–L2 in adults, the spinal tap is performed below that level. The level of the tap is usually in the third or fourth lumbar interspace for adults and the fourth or fifth interspace for children.

CEREBROSPINAL FLUID PRESSURE. Once the needle is in the subarachnoid space, the pressure of the fluid is measured with a manometer attached to the needle. If the pressure is in the normal range, a specimen of up to 20 ml can be removed. After the removal of 10 to 20 ml of cerebrospinal fluid in a normal spinal tap, the closing pressure is normally 45 to 90 mm H_2O.

Since children have less total fluid in proportion to age and body size, the specimen sample must be considerably smaller. If the child's opening pressure is higher or lower than normal, a specimen of only 1 to 2 ml can be removed. This limitation is imposed because there is a risk of cerebellar herniation or spinal cord compression.

ANALYSIS OF THE CEREBROSPINAL FLUID

Appearance. The normal cerebrospinal fluid is clear and colorless, with a viscosity similar to that of water. Cloudy fluid, called *pleocytosis*, is caused by an increased number of cells in the fluid. There may be an increase in erythrocytes, leukocytes, microorganisms, or protein. The cloudiness is sometimes measured on a scale of 0 to 4+ (from clear to cloudy).

Discoloration of the fluid, called *xanthochromia*, indicates that there are abnormal components present in the fluid. The fluid may appear pink, orange, or yellow. The abnormal components include oxyhemoglobin, carotene, bilirubin, and other substances. Gross blood may be present and is caused by a traumatic tap, a subarachnoid hemorrhage, or an intracerebral hemorrhage. The increased viscosity of the fluid may be caused by a metastatic mucin-secreting adenocarcinoma.

Microscopic Examination. The normal total cell count is low in adults and in children of all ages. There is a slight increase in the monocytes in the normal neonate. When there is a high elevation of leukocytes, the cause is often bacterial meningitis, but the count varies among infected patients. A cloudy specimen is associated with a white blood cell count of more than 200 cells per µl and a very high count may be greater than 50,000 cells per µl. The erythrocyte count is of little diagnostic value because the source of the red blood cells is usually the peripheral blood or a traumatic tap.

Differential Cell Count. Normally, lymphocytes and monocytes are the predominant cells in cerebrospinal fluid. In bacterial meningitis, the neutrophil count is greatly elevated. In other causes of meningitis—including viral, tubercular, fungal, and syphilitic infection—there is an increased lymphocyte count.

Other cells may be present and indicate abnormality. The presence of plasma cells can be due to acute viral infection, a chronic inflammatory condition, or multiple sclerosis. A large increase in eosinophils is indicative of a parasitic or fungal infection but may also occur with a malfunctioning intracranial shunt or an intrathecal injection of medication or contrast medium. Malignant cells indicate a primary or metastatic tumor. Metastases are commonly from melanoma, leukemia, lymphoma, or cancer of the breast, lung, or gastrointestinal tract.

CHEMICAL ANALYSIS

Lactate. The lactate level increases in conditions of anaerobic metabolism, tissue hypoxia, and decreased oxygenation of the brain. The problem may be systemic and interfere with oxygen transport to the brain and central nervous system, or it may be a problem within the brain itself.

Glucose. The glucose concentration is proportionate to the level of blood glucose. Within a period of 2 hours before the spinal tap, the glucose level in the cerebrospinal fluid is normally 60 to 70% of the blood level. To interpret the glucose level of the cerebrospinal fluid correctly, a blood specimen must be drawn 30 to 60 minutes before the spinal tap is performed. Higher than normal values of glucose in the cerebrospinal fluid reflect hyperglycemia. Lower than normal values (<40 mg/dl) of glucose in the cerebrospinal fluid occur with many forms of meningitis, neoplasm, inflammatory disorder, and other conditions.

Protein. Some protein is normally present in the cerebrospinal fluid, but an excessive increase or decrease is indicative of a problem. The increased level may be the result of increased permeability of the blood-brain barrier, allowing protein to pass into the cerebrospinal fluid. It may also be the result of poor resorption of the protein or an increase in immunoglobulin synthesis. Decreased protein values occur when there is an increase in water resorption, such as with increased intracranial pressure or with leakage of the cerebrospinal fluid as the result of head trauma.

Albumin. Among the different proteins that compose the total protein value, albumin is the largest component. It enters the cerebrospinal fluid by crossing the blood-brain barrier. Therefore, the albumin level monitors its permeability.

IgG. Increased amounts of IgG may result from increased production of the antibody within the central nervous system or from an increase in the transport of the antibody across the blood-brain barrier. Elevated values are indicative of multiple sclerosis and other inflammatory disorders of the central nervous system.

PROTEIN ELECTROPHORESIS. This test reveals the specific composition and distribution of the cerebrospinal fluid proteins. The primary purpose of this test is to identify *oligoclonal bands* in the gamma region. The presence of these bands is highly indicative of multiple sclerosis. Serum protein electrophoresis is performed on the patient's blood, which is drawn at the same time the lumbar puncture is performed. In 90% of patients with multiple sclerosis, the oligoclonal bands are not present in the serum specimen, but they are present in the cerebrospinal fluid at some point during the course of the disease.

MYELIN–BASIC PROTEIN. Myelin–basic protein is one of the proteins of the myelin sheath that surrounds axons of nerves. In multiple sclerosis and other demyelinating diseases, the myelin–basic protein is released into the cerebrospinal fluid during an acute exacerbation of the disease and deterioration of the myelin sheaths. The test is used to monitor the disease and to identify patients who have multiple sclerosis but who do not demonstrate oligoclonal banding.

MISCELLANEOUS TESTS. In addition to the standard tests, the cerebrospinal fluid may be cultured to identify the infectious agent. The common aerobic pathogens that cause meningitis are *Haemophilus influenzae*, *Neisseria meningitidis*, and *Streptococcus pneumoniae*. Other agents are fungal, parasitic, bacterial, tubercular, or viral in origin.

Immunologic examination may also be performed to detect the specific microbial antigen that is present in bacterial or fungal meningitis. Immunologic testing may include the testing performed to confirm neurosyphilis.

Cytologic examination may be performed to identify the cells of the primary or metastatic tumor. The malignant cells are shed from a malignant tumor that has extended into the ventricles or subarachnoid space.

Purpose of the Test

Lumbar puncture is performed to measure the pressure of the cerebrospinal fluid and to detect obstruction in the circulation of this fluid.

Analysis of the cerebrospinal fluid is performed to confirm the diagnosis of infection in the central nervous system or to identify a tumor or hemorrhage in the brain, spinal cord, or surrounding lining of the tissues. It may be performed to confirm a chronic central nervous system infection such as neurosyphilis.

Procedure

Lumbar Puncture: Under sterile conditions and using local anesthesia, a spinal needle is inserted between the lower lumbar vertebrae and into the subarachnoid space (Fig. 22–2). After pressure measurements, 15 to 20 ml of cerebrospinal fluid is collected in three or more sterile tubes.

Findings

ELEVATED VALUES

Cells

Leukocytes
Bacterial meningitis

Neutrophils
Bacterial meningitis
Encephalomyelitis

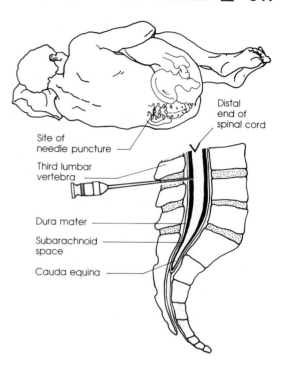

Distal
end of
spinal cord

Site of
needle puncture

Third lumbar
vertebra

Dura mater

Subarachnoid
space

Cauda equina

FIGURE 22–2. Patient position for lumbar puncture. The flexion of the lumbar spine widens the intervertebral spaces so that the needle can be inserted into the subarachnoid space more easily. (Reproduced with permission from Dewit, S.C. [1992]. *Keane's essentials of medical surgical nursing* [3rd ed., p. 330]. Philadelphia: W.B. Saunders.)

Lymphoctyes
Meningitis
Parasitic infection

Plasma Cells
Multiple sclerosis
Guillain-Barré syndrome

Malignant Cells
Leukemia
Lymphoma
Medulloblastoma
Metastatic carcinoma

Chemistry

Lactate
Low arterial P_{O_2}
Hypotension
Stroke
Hydrocephalus
Brain trauma
Cerebral edema
Meningitis
Cerebral arteriosclerosis

Cerebral abscess
Cerebral hemorrhage
Cerebral infarction
Tumor

Eosinophils
Parasitic infection
Fungal infection
Allergic reaction within the central
  nervous system

Glucose
Hyperglycemia

Total Protein
Meningitis
Stroke
Extradural abscess
Endocrine disorder
Trauma
Tumor
Herniated disc
Multiple sclerosis
Neurosyphilis

Protein Electrophoresis

Alpha$_2$-Globulin
Severe craniocerebral trauma

Gamma Globulin
Multiple sclerosis

Oligoclonal Bands
Multiple sclerosis
Subacute sclerosing panen-
  cephalitis
Jakob-Creutzfeldt disease
Encephalitis
Guillain-Barré syndrome
Neurosyphilis
Cerebrovascular accident
Cerebral vasculitis
Neoplasm

DECREASED VALUES

Glucose
Acute, chronic meningitis
Meningoencephalitis
Systemic hypoglycemia
Subarachnoid hemorrhage
Neurosyphilis
Sarcoidosis (meningeal)
Carcinomatous meningitis

Albumin
Viral meningitis
Guillain-Barré syndrome
Collagen diseases

IgG
Multiple sclerosis
Sclerosing panencephalitis
Neurosyphilis

Myelin-Basic Protein
Multiple sclerosis
Head trauma
Cerebrovascular accident
Leukemia
Neurosyphilis
Systemic lupus erythematosus
Guillain-Barré syndrome

Total Protein
Trauma, dural tear
Increased intracranial pressure

Interfering Factors

- Infection of skin or epidural abscess at the site of the proposed spinal tap
- Increased intracranial pressure
- Spinal block (incomplete or complete)
- Bleeding disorder

Nursing Implementation

Pretest

Obtain written consent from the patient or the person legally responsible for the patient's health care decisions.

Ask the patient about any history of hemophilia, thrombocytopenia, other bleeding disorder, or anticoagulation therapy. Because these problems will result in prolonged bleeding into the tissues or cerebrospinal fluid, they are a relative contraindication to lumbar puncture.

Assist the patient in removing all clothing and putting on a hospital gown.

Take and record vital signs.

Place the patient in a lateral recumbent position with his or her back at the edge of the bed or examining table. Flex the patient's neck and knees toward the chest (Fig. 22–2). The flexion of the spine widens the intervertebral spaces.

During the Test

Assist with the preparation of the equipment and sterile field, the antiseptic cleansing of the skin, and the preparation of the local anesthetic. Usually, lidocaine, 1 to 2 ml, is administered subcutaneously by the physician.

Instruct the patient to remain absolutely still during the insertion of each needle. Hold the patient in position to help prevent movement.

Critical Thinking: As the patient is positioned for lumbar puncture, she tells you that she is very frightened. Before and during the procedure, what nursing interventions can you use to help her?

Provide reassurance to the patient as the needles are inserted. The administration of the anesthetic causes a stinging sensation. There is brief pain as the spinal needle penetrates the dura and enters the subarachnoid space.

Assist the patient in placing the legs in extension for the pressure reading.

Assist with the collection of the cerebrospinal fluid.

Mark the tubes "1, 2, 3," and so on in the order that they are collected.

QUALITY CONTROL

The first tube is used for chemical and immunologic analysis because blood or tissue fluid will not alter these test results. The second tube is used for microbial analysis, and the third tube is used for microscopic examination of cells. If only a small amount of fluid is drawn, it is placed in a single tube and the physician prioritizes the tests.

Arrange for immediate delivery of the specimen to the laboratory.

QUALITY CONTROL

With delay, lysis of the white blood cells results in a false decrease in the cell count. Additionally, glycolysis causes a false rise in the lactate value and the microbial organisms may be destroyed. If there is an unavoidable delay in the laboratory, tube No. 1 (chemical and immunologic tests) is frozen. Tube No. 2 (microbiologic tests) is kept at room temperature, and tube No. 3 (cell counts and cytologic study) is refrigerated (Brunzel, 1994).

Posttest

Take vital signs at regular and frequent intervals until they are stable. At the same time, assess the patient's level of consciousness and responsiveness.

Assess the puncture site for swelling, redness, or leakage of cerebrospinal fluid.

Instruct the patient to lie flat in a supine position for 1 to 6 hours. This helps prevent headache following lumbar puncture. If headache occurs, bedrest is extended to 12 hours.

Administer extra fluids to help the patient replace the volume of fluid in the subarachnoid space and to help prevent headache.

Administer the prescribed pain medication, as needed.

At regular intervals, assess the patient's motor ability in the lower legs (Mason, 1992). If there is spinal blockage and severe compression of the cord following the procedure, paresis can turn into paralysis. In addition, massive hematoma can occur within the subarachnoid space. This would compress the cauda equina and result in paralysis (Guberman, 1994).

Complications

The most frequent complication of a lumbar puncture is headache. Infection, hematoma, and bleeding can also occur. Although it is an infrequent complication, increased intracranial pressure can occur as the result of a complete spinal block and the resultant interference with the circulation of cerebrospinal fluid. The increase in the intracranial pressure can also be caused by meningitis or the patient's illness.

A summary of the complications of a lumbar puncture is presented in Table 22–1.

DIAGNOSTIC PROCEDURES

TABLE 22–1
COMPLICATIONS OF LUMBAR PUNCTURE

Complication	Nursing Assessment
Spinal headache	Severe head pain
Increased intracranial pressure	Deteriorating level of consciousness (deepening stupor to coma)
	Bradycardia
	Elevated blood pressure
	Slowed or irregular respirations
	Pupillary changes
Infection (meningitis)	High fever
	Headache
	Myalgia
	Back pain
	Photophobia
	Deteriorating level of consciousness
	Meningeal irritation (muscle stiffness or spasm in neck and other extensor muscles, positive Kernig sign, positive Brudzinski sign)
	Seizures
Complete spinal block	Paresis (weakness of the lower legs)
	Paralysis of the lower legs
	Signs of increased intracranial pressure
Bleeding, hematoma	Oozing of blood or cerebrospinal fluid from the puncture site
	Localized swelling-edema
	Bruising-ecchymosis near the puncture site

ANGIOGRAPHY, BRAIN, HEAD, AND NECK

(RADIOGRAPHY)

Synonym:

cerebral angiography

——————————— **NORMAL VALUES** ———————————

No abnormalities of the tissue or vasculature are visualized.

Background Information

Angiography of the brain, head, and neck provides clear imaging of intracranial and extracranial vascular abnormalities and their locations. Although the less invasive procedure of computed tomography (CT) has surpassed

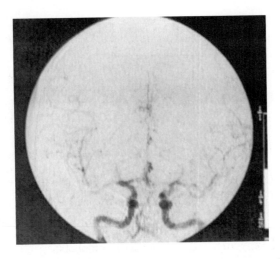

FIGURE 22–3. Digital cerebral angiogram. Vessels appear dark because of computer manipulation. (Courtesy of David Skarbek.)

angiography for the imaging of tumors and trauma to the brain, angiography remains a mainstay in the investigation of the cerebral vasculature. There are several different types of cerebral angiography that can be performed.

CEREBRAL AND ARCH ANGIOGRAPHY. In this type of angiography, a thin catheter is inserted via the femoral artery and passed up the aorta. At the aortic arch, the catheter is passed into the innominate, common carotid, or left subclavian artery, and then into the vertebral, internal, or external carotid artery. Once the catheter is in place, iodinated radiopaque contrast medium is injected under pressure, and rapid serial x-rays are taken. The contrast material provides visualization of the extracranial and intracranial circulation. In selected cases, a catheter is not passed through the arterial system. Instead, the contrast medium is introduced by a direct puncture of the common carotid artery or by a retrograde injection of contrast material into the brachial artery. The angiography procedure is sometimes called plain film angiography because of the use of simple x-ray or plain films for the imaging process.

DIGITAL SUBTRACTION ANGIOGRAPHY. In this newer methodology, the visualization of the contrast medium and the vasculature is enhanced by computer resolution that subtracts out the images of bone and other overlying tissues that interfere with the visualization of the arteries. Digital subtraction angiography is particularly useful in the investigation of extracranial blood vessels. When the contrast material is injected into an artery, the procedure is called *intraarterial digital subtraction angiography* (Fig. 22–3). The femoral artery is commonly used. With the assistance of computer resolution, the images are clearer and more magnified. When the contrast medium is injected into a vein, the procedure is called *intravenous subtraction angiography.* An antecubital vein is commonly used. Although the venous route is technically easier and there are fewer complications or arterial emboli, the imaging is less clear. In addition, there are a greater number of other complications, including allergy or toxicity to the contrast medium (Snopek, 1992).

In addition to the visualization of the vasculature of the head, neck, and brain, cerebral angiography demonstrates the location and characteristic vascular patterns of different types of brain tumors. It locates and defines the source of a subarachnoid hemorrhage and also identifies vascular malformation. Thrombosis, embolic occlusion, or atheromatous stenosis can be seen when it occurs in a major extracranial or intracranial artery. Subdural hematoma is also visualized because there is no contrast material circulating in the space between the skull and the displaced brain tissue.

There are infrequent, but devastating, complications that can occur with cerebral angiography. Many of the patients are elderly and in poor general health, with extensive arteriosclerotic disease or heart disease, or both. These problems make them more vulnerable to complications following the procedure. The incidence and seriousness of the complications have lessened considerably in recent years. This is partially because of improvements in the catheter materials and the lower toxicity of the contrast media (Kim and Orron, 1992; Dublin, 1989).

Purpose of the Test

Cerebral angiography identifies abnormalities of the vasculature and the blood flow in the neck and brain.

Procedure

Iodinated radiopaque contrast material is injected arterially or intravenously. Rapid serial x-ray films are taken to image the bolus of contrast medium as it moves through the circulation of the neck and extracranial and intracranial blood vessels.

Findings

ABNORMAL VALUES

Brain tumor
Arteriovenous malformation
Arteriosclerosis
Vasospasm, arteritis
Cerebral edema
Stenosis
Vascular occlusion

Fistula
Obstruction of the cerebrospinal fluid
Atherosclerotic plaque
Cerebral aneurysm
Subarachnoid hemorrhage

Interfering Factors

• Movement of the head during imaging
• Metal objects in the x-ray field

- Vomiting during the imaging process
- Allergy to iodine

Nursing Implementation

Pretest

Ask the patient about history of previous allergy to iodine, including an allergic reaction to seafood, shellfish, or iodine during previous x-ray studies using contrast medium.

Obtain written consent from the patient or the person who has legal responsibility for the patient's health care decisions.

Instruct the patient regarding the food and fluid restrictions before the test. Because there are some variations among institutions, verify the protocol that is to be used by the particular radiology department.

- Instruct the patient to discontinue food intake for 6 to 8 hours before the test. The contrast medium can cause nausea. If there is food in the stomach, the vomiting would result in head movement during the imaging process and blurring of the photographic results.
- Most institutions permit the intake of clear fluids during the fasting period (Snopek, 1992). Some limit the amount and others encourage extra intake of fluids to promote hydration and renal excretion of the contrast medium (Torres, 1993). For the patient who has fluid restrictions, intravenous fluids are started early in the test period so that renal function is optimal.
- When this test is to be performed on an outpatient or ambulatory basis, instruct the patient to have a responsible person available for transportation home after the test. The sedative effects of the medications will remain for several hours after the test is completed.

Assist the patient in removing all clothing and putting on a hospital gown. All metal objects and jewelry are removed from the head, hair, neck, and upper torso.

Take the baseline vital signs and assess the peripheral pulses. Record the results.

Administer the prescribed pretest sedative and analgesic medications. The purposes of the medications are to decrease central nervous system activity, anxiety, tension, physical activity, and potential agitation. Some of the medications also reduce nausea and the potential for vomiting. The particular combination of drugs varies with the institutional protocol or choice of the physician. Drugs with a sedative or calming effect include phenobarbital (Nembutal), hydroxyzine hydrochloride (Vistaril), promethazine hydrochloride (Phenergan), diphenhydramine (Benadryl), and diazepam (Valium). Choices of analgesics include morphine sulfate, meperidine (Demerol), and fentanyl (Sublimaze) (Snopek, 1992).

During the Test

Establish an intravenous line for fluid replacement and the electrocardiographic leads for monitoring the heart rate and rhythm. Take vital signs at appropriate intervals.

Instruct the patient to keep the head and neck absolutely still during the injection of contrast material and the imaging sequence. Restraints may be used to prevent movement.

Inform the patient that he or she may feel a temporary flushing or burning sensation, a salty taste, headache, or nausea as the contrast medium is injected.

Posttest

Once the catheter is removed from the artery, use sterile gauze to apply digital pressure to the puncture site for 10 minutes. This should prevent bleeding or hematoma formation. If swelling or redness occurs, apply ice to the area.

Continue to monitor vital signs at frequent intervals until they are stable and in a normal range.

Assess the extremity that is distal to the arterial injection site. There should be adequate circulation and mobility and intact neurologic function.

Assess the patient's mental status, observing for clarity of thinking, alertness, and intact neurologic function.

Critical Thinking: One hour after cerebral angiography, you note that the patient has one pupil that is sluggish in response to light. What other immediate nursing assessments are indicated?

Prior to discharge, instruct the patient to remain on bedrest for the remainder of the day. The extremity used for the arterial injection should be maintained in extension. By the next day, most physical activities may be resumed, but vigorous exercise should be avoided for an additional day or two.

Complications

After cerebral angiography, the overall incidence of complication is 0.3 to 1% and includes neurologic deficit, stroke, leg ischemia, excessive bleeding, and a reaction to the contrast medium. In most instances, the complications occur within 1 to 2 hours after the test.

COMPUTED TOMOGRAPHY, CRANIAL, SPINAL

(TOMOGRAPHY)

Synonyms:

The CT scan is an effective primary diagnostic procedure. It is used to investigate intracerebral, extracerebral, and spinal lesions. The abnormalities may be congenital, degenerative, inflammatory, vascular, or tumorous in origin.

Because the scan produces tomographic axial slices for viewing, the precise location, size, and characteristics of the abnormality can be seen. The procedure is performed with or without the use of contrast material.

Intracranial lesions that are identified by CT are hydrocephalus and aqueduct stenosis, cerebral atrophy, hemorrhage, hematoma, infarction, and edema of the brain. Tumors within the cranium may be (1) intracerebral and often malignant or (2) extracerebral and probably benign. Extracerebral tumors include meningiomas, acoustic neuromas, epidermoid tumors, dermoid tumors, craniopharyngiomas, and pituitary tumors. An extracerebral hematoma can also be identified, and its relationship to a fracture of the skull is visible.

In the spinal column, the CT scan demonstrates the bony and soft tissue abnormalities that compress the cord and nerve roots. It visualizes the bulge in a disc, a degenerative change, the alignment and structure of the vertebrae, spinal infection, and hypertrophy of the ligaments. In addition, the diameter of the spinal cord can be measured. CT is often used to confirm spinal stenosis as a cause of spinal cord disorder (Chase, 1991).

A detailed discussion of CT is presented in Chapter 12.

ELECTROENCEPHALOGRAPHY

(ELECTROPHYSIOLOGY)

Synonyms:

electroencephalogram, EEG

--- **NORMAL VALUES** ---

Normal patterns of electric brain activity are seen.

Background Information

Electroencephalography records the spontaneous brain activity that originates from the cortical pyramidal cells on the surface of the brain. The electric activity, called action potential, comes from the depolarization along nerve cell membranes. The fluctuations of electric activity from the larger cortical areas of the brain are detected on the electroencephalogram (EEG) (Mason, 1992).

Using the older electroencephalographic methodology, the fluctuations in electric activity are recorded on a moving paper by a series of pens. In several of the newer methodologies, the data are computerized and displayed on a monitor. In the process of *electric brain mapping*, the computer demonstrates trends in particular areas of brain activity. Another alternative electroencephalographic methodology uses the *video electroencephalography monitor*. It combines the recording of the EEG waveforms with videotaping to correlate the behavioral events with electroencephalographic seizure activity. This method is particularly useful with neonates in the neonatal intensive care unit (Squires, 1992). The video electroencephalography monitor may also be used for older children or adults. The recording and imaging are often performed continuously for a 7 to 8 hour period. The patient can move and walk around the room at intervals without interfering with the monitoring procedure. *Ambulatory monitoring*, another variation in methodology, uses a small portable cassette recording device. It is useful for small children who have seizures in school.

During the recording of the EEG, *sensory evoked potentials* can be measured. These are the electric brain responses that occur when there is a visual, auditory, or somatosensory stimulus. One type of visual stimulus is a strobe light, and the response to this stimulus is recorded by an electrode placed over the occipital lobe. The auditory stimulus is a clicking noise, and it may be used to evaluate the integrity of the eighth cranial nerve during surgery to remove an acoustic neuroma. The somatosensory stimulus is an electric shock delivered to the posterior tibial nerve or median nerve. It is used to assess the lower extremity for movement in the paralyzed individual. It may also be used to assess the function of other specific neural pathways. Sensory evoked potentials may also be used to determine cerebral death.

The rhythms of the electroencephalographic recording are identified as delta (the slowest), theta, alpha, and beta (the fastest). The interpretation of the EEG considers the frequency of the predominant rhythm, amplitude, abnormal waves or wave groups, and asymmetry between the right and left hemispheres.

Purpose of the Test

The major applications of the EEG are in the diagnosis of epilepsy, the determination of the type of epilepsy, the diagnosis of metabolic encephalopathy, and in helping to detect brain injury.

Procedure

In adults, 21 recording needle electrodes are applied to the scalp in particular groupings, using electric paste to promote conduction. The electrode wires are connected to the electroencephalograph recorder. In neonates, fewer electrodes are used because of the smaller head size (Squires, 1992) (Fig. 22–4). The electroencephalography procedure usually takes several hours, but the sleep EEG is recorded all night. For the neonate, the test is usually performed in the isolette in the neonatal intensive care unit.

Findings

ABNORMAL VALUES

Epilepsy (grand mal, focal, temporal lobe, myoclonal, petit mal)
Cerebral infarct

Intracranial hemorrhage
Mental retardation
Hypoxic, ischemic encephalopathy

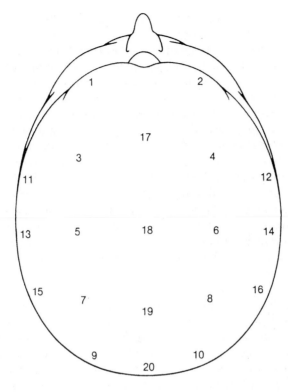

FIGURE 22–4. Placement of electroencephalogram electrodes in the infant. (Reproduced with permission from Squires, L.A. [1992]. Neonatal seizures. *Critical Care Clinics of North America, 4,* 497.)

Hypocalcemia
Hypoglycemia
Meningitis
Brain tumor

Drug withdrawal
Toxoplasmosis, rubella, cytomegalovirus, herpes simplex (TORCH) infection

Interfering Factors

- Caffeine
- Movements of the hands, body, or tongue
- Muscle contractions
- Drug intoxication (heroin, cocaine, marijuana, crack, lysergic acid diethylamide [LSD])
- Particular medications (narcotics, sedatives, tranquilizers, monoamine oxidase inhibitors, anticonvulsants, antihistamines)

Nursing Implementation

Pretest

Instruct the patient to avoid caffeine before the test because stimulants alter the electroencephalographic activity. A light meal and fluid intake are encouraged because a low blood glucose level can also alter the electroencephalographic results.

Instruct the patient to wash his or her hair thoroughly before the test. Hair spray, creams, or oils interfere with the recording of results.

If a sleep-deprived EEG is performed to evaluate sleep disorder or seizures that occur during sleep, advise the patient not to sleep on the night before the test. At the time of the test, a sedative may be given to promote sleep. If this form of EEG is used, advise the patient to have a responsible person available to drive him or her home after the test is completed.

Since anticonvulsant and other sedative medications alter the electric activity of the brain, these medications may be withheld for 24 to 48 hours before the test begins, as determined by the physician. If the medications cannot be withheld because of the seriousness of the patient's seizure disorder, all medications taken in the 24- to 48-hour pretest period are documented on the requisition slip.

During the Test

Help the patient to relax in the reclining chair or bed.

Inform the patient that a prickly sensation or temporary pain is felt as the electrodes are attached to the scalp. Reassure the patient that the electrodes and wires will not cause a shock or harm the patient.

Instruct the patient not to move the head or body and not to talk during the test. These muscle movements alter the electroencephalographic readings. For the neonate, place the head in a midline alignment.

Reassure the patient that the nurse is nearby, with full visibility of the patient during the procedure. If a seizure occurs, the nurse is prepared to provide care during the episode.

Posttest

Observe the patient for seizure activity.

Remove the electrodes. The electrode paste is cleaned from the hair and scalp by using acetone and cotton balls. Acetone is not used in the isolette because of the limited circulation of air (Squires, 1992).

Anticonvulsant medications that were withheld for the test are not automatically restarted at the same dosage. The previous orders are reviewed by the physician and a new set of orders are written.

ELECTROMYOGRAPHY—NERVE CONDUCTION STUDIES

(ELECTROPHYSIOLOGY)

Synonyms:

EMG, NCS, electrodiagnostic studies

─────────────── **NORMAL VALUES** ───────────────

The muscle shows minimal activity at rest. Nerve conduction time is within normal limits.

Background Information

Muscle fibers are innervated by a terminal branch of an axon, located near the midpoint of a muscle. With nerve stimulation, there is depolarization of the nerve, release of acetylcholine by the nerve terminals, and diffusion of the stimulus across the synapse to contract the muscle membrane. As the muscle contracts, there is movement of the body and the performance of work.

When a patient complains of muscle weakness, muscle spasms, or paralysis, the cause may be disease of the muscle or nervous system or a problem with neuromuscular transmission at the junction between the nerves and the muscle fibers. Electromyography (EMG) and nerve conduction studies are two diagnostic tests that help identify the physiologic location of the problem.

ELECTROMYOGRAPHY. This procedure records the electric potential of various muscles in a resting state and during voluntary contraction of the muscles. The linear recordings are comparable to electrocardiographic recordings. The normal tracings of muscle potential demonstrate characteristic patterns at rest and during a strong voluntary muscle contraction. The recordings of "motor unit potentials" are examined for amplitude, duration, form, and abundance. Characteristic abnormal patterns are seen when the problem is neurologic in origin, such as denervation, or muscular, such as muscle inflammation.

NERVE CONDUCTION STUDIES. These studies measure motor conduction velocity and sensory conduction. Motor conduction velocity is the timed measurement of conduction along a nerve between two points, as measured by the stimulating and recording electrodes that are applied on the nerve's pathway. Sensory conduction measures the voltage or strength of the nerve stimulus in sensory nerve endings, as measured by recording electrodes applied to a distal area of tissue.

Carpal tunnel syndrome provides an illustration of how nerve conduction studies are used. In this disorder, the median nerve is trapped in the bony canal of the wrist. Because of the compression, there is some loss of nerve conduction and diminished nerve stimulation of specific muscles in the hand and fingers. In nerve conduction studies, the nerve stimulus is applied above the area of entrapment and recorded in the distal electrodes of the digits. Because of the nerve entrapment, the time and analysis of the tracings demonstrate a slowing of the impulses and lower voltage (a decrease in stimulation) in the digits.

The electrodiagnostic tests are somewhat painful, and they provoke some anxiety. The discomfort is sharp, but it is brief and temporary. The pain is caused by the needle insertions and the electric stimuli. Sedation is not recommended because it interferes with voluntary muscle activity. Adult patients who draw on coping strategies such as confidence in their own ability to manage or control pain seem to be more effective in the management of anxiety, even though most coping attempts do not diminish the pain (Buckelew, 1992).

For infants and children, the process of testing is similar to that of adults, with some modifications because of the smaller body size. The infant or child may have a focal nerve deficit, such as paralysis from a brachial plexus injury that occurred during birth. Other types of problems can include generalized hypotonia and weakness that may be congenital or acquired and involve a systemic or muscular disorder.

Critical Thinking: A 9-year-old child is scheduled for nerve conduction studies. Develop a pretest plan that will promote the cooperation of the child during the test.

When nerve conduction studies must be performed on the infant or small child, the parent may wish to stay and hold the child during the procedure. The presence of a supportive parent can be a comfort to the child. Children older than 5 years are often able to cooperate and participate in the test, thus reducing their anxiety. If the small child cannot cooperate because of the high level of fear or anxiety, sedation with an oral dose of chloral hydrate, 50 to 75 mg/kg, is used for nerve conduction studies (Jablecki, 1991).

Purpose of the Test

These tests help distinguish among the causes of weakness and paralysis, differentiating nerve involvement from a muscle disorder. The tests are also used to identify the particular nerve or muscle group that is involved, localize the site of the abnormality, evaluate the severity, and distinguish sensorimotor nerve disorder from pure motor disorder.

Procedure

Needle electrodes are inserted into muscles and connected to stimulator and recorder devices (Fig. 22–5). As the electric stimulus is initiated, the results appear on an oscilloscope or video screen or are photographed. Linear tracings of the electromyography are made by the electromyograph equipment.

Findings

ABNORMAL FINDINGS

Amyotrophic lateral sclerosis	Botulism
Muscular dystrophy	Herniated lumbar disc
Myasthenia gravis	Guillain-Barré syndrome
Poliomyelitis	Carpal tunnel syndrome
Inflammatory myositis	Brachial plexus injury
Myopathy (endocrine, metabolic, toxic, congenital)	Lumbosacral plexus injury
	Nerve trauma
Hypothyroidism	Glycogen storage disease

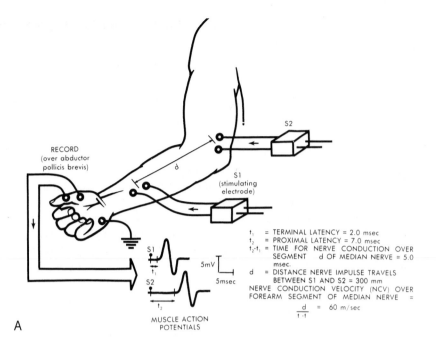

RECORD
(over abductor
pollicis brevis)

S1
(stimulating
electrode)

t_1 = TERMINAL LATENCY = 2.0 msec
t_2 = PROXIMAL LATENCY = 7.0 msec
t_2-t_1 = TIME FOR NERVE CONDUCTION OVER
SEGMENT   d OF MEDIAN NERVE = 5.0
msec.
d = DISTANCE NERVE IMPULSE TRAVELS
BETWEEN S1 AND S2 = 300 mm
NERVE CONDUCTION VELOCITY (NCV) OVER
FOREARM SEGMENT OF MEDIAN NERVE =

$$\frac{d}{t \cdot t} = 60 \text{ m/sec}$$

5mV

5msec

MUSCLE ACTION
POTENTIALS

A

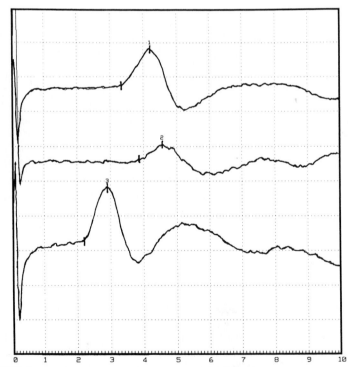

B

FIGURE 22–5. Peripheral nerve conduction studies. *A,* The technique of measurement of motor nerve conduction velocity in the forearm. *B,* The results of sensory nerve conduction velocity. The results are of median nerve (*upper two tracings*) and ulnar nerve (*lower tracing*) conduction in carpal tunnel syndrome. The compression of the median nerve resulted in nerve impairment, with delayed response and low voltage (*second tracing*). (Reproduced with permission from Guberman, A. [1994]. *An introduction to clinical neurology.* Boston: Little, Brown.)

Interfering Factors

- Smoking
- Caffeine
- Acute anxiety

Nursing Implementation

Pretest

Obtain written consent from the patient or person legally responsible for the patient's health care decisions.

Instruct the patient to refrain from smoking for 24 hours before the test and to avoid caffeine (coffee, tea, cola) for 2 to 3 hours before the test.

Inform the patient that the insertion of the needles can be painful and that the small shocks are also painful.

Reassure the patient that these sensations are brief and temporary and can be tolerated.

If possible, encourage the parent to comfort the child during the procedure.

During the Test

Cleanse the skin with antiseptic before inserting the electrodes.

As the electrodes are inserted, again reassure the patient to help reduce anxiety.

For grounding, place a metal plate under the patient's body.

At appropriate intervals during EMG, ask the patient to perform various voluntary muscle contractions.

Posttest

To avoid additional pain, remove the needle electrodes gently and slowly.

If pain persists at the puncture sites, instruct the patient to apply warm compresses.

MAGNETIC RESONANCE IMAGING, BRAIN, SPINAL CORD

(MAGNETIC FIELD SCAN)

Synonym:

MRI

Magnetic resonance imaging (MRI) is particularly valuable for assessment of the soft tissue of the brain and spinal cord. Although it cannot image the bones of the skull and vertebrae, there is clear imaging of the organs and tissues contained within these bones. MRI uses magnetic frequencies and radiofrequency waves to assess the movement of concentrations of protons within magnetic fields. The signals emitted from tissues are converted to images. Images from transverse, coronal, and sagittal planes can be obtained to provide additional information.

In the study of the brain, MRI visualizes tumors, cerebral edema, and multiple sclerosis. In the study of the spinal cord, MRI visualizes disc degeneration, spinal cord tumor, epidural fat, and postoperative scar tissue that impinges on the cord or its nerve roots.

A complete discussion of MRI is presented in Chapter 12.

MYELOGRAPHY

(RADIOGRAPHY)

Synonyms:

myelogram, low-dose myelography, LDM

─────────────────── **NORMAL VALUES** ───────────────────

No obstruction or structural abnormalities of the spinal canal, discs, cord, or nerve roots are noted.

Background Information

As a single procedure, myelography is a radiographic study that uses plain x-ray film with contrast medium to evaluate spinal disorders. More commonly, it is combined with CT *(CT myelography)* in the detection of pathologic conditions of the spine. The combination procedure is particularly useful when the CT examination has not resulted in a clear diagnosis.

Although CT and MRI have replaced myelography in most instances, myelography is still useful in the evaluation of the postoperative spinal surgery patient, the obese patient, and the patient who has a mobile herniated disc that is demonstrated only in a weight-bearing or flexion-extension position.

In myelography, the radiopaque contrast material is instilled in the subarachnoid space using a lumbar puncture needle. The patient is then placed in a prone position with the table tilted to a head-down position. This positioning allows the contrast medium to move up the spinal column. Once the contrast material is in place, the spinal cord, spinal nerve roots, and thecal sac appear radiolucent (Fig. 22–6). X-ray films or a CT scan is used for imaging. The area of the spinal pathology can be anywhere along the spinal column, and the regions are identified as cervical, lumbothoracic, or lumbar.

Several iodinated contrast media are available for use. In the past, an oil-based medium was used and was removed by needle aspiration at the end of the procedure. This contrast material had frequent side effects, including encephalopathy and seizures. Today, a water-soluble contrast medium is used most

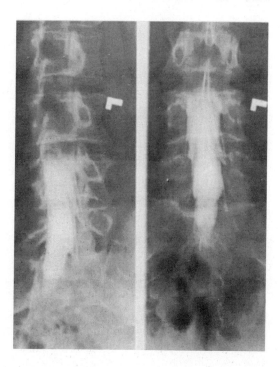

FIGURE 22–6. Lumbar myelogram. Posteroanterior (PA) and oblique views of the spinal column. The contrast material is in the subarachnoid space. (Reproduced with permission from Adler, A.M., & Carlton, R.R. [1994]. *Introduction to radiography and patient care* [vol. 1, Slide 206]. Philadelphia: W.B. Saunders.)

frequently. It is better tolerated by the patient; the side effects are nausea, vomiting, and headache.

Purpose of the Test

Myelography is performed to identify an obstruction or abnormality that impinges on the spinal cord or its nerve roots.

Procedure

Under local anesthesia and guided by fluoroscopy, iodinated contrast material is instilled into the lumbar subarachnoid space using a lumbar puncture needle. Once the contrast medium has filled the subarachnoid space or the whole spinal column, the images are taken at the appropriate level. The procedure takes 1 to 2 hours.

Findings

ABNORMAL VALUES

Protrusion of an intervertebral disc
Herniated intervertebral disc
Cervical spondylosis
Lumbar stenosis
Epidural mass or tumor

Spinal nerve root injury
Syringomyelia
Tumor of the spinal cord
Arachnoiditis

Interfering Factors

- Allergy to iodine
- Incorrect placement of the needle
- Failure to maintain a nothing-by-mouth status

Nursing Implementation

Pretest

Obtain a written consent from the patient or person who is legally responsible for the patient's health care decisions.

Ask the patient about a history of allergy to iodine or shellfish or a reaction to contrast material during a previous x-ray study.

When this procedure is performed in an outpatient setting, instruct the patient to have a responsible adult present to provide transportation home at the end of the procedure.

Instruct the patient about pretest modifications of food and fluid intake. For 8 hours before the test, most institutions require a fast from food and also require that the patient drink extra fluids to maintain the hydration status (Torres, 1993). Because there is some variation among institutions regarding the fluid intake and period for the modifications, the protocol of the individual radiology department is followed.

Help the patient to undress completely and put on a hospital gown. Also assist the patient in moving into the desired positions on the examining table. Most of these patients have problems with back pain and limited mobility because of their spinal injury or disease.

Take baseline vital signs and record the results.

If the patient is extremely anxious or has muscle spasm, administer diazepam (Valium), 5 mg, by mouth or intravenously, as prescribed. Most patients do not require pretest medication.

During the Test

Position the patient according to the requirements of the radiologist or anesthesiologist who administers the local anesthesia and performs the lumbar puncture. Alternative positions include (1) seated at the edge of the table with the legs dangling and the back somewhat flexed, (2) a lateral position with the head and knees flexed toward the chest, and (3) prone, with a small pillow under the abdomen.

If there is hair on the lower back, the skin is shaved before cleansing the skin. Assist the physician with the skin preparation, draping, and preparation of the local anesthetic.

Prepare the sterile lumbar puncture tray for the intrathecal administration of contrast medium.

Reassure the patient during the injection of the local anesthetic. It causes stinging pain as it is injected subcutaneously.

Help the patient remain still as the lumbar puncture needle is inserted. There is usually brief pain as the needle penetrates the thecal sac.

After the contrast medium has been instilled, place the patient in a prone position, with a shoulder harness and footrest in place. These are used to help the patient maintain position as the table is tilted.

Posttest

Place the patient in a slight semi-Fowler position to ease the lumbar pain.

Take vital signs at regular, frequent intervals for 1 hour or until the results are stable in a normal range.

Instruct the patient who received water-based contrast medium to remain on bedrest at home for 8 to 10 hours. Two pillows are used to elevate the upper torso and head. For the patient who received an oil-based contrast material, the period of bedrest is 8 to 24 hours. Bedrest eases the backache, and the pillows prevent the contrast medium from rising up to the head and causing headache.

Encourage the patient to drink extra fluids for the next day or two. The water-based contrast medium eventually diffuses out of the subarachnoid space and is excreted in the urine. Alcohol and caffeine intake are not permitted for 24 hours, however, because they promote rapid diuresis.

Instruct the patient to notify the physician if there is a problem because of inability to urinate or if there is onset of fever, drowsiness, stiff neck, paralysis, or seizures.

SINGLE PHOTON EMISSION COMPUTED TOMOGRAPHY SCAN, BRAIN

(RADIONUCLIDE SCAN)

Synonyms:

SPECT brain imaging, cerebral single photon emission computed tomographic imaging; SPECT scan, brain

━━━━━━━━━━━━━━━━ **NORMAL VALUES** ━━━━━━━━━━━━━━━━

No abnormalities of the brain or its structures are noted.

Background Information

Cerebral single photon emission computed tomography (SPECT) imaging uses a radionuclide that emits gamma rays and a multidetector rotary camera to produce tomographic images of the brain. In an earlier and simpler procedure, this was called a brain scan. In more recent years, with the development of new radiopharmaceuticals and better scanning equipment, the SPECT scan produces clear imaging and a shorter imaging time. The results of the SPECT scan are usually compared with the results of the CT or MRI scan to provide additional information about the changes in the patient's brain tissue (Van Heertum et al., 1993). Additional discussion about nuclear scans and the SPECT scan is presented in Chapter 10.

In cerebral studies, the radiopharmaceutical technetium-99m hexamethyl propylenamine oxime is most widely used. Once it is injected into the vascular system it travels rapidly to the head, crosses the blood-brain barrier, and perfuses into the brain tissue. The tracer undergoes some decomposition so that it cannot recross the blood-brain barrier, and it remains trapped in the brain tissues. The radioactive capability of this tracer has a short half-life of 6 hours.

The imaging is performed about 1½ to 2 hours after the radiopharmaceutical is introduced. This interval allows maximal absorption of the radiopharmaceutical into the brain. The normal imaging time is 20 to 30 minutes. From the data received by the SPECT camera, the SPECT computer can produce the images along transaxial, coronal, and sagittal planes, providing visualization of all lobes, tissues, and structures of the brain.

In the investigation of cerebrovascular disease, SPECT can be used for the detection of acute ischemia, the cause of stroke, and assessment of a transient ischemic attack. In the study of dementia, this method can help identify the cause and distinguish among Alzheimer disease, multiinfarct dementia, and frontal lobe dementia. In epilepsy, this test can help identify the seizure focus in conjunction with other neurologic procedures. In cases of head trauma, SPECT can identify mild head injury that is not visible on the CT scan.

Purpose of the Test

The SPECT scan is used to investigate cerebrovascular diseases, dementia, epilepsy, and head trauma. It may be used to assess and diagnose the disorder as well as evaluate the brain's response to treatment.

Findings

ABNORMAL VALUES

Stroke
Intracranial hemorrhage
Transient ischemic attack
Hypertensive encephalopathy
Alzheimer disease

Human immunodeficiency virus encephalopathy
Multiinfarct dementia
Epilepsy
Intracranial trauma

Interfering Factors

- Movement of the head during imaging
- Failure to remove metal objects from the imaging field

Nursing Implementation

Pretest

Critical Thinking: An elderly female with dementia is placed on the table for a SPECT scan. She has been given pretest instructions, but she continues to look around and lifts her head and upper body repeatedly. How can you help her lie quietly?

Instruct the patient to avoid caffeine intake (coffee, tea, cola) for 24 hours before the test.

Obtain a written consent from the patient or the person legally responsible for the patient's health care decisions.

Assist the patient in removing all clothes and putting on a hospital gown. All jewelry and metal objects are removed from the head, hair, and neck.

Place the patient in a recumbent position on the scanning table. Apply a minimal restraint to prevent a fall from a table that has no side rails.

The person who needs a SPECT scan is usually elderly and suffering from dementia, or it is a person who has residual trauma to the brain. The strange room and the procedure may be confusing or frightening to this type of individual. Instructions may be difficult to follow. If these conditions exist, give simple instructions and close guidance to the patient. Since there is no radiation hazard, a member of the family or a familiar person can be in the room with the patient at all times.

Remind the patient to keep the head still during the injection of the radiopharmaceutical and imaging procedure.

Explain that the room will be kept calm for 10 minutes before and after the radiopharmaceutical is administered. During this quiet time, the patient should keep his or her eyes open. Blinking is allowed. Earplugs are unnecessary (Van Heertum, 1993).

QUALITY CONTROL

The quiet, stimulus-free environment promotes a resting basal state of brain activity. The patient keeps his or her eyes open during administration of the radionuclide so that the occipital lobes are more clearly visible.

During the Test

Position the patient's head in body alignment.

Establish the intravenous line for the administration of the radiopharmaceutical.

To maintain a quiet environment, dim the lights in the room, keep noise to a minimum, and prevent traffic in the room.

During the scanning process, the patient will hear the quiet sounds of the scanner, but there is no pain or discomfort.

Posttest

Remove the intravenous line and apply a small bandage to the venipuncture site.

Since the kidneys will remove the radionuclide from the blood and excrete it in the urine, instruct the patient to wash his or her hands after voiding. This prevents radioisotopes from remaining on the skin. By 6 hours after the test, the radioactivity level of the isotope is minimal to none.

No further intervention is needed.

SINGLE PHOTON EMISSION COMPUTED TOMOGRAPHY SCAN, SPINE

(RADIONUCLIDE SCAN)

Synonym:

SPECT scan, spine

Bone SPECT imaging is one of the more common uses for the SPECT scan. This radionuclide is superior to the regular bone scan in regions where there is overlapping of bones such as the vertebral body and neural arch of the spine. It is particularly useful in the investigation of low back pain when the bone abnormality impinges on the nerve roots or the spinal cord (Yudd et al., 1992).

Abnormalities identified by the SPECT scan include benign or malignant spinal disease, discitis, ankylosing spondylitis, and septic arthritis. In a sports injury, it investigates the cause of low back pain produced by an acute stress injury.

Additional discussion of the SPECT scan is presented in Chapter 10.

ULTRASOUND, CRANIAL, NECK

(ULTRASONOGRAPHY)

Synonyms:

In infants, the anterior fontanelle serves as a window for the passage of ultrasound waves into the brain (Fig. 22–7). Ultrasound imaging can identify hydrocephalus, hemorrhage, cystic or solid tumors, or infections such as toxoplasmosis, rubella, cytomegalovirus, and herpes simplex (TORCH). This diagnostic procedure is often used in the neonatal intensive care unit when the infant has a suspected intracranial hemorrhage, a low Apgar score, suspected congenital malformations, or an abnormal neurologic examination.

With newer Doppler techniques, ultrasound may be used to evaluate the circulation of the major intracranial arteries. The Doppler probe is placed over the thin layer of temporal bone, the bony orbits, and the foramen magnum. This technique provides visualization of a stenosis of the internal carotid artery and its branches, the vertebral artery, and the basilar artery. It may also identify a vasospasm caused by a subarachnoid hemorrhage or an arteriovenous malformation (Guberman, 1994).

Doppler ultrasound is also useful in the assessment of the arteries of the neck. The procedure demonstrates the velocity of blood flow, turbulence, direction of flow, and patency of the arteries. It is particularly helpful in the investigation of

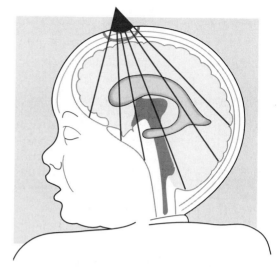

FIGURE 22–7. Pediatric ultrasound. The anterior fontanelle provides the window for imaging the brain of the infant. (Redrawn with permission from Blickman, J. [1992, May]. The inroads of ultrasound, CT, and MR in pediatric imaging. *Applied Radiology*, 39.)

transient ischemic attacks and the determination of arterial patency after a carotid thromboendarterectomy or arteriotomy with anastomosis (Foldes, 1993).

A complete discussion of ultrasound is found in Chapter 8 of this text.

X-RAY, SKULL

(RADIOGRAPHY)

Synonym:

skull series

Plain x-rays of the skull demonstrate changes in the bony tissue and may demonstrate changes in the brain tissue. A skull fracture can be identified, located, and described. The bone tissue may show erosion or thinning because of chronically increased intracranial pressure or a cerebral tumor. In children, the increased intracranial pressure causes separation of the sutures. Tumors can cause a localized thickening of the bony tissue. Abnormalities of the brain can be visualized when the tissue is calcified, such as in some types of tumor or the displacement of the pineal gland.

Because the skull x-ray series is helpful but does not provide detailed data, other specialized tests such as the CT scan, MRI, or isotope scan are used to obtain better information.

A complete discussion of x-ray studies is presented in Chapter 9.

X-RAY, SPINE

(RADIOGRAPHY)

Synonyms:

The plain x-ray film of the spine can provide helpful data regarding the cause of neurologic disability. Spinal abnormalities include inflammatory lesions such as tuberculosis of the spine, malignant tumor or metastasis, or congenital abnormality of the cervical spine. Fractures and dislocations are also apparent on x-ray film. When there are bone abnormalities such as these, there may be resultant neurologic abnormality as the spinal cord or nerve roots are compressed. In radiologic views of the soft tissues, a protruding disc can be seen along with the narrowing or bony sclerosis of the vertebrae. Intraspinal tumor with erosion of the vertebral body is also evident.

As with the x-ray series of the skull, the x-ray film of the spine does not provide sufficient detail about the neurologic problem. Follow-up with myelography, CT, or MRI provides better visualization and accurate diagnosis of a spinal pathologic condition.

A complete discussion of radiology is presented in Chapter 9.

REFERENCES

Blickman, J.G. (1992). The inroads of ultrasound, CT, and MRI in pediatric imaging. *Applied Radiology 21*, 38–47.

Brunzel, N.A. (1994). *Fundamentals of urine and body fluid analysis.* Philadelphia: W.B. Saunders.

Buckelew, S.P., et al. (1992). Spontaneous coping strategies to manage acute pain and anxiety during electrodiagnostic studies. *Archives of Physical Medicine and Rehabilitation, 73*, 594–598.

Chase, J.A. (1991). Spinal stenosis. *Nursing Clinics of North America, 26*, 53–64.

Chestnut, R.M. (1994). Computed tomography of the brain: A guide to understanding and interpreting normal and abnormal images in the critically ill patient. *Critical Care Nursing Quarterly, 7*, 33–50.

Dublin, A.B. (1989). *Outpatient invasive radiologic procedures: Diagnostic and therapeutic.* Philadelphia: W.B. Saunders.

Foldes, M. (1993). The role of duplex and color Doppler imaging in the operating room. *Journal of Vascular Nursing, 11*, 108–110.

Guberman, A. (1994). *An introduction to clinical neurology.* Boston: Little, Brown.

Jablecki, C.K. (1991). Pediatric electrodiagnosis. *Physical Medicine Rehabilitation Clinics of North America, 2*, 917–929.

Kim, D., & Orron, D.E. (1992). *Peripheral vascular imaging and intervention.* St. Louis: Mosby-Yearbook.

Mason, P.J.B. (1992). Neurodiagnostic testing in critically injured adults. *Critical Care Nurse, 12*, 64–73, 75.

Moss, A.A., Gamsu, G.G., & Genant, H.C. (Eds.). (1992). *Computed tomography of the body, with magnetic resonance imaging* (2nd ed., vol. 2, Bone and joint). Philadelphia: W.B. Saunders.

Nadalo, L.A. (1991). The neuroradiology of visual disturbances. *Neurologic Clinics, 9*, 1–35.

Osborne, A.G. (1994). *Diagnostic neurology.* St. Louis: C.V. Mosby.

Snopek, A.M. (1992). *Fundamentals of Special Radiographic Procedures* (3rd ed.). Philadelphia: W.B. Saunders.

Squires, L.A. (1992). Neonatal seizures. *Critical Care Nursing Clinics of North America, 4*, 495–506.

Torres, L.S. (1993). *Basic medical techniques and patient care for radiologic technologists.* Philadelphia: J.B. Lippincott.

Van Heertum, R.L., et al. (1993). SPECT brain imaging in neurologic disease. *Radiologic Clinics of North America, 31*, 881–904.

Yudd, A.P., et al. (1992). Bone scintigraphy: Lumbar SPECT imaging. *Applied Radiology, 21*, 45–51.

Musculoskeletal Function

The musculoskeletal system consists of bones, joints, cartilage, ligaments, tendons, muscle, fascia, and bursae. An integrated system, the skeleton, muscle, and connective tissue function to provide support, protection, movement, and blood formation for the body. The musculoskeletal system is subject to many disorders caused by trauma, malignancy, inflammation, metabolic change, degeneration, or vascular deficiency.

In this chapter, the section on laboratory tests examines the blood and synovial fluid. In many cases, there is no one test that diagnoses an autoimmune disorder or cause of inflammation. The diagnosis is confirmed or excluded by a combination of laboratory tests, diagnostic procedures, and clinical findings. The laboratory tests are also used to evaluate the severity of disease and to monitor the effects of treatment.

Most of the diagnostic procedures in this chapter allow visualization of the bones or joints. Other procedures are used to obtain samples of tissue or fluid. These specimens are stained or cultured and analyzed microscopically. The

LABORATORY TESTS

diagnostic procedures provide specific data regarding the cause or extent of pathologic change in the bone or joint.

ANTI-DNA ANTIBODY

(SERUM)

Synonyms:

antibody to double-stranded DNA, anti-ds-DNA, antibody to native DNA, DNA antibody, n-DNA, ssDNA

─────────────── **NORMAL VALUES** ───────────────

NEGATIVE
<10% binding (radioimmunoassay method)
<250 U/L (enzyme immunoassay method)
<1:10 (indirect immunofluorescent method)

Background Information

In autoimmune disease, antibodies attach to and destroy nuclear or cytoplasmic antigens of one's own body tissue. The autoimmune response causes inflammation, fibrosis, and destruction of a single target organ, or the process becomes disseminated and affects many different organs or tissues of the body.

The anti-DNA antibody test is one of the specific antinuclear antibody (ANA) tests. Antibodies to single-stranded or double-stranded DNA are found in the serum of 65 to 80% of patients with active systemic lupus erythematosus (Henry, 1991). It is present to a much lesser degree in patients with other collagen vascular or autoimmune diseases.

Among the different laboratory methods, all use binding assay to detect the antibodies in the serum. Although the normal values are expressed differently according to the method of analysis, high levels of antibodies are abnormal and confirm the diagnosis of systemic lupus erythematosus. By radioimmunoassay technique, the abnormal level is greater than 20% binding. By enzyme-linked immunosorbent assay, greater than 800 U/L is specific for systemic lupus erythematosus. By the indirect immunofluorescent technique, the antibody is detected in a titer with a dilution greater than 1:10.

The laboratory technique of indirect immunofluorescence visually demonstrates the presence of ANA in the serum (Fig. 23–1) and provides quantitative data regarding the concentration of antibody in the serum. The serum is placed on a microscopic slide that contains mouse liver substrate, the laboratory source of nuclear antigen. If ANA is present in the serum, it will bind to the antigen, forming antigen-antibody complexes. Fluorescein-labeled antiglobulin is added to give a fluorescent stain to the newly formed complexes. The patterns of fluorescence of the nuclei are demonstrated under fluorescent microscopy.

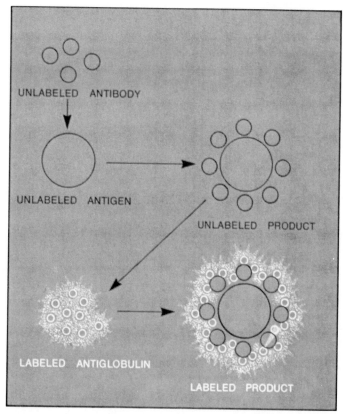

FIGURE 23–1. Indirect fluorescent antibody procedure. (Reproduced with permission from Bryant, N.J. [1986]. *Laboratory immunology and serology* [2nd ed., p. 55]. Philadelphia: W.B. Saunders.)

Purpose of the Test

The anti-DNA antibody test confirms the diagnosis of systemic lupus erythematosus. It is also used to monitor the response to treatment.

Procedure

A red-topped tube is used to collect 5 to 10 ml of venous blood.

Findings

ELEVATED VALUES
Active systemic lupus erythematosus
Discoid LE
Rheumatoid arthritis

Other collagen vascular or rheumatic disorders
Chronic active hepatitis (lupoid hepatitis)
Infectious mononucleosis
Biliary cirrhosis

Interfering Factors

- Administration of radioactive isotopes in the preceding 7 days
- Warming of the specimen

Nursing Implementation

Pretest

Schedule this test before any radioactive isotope test.

Posttest

Arrange for prompt transport of the specimen to the laboratory.

QUALITY CONTROL

The serum must be chilled to 56° C to prevent false-positive results.

ANTINUCLEAR ANTIBODY

(SERUM)

Synonyms:
ANA, fluorescent antinuclear antibody, FANA, ANF

─────────────── **NORMAL VALUES** ───────────────

Negative at a 1:20 dilution

Background Information

Autoimmune diseases are disorders that produce tissue injury because of an immunologic reaction against one's own tissue antigens. When the antibodies attack one or more antigens in the cell nuclei, the antibodies are called antinuclear antibodies or ANA. Of the many different autoimmune disorders, some affect cell nuclei of a single organ and others cause systemic disease, affecting the cell nuclei of many tissues.

In disorders that are organ-specific, the autoimmune response is directed at the antigen of DNA, other nuclear antigens, and the mitochondria within the nuclei. Organ-specific autoimmune diseases can affect the blood; the endocrine, neurologic, or intestinal systems; kidney; liver; muscle; eye; skin; or other target organs.

In systemic autoimmune diseases, the pathophysiologic process deposits immune complexes in the capillaries of multiple organs. These complexes contain tissue components and complement. The presence of complement results in inflammatory reactions and tissue destruction. Systemic lupus erythematosus and other collagen vascular diseases are all systemic autoimmune disorders.

In the ANA test, the analysis consists of microscopic examination of the serum for the presence of immunofluorescent-stained antigen-antibody complexes. Additionally, the amount of antibody is measured by the presence of a high serum titer (Table 23–1). Positive ANA results identify the presence of the antitissue antibodies of autoimmune disease, but it cannot identify the specific disease. As a screening tool, however, ANA is particularly relevant in the detection of systemic lupus erythematosus because of a greater that 95% accuracy rate in detection of this particular antibody (Henry, 1991). Conversely, a negative result is considered strong evidence for ruling out the presence of this collagen vascular disease.

The ANA immunofluorescence test can produce false-positive results because of medications, including penicillin, procainamide, and hydrazaline. It sometimes produces false-positive results in normal individuals, and the results can be elevated in up to 40% of normal elderly individuals (Bryant, 1986).

Purpose of the Test

The ANA test is used as a screen to detect autoimmune disease or systemic lupus erythematosus, or both. It is also used to monitor the effectiveness of medication in the treatment of systemic lupus erythematosus.

Procedure

A red-topped tube is used to collect 7 to 10 ml of venous blood.

QUALITY CONTROL

Venipuncture technique must be smooth, with a blood flow that fills the vacuum tube rapidly. If the blood has excessive turbulence because of flawed venipuncture technique, the hemolysis of the erythrocytes will alter test results.

TABLE 23–1

POSITIVE REACTIONS USING RECOMMENDED PROCEDURE FOR ANTINUCLEAR ANTIBODY IN SYSTEMIC LUPUS ERYTHEMATOSUS, PROGRESSIVE SYSTEMIC SCLEROSIS, AND RHEUMATOID ARTHRITIS

Titer	Normal Population	Systemic Lupus Erythematosus	Progressive Systemic Sclerosis	Rheumatoid Arthritis
Negative Tests				
1 : 10 (or lower)	96	1	4	15
Positive Tests				
1 : 20	0	0	2	0
1 : 49–1 : 80	0	2	4	4
1 : 160–1 : 320	0	4	3	1
1 : 640–1 : 1280	0	7	4	0
1 : 2560 (or higher)	0	6	0	0
Per cent positive		95	76	25

Reproduced with permission from Bryant, N.J. (1986). *Laboratory immunology and serology* (2nd ed., p. 134). Philadelphia, W.B. Saunders.

Findings

ELEVATED VALUES

Systemic Autoimmune Diseases

Systemic lupus erythematosus
Rheumatoid arthritis
Ankylosing spondylitis
Necrotizing angiitis
Polymyositis
Dermatomyositis
Progressive systemic sclerosis
Mixed connective tissue disease
Sjögren syndrome

Autoimmune Diseases of Blood and Target Organs

Hashimoto thyroiditis
Myxedema
Thyrotoxicosis
Hepatic or biliary cirrhosis
Leukemia
Chronic renal failure
Multiple sclerosis
Pernicious anemia
Regional ileitis
Ulcerative colitis
Gluten-sensitive enteropathy
Pemphigus vulgaris

Interfering Factors

• Hemolysis of the blood specimen

Nursing Implementation

Pretest

List any medications taken by the patient.

Posttest

Arrange for prompt transport of the specimen to the laboratory. The cells must be extracted from the serum promptly to prevent contamination of the specimen because of hemolysis.

C-REACTIVE PROTEIN

(SERUM)

Synonym:
CRP

NORMAL VALUES

<1 mg/dl *or* SI <10 mg/L

Background Information

C-reactive protein is a globulin, a serum protein that is synthesized by the liver. Normally, it is not present in the blood, except when there is tissue necrosis, trauma, inflammation, or infection. Its synthesis and rise in serum values are triggered by the presence of antigens, immune complexes, bacteria, and fungi. Once it enters the blood, this protein attaches to the surface of many bacteria, fungi, or other microorganisms and initiates the pathway of complement as part of the immunologic response. It is believed that the function of C-reactive protein is to act as an early defense mechanism against infection or to detoxify and remove products of tissue degradation (Teitz, 1990).

The serum level of C-reactive protein rises rapidly in response to bacterial infection and acute inflammation. The progressive rise in value reflects increasing infection, inflammation, or tissue damage. Equally, the progressive fall in the serum value indicates healing or the effectiveness of antibiotic or antiinflammatory medication. In a normal postoperative response, the C-reactive protein value demonstrates a sharp rise by the third postoperative day. If no bacterial sepsis is present, the value falls by the seventh day.

Serial testing for C-reactive protein may be used to monitor for postoperative infection. Because the protein level does not rise in the presence of viral infection, the test may be used to differentiate between viral and bacterial sources of infection, as in meningitis. Because it responds to necrosis, it may be used to detect reinfarction or the extension of a myocardial infarction.

Purpose of the Test

C-reactive protein is used as a nonspecific indicator of infection or inflammation and also to monitor the response to antibiotic or antiinflammatory medication. It is commonly used to help with the diagnosis of rheumatoid arthritis and rheumatic fever, particularly when the erythrocyte sedimentation rate (ESR) and other test results are inconclusive.

Procedure

A red-topped tube is used to collect 5 to 10 ml of venous blood.

QUALITY CONTROL

Venipuncture technique must be smooth, with a blood flow that fills the vacuum tube readily. If the blood has excessive turbulence because of flawed venipuncture technique, the hemolysis of the erythrocytes will alter the test results.

Findings

ELEVATED VALUES

Rheumatoid arthritis

Rheumatic fever

Systemic lupus erythematosus
Tuberculosis
Crohn disease

Bacterial sepsis
Pneumococcal pneumonia
Myocardial infarction

Interfering Factors

- Oral contraceptives
- Intrauterine device
- Hemolysis

Nursing Implementation

Pretest

Instruct the patient to fast from food for 4 to 8 hours before the test. Fluids are permitted (Norris, 1992). Fasting is required, because for accurate results, the blood should have a level of serum lipids that is as low as possible.

Posttest

No specific intervention is necessary.

ERYTHROCYTE SEDIMENTATION RATE

(BLOOD)

Synonyms:
ESR, sed rate

NORMAL VALUES

Adult <50 Years	
Male:	0–15 mm/hour
Female:	0–20 mm/hour
Adult >50 Years	
Male:	0–20 mm/hour
Female:	0–30 mm/hour
Child:	0–10 mm/hour

Background Information

The ESR is a nonspecific measurement of infection or inflammation in the body. The rate particularly rises when elevated levels of fibrinogen or globulins, or both, are present in the blood.

When venous blood is placed in a vertical tube, the erythrocytes act like sediment; over time, they fall to the bottom of the tube. In normal conditions, as the erythrocytes settle, they exhibit a characteristic *rouleau formation*, meaning that they form a stack. In conditions that produce greater amounts of fibrinogen or globulins, the rouleau formation is greater, the sedimentation rate is faster, and the ESR is elevated. Anemia also increases the ESR because there are fewer erythrocytes in the plasma.

Microcytes have a slower sedimentation rate than do macrocytes. Additionally, erythrocytes with irregularities or abnormal shape exhibit less rouleau formation. They demonstrate less sedimentation and the ESR is lower than normal.

Purpose of the Test

The erythrocyte sedimentation test is useful in identifying and monitoring disease activity in infectious, inflammatory, and neoplastic conditions. It is especially useful in rheumatic and collagen diseases.

Procedure

A purple- or blue-topped tube is used to collect 5 to 10 ml of venous blood.

QUALITY CONTROL

Venipuncture technique must be smooth, with a blood flow that fills the vacuum tube readily. If the blood has excessive turbulence because of flawed technique, the hemolysis of erythrocytes will alter the test results.

Findings

ELEVATED VALUES

Rheumatoid arthritis
Rheumatic fever
Inflammation
Temporal arteritis
Polymyalgia rheumatica

Multiple myeloma
Waldenström macroglobulinemia
Anemia
Pregnancy

DECREASED VALUES

Sickle cell anemia
Spherocytosis

Polycythemia
Hypofibrinogenemia

Nursing Implementation

Pretest

Since many medications, including salicylate, can alter laboratory values, list all medications taken by the patient on the requisition slip. In some cases, the medication may be withheld until after the test.

Posttest

Ensure that the specimen is sent promptly to the laboratory. The specimen must be analyzed within 4 hours of collection.

HUMAN LEUKOCYTE ANTIGEN B27

Synonym:

HLA B27

The human leukocyte antigens (HLA) are derived from specific loci on the short arm of the sixth chromosome. Their loci are labeled A, B, C, and D. These antigens appear on all nucleated cells and are the major antigens of white blood cells and platelets. It is believed that the HLA antigens play a major role in immune surveillance (Henry, 1991). HLA B27 is one of many different antigens in the HLA group.

HLA B27, an inherited antigen, has a statistically high correlation with ankylosing spondylosis (Marie Strümpell disease) and Reiter syndrome. Ninety-six per cent of patients with ankylosing spondylosis have the inherited antigen HLA B27, confirming the genetic linkage to this disorder (Bryant, 1986). Although there is also statistical linkage of this antigen with Reiter syndrome, it is less strong.

The significance of this genetic marker antigen is not well understood. Although HLA B27 is not the cause of the disease, it is a marker of disease susceptibility. Infection or environmental stimuli may alter HLA B27 and initiate a complex autoimmune response. Ultimately, there is injury or destruction of the tissue of one's own target cells, such as synovial or cartilage tissue.

HLA B27 may be used clinically to assess the disease state of ankylosing spondylosis. A heparinized, green-topped tube is used to collect 7 to 10 ml of venous blood.

A complete discussion of the HLA antigens is presented in Chapter 16.

LE TEST

Synonyms:

LE prep, LE slide cell test, lupus test, lupus erythematosus cell test

Background Information

In autoimmune disease, the serum contains the antibodies that are directed against cell nuclei of one's own body tissues. In systemic lupus erythematosus, the antinuclear antibody is usually IgG and is called the *LE factor*. The antibody reacts with the deoxyribonucleoprotein of leukocytes by attaching to the nucleus and infiltrating it. After infiltration, the altered cell becomes a homogeneous

—————— **NORMAL VALUES** ——————

Negative; No LE cells are present.

mass of cytoplasm and is then called an *LE body*. Other neutrophils and phagocytes surround the LE body and engulf it by phagocytosis. After phagocytosis, the final cell, the *LE cell*, is a polymorphonuclear leukocyte with a lysed nucleus as an inclusion body (Bryant, 1986). In systemic lupus erythematosus, the LE cells are found in the bone marrow and peripheral blood.

In the LE test, the laboratory sample blood cells are ruptured by using glass beads to release nuclear material. The patient's serum is then mixed and incubated with this nuclear material. If the LE factor is present, the antibody interacts with the sample nuclear material and the altered nuclei undergo phagocytosis. The specimen is stained and prepared for microscopy. The presence of lavender-stained LE cells is considered a positive result.

The LE test is an indirect measure used to detect one of the antinuclear antibodies. The value of the test is limited because it is less sensitive than the fluorescent ANA test. A positive LE test is useful in the diagnosis of lupus erythematosus, but many patients who are acutely ill with this disease have negative test results. Additionally, there are numerous medications, including phenytoin (Dilantin), that produce a false-positive result. The LE test is rarely used today because of time-consuming methodology and the insensitivity of the test.

Purpose

The LE test is used to help diagnose lupus erythematosus and to monitor the response to treatment.

Procedure

A green-topped tube is used to collect 7 to 10 ml of venous blood.

Findings

POSITIVE VALUES
Systemic lupus erythematosus
Rheumatoid arthritis
Chronic active hepatitis (lupoid hepatitis)
Scleroderma
Drug hypersensitivity
Drug-induced lupus syndrome

Interfering Factors

- Severe leukopenia, neutropenia
- Heparin
- Inadequate volume of blood (<6 ml)

Nursing Implementation

Pretest

If heparin has been administered, schedule the test 2 days after the heparin is discontinued.

On the laboratory requisition slip, list the medications taken by the patient.

Posttest

Arrange for transport of the specimen to the laboratory within 30 minutes.

RHEUMATOID FACTOR

(SERUM, SYNOVIAL FLUID)

Synonyms:

RF, RA factor

NORMAL VALUES

Negative

Background Information

Rheumatoid factor is a group of immunoglobulins that are directed against the Fe fragment of IgG molecules. Stated in a simpler way, rheumatoid factor is an antiantibody.

Rheumatoid factor is present in the serum of the majority of patients with rheumatoid arthritis and other inflammatory conditions. Even though there is a high correlation between the presence of rheumatoid factor and rheumatoid arthritis, the exact nature of the relationship is unknown. If rheumatoid arthritis is an autoimmune disorder, the antigen is probably present on the patient's IgG antibodies. Perhaps the antibody molecules must be altered before an antigen-antibody response can occur. It is also possible that rheumatoid factor is not the cause of disease but is produced in response to an infectious or inflammatory disorder (Jacobs, 1990).

Rheumatoid factor can be detected by the latex fixation method or the sheep cell agglutination method. In the latex fixation method, latex beads are coated with human IgG. In the sheep cell agglutination test, sheep erythrocytes are coated with rabbit IgG. Either of these two antigens is mixed with diluted serum from the patient. If the serum has antibody against IgG, a visible agglutination (clumping) indicates a positive result. Synovial fluid can also be analyzed for rheumatoid factor, using the patient's joint fluid instead of serum. The test results are comparable.

Critical Thinking: Venipuncture from a vein in the antecubital fossa is impossible because the patient has severe bilateral contractures of her hands and elbows. What alternatives can be used?

The titer is the highest dilution in which there is agglutination or a positive result. In rheumatoid arthritis, the highest titers occur in patients who have severe active disease. Additionally, Sjögren syndrome demonstrates high titers of rheumatoid factor. Positive results at low titers occur in normal elderly individuals, those with infectious mononucleosis, or those with acute inflammation from another cause.

Purpose of the Test

The test for rheumatoid factor is used in the diagnosis and prognosis of rheumatoid arthritis.

Procedure

A red-topped tube is used to collect 7 to 10 ml of venous blood.

Findings

POSITIVE VALUES

Rheumatoid arthritis
Systemic lupus erythematosus
Scleroderma
Waldenström disease
Infectious mononucleosis
Tuberculosis
Chronic liver disease

Sjögren syndrome
Dermatomyositis
Polymyositis
Sarcoidosis
Subacute bacterial endocarditis
Chronic lung disease

Interfering Factors

- Severe lipemia
- Circulating immune complexes

Nursing Implementation

No special nursing measures are required.

SYNOVIAL FLUID ANALYSIS

(SYNOVIAL FLUID)

Synonym:

joint fluid analysis

NORMAL VALUES

Appearance:	crystal clear, transparent, pale yellow
Viscosity:	high
Volume:	<3.5 ml
Red blood cells:	absent
White blood cells:	0–200/mm^3 *or* SI 0–200 × 10^6/L
Nucleated cell count:	<200 cells/μL *or* SI <200 × 10^6 cells/L
Granulocytes:	<25% of nucleated cells
Protein:	3 g/dl *or* SI 30 g/L
Uric acid:	<8 mg/dl *or* SI 476 μmol/L
Glucose (fasting):	70–110 mg/dl *or* SI 3.9–6.1 mmol/L
Blood-synovial fluid glucose difference:	<10 mg/dl *or* SI <0.56 mmol/L
Fibrin clot:	negative or absent
Mucin clot:	positive or abundant
String test:	formation of a long string
Culture:	no growth

Background Information

Arthrocentesis, needle aspiration of the joint, is used to obtain a sample of synovial fluid. Normally, the joint contains little fluid volume. In inflammation, infection, trauma, or irritation of the joint, cartilage, or synovial membrane, the fluid fills or distends the joint capsule. Analysis of the aspirated fluid provides data regarding the cause of the swelling and increased fluid production.

There should be few to no red blood cells in the fluid. If the specimen is grossly bloody, it indicates hemorrhage into the joint such as from fracture, hemophilia, trauma, or a traumatic tap.

An abnormal leukocyte count can be mildly to dramatically elevated. Virtually all the diseases listed in the Findings section demonstrate a high white blood cell count in the synovial fluid.

Protein increases in the synovial fluid because of inflammation. When the patient has gout, the uric acid level is elevated. The glucose level should be equivalent to or less than a 10-mg difference between the blood value and the synovial fluid value. A decrease in the synovial fluid glucose level is indicative of inflammatory arthritis. For the glucose analysis, the patient is usually in a fasting state before the test is performed. This provides a stable baseline value for both the blood and synovial fluid.

There should not be a fibrin clot because normal synovial fluid has no fibrinogen. When clotting occurs, it is a sign of inflammation. A mucin clot and a favorable string test are indications of normal viscosity. Inflammation and excessive synovial fluid lessen the viscosity. When the fluid is poured, only a short string can be formed.

Culture of the fluid may identify the pathogen that caused the infection. Microscopic examination of the fluid is also performed to identify cells, sediment, or crystals in the fluid.

Purpose of the Test

Synovial fluid analysis helps in the diagnosis of rheumatic diseases, infection, or other diseases that cause swelling of the joint, increased production of fluid, or damage to the joint space.

Procedure

Joint: Under sterile conditions, an aspiration needle is inserted into the joint space and fluid is withdrawn. The fluid specimen is placed into one green-topped tube with heparin and two red-topped tubes.

Blood: A red-topped tube is used to obtain 7 to 10 ml of venous blood for a serum chemistry profile. If additional tests are to be performed, a second red-topped tube is filled. The blood is drawn in the same period as the joint aspiration.

Culture: If *Gonococcus* is suspected, some synovial fluid is inoculated onto a plate that contains Thayer-Martin medium. This is carried out immediately after the arthrocentesis is completed. Other cultures are started in the laboratory.

Findings

ABNORMAL VALUES

Rheumatoid arthritis
Infectious arthritis
Traumatic arthritis
Osteoarthritis
Hemophilic arthritis
Systemic lupus erythematosus

Rheumatic fever
Tuberculosis
Lyme disease
Gout
Pseudogout

Interfering Factors

• Failure to maintain a nothing-by-mouth status

Nursing Implementation

Pretest

Inform the patient about the procedure and obtain written consent from the patient or person legally designated to make health care decisions for the patient.

Instruct the patient to fast for 6 to 8 hours before the test.

Inform the patient that the procedure is performed with local anesthesia. Mild discomfort may be felt as the anesthetic is injected and as the joint capsule is penetrated.

During the Test

Assist with positioning of the extremity. The skin is cleansed with antiseptic and the area is covered with a sterile drape.

Assist with the preparation of the local anesthetic and the collection of all specimens.

Posttest

After the needle is withdrawn, apply a pressure dressing to the aspiration site to prevent hematoma.

An elastic binding may be applied to the joint for 8 to 24 hours to increase the stability of the joint.

Instruct the patient to apply a cold pack to the joint for 24 to 36 hours to decrease the swelling. The extremity may be elevated on pillows.

Teach the patient to avoid excessive use of the joint for 2 to 3 days. This will help prevent stiffness, pain, and swelling.

Arrange for immediate transport of the specimens to the laboratory.

Complications

Infection is a possible complication of arthrocentesis or any other procedure that opens the joint capsule. The infection can be introduced from environmental contamination or from aggravation of infection already present in the joint tissues. The drainage is purulent and the dressing is contaminated by the secretions. The nursing assessment for complications of arthrocentesis is presented in Table 23–2.

URIC ACID

(SERUM)

Synonym:

urate

TABLE 23-2
COMPLICATIONS OF ARTHROCENTESIS, ARTHROSCOPY, AND SYNOVIAL BIOPSY

Complication	Nursing Assessment
Infection of the joint	Fever
	Joint swelling
	Pain
	Purulent, malodorous drainage

NORMAL VALUES

Adult	
Male:	4.5–8 ng/dl *or* SI 0.27–0.47 mmol/L
Female:	2.5–6.2 ng/dl *or* SI 0.15–0.37 mmol/L
Child <12 Years:	2–5.5 ng/dl *or* SI 0.12–0.32 mmol/L
Adult >60 Years:	
Male:	4.2–8 ng/dl *or* SI 0.25–0.47 mmol/L
Female:	2.7–6.8 ng/dl *or* SI 0.16–0.40 mmol/L

Background Information

Uric acid is the end product of protein metabolism and is excreted from the body by the kidneys and bowel. The production of uric acid comes from a combination of dietary intake of protein and purine foods, purine biosynthesis, and catabolism of body tissues. The normal excretion of uric acid by the kidneys should eliminate two thirds of the uric acid from the blood daily. The remaining one third is in the bile and intestinal secretions. The intestinal bacteria act on the secretions by uricolysis, and the wastes are excreted in feces. The level of uric acid in the blood is maintained by a balance between the amount that is produced and the amount that is excreted (Fig. 23–2).

Under normal conditions, a temporary rise in the serum uric acid level can occur after ingestion of foods that are rich in purine (organ meats, legumes, meat, and some fish), after strenuous exercise or heavy alcohol ingestion, or during periods of stress. This type of rise is temporary and the blood level returns to normal within a day.

Hyperuricemia, an elevated level of uric acid in the blood, results from excessive production of uric acid or impaired excretion of uric acid, or a combination of the two causes. The conditions of abnormal overproduction include the abnormal metabolism of purines and amino acids, excessive catabolism of body tissues, destruction of nucleoproteins, some cancers before and after chemotherapy or radiation, some endocrine and hemolytic disorders,

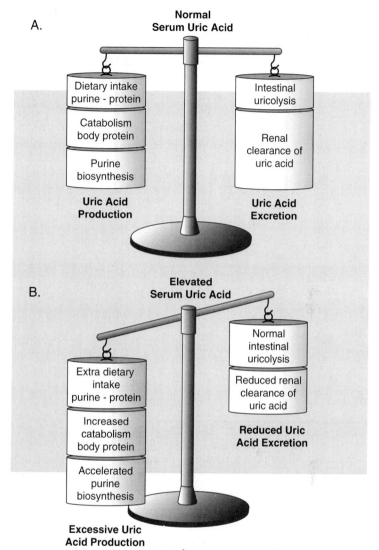

FIGURE 23–2. Uric acid production and excretion. *A,* Normal physiology. *B,* Pathophysiology of hyperuricemia.

and conditions that cause acidosis or lactic acidosis. Impaired excretion or urate retention is usually due to renal disease that affects tubular secretion and reabsorption. It may also be caused by reduced renal blood flow and decreased renal filtration of the blood.

Gout is a genetic disorder of purine metabolism that usually produces a high level of uric acid in the blood and monosodium urate crystal deposits throughout the body. The deposits are located in the joints, cartilage, bone, bursae, and subcutaneous tissue. Some patients, however, develop gout with lower elevations of serum uric acid, and some patients have high levels of serum uric acid and do not acquire this inflammatory disease. The urate crystals can also accumulate in the renal pelvis and cause uric acid kidney stones to form.

Severe hyperuricemia, as indicated by serum uric acid levels of 12 mg/dl (SI, 0.714 mmol/L) or more can be dangerous because the urate crystals can accumulate in the renal tubules and ureters, resulting in obstruction and renal failure. This crisis can occur when leukemia is treated with cytotoxic drugs or a malignancy is irradiated. Both of these treatments cause rapid necrosis of tissue and excess catabolism of nucleoproteins.

Hypouricemia, the abnormally low level of uric acid in the blood, usually results from defects in renal tubular absorption. The disorder can be congenital or acquired, but there is an increased urinary loss of urate and therefore a low level of uric acid in the blood.

Purpose of the Test

The elevated level of uric acid is used to confirm the diagnosis of gout and helps detect renal impairment that causes prerenal azotemia and renal failure.

Procedure

A red-topped tube is used to collect 5 to 10 ml of venous blood.

Findings

ELEVATED VALUES

Gout	Diabetic ketoacidosis
Renal failure	Shock
Polycystic kidney disease	Down syndrome
Leukemia	Glycogen storage disease
Lymphoma	Lesch-Nyhan syndrome
Toxemia of pregnancy	Hemolytic anemia
Lead poisoning	Polycythemia vera
Psoriasis	Pernicious anemia
Tumor lysis syndrome	

DECREASED VALUES

Falconi syndrome	Wilson disease
Hodgkin disease	Multiple myeloma
Bronchogenic carcinoma	Xanthinuria

Interfering Factors

- Starvation
- High purine diet

- Stress
- Caffeine or vitamin C ingestion

Nursing Implementation

Pretest

When the laboratory protocol specifies a fasting specimen, instruct the patient to discontinue all food and fluid for 8 hours.

On the requisition slip, list all medications taken by the patient. Many drugs cause either a false-positive or false-negative result.

Posttest

No specific nursing intervention is required.

DIAGNOSTIC PROCEDURES

ARTHROGRAPHY

(RADIOLOGY)

Synonyms:

─────────────── **NORMAL VALUES** ───────────────

Normal joint capsule and ligament structure; no abnormalities noted

Background Information

The articulating bones, cartilage, and ligaments form the joint and its capsule. The inner surface of the joint capsule is lined by cartilage and synovium. The small amount of synovial fluid provides lubrication for easy joint motion.

The knee and shoulder are joints that are heavily bound by ligaments and tendons. They are subject to injury or trauma when they are forced beyond the normal range. Injury to the muscles, ligaments, tendons, bursae, synovial tissue, cartilage, or bone alters the structure of the joint capsule and limits the function of the joint.

Purpose of the Test

Arthrography is performed to evaluate suspected adhesion, cartilage tear, or other abnormality of the joint capsule.

Procedure

Using sterile technique and local anesthesia, a needle is inserted into the joint space to remove the synovial fluid and to inject air and iodinated contrast material. Fluoroscopy is used to guide the placement of the needle, and x-ray films are taken to document the interior structure of the joint capsule. The time needed for this test is 1 to 2 hours.

Findings

ABNORMAL VALUES

Damage or deterioration of the cartilage
Disruption of the joint capsule
Torn collateral or cruciate ligaments of the knee
Tear or laceration of the medial meniscus of the knee
Rotator cuff tear of the shoulder
Synovial abnormality
Adhesions of the joint capsule
Tenosynovitis
Osteochondritis dissecans
Osteochondral fracture
Chondromalacia patellae

Interfering Factors

- Incomplete removal of synovial fluid
- Incorrect placement of the contrast medium
- Allergy to iodine

Nursing Implementation

Pretest

Ask the patient about any history of allergy to iodine or shellfish or a reaction to a previous x-ray test that used dye.
Explain the procedure and obtain written consent from the patient or person legally designated to make the patient's health care decisions.

Inform the patient that the procedure is performed with local anesthesia. Mild pain is felt as the anesthetic is injected, and a tingling or sensation of pressure is felt when the contrast medium is injected. Once the needle is removed, the patient will be asked to move the joint to various positions. This distributes the contrast material until all structures are visible on x-ray film.

During the Test

Place the synovial fluid in a sterile specimen container and send it to the laboratory for analysis.

Posttest

Take the patient's vital signs to ensure that the blood pressure and pulse readings are within normal limits.

Determine that the pressure dressing or elastic bandage is intact and dry.

Instruct the patient to rest the joint for 12 hours.

Apply ice packs to the joint to reduce the swelling.

Mild pain medication may be taken to relieve any discomfort.

Advise the patient that a crackling sensation (crepitus) in the joint is expected for 1 to 2 days until the air contrast is fully absorbed. The iodinated contrast material is a water-soluble medium and is quickly absorbed from the joint by normal body processes.

ARTHROSCOPY

(ENDOSCOPY)

Synonyms:

────────────────── **NORMAL VALUES** ──────────────────

No tissue or structural abnormalities of the joint space are noted.

Background Information

An arthroscope—a thin, flexible fiberoptic endoscope—provides direct visualization of the joint structures and tissues in the joint space (Fig. 23–3). The instrument has light, fiberoptics, and lenses to allow inspection of the interior of the joint and any abnormalities that are present. The arthroscope is attached to a video camera so that the images can be shown on a monitor and videotaped for further study. The arthroscope contains a small camera that can photograph areas

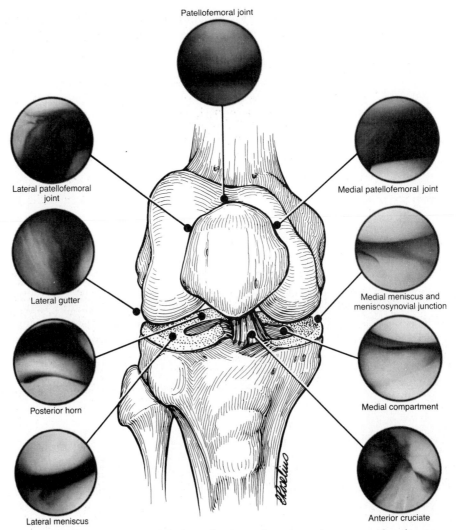

Patellofemoral joint

Lateral patellofemoral joint

Medial patellofemoral joint

Lateral gutter

Medial meniscus and meniscosynovial junction

Posterior horn

Medial compartment

Lateral meniscus

Anterior cruciate

FIGURE 23–3. Anterior view of the knee showing each section as it appears with arthroscopy. (Reproduced with permission from Scott, W.N. [1990]. *Arthroscopy of the knee: Diagnosis and treatment* [p. 63]. Philadelphia: W.B. Saunders.)

of interest. The special accessory instruments can be used to obtain biopsy specimens or to aspirate synovial fluid.

The joint, its interior ligaments, structures, synovial lining, and bony surfaces can develop infection, inflammation, tumor growth, or injury from trauma. When the pathologic change in the joint is not fully explained by more simple laboratory tests and diagnostic procedures, arthroscopy may be needed to confirm the diagnosis and evaluate the extent of the problem. The knee is the most common joint to be examined by arthroscopy, but the shoulder and other joints also can be examined by this method.

Diagnostic arthroscopy is performed as a same-day surgical procedure. Either local or general anesthesia may be used. Arthroscopy is an invasive procedure because surgical openings are made into the joint capsule to allow the insertion of the endoscope. Following the diagnostic phase, arthroscopic surgical repair of the torn or damaged tissue may be performed.

Purpose of the Test

Arthroscopy provides direct visualization of the interior of the joint and tissue surfaces. It is used to detect torn ligament, injured meniscus, and damaged cartilage.

Procedure

Two surgical incisions are made in the skin. A trochar is inserted into the joint capsule through one incision, followed by the insertion of the arthroscope. A probe or the accessory instruments are inserted through the other incision. The joint capsule is filled and distended with saline or Ringer's lactate to promote visualization. Additional incisions may be needed to visualize all aspects of the joint. Tissue and fluid samples may be collected for laboratory analysis. Once the fluid is drained and the instruments removed, sutures or tape strips are used to close the incisions (Folick, 1991). The total time needed for the procedure is 2 to 3 hours.

Findings

ABNORMAL RESULTS

Torn anterior cruciate or tibial collateral ligaments of the knee
Torn medial or lateral meniscus of the knee
Degenerative articular cartilage
Synovitis
Loose bodies
Subluxation, fracture, or dislocation of the bone
Chondromalacia
Osteochondritis dissecans
Arthritis
Gout or pseudogout
Ganglion or Baker cyst

Interfering Factors

• Failure to maintain a nothing-by-mouth status

Nursing Implementation

Pretest

Explain the procedure and obtain a written consent from the patient or person legally designated to make health care decisions for the patient.

Instruct the patient to discontinue all food and fluids for 8 hours before the procedure.

Give instructions for the patient to have a responsible person available to provide transportation after the procedure.

Take baseline vital signs and record the results.

Posttest

Critical Thinking: During the discussion of the posttest activity restrictions, your patient tells you that his bathroom and bedroom are on the second floor of his house. What suggestions can you make to help him modify the ambulation activity appropriately?

If general anesthesia has been administered, take vital signs immediately and thereafter every 15 minutes for 2 hours, every 30 minutes for 1 hour, and every hour for 2 hours or until discharge from the postanesthesia unit.

If local anesthesia has been administered, take initial vital signs and repeat them at regular intervals thereafter.

Assess for pain and provide the prescribed medication for relief of pain, as needed.

Check the elastic compression dressing for any signs of excessive bleeding, constriction, or excessive swelling of the joint or distal extremity.

Inform the patient that walking is permitted, but there should be no exercise or excessive use of the joint for 24 hours.

Provide the prescriptions for medications to be taken at home. Pain is usually minimal and can be relieved by nonsteroidal, antiinflammatory medications and nonnarcotic analgesics.

Complications

The complications of diagnostic arthroscopy are rare, but infection can occur. Instruct the patient to report any sign of infection to the physician. The complications of arthroscopy are found in Table 23–2.

BONE BIOPSY

(TISSUE BIOPSY)

Synonym:
bone needle aspiration cytology

———————— **NORMAL VALUES** ————————

Bone tissue is normal with no tumor cells present.

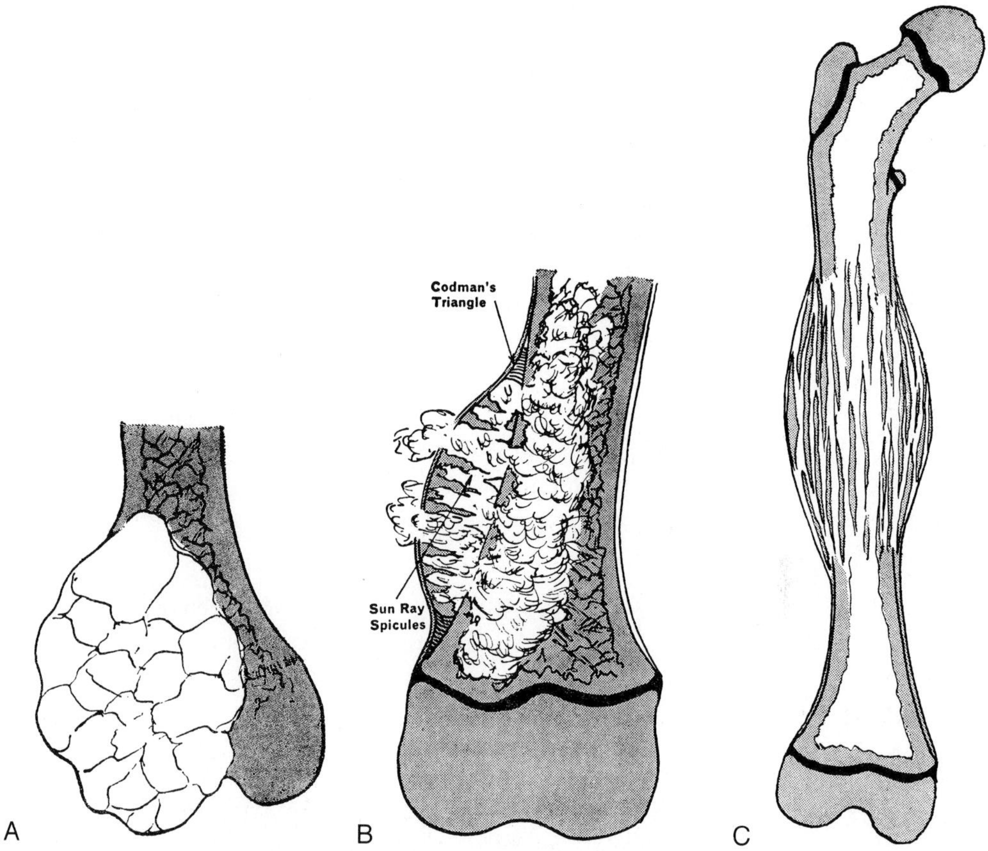

FIGURE 23–4. Tumors of the bone. *A*, Giant cell tumor. *B*, Osteogenic sarcoma. *C*, Malignant endothelioma (Ewing's tumor). (Reproduced with permission from Hughes, S. [1983]. *A short textbook of orthopedics and traumatology* [3rd ed.]. New York: Arco.)

Background Information

Benign bone tumors are characterized by their uniform density and well-defined margins. The most common benign tumor is the giant cell tumor, often located in the end of a long bone near a joint.

Malignant primary bone tumors are characterized by borders that extend outward into surrounding fat or muscle tissue or inward into the marrow and medullary cavity, or both (Fig. 23–4). The most common primary bone malignancy is osteogenic sarcoma, often located in the region of the knee.

Malignant bone tumors may also be metastatic tumors, with the primary site located elsewhere in the body (Table 23–3). Ninety per cent of bone metastases are in multiple sites, usually located in the vertebrae, ribs, sternum, or pelvis (Datz, 1988; Moss et al., 1992).

When bone tumor is suspected, a bone scan or computed tomography (CT) scan is performed first. These preliminary tests are used to verify the presence

TABLE 23–3
PRIMARY SITES OF METASTATIC BONE TUMORS
Breast
Lung
Prostate
Lymphoma
Thyroid
Kidney
Neuroblastoma

of the tumor and identify the site for bone biopsy. These preliminary tests are also used to identify additional metastatic sites and help assess the extent of growth or invasion of the tumor. Unlike biopsy, the preliminary tests cannot distinguish benign from malignant disease.

Purpose of the Test

Bone biopsy is performed to examine a specimen of bone tissue for its cell type and to distinguish benign from malignant bone tumor.

Procedure

With local anesthesia, a small incision is made in the skin, and a bone biopsy needle is drilled or pushed into the bone. Once it is in place, the biopsy needle is rotated 180 degrees to obtain a core sample of the tissue. The specimen is placed on a slide with fixative or in a specimen jar with 95% alcohol as a fixative, or both procedures are carried out. The time needed for this procedure is 30 minutes or more.

Findings

ABNORMAL VALUES

Malignant	Benign
Osteogenic sarcoma	Giant cell tumor
Ewing sarcoma	Osteoma
Reticulum cell sarcoma	Osteoid osteoma
Angiosarcoma	Chondroma
Multiple myeloma	
Metastatic tumor	

Interfering Factors

* Failure to obtain an adequate sample of tissue
* Failure to send the specimen to the laboratory immediately

Nursing Implementation

Pretest

Explain the procedure to the patient and obtain written consent from the patient or person legally designated to make the patient's health care decisions.

Instruct the patient to remove all clothing and put on a hospital gown.

Take baseline vital signs and record the results.

Shave the skin at the biopsy location and cleanse it with antiseptic.

During the Test

Provide support to the patient as the skin and subcutaneous tissue are anesthetized and as the biopsy needle is inserted. Despite the local anesthetic, momentary pain is experienced as the needle penetrates the periosteum and enters the bone.

Label all specimen containers and slides with the patient's name and the tissue source.

Complete the requisition form for a tissue cytologic study. The requisition slip states the patient's name, age, any history of carcinoma or infection, and the site of biopsy.

Send the slides or specimen, or both, to the laboratory without delay.

QUALITY CONTROL

The final preparation of the slides must be performed within 6 hours to prevent deterioration of the tissue.

Posttest

Take vital signs and monitor them at regular intervals until they are stable. Determine that the adhesive bandage is clean, dry, and intact.

Complications

Infection of bone is a possible complication. Instruct the patient to notify the physician if untoward symptoms occur. The complications of bone biopsy are presented in Table 23–4.

BONE SCAN

(RADIONUCLIDE SCAN)

Synonyms:

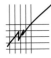

TABLE 23–4
COMPLICATIONS OF BONE BIOPSY

Complication	Nursing Assessment
Infection of bone	Fever
	Bone pain
	Headache
	Pain on movement
	Redness
	Drainage
	Purulence or abscess
	Elevated leukocyte count

—— **NORMAL VALUES** ——

There is symmetry of uptake of the radionuclide, with no bone abnormalities noted.

Background Information

Radionuclide bone studies produce sensitive, high-resolution images of the skeleton and joints. Because of the effectiveness of bone-seeking radiopharmaceuticals, the bone scan is sensitive to changes in bone. It can detect early stages of bone disease before other radiologic procedures can.

The basic structure of bone is a crystalline lattice of calcium, phosphate, and hydroxyl ions. The other components include collagen, ground substance, and additional minerals. Bone tissue is metabolically active, with a large number of nutrients exchanged in the blood vessels that supply the bones. There is a continual renewal of bone tissue that is maintained by a balance between *osteogenesis*, the manufacture of new bone, and bone reabsorption. This renewal process is called *bone turnover*.

The bone scan procedure uses the physiology of bone turnover to ensure uptake of the radiopharmaceutical into the bone. Technetium-99m is a radioisotope that can be combined with an analog of calcium, hydroxyl group, or phosphate to become a bone-seeking radioisotope. Once this radioactive substance is in the blood, it will be taken up by the bones and detected by the scintillation camera or scanner. To achieve adequate uptake by the bones, there must be (1) adequate blood supply and (2) metabolic activity (bone turnover).

BONE IMAGING. The normal scan demonstrates symmetric activity throughout the skeleton. In children, there is greater uptake in the growth regions of the epiphyses, cranial sutures, and joints of the pelvic bones.

The abnormal scan presents "hot" spots or "cold" spots and an asymmetric uptake of the radiopharmaceutical. A hot spot is an area of increased uptake of

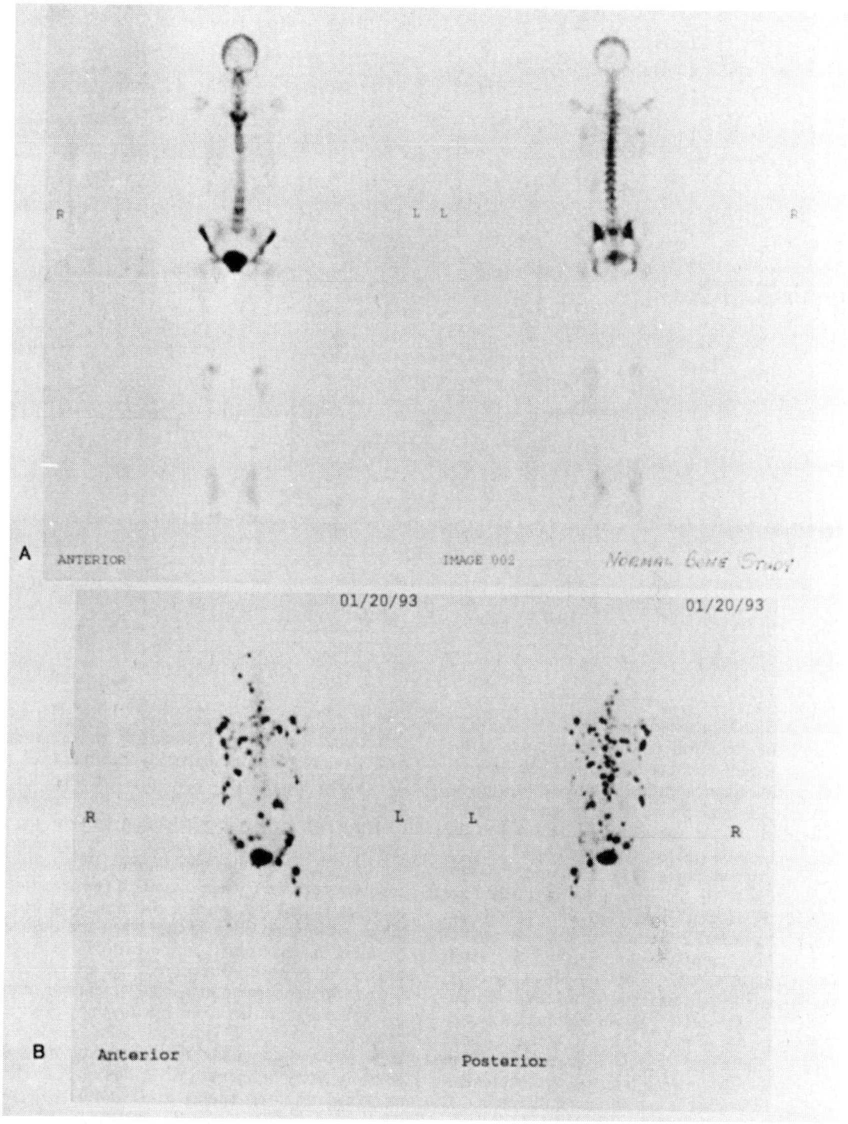

FIGURE 23-5. Bone scans. *A*, A normal nuclear medicine bone image. *B*, A nuclear medicine bone image of a patient with metastatic bone cancer. (Reproduced with permission from Thompson, M.A., et al. [1994]. *Principles of imaging science and protection* [vol. 2, Slide 392]. Philadelphia: W.B. Saunders.)

the radiopharmaceutical that indicates increased osteogenic activity (Fig. 23–5). The cause may be a primary or metastatic malignancy, infection, healing activity in the repair of a fracture, or other conditions that accelerate osteogenesis. A cold spot indicates decreased uptake because of an absence of osteogenic activity. Causes of decreased or absent activity include a lack of blood supply to the area of bone or destruction of bone tissue by tumor, an inflammatory mass, or irradiation.

JOINT IMAGING. Because joints can be imaged, the bone scan can evaluate inflammatory joint disease. The radionuclide collects in tissues with increased blood flow, such as in the increased vascularity of synovitis or degenerative arthritis. Often, early joint inflammation is detected by radionuclide scan before it can be seen on x-ray film.

Purpose of the Test

The bone scan is used to detect the presence and extent of metastatic disease of the bones. In addition, it is used to monitor degenerative bone diseases, detect osteomyelitis, determine bone viability, identify bone biopsy sites, and evaluate difficult fractures or fractures in battered children.

Procedure

An intravenous injection of a technetium radiopharmaceutical is followed by scanning with a gamma camera 1 to 4 hours later. The time variable depends on the type of radiopharmaceutical that is used. Scans are taken of anterior and posterior views. The images are seen on the monitor and are photographed for further study. The scanning process takes 1 hour to complete.

QUALITY CONTROL

When administering the radiopharmaceutical, the needle must be placed correctly in the vein lumen. If there is leakage into surrounding tissue, the scanner detects the pooled isotopes. The localization may be interpreted as a false-positive finding.

Findings

ABNORMAL VALUES

Primary malignant bone tumor
Metastatic tumors
Fractures
Loose prostheses
Aseptic necrosis

Osteomyelitis
Paget disease
Arthritis
Soft tissue activity
Following radiation therapy

Interfering Factors

* Metallic objects
* Full or enlarged bladder
* Pregnancy

Nursing Implementation

Pretest

Explain the procedure to the patient and obtain a written consent from the patient or the person legally designated to make health care decisions for the patient. Ensure that the patient is not pregnant because the radio-activity presents a potential danger for the fetus.

The radiopharmaceutical is a radioactive substance, but it is of low dosage and has a short half-life. The phosphate radiopharmaceutical is excreted rapidly from the body by the kidneys and bladder so that radiation exposure is minimal.

Instruct the patient to remove all clothing and jewelry and put on a hospital gown. The bladder must be emptied before the start of the procedure because retained urine will contain the radiopharmaceutical and prevent a clear view of the pelvis.

During the Test

The radiopharmaceutical is injected intravenously, usually in the arm.

Help the patient drink several glasses of water after the injection before the scanning process begins. These extra fluids will help the patient void at the end of the procedure.

Posttest

If the venipuncture site is sore or swollen, instruct the patient to apply moist compresses every 2 to 4 hours.

COMPUTED TOMOGRAPHY, BONES AND JOINTS

(TOMOGRAPHY)

Synonym:

CT scan

In orthopedics, the CT scan is particularly useful because the bone tissue is dense and absorbs many of the x-ray photons. Thus, the image of the bones appears white or bright on the film. The scan gives accurate definition of the structure of the bones and demonstrates subtle pathologic changes such as the small linear fracture, stenosis of a bony canal, or erosion of the bone (Shankar and Montanera, 1991).

Another CT application is quantitative CT used to measure or quantify the density of specific bone tissue. This specialized analysis uses the CT scan and mathematical calculations to assess the bone mineral content of the vertebrae in the lower back (T4–L3). The quantitative analysis may be used to assess os-teoporosis or to evaluate the results of medical therapy and its effect on the bones.

CT may also be used to assess the spinal column, confirming the presence of bony or soft tissue changes that affect the vertebrae or spinal canal. CT detects congenital malformation, bony overgrowth, bone spurs, lumbar stenosis, cervical spondylosis, degenerative changes, a bulging disc, and ligament hypertrophy (Chase, 1991).

The complete discussion of CT is presented in Chapter 12.

MAGNETIC RESONANCE IMAGING, BONES

(TOMOGRAPHY)

Synonym:

MRI

Magnetic resonance imaging (MRI) has limited use in orthopedics because the bone tissue produces a weak signal and therefore a poor image. MRI is used, however, in the evaluation of ligaments of the knee. It can demonstrate a tumor or other abnormalities of the anterior or posterior cruciate ligaments (Folick, 1991). MRI can also be used to diagnose spinal stenosis and to evaluate the soft tissues of the spine (Chase, 1991). MRI demonstrates degenerative disc changes, epidural fat, and postoperative scar tissue that affects spinal or neural function.

A complete discussion of MRI is presented in Chapter 12.

ROENTGENOGRAPHY, BONES AND JOINTS

(RADIOLOGY)

Synonym:

x-ray

Critical Thinking: During your first home visit to your elderly patient, you note a possible fracture of the nose and some bruises that are in different stages of healing. The injuries are not consistent with the explanation that he has given. You suspect possible elder abuse. What additional nursing assessments are needed before you can make a diagnosis?

X-ray films of bones and joints can identify fractures and monitor the degree of healing. This radiology procedure also demonstrates pathologic changes in bone such as abnormal structure, decreased bone density, tumor, arthritic change, and avascular necrosis (Fig. 23–6). Changes in the joints include narrowing of the joint spaces, bony overgrowth, loose bodies, erosion of the joint margins, subluxation, and dislocation. A complete discussion of roentgenography is presented in Chapter 9.

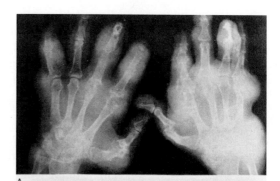

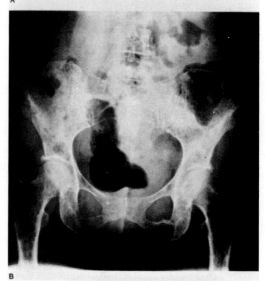

FIGURE 23–6. Radiographic visualization of osteolytic changes in bones. *A*, Osteolytic changes have resulted from bone destruction due to the disease process known as gout. Note the soft tissue swelling and bone destruction in the joints of both hands. *B*, Multiple myeloma produces osteolytic changes as the result of metastases. Radiolucent areas can be seen throughout the pelvis. (Reproduced with permission from Thompson, M.A., et al. [1994]. *Principles of imaging science and protection* [vol. 2, Slide 293]. Philadelphia: W.B. Saunders.)

SYNOVIAL MEMBRANE BIOPSY

(TISSUE BIOPSY)

Synonyms:

──────────────── **NORMAL VALUES** ────────────────

Normal cells of the synovial membrane

Background Information

The synovial membrane forms the inner lining of the joint capsule and secretes small amounts of synovial fluid within the joint cavity. The fluid is a thickened liquid that lubricates the joint surfaces and provides nourishment to the joint cartilage. The volume of synovial fluid is minimal because the surrounding tissue absorbs the excess fluid and electrolytes on a continual basis.

The synovium is subject to inflammation, granulation, or degeneration from a variety of causes, including infection, trauma, and inflammatory or arthritic changes of the joint itself. When the synovium is infected or inflamed, there is excess production of fluid. The edema and congestion in the joint tissues prevent the absorption of the fluid, and the joint capsule becomes swollen and painful. Following the inflammatory stage, granulation and fibrosis develop as the synovial tissue heals. Eventually, the synovial tissue can be destroyed by an ongoing pathologic process.

The synovial membrane biopsy procedure can be performed on the affected knee, elbow, wrist, ankle, or shoulder joint. From the tissue specimen, histologic examination looks for evidence of inflammation. Synovial fluid is collected during the procedure and is sent for culture.

Purpose of the Test

Synovial membrane biopsy is used to help differentiate among the various types of arthritis, collagen diseases, infections, and other disorders that cause inflammation of the joint and its synovial lining.

Procedure

Using sterile technique and local anesthesia, a trochar is pushed into the joint capsule. A special synovial biopsy needle is inserted through the trochar and a small sample of synovial tissue is aspirated into a syringe. The tissue is sent to the laboratory for analysis. The procedure requires 30 minutes to complete.

Findings

ABNORMAL VALUES

Coccidioidomycosis
Lyme disease
Rheumatoid arthritis
Synovitis
Tumor

Gout
Pseudogout
Reiter disease
Sarcoidosis
Systemic lupus erythematosus

Interfering Factors

- None

Nursing Implementation

Pretest

Explain the procedure to the patient and obtain a written consent from the patient or person legally designated to make the patient's health care decisions.

Inform the patient that the local anesthetic is injected and the procedure is not started until the tissue is numb. Brief pain is felt, however, as the trochar is inserted into the joint capsule.

Take baseline vital signs and record the results.

During the Test

Assist with the positioning of the patient's extremity, the cleansing of the skin, application of the drape, and instillation of the anesthetic.

Place the biopsy tissue in a sterile container with preservative. Label the container with the patient's name and date and the source of the tissue.

Posttest

Critical Thinking: During the early postoperative period, the patient complains of "burning pain along the shinbone, below the kneecap." To obtain complete information, what additional nursing assessments are needed?

Take the patient's vital signs at regular intervals until they are stable.

Check the compression dressing. The elastic bandage should be intact but without constricting the circulation in the extremity. There should be no evidence of swelling or bleeding, and distal pulses should be present.

Send the specimen and requisition slip to the laboratory.

Instruct the patient to rest the joint for 24 hours to prevent hemorrhage or effusion.

Advise the patient to notify the physician about excessive swelling, pain in the joint, or bleeding, because hemorrhage or effusion can occur. Infection in the joint can also occur, and the patient must report any problems of fever, malodorous drainage, or purulent drainage. The complications of synovial biopsy are presented in Table 23–2.

REFERENCES

Baumann, G.P., & Hurtubise, P. (1988). Anti-ideotypes and autoimmune disease. *Clinics in Laboratory Medicine, 8,* 373–384.

Braun, W.E., & Zachary, A.A. (1988). The HLA histocompatibility system in autoimmune states. *Clinics in Laboratory Medicine, 8,* 351–372.

Bryant, N.J. (1986). *Laboratory immunology and serology* (2nd ed.). Philadelphia: W.B. Saunders.

Chase, J.A. (1991). Spinal stenosis. *Nursing Clinics of North America, 26,* 53–64.

Datz, F.L. (1988). *Nuclear medicine.* Chicago: Yearbook Medical.

Folick, M.A. (1991). Meniscal injuries. *Nursing Clinics of North America, 26,* 181–198.

Henry, J.B. (Ed.). (1991). *Clinical diagnosis and management by laboratory methods* (18th ed.). Philadelphia: W.B. Saunders.

Jacobs, D.S., et al. (Eds.). (1990). *Laboratory test handbook* (2nd ed.). Baltimore: Williams & Wilkins.

Marino, C., & McDonald, E. (1992). Diagnostic joint aspiration: When is it necessary? *Emergency Medicine, 24,* 67.

Mettler, F.A., & Guiberteau, M.L. (1991). *Essentials of nuclear medicine imaging* (3rd ed.). Philadelphia: W.B. Saunders.

Moss, A.A., Gamsu, G., & Genant, H.K. (1992). *Computed tomography of the body with magnetic resonance imaging* (vol. 2, Bone and joint). Philadelphia: W.B. Saunders.

Norris, M.K.G. (1992). Evaluating C-reactive protein levels. . . lab test tips. *Nursing, 22,* 119.

Raatikainen, T., et al. (1992). Arthrography. Clinical examination and stress radiograph in the diagnosis of acute injury to the lateral ligaments of the ankle. *American Journal of Sports Medicine, 20,* 2–6.

Shankar, L., & Montanera, W. (1991). Computed tomography versus magnetic resonance imaging and three-dimensional applications. *Medical Clinics of North America, 75,* 1355–1366.

Shmerling, R.H., et al. (1990). Synovial fluid tests: What should be ordered? *JAMA, 264,* 1009.

Speer, K.P., et al. (1991). Magnetic resonance imaging of traumatic knee articular cartilage injuries. *American Journal of Sports Medicine, 19,* 396–402.

Teitz, N.W. (Ed.). (1990). *Clinical guide to laboratory tests* (2nd ed.). Philadelphia: W.B. Saunders.

Zosche, D.C. (1992). Is it Lyme disease? How to interpret the results of laboratory testing. *Postgraduate Medicine, 91,* 46.

CHAPTER **24**

Sensory Function

This chapter contains the diagnostic procedures that assess the sensory organs of the eyes, ears, and skin. Because of the distinctly different nature of these diagnostic procedures, they are organized in sections that reflect the individual organ systems.

The diagnostic procedures are used to identify and locate abnormality as well as assess the extent of change or impairment. The abnormality is caused by a change in the structure or function of the organ system, or both. Many of these tests can provide data early in the course of the disorder. This provides accurate information and guidance for prompt treatment. In some conditions, the treatment results in cure. In other conditions, early diagnosis and treatment minimize the deficit or loss of sensory function.

DIAGNOSTIC PROCEDURES

—————————————— **EYE TESTS** ——————————————

COMPUTED TOMOGRAPHY, EYE, ORBITS

(TOMOGRAPHY)

Synonym:

CT scan

The computed tomography (CT) scan with contrast medium is the primary imaging procedure used to examine the eye orbits and their contents. It provides visual information about the bones and soft tissues. The use of the tomographic slices and different visual planes allows the assessment of the parts in a complex anatomic area (Squire and Novelline, 1990). The procedure has an additional advantage because it can be performed rapidly. This is beneficial when a small child or an uncooperative patient requires an examination but cannot remain still for a long period of imaging.

In imaging the bones of the orbits, the CT scan identifies abnormalities caused by calcification, fracture, trauma, and metastatic lesion. In the assessment of the orbital contents, the CT scan can image the globe, lens, ocular muscles, and the optic nerve. Abnormalities that are clearly defined include retinoblastoma, meningioma, granuloma, penetrating foreign bodies, orbital hematoma, some vascular lesions, and the muscle changes associated with the exophthalmos of Graves disease.

A complete discussion of CT is presented in Chapter 12.

FLUORESCEIN ANGIOGRAPHY

(PHOTOGRAPHY WITH CONTRAST)

Synonyms:

intravenous fluorescent angiography, IVFA

—————————————— **NORMAL VALUES** ——————————————

Retinal blood vessels are intact with normal circulation and no evidence of leakage.

Background Information

The normal circulation of the retina consists of the central retinal artery and the central retinal vein, their four main branches, arterioles, venules, and capillaries. Behind the retina is the vascular choroid layer that allows the retinal exchange of oxygen, nutrients, and metabolic waste products. When local or systemic disease alters the retinal circulation, the changes can be seen in the retina and blood vessels. Fluorescein angiography photographs the changes to document the location and extent of the circulatory abnormality.

The dye used in the examination illuminates the blood vessels by its fluorescence. When there is rupture or leakage of the blood vessel, the dye leaks into the vitreous humor, producing a hyperfluorescent area. Retinal arterial stenosis or occlusion demonstrates an area of hypofluorescence or prolonged venous drainage. Abnormal vascular patterns are characteristic of other retinal and circulatory problems, and the findings are used to diagnose the retinal condition.

Purpose of the Test

This test is used to highlight the retinal circulation as part of the evaluation of retinopathy. The retinopathy is the result of a systemic, intraocular, or retinal pathologic change.

Procedure

After pupillary dilation, the fluorescent dye is injected intravenously. A rapid series of 20 to 30 photographs is taken at 1- to 2-second intervals to document the retinal circulation. After a rest period, a second series of photographs may be obtained to document the retinal findings.

Findings

ABNORMAL VALUES

Microaneurysm
Occlusion (arterial, venous)
Tortuosity of blood vessels
Hypertensive retinopathy
Edema (retinal, macular)
Papilledema

Arteriovenous shunt
Neovascularization
Capillary hemangioma
Tumor
Ruptured blood vessel

Interfering Factors

- Allergy to the iodinated contrast medium
- Cataracts
- Insufficient dilation of the pupils
- Movement of the head, eyes, eyelids

Nursing Implementation

Pretest

Obtain a written consent from the patient or person who is legally responsible for the patient's health care decisions.
Inquire about past history of allergy to iodine or seafood or a previous reaction to contrast material during a radiographic examination.

If the patient has glaucoma, instruct him or her to omit eye drop medication on the morning of the test. Glaucoma medication constricts the pupils. The pupillary dilation needed for the test would be difficult to accomplish.

Take the patient's baseline vital signs and record the results.

During the Test

Dilate the pupils with mydriatic eye drops.

Insert the intravenous line into a vein of the antecubital fossa. A scalp vein needle commonly is used.

Instruct the patient to sit in the chair with the chin and forehead resting against supports. The camera is positioned in front of the eye and is focused on the retina.

Instruct the patient to keep the head immobile and to stare straight ahead. Normal breathing and blinking are carried out during the photography phase.

Inform the patient that there may be a sensation of nausea, hot flashes, or warmth as the fluorescein dye is injected. Vomiting can occur.

After the photographs are taken, remove the intravenous needle and instruct the patient to rest for 20 to 60 minutes. If a second series of photographs is taken after the rest interval, no additional dye is needed. The dye has recirculated so that the retina is clearly visible.

Posttest

Critical Thinking: At the urban diagnostic eye center, the patient has just completed a fluorescein angiography examination. She tells you that she and her friend are now going to shop and then have lunch. What precautionary advice can you provide?

Inform the patient that the skin and sclera may appear yellow because of the dye circulation, but that the yellow color disappears in 4 to 6 hours. The urine will be fluorescent yellow-orange for about 24 hours, as the dye is excreted from the body.

Instruct the patient to drink extra fluids to help with the renal clearance of the dye.

Since the pupils remain dilated for a few hours, instruct the patient to wear sunglasses to protect the eyes from the glare of sunlight. Instruct the patient to avoid driving a car until the vision is clear.

MAGNETIC RESONANCE IMAGING, EYE

(TOMOGRAPHY)

Synonym:

MRI

Although magnetic resonance imaging (MRI) cannot image the bones or calcification of the orbits, it provides exceptional visualization of the soft tissue structures of the eye. It is often used as a supplement to the CT scan, particularly in the evaluation of a soft tissue tumor, the extraocular muscles, or the optic nerve. MRI can distinguish among solid tumor, subretinal fluid, and effusion. It is also useful in determining the cause of visual disturbance when the origin of the problem is brain infarct, brain tumor, inflammation of the brain, and demyelinating disease (Nadalo et al., 1991).

A complete discussion of MRI is presented in Chapter 12.

ORBITAL RADIOGRAPHY

(RADIOGRAPHY)

Synonym:

x-ray of orbits

Plain radiography of the bony orbits may be used to investigate possible orbital fracture. When resulting from facial trauma, the fracture may be linear or with displacement of bone fragments. Severe facial fracture may result in a widening of the protective bones that surround the eyes, which can be seen on x-ray film. Increased bone density is indicative of metastatic cancer, Paget disease, or meningioma. Because of the superior ability of the CT scan to provide images from many tomographic planes, it is the preferred modality to investigate problems of the bony orbits.

A complete discussion of radiography is found in Chapter 9.

ULTRASONOGRAPHY, EYE

(ULTRASOUND)

Synonyms:

Ultrasonography of the eye and orbit provides an accurate assessment of retinal and choroidal detachment and can detect fluid leakage or hemorrhage within the eye or behind the retina. It can identify the presence of an intraocular tumor and differentiate among the different types with 98% accuracy (Coleman et al., 1992). Ultrasound may be used to assess and measure extraocular muscles or other eye structures that are altered because of inflammation, infection, or edema. It is also used to locate a foreign body in the eye. This examination is useful in the preoperative period or with a complication that occurs during the operative period.

A complete discussion of ultrasound is presented in Chapter 8.

VISUAL ACUITY TESTS

(VISION TESTS)

Synonym:

VA

——————————————— **NORMAL VALUES** ———————————————

Distance Vision:	20/20 vision or better in each eye
Near Vision:	14/14 vision or better in each eye
Astigmatism:	All lines are seen as clear and of equal blackness

Background Information

Central vision is a function of the fovea in the center of the macula. This retinal tissue provides the sharp image of both distant and near objects, aided by the functions of the cornea and lens.

DISTANCE VISION. This type of vision is assessed by the use of the Snellen chart (Fig. 24–1). Each eye is tested separately, without and then with the use of corrective lenses. By tradition, the right eye is tested first.

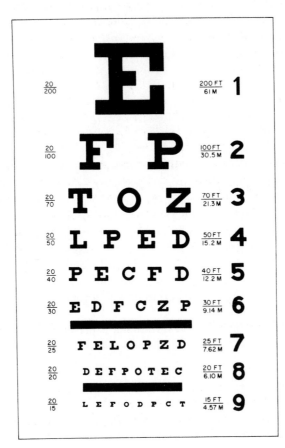

FIGURE 24–1. The Snellen chart. This chart is used to assess distance vision.

The test results are written in a fraction form, such as 20/20 vision. The first number, or the numerator, represents the distance between the patient and the Snellen chart. The second number, or the denominator, represents the lowest line on the Snellen chart that is read correctly by the patient. When the patient stands at a distance of 20 ft from the chart and with one eye reads line 20 correctly, the result is recorded as 20/20 for that eye. The interpretation is that the patient sees at 20 ft what other individuals see at 20 ft. If the patient has a result of 20/80 in one eye, it means that the patient sees at 20 feet what other individuals see at 80 feet.

The legal definition of blindness is 20/200 or worse with corrective lenses. If the patient cannot see the large letter E (line 200) at a distance of 20 ft, the patient is retested at a distance nearer the chart. Thus, when the patient can see the letter E at a distance of 10 ft, the result is 10/200.

For the patient who cannot see the letter E at any distance, additional assessment is performed. The patient may be able to count fingers (CF) that are 1 ft in front of his or her face. The recording of the vision is 1/CF. If this is unsuccessful, the patient may be able to see hand movement (HM) at a 1-ft distance. The information is written as 1/HM. If this is unsuccessful, light perception (LP) is tested. When a bright light shines in the eye, the patient is asked to state if the light is off or on. The affirmative response is recorded as 1/LP, meaning that there is light perception at a 1-ft distance. The negative response is recorded as no light perception (NLP).

NEAR VISION. This is tested to determine the patient's ability to focus on small details that are in close range. At rest, the normal eye is adapted for distance vision. If there is a need to focus on fine details, the eye must accommodate or change. This is carried out by contraction of the ciliary muscles and a change in the shape and thickness of the lens. Patients older than 40 years of age may have a loss of elasticity of the lens, resulting in difficulty with accommodation, or presbyopia. Near vision testing assesses the power of accommodation and is performed by reading small print or focusing on small objects.

ASTIGMATISM. This is the blurring of vision caused by the irregular curvature of the cornea or lens. Because of the irregularity, part of the view is clear and part is blurred. The astigmatism test chart is used to measure the clarity of vision in different axis areas of the cornea and lens. When astigmatism is present, the patient sees some of the axis lines as blurred or distinctly darker than other lines.

Purpose of the Test

Visual acuity testing is performed to assess the sharpness of central vision.

Procedure

Distance Vision: Testing each eye separately, the patient is asked to read the lines of the Snellen chart from a distance of 20 ft.

Near Vision: From a distance of 14 in., the patient is asked to read the small print or identify the location of the opening in each letter C.

Astigmatism: The patient looks at the chart and identifies any lines that are blurred or darker in tone.

Findings

ABNORMAL VALUES

Hyperopia
Myopia
Presbyopia
Retinal detachment

Macular degeneration
Corneal opacity
Advanced cataracts
Optic nerve impairment

Interfering Factors

- Failure to bring corrective lenses to the test
- Using improperly prescribed or outdated lenses

Nursing Implementation

Pretest

Snellen Chart

Critical Thinking: A German patient requires testing for visual acuity, but he speaks no English at all. What modifications of the testing process can be made to obtain accurate information?

Place the patient 20 ft from the chart. The patient may stand or sit for the test. Plan to test the vision without corrective lenses first and then with the corrective lenses used for distance vision.

During the Test

Have the patient occlude the left eye and begin testing the right eye.

Ask the patient to read the letters for each line, starting at the top or starting at a lower line where the patient can see the letters clearly.

If the chart uses the letter E, ask the patient to position the fingers in the same direction as the E on a particular line of the chart. If the chart has numbers or objects, the patient identifies them.

Ask the patient to continue reading the progressively smaller lines until errors are made on more than half the letters or until the line marked 20 is completed.

Repeat the test for the other eye.

If the patient with corrective lenses cannot see the line marked 400 (the large E) from 20 ft away, walk the patient toward the chart until the letter can be identified. Record the distance from the chart. If necessary, assess the ability of the patient to count fingers, see hand movement, or perceive light, usually from a distance of 1 ft.

Near Vision

Request that the patient use the corrective lenses to read a sample of tiny print from a distance of 14 in. As an alternative, ask the patient to use a finger to point in the same direction as the opening of the letter C. Each eye is tested separately.

Astigmatism

Test each eye separately, first without and then with corrective lenses.
Instruct the patient to look at the center of the figure with the radial black lines.
Ask the patient to identify any blurred lines or any lines that look darker than the others.

Posttest

Record the results for each eye, without and then with the corrective lenses.

VISUAL FIELD TESTING

(VISION TESTS)

Synonyms:

NORMAL VALUES

Amsler Grid: There is ability to see the black dot, four sides of the grid, and all squares within the grid.
Tangent Screen
Examination: The test object remains visible in all areas of central vision.

Background Information

The visual field is the total extent of vision out to the periphery. The two areas that combine to make the total are the central and the peripheral areas of the visual field. The central portion contains the fovea centralis, the retinal area of visual acuity. It provides sharp focus in an area of 25 degrees surrounding a fixation point. The peripheral visual field is the larger area that has vision but little acuity or focus. The peripheral field extends out to 60 degrees on the nasal side and 85 degrees on the temporal side of each retina.

AMSLER GRID. This is a screening test that assesses the central portion of the total visual field (Fig. 24–2A). When there is deterioration or damage to the central visual field, the fovea centralis, or the macula, the patient may be unable to see the central black dot or may not see all four sides of the grid (Fig. 24–2B). Some of the grid may be seen as blurred or distorted instead of the horizontal and vertical black lines that form squares.

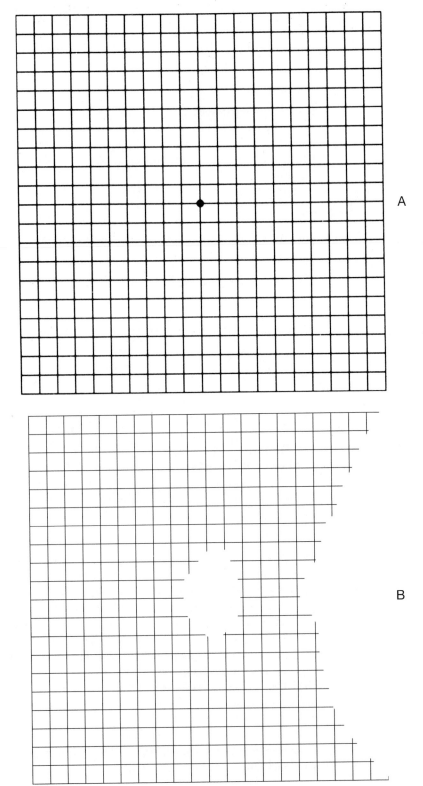

FIGURE 24-2. *A,* Amsler grid. *B,* Loss of visibility of some lines or the dot indicates retinal abnormality, particularly in the area of the macula.

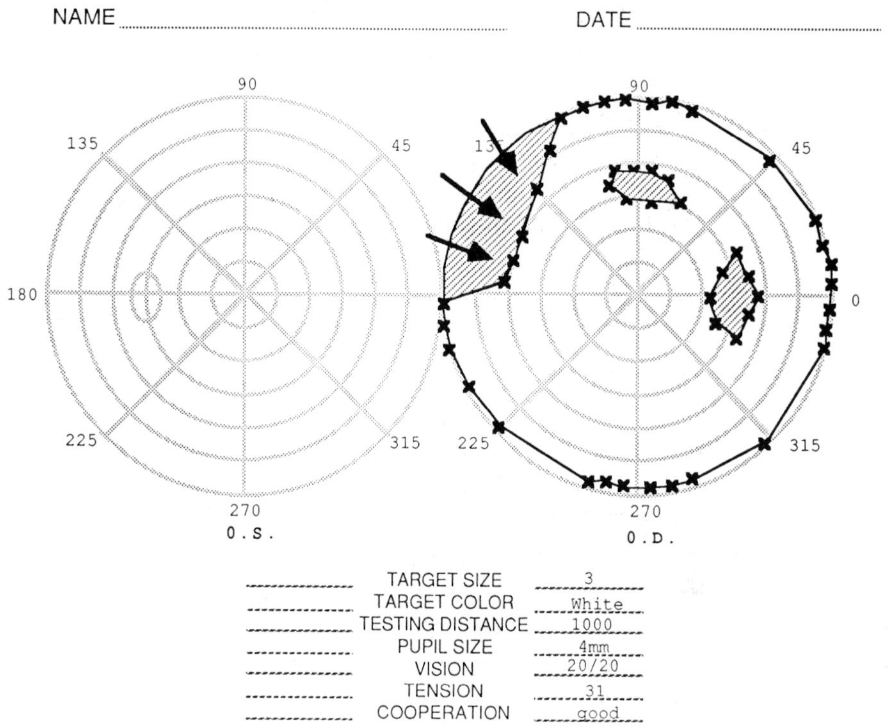
NAME
DATE
90
135
45
180
225
315
270
O.S.
90
45
0
315
225
270
O.D.
TARGET SIZE 3
TARGET COLOR White
TESTING DISTANCE 1000
PUPIL SIZE 4mm
VISION 20/20
TENSION 31
COOPERATION good

FIGURE 24–3. A tangent screen recording sheet. The test provides a mapping of the visual field of each eye. For the left eye (OS), a record has not yet been made on the chart. For the right eye (OD), the chart is filled in and shows a superior nasal step, an arcuate scotoma, and vertical enlargement of the blind spot such as might be found in glaucoma. (Reproduced with permission from Carlson, N.B., et al. [1990]. *Clinical procedures for ocular examination* [p. 205]. Norwalk, CT: Appleton & Lange.)

TANGENT SCREEN TEST. This measures the central portion of the visual field by mapping the boundaries of the central vision of each eye (Fig. 24–3). After mapping the perimeter, the optic disc area is located and its boundary is mapped. Since the optic disc has no photoreceptors, it acts like a small blind spot in the central visual field. Once the mapping of the outer and inner boundaries is completed, each eye is tested to verify that there is visual acuity in all areas within the boundaries. This method can provide some data, but in patients who have a deficit in central visual acuity, more precise automated or computerized equipment is used to measure the abnormality.

Purpose of the Test

These tests detect a loss of acuity in part of the central visual field and estimate the location and extent of the retinal change.

Procedure

The Amsler grid is placed 13 to 14 in. from the patient, and the vision of each eye is tested separately. The patient is asked to describe what is seen.

The tangent screen hangs on a wall, 40 in. from the patient, and the vision of each eye is tested separately. The patient states when he or she sees the test object, which is a disc with a black side and a white side. Use the black side when the tangent screen has a white background and the white side when the screen has a black background. The results are mapped to define the perimeters of the central visual field and any areas of deficit within the normal field.

Findings

ABNORMAL VALUES

Macular degeneration
Pituitary tumor
Cerebral aneurysm
Glaucoma
Retinitis pigmentosa

Hemianopsia
Meningioma
Cerebral vascular accident
Retinal detachment

Interfering Factors

- Severe loss of vision or blindness
- Failure to focus on the central dot or object on the map

Nursing Implementation

Pretest

Instruct the patient to wear corrective lenses for each of these tests.
Provide an occluder or a folded tissue to cover one eye as the other eye is tested.

During the Test

Amsler Grid

Place the patient about 13 in. from the Amsler grid.
Request that the patient keep his or her eye focused on the black dot.
Ask the patient:
- Is the black dot visible?
- Are the four sides of the grid visible?
- Are all lines and squares visible?
Repeat the test on the other eye.

Tangent Screen

Ask the patient to sit down for the examination. The chair is placed 40 in. from the wall where the screen is hung.

Stand at the side of the screen and observe that the patient's eye remains centered and does not search for the test object.

Ask the patient to fix his or her eye on the center of the screen and state when the test object first comes into view on the screen.

Use a hand-held wand with the test object on the tip to do the mapping. Along each tangent line, bring the object into view, from the periphery toward the center.

Place a pin on each tangent line where the patient states the test object is first seen. These pins mark the outer boundary of the central visual field.

Identify and map the boundaries of the optic disc. In a small area on the nasal side of each visual field, the patient sees the disc along several tangent lines; first it disappears and then reappears. Mark the places of disappearance and reappearance until the circular area is completed. This is the area of the optic disc.

Now that the boundaries are completed, use the test object to confirm visual acuity throughout the visual field. In each sector defined by the tangent lines, place the black test object on the black field. Turn the test object so that the white side shows. Ask the patient to state when the object appears. Repeat this maneuver in each sector.

If an area is not identified, repeat the maneuver with a test object of a different color or one of a larger size.

Record the results on the special test sheet and then repeat the test on the other eye.

Posttest

No special nursing intervention is required.

--- **EAR TESTS** ---

AUDIOMETRY

(HEARING TEST)

Synonyms:

hearing test, audiometric test, audiogram

Background Information

Hearing occurs by bone, air, and nerve conduction of the sound waves. *Conductive hearing loss* occurs when there is interference with air conduction caused by problems in the external or middle ear. *Sensorineural hearing loss* occurs because of interference with nerve transmission caused by problems of the inner

―――――――― **NORMAL VALUES** ――――――――

Pure Tone Average:	0–20 dB
Speech Reception Threshold:	Ability to repeat 50% of the words correctly, in a range of 0–20 dB
Word Discrimination Test:	>90% of the words are repeated correctly

ear, cochlea, or acoustic nerve, or a combination. A *mixed hearing loss* involves some impairment of bone and air conduction.

Audiometry is a test that measures the degree of hearing or hearing loss in response to pure tones and speech. The audiometer is the diagnostic instrument that produces sounds in different intensities (degrees of loudness) and different frequencies (degrees of pitch). Intensity is measured in decibels (dB) and frequency is measured in hertz (Hz) or cycles per second.

PURE TONE AUDIOMETRY. In this method of testing, the audiometer emits a series of tones at different frequencies. For the assessment of air conduction, the patient wears headphones and indicates when the different tones are heard. For the assessment of bone conduction, a vibrator is placed at the mastoid bone and emits the different tones. The tones that are heard identify the patient's hearing thresholds. A hearing threshold is the lowest decibel level at distinct frequencies when at least 50% of the tones are heard.

As the patient indicates that a sound is heard, the examiner plots the response on an audiogram (Fig. 24–4). The normal range of hearing is 0 to 20 dB at all tested frequencies. The patient with a hearing loss requires a higher decibel level to obtain a threshold response. Impaired hearing is measured in terms of a decibel loss, such as a 40-dB loss. Some patients have a decibel loss only at particular frequencies. These are usually the higher level frequencies. Each ear is tested separately, starting with the better ear.

In sensorineural hearing loss, both air and bone conduction thresholds demonstrate higher decibel ratings (or a greater decibel loss). In conductive hearing loss, the air conduction threshold has a higher decibel rating (or a greater decibel loss), but bone conduction is normal. In a mixed type of hearing loss, both air and bone conduction have higher decibel ratings, but air conduction is worse than bone conduction.

SPEECH AUDIOMETRY. Hearing for speech measures the *speech reception threshold* and the *word discrimination score*. The speech reception threshold is a spoken word test that measures sound intensity. It helps detect conduction hearing loss. The word discrimination threshold measures the client's ability to understand spoken words. It helps detect sensorineural hearing loss.

The speech reception threshold measurement uses *spondee* words. These are easily understood words of two syllables, such as *airplane, hardware, woodchuck,* and *birthday.* The speech reception threshold identifies the decibel level at which

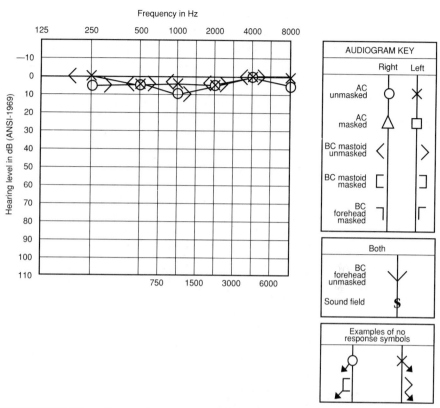

Frequency in Hz

FIGURE 24–4. The audiogram. Audiometry provides precise measurement of hearing of pure tones and speech for each ear. (From Newby, H.A., & Popelka, G.R. [1985]. *Audiology* [5th ed., pp. 146, 151, 152, and 155]. Needham Heights, MA: Allyn & Bacon. Copyright 1985 by Allyn and Bacon. Adapted by permission. With permission from Ignatavicius, D.D., et al. [1995]. *Medical-surgical nursing* [2nd ed., p. 1362]. Philadelphia: W.B. Saunders.)

the patient can repeat 50% of the words accurately. The decibel level of the speech reception threshold is usually similar to the results of tone testing for air conduction hearing.

The word discrimination test uses familiar, one-syllable words that are balanced phonetically, such as *day*, *stove*, and *run*. The patient hears the words at an intensity of about 30 dB above the speech reception threshold and repeats the words. The normal score is greater than 90% accuracy, but individuals with normal hearing often have 95 to 100% accuracy.

The patient with sensorineural hearing loss has a below normal score on the word discrimination test no matter what decibel level is used. This patient might describe the hearing loss as "hearing the sounds but having difficulty in understanding the words." In contrast, the patient with conductive hearing loss will have a good response on this test at the higher decibel levels. This patient might describe the hearing loss as "hearing the words as long as they are loud enough."

Purpose of the Test

Audiometry tests determine the type and extent of hearing loss.

Procedure

Pure Tone Audiometry: Sounds of differing intensity and frequency are emitted through earphones and a vibrator that is placed on the mastoid bone. When they are heard, the patient's responses are charted on an audiogram.

Speech Audiometry: Words are spoken through earphones at different decibel levels. As the patient repeats the words, the accuracy is recorded and the overall measurement is calculated in percentage of accurate answers.

Findings

ABNORMAL VALUES

Otitis media
Otosclerosis
Ruptured tympanum
Acoustic neuroma
Meniere disease
Infection, inflammation
Hypothyroidism

Cerebral infarction
Kernicterus
Multiple sclerosis
Mastoiditis
Labyrinthitis
Ototoxicity

Interfering Factors

- Impacted cerumen in the external auditory canal
- Background noise
- Inattention or mental confusion
- Extraneous cues from the examiner
- Recent ear or upper respiratory tract infection

Nursing Implementation

Pretest

Examine the external auditory canal and remove any impacted cerumen. Provide an overview of the examination including what to expect and how to respond. This promotes the patient's cooperation and responsiveness. Instruct the patient to remove hearing aid, hat, and eyeglasses and then to sit in the soundproof booth or room.

During the Test

Place the headphones on the patient and adjust them to fit properly.

Prior to each test, repeat the specific instructions so that the patient knows how to respond.

Posttest

No specific nursing interventions are needed.

COMPUTED TOMOGRAPHY, LABYRINTH SYSTEM

(TOMOGRAPHY)

Synonym:

CT scan

The CT scan is used to evaluate the labyrinth system as part of the investigation of dizziness. It provides visualization of congenital abnormality, tumor, abscess, bony changes, temporal bone fracture, and inflammatory disease. A complete discussion of CT is presented in Chapter 12.

ELECTRONYSTAGMOGRAPHY

(ELECTRIC MONITORING)

Synonym:

ENG

NORMAL VALUES	
Electronystagmography:	Normal waveform patterns; no nystagmus present
Caloric Test:	Normal waveform pattern
Cold Stimulation:	Nystagmus present in the opposite ear
Warm Stimulation:	Nystagmus present in the same ear

Background Information

Electronystagmography is used to help determine the cause of dizziness, vertigo, tinnitus, and unexplained hearing loss. Some sources of these symptoms are an abnormality in the labyrinth system, the eighth cranial (acoustic) nerve, cerebellum, or brain stem.

The interaction between the vestibular system and oculomotor function is regulated by the vestibuloocular reflex. The regulation allows the eyes to maintain visual fixation while the head turns. In normal function, lateral nystagmus occurs only when the head is turned to an extreme lateral position, or when the eyes move in to an extreme lateral position. The eyes then return rapidly to a normal position with no further nystagmus. Abnormal nystagmus

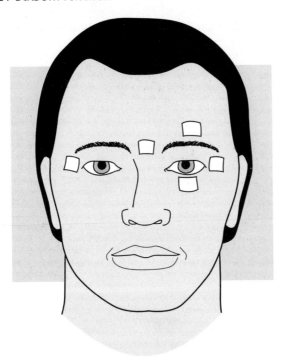

FIGURE 24–5. Placement of the electrodes for electronystagmography. The needle electrodes are inserted under the skin and are held in place with squares of adhesive tape. During the testing process, these electrodes transmit data that identify horizontal or vertical nystagmus.

occurs at rest (spontaneously), or it persists after head turning or other evoked stimulus.

The measurement of eye movements is based on the recording of changing electric potentials. The cornea of the eye has a positive electric charge and the retina has a negative electric charge. The electrodes detect the changing position of the eyes, and the results are recorded as linear patterns on graph paper.

An electrode is placed near the outer canthus of each eye to detect lateral nystagmus. Additional electrodes are placed above and below one eye to detect vertical nystagmus. One electrode is placed above the bridge of the nose to minimize noise interference (Fig. 24–5).

Purpose of the Test

These tests are used to verify the problem of dizziness and vertigo and to help identify the location of the abnormality.

Procedure

There are a number of different test maneuvers that are performed during the examination. Most are carried out with the patient in a seated position and involve having the patient move the eyes, fix on or follow a light, move the head, or move the body. The test battery includes the *spontaneous nystagmus test, gaze nystagmus, position tests, pendulum tracking test, optokinetic test,* and *caloric test.*

In the caloric test, the patient lies supine with the head elevated 30 degrees. Cool water (30° C) and then warm water (44° C) is instilled in each ear.

Findings

ABNORMAL VALUES

Meniere disease

Lesion, tumor of the cerebello-
pontine angle

Infection, inflammation

Head injury

Ototoxicity

Otosclerosis

Acoustic nerve tumor

Congenital malformation

Multiple sclerosis

Cerebral infarction

Ischemic neuritis

Posterior fossa mass, deformity

Temporal lobe epilepsy

Hypothyroidism

Labyrinthitis

Interfering Factors

- Perforated tympanum
- Cardiac pacemaker
- Intake of caffeine or alcohol
- Poor eyesight
- Inability to comply with test instructions
- Back or neck disorder

Nursing Implementation

Pretest

Ask if the patient has a pacemaker, neck or back disorder, ruptured eardrum, or other problem that would interfere with the procedure.

Obtain written consent from the patient or person legally responsible for the patient's health care decisions.

Instruct the patient to avoid a heavy meal and the intake of alcohol and caffeine on the day of the test. The alcohol and caffeine alter the nerve potentials and the heavy meal is avoided because the test can cause nausea and vomiting.

Many medications subdue the neurologic responses and are often omitted for 24 to 48 hours before the test. These include antivertigo and antiinflammatory drugs, aspirin, depressants, tranquilizers, sedatives, and stimulants. If the patient has been instructed by the physician to continue with these medications, record them on the requisition slip.

If a caloric test is planned, use the otoscope to examine the external auditory canal for a perforation of the tympanum and the presence of cerumen. An opening in the tympanum is a contraindication for this test. If there is an impaction, the cerumen must be removed.

Explain that dizziness and nausea can occur during the tests but that they subside after the tests are completed.

Provide reassurance that the examiner or nurse will remain nearby to prevent a fall. Position the patient comfortably in the chair.

During the Test

Prior to the placement of the electrodes, cleanse the skin with alcohol to reduce the electric impedance caused by skin oil.

To improve conduction, apply the electrode paste to the five sites. Insert the skin electrodes. Inform the patient that the electrodes on the face will feel uncomfortable.

As each test is ready, provide specific instructions to the patient. These instructions include looking at the light, following the light, opening or closing the eyes, and changing the head or body position.

Assess the patient for nausea, dizziness, weakness, or vomiting throughout the test period.

Posttest

Remove the electrodes and paste from the skin.

Assist the patient to a chair or couch to rest until the symptoms subside.

SKIN TESTS

BIOPSY, SKIN

(TISSUE BIOPSY)

Synonym:

gross and microscopic pathology, skin

NORMAL VALUES

Benign; no malignant cells are present. No infectious organisms are present.

Background Information

When a skin lesion is present and the clinical diagnosis is uncertain or must be verified, a skin biopsy is carried out to determine the cellular composition of the lesion or the presence of infection. Skin biopsy can be performed by three different types of technique, all of which cause minimal amounts of discomfort,

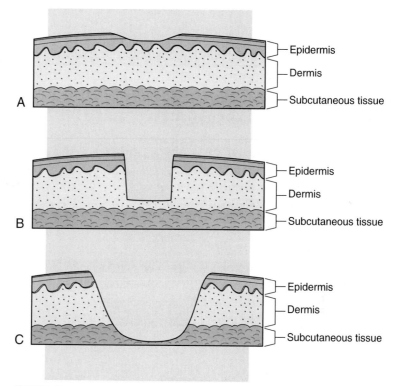

FIGURE 24–6. Skin biopsy. The depth of tissue removal for *(A)* shave biopsy, *(B)* punch biopsy, and *(C)* elliptical incision biopsy.

scarring, and bleeding. The methods are *shave biopsy*, *punch biopsy*, and *elliptical excision* (Fig. 24–6).

SHAVE BIOPSY. This procedure is used when there is a small, raised growth or lesion. The scalpel is placed parallel to the surface of the growth, and a shallow cut is used to remove some of the superficial tissue layers.

PUNCH BIOPSY. This technique is used when the lesion extends into the middle to lower portion of the dermis. A circular cutting tool is rotated with downward pressure to cut and remove a core sample of the tissue. The small hole may be closed with a suture or allowed to heal by granulation.

ELLIPTICAL INCISIONAL BIOPSY. This method is used when the lesion or growth is greater than 4.5 mm in diameter or is thought to extend deeper than the middermis. A scalpel is used to excise the tissue to a depth that includes some subcutaneous fat. The tissue defect is closed with sutures.

Critical Thinking: The skin biopsy result identifies the patient's lesion as a squamous cell carcinoma. Prepare a teaching plan that will help the patient protect herself from additional exposure to sunlight.

Purpose of the Test

Skin biopsy is performed to differentiate a benign from a malignant growth. It is sometimes used to diagnose particular bacterial or fungal infections.

Procedure

After local anesthesia, a small sample of skin tissue is removed surgically for histologic and microbiologic examination.

Findings

ABNORMAL VALUES

Malignant melanoma
Basal cell carcinoma
Squamous cell carcinoma
Neurofibroma
Dermatofibroma
Mole

Seborrheic dermatitis
Keloid
Cyst
Bacterial infection
Fungal infection

Interfering Factors

- Failure to identify the specimen
- Failure to identify the specimen accurately

Nursing Implementation

Pretest

Obtain signed consent from the patient or person legally responsible for the patient's health care decisions.

Instruct the patient to remove the clothing necessary to expose the biopsy site. A hospital gown may be worn as needed.

Take the patient's vital signs and record the results.

Depending on the site of the lesion, instruct the patient to sit or lie down on the examining table.

During the Test

Cleanse the skin site with a surgical antiseptic.

Assist with the application of the surgical drape and the preparation of the local anesthetic (lidocaine 1%).

Once the tissue sample has been removed, place it in a sterile, covered container with formalin or other tissue preservative.

If a tissue sample is needed for culture, place a small amount of tissue in a sterile container *without preservative*.

Close and label each container accurately, including the patient's name, the date, and the tissue source. Place the same information on the requisition slip.

After the bleeding ceases, place a small sterile dressing over the biopsy site.

Posttest

Take the patient's vital signs and record the results.

Assess the dressing for signs of bleeding. It should be clean, dry, and intact.

Ensure that the specimens are transported to the laboratory promptly. Microbiologic specimens must be sent immediately because they can dry out. The specimens in preservative are sent on a routine basis.

Instruct the patient to keep the dressing clean and dry.

If sutures are in place, instruct the patient to return to the physician for their removal. Facial sutures are removed in 3 to 5 days. For other sites, the time of removal is 7 to 14 days.

PATCH TEST, SKIN

(SKIN SENSITIVITY TESTS)

Synonyms:

──────────────── **NORMAL VALUES** ────────────────

Negative: No abnormal skin reactions are noted.

Background Information

Allergic contact dermatitis is an eczematous skin change that occurs as an inflammatory response to contact with a particular antigen. The person is sensitized to the antigen over time, without the immediate development of a skin reaction. Eventually, reexposure to the antigen induces a vigorous cell-mediated immune (allergic) response at the site of contact with the antigen (Lynch, 1994).

Since one part of the treatment of the skin eruption is to remove the patient from further contact with the antigen, the antigen must be identified. In some cases, a patch test is used to identify one or more suspected antigens by evoking a skin reaction.

The patch test may be carried out by placing the suspected allergen—such as a small piece of clothing, a bit of the cosmetic substance, or a diluted solution of chemical components—on the skin. The most common antigens are listed in the findings section. Industrial substances or laboratory chemicals are never used because they can produce an irritant dermatitis or a chemical burn.

A positive reaction is a red, raised, pruritic area of skin where a particular allergen was placed. An undecided result is a red but flat lesion. A negative reaction demonstrates no change.

Purpose of the Test

This test is used to determine the cause of contact dermatitis by identifying the particular allergen. It is also used to differentiate contact dermatitis from other causes of eczematous disease.

Procedure

Samples of selected allergens used by the patient or a number of standard allergens are taped to the patient's skin for 48 hours of contact (Fig. 24–7). The readings of the results are performed at 48 hours and again at 72 hours to 7 days, as prescribed.

Findings

ABNORMAL VALUES

Nickel (snaps, belt buckle, rings, watch bands, bracelets, earrings)
Topical medication with neomycin, benzocaine, ethylenediamine

Formaldehyde (permanent press clothing)
Chromates (cement, cutting oil)
Epoxy resins

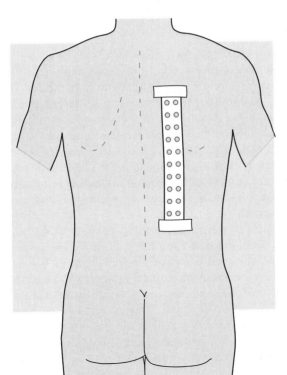

FIGURE 24–7. Patch test. Various allergens are applied to the skin of the patient's back. Those allergens that cause an allergic skin response are identified as the sources of contact dermatitis.

Chemicals in sunscreen ointment
Permanent wave solutions

Fragrances in perfumes, soaps, deter-
gents

Interfering Factors

- Concurrent dermatitis from another source
- Exposure of the patch site to water or excessive perspiration
- Inaccurate interpretation of the results
- Inaccurate timing for the reading of results

Nursing Implementation

Pretest

Schedule this test after the acute dermatitis has subsided and after the treatment with corticosteroids has ceased.

If the products the patient uses are to be tested, instruct the patient to bring them in beforehand. The patch test must be prepared and a detailed list of the ingredients written.

Obtain a signed consent from the patient or the person legally designated to make the patient's health care decisions.

During the Test

Tape the allergen patch to the patient's upper back between the scapula and the spinal column (Fig. 24–7).

Make a diagram on paper to identify the location of each allergen.

Posttest

Instruct the patient to refrain from showers and physical exercise during the next 48 hours. Water and perspiration would loosen the tape of the patch.

Inform the patient that the itching is usually caused by the tape. If, however, there is burning or pain under one of the discs of allergen, it may be removed from that one area.

Instruct the patient to return in 48 hours for the first evaluation of the results. The patch is removed at that time. After a 30-minute to 1-hour wait, the skin is assessed for any reaction in the area of the allergens (Swartz and Sherertz, 1993).

Instruct the patient to return for the second appointment to reevaluate the skin. This is scheduled to be performed 72 hours to 7 days after the patch is applied.

Teach the patient that exercise and showers are permitted while waiting for the second evaluation, but there can be no use of soap and no scrubbing, scratching, or rubbing the skin in the test area.

REFERENCES

Carlson, N.B., et al. (1990). *Clinical procedures for ocular examination.* Norwalk, CT: Appleton & Lange.

Coleman, D.J., et al. (1992). Ophthalmic ultrasonography. *Radiologic Clinics of North America, 30,* 1105–1110.

Lynch, P. (1994). *Dermatology* (3rd ed.). Baltimore: Williams & Wilkins.

Nadalo, L.A., et al. (1991). The neuroradiology of visual disturbances. *Neurologic Clinics, 9,* 1–35.

Siebert C., & Dreisbach, J.N. (1990). Neuroradiology of vestibular pathways. *Neurologic Clinics, 8,* 375–394.

Sigler, B.A., & Schuring, L.T. (1993). *Ear, nose and throat disorders.* St. Louis: C.V. Mosby.

Silverstein, H., et al. (1992). Diagnosis and management of hearing loss. *Clinical Symposia, 44,* 2–32.

Squire, L.F., & Novelline, R.A. (1990). *Fundamentals of radiology* (4th ed.). Cambridge, MA: Harvard University Press.

Swartz, S.M., & Sherertz, E.F. (1993). The technique of patch testing: The role of the office staff. *Dermatology Nursing, 5,* 133–137, 144.

Therapeutic Drug Monitoring

Therapeutic drug monitoring provides exact information about the quantity of medication that is in the blood. This testing is performed for several reasons. In the patient with a normal metabolism, the standard dose and schedule of a particular medication usually results in a therapeutic blood level of the medication within a specific period. In other patients, such as elderly individuals, neonates, and obese persons, the standard dose may produce a diminished or excessive clinical result because of abnormal metabolism or diminished renal or hepatic function. Therapeutic drug monitoring is used to adjust the dose and schedule of medications, as needed.

For a variety of reasons, many patients do not take their medication in the same amount that was prescribed. The result of therapeutic drug monitoring provides data to alert the physician or nurse about the need to investigate the cause of the problem.

Some medications have a narrow range of values for a therapeutic effect. If there is a small increase beyond that range, a toxic result can occur. Therapeutic drug monitoring is carried out to protect the patient from the harm of excess medication.

In the case of overdose (accidental or deliberate), the laboratory tests can identify the medication and the amount that is in the blood. The patient may be comatose, psychotic, or agitated from the effect of the overdose and cannot describe what was ingested. The test results provide data for corrective action.

Table A-1 provides the range of blood values of selected medications to measure for therapeutic effect and for toxicity. For therapeutic drug monitoring, the tests are ordered at planned intervals to establish and maintain an effective medication level in the blood. To identify a problem of toxicity, the laboratory test may be ordered when the patient demonstrates side effects to the medication or when there is an unexplained change of behavior, such as loss of consciousness, that indicates an overdose of medication or drug.

TABLE A–1
THERAPEUTIC DRUG MONITORING

Drug	Collection Tube Stopper	Therapeutic Dose	Toxic Dose
Acetaminophen (Anacin-3, Datril)	Red	10–30 µg/ml SI: 7–200 µmol/L	>150 µ/ml SI: >990 µmol/L
Amikacin (Amikin)	Red	2–25 µg/ml SI: 34–43 µmol/L	>35 µg/ml SI: >60 µmol/L
Amitriptyline (nortriptyline, Elavil, Endep)	Red or green	100–250 ng/ml SI: 360–900 nmol/L	>300 ng/ml SI: >1080 nmol/L
Carbamazepine (Tegetrol)	Red	6–12 µg/ml SI: 25–51 µmol/L	>12 µg/ml SI: >51 µmol/L
Chloramphenicol (Chloromycetin)	Red	10–25 µg/ml SI: 31–77 µmol/L	>25 µg/ml SI: >77 µmol/L
Chlordiazepoxide (Librax, Librium)	Gray	0.1–3 µg/ml SI: 0–10 µmol/L	>23 µg/ml SI: >77 µmol/L
Diazepam (Valium)	Red or lavender	0.2–1.5 µg/ml SI: 0.7–5.3 µmol/L	>5 µg/ml SI: >18 µmol/L
Digitoxin (Digitaline)	Red or lavender	20–35 ng/ml SI: 26–46 nmol/L	>45 ng/ml SI: >59 nmol/L
Digoxin (Lanoxin)	Red, green, or lavender	1–2 ng/ml SI: 1.3–2.6 nmol/L	>2 ng/ml SI: >2.6 nmol/L
Disopyramide (Norpace)	Red, green, or lavender	2–5 µg/ml SI: 5.9–14.7 µmol/L	>7 µg/ml SI: 20.6 µmol/L
Fluoxetine (Prozac)	Red or green	100–800 ng/ml SI: 289–3214 nmol/L	>2000 ng/ml SI: >5784 nmol/L
Haloperidol (Haldol)	Red or green	6–245 ng/ml SI: 16–652 nmol/L	Not defined Not defined
Imipramine (Tofranil)	Red or green	150–250 ng/ml SI: 530–890 nmol/L	>300 ng/ml SI: >1070 nmol/L
Lidocaine (lignocaine, Xylocaine)	Red, green or lavender	1.5–4 µg/ml SI: 6.4–17.1 µmol/L	>6 µg/ml SI: >25.6 µmol/L
Lithium (Eskalith)	Red	0.6–1.2 mEq/L SI: 0.6–1.2 mmol/L	>2 mEq/L SI: >2 mmol/L
Methotrexate (Mexate)	Green or lavender	Variable SI: Variable	>2.27 µg/ml SI: >5 µmol/L
Phenobarbitol (Luminal)	Red, green, or lavender	20–40 µg/ml SI: 86–172 µmol/L	>40 µg/ml SI: >172 µmol/L
Phenytoin (Dilantin)	Red or lavender	10–20 µg/ml SI: 40–79 µmol/L	>20 µg/ml SI: >79 µmol/L
Procainamide (Pronestyl)	Red, gray, or lavender	4–10 µg/ml SI: 17–42 µmol/L	10–12 µg/ml SI: 42–51 µmol/L

Table continued on following page

TABLE A-1
THERAPEUTIC DRUG MONITORING *Continued*

Drug	Collection Tube Stopper	Therapeutic Dose	Toxic Dose
Propoxyphene (Darvocet-N, Darvon)	Red	0.1–0.4 µg/ml SI: 0.3–1.2 µmol/L	>0.5 µg/ml SI: >1.5 µmol/L
Propranolol (Inderal)	Determined by the laboratory	50–100 ng/ml SI: 190–390 nmol/L	>1000 ng/ml SI: >3860 nmol/L
Salicylate (acetylsalicylic acid, aspirin)	Red or lavender	<100 µg/ml SI: 0.72 mmol/L	>500 µg/ml SI: >3.62 mmol/L
Theophylline (aminophylline, Elixophyllin)	Red, green, or lavender	10–20 µg/ml SI: 56–111 µmol/L	*Adult:* >20 µg/ml SI: >111 µmol/L *Neonate:* >10 µg/ml SI: >111 µmol/L
Thiocyanate (nitroprus- side, Nipride)	Red or lavender	1–4 µg/ml SI: 0.02–0.07 mmol/L	>35 µg/ml SI: >0.06 mmol/L
Verapamil (Isoptin)	Red or green	50–200 ng/ml SI: 100–410 nmol/L	>400 ng/ml SI: >815 nmol/L
Warfarin (Coumadin, Panwarfarin)	Red or lavender	2–5 µg/ml SI: 6.5–16.2 µmol/L	>10 µg/ml SI: 32.4 µmol/L

Toxic Substances

Screening for toxic substances is performed to identify the agent responsible for an acute, chronic, or possibly life-threatening illness. Some of these toxic substances are the source of substance abuse and have been taken in an unknown quantity. The clinical effect of the substance varies among individuals who are occasional or habitual users. It can also vary with the preparation or mixture that was inhaled, injected, or eaten.

Some toxic substances are ingested by small children. The poisons that are commonly ingested include rat poison, antifreeze, and insecticide. Other toxic substances that can be identified by laboratory test are toxic chemicals and metals that poison the individual from an environmental source, including hazardous industrial wastes. When the individual is acutely ill from any of these toxic substances, it is essential to identify the cause. Appropriate action can then be taken to reverse the effect and protect the organs from further damage. Some of the toxins pose a long-term threat because they cause mutation and eventual malignancy.

In Table B-1, the values for the normal range of a toxic substance vary from none to minute amounts. The values for toxicity levels are not always defined. The toxicity may vary among individuals, or its very presence is considered toxic.

TABLE B–1
TOXIC SUBSTANCES

Substance	Specimen Source	Collection Container or Tube	Normal Value	Toxic Level
Alcohol (ETOH, ethanol)	Blood	Red- (clotted), blue-, green-, or gray-topped tube	Negative	>300 mg/dl SI: 65.1 mmol/L
Amphetamines	Urine (50–60 ml)	Plastic urine cup	Negative	Not defined
Arsenic	Blood (20 ml)	Trace metal–free, metal container	<7 μg/dl SI: 93.5 nmol/L	>60 μg/dl SI: 801 nmol/g
	Urine (24-hour)	Plastic, acid-washed container	0–100 μg/L	>850 μg/L
Cadmium	Blood	Metal-free tube	SI: 0–1.3 μmol/L <1 μg/L SI: 8.9 μmol/L	SI: >11.3 μmol/L >10 μg/L SI: 8.8–9.7 μmol/L
	Urine (24-hour)	Plastic, acid-washed container	<1 μg/L SI: 8.9 μmol/L	10–20 μg/L SI: 89–178 μmol/L
Cannabis (marijuana, hashish)	Urine (random)	Plastic urine cup	Negative	Not defined
Cocaine	Blood	Red- or gray-topped tube	Negative	Not defined
	Urine (50–60 ml)	Plastic urine cup	Negative	Not defined
Cyanide	Blood	Green-, gray-, or lavender-topped tube	<2 μg/ml SI: <8 μmol/L	>2 μg/ml SI: >8 μmol/L
Ethylene glycol	Blood	Red-, or green-topped tube	Negative	0.3–4 g/L
Fluoride	Blood	Red-topped tube	1.9–7.6 μg/dl SI: 1–4 μmol/L	>28.5 μg/dl SI: >15 μmol/L
Lead	Blood	Special lead-free tube with heparin	<20 μg/dl SI: 0.97 μmol/L	>80 μg/dl SI: >3.86 μmol/L
Mercury	Blood	Special metal-free tube	<0.005 μg/ml SI: 0 μmol/L	>0.05 μg/ml SI: >0 μmol/L
Opiates (codeine, morphine)	Urine (24-hour)	Plastic, acid-washed container	0–20 μg/24 hours SI: 0.1 μmol/24 hours	>50 μg/24 hours SI: >25 μmol/24 hours
	Urine (random)	Plastic urine cup	Negative	Not determined

Abbreviations Associated with Laboratory and Diagnostic Testing

A/G	Albumin-globulin ratio
A-a	Alveolar-arterial
ABI	Ankle brachial index
ACE	Angiotensin-converting enzyme
ACTH	Adrenocorticotropic hormone
ADH	Antidiuretic hormone
AFAFP	Amniotic fluid alpha$_1$-fetoprotein
AFP$_1$	Alpha$_1$-fetoprotein
AFP$_2$	Alpha$_2$-fetoprotein
AGT	Antiglobulin test
ALB	Albumin
ALP	Alkaline phosphatase
ALT	Alanine aminotransferase
ANA	Antinuclear antibody
Anti-HAV	Hepatitis A antibody
Anti-HBc	Hepatitis B core antibody
Anti-HBe	Hepatitis Be antibody
Anti-HCV	Hepatitis C antibody
Anti-HDV	Hepatitis Delta antibody

ApTT	Activated partial thromboplastin time
ART	Automated regin test
AST	Aspartate aminotransferase
BAO	Basal acid output
BUN	Blood urea nitrogen
C & S	Culture and sensitivity
Ca^{++}	Calcium
CA 19-9	Carbohydrate antigen 19-9
CA 125	Cancer antigen 125
CAT	Computed axial tomography
CBC	Complete blood count
CCR	Creatinine clearance
CEA	Carcinoembryonic antigen
CH_{50}	Complement, total
CK	Creatine kinase
Cl^-	Chloride
CO_2	Carbon dioxide
CPK	Creatine phosphokinase
CRP	C-reactive protein
CSF	Cerebrospinal fluid
CST	Contraction stress testing
CT	Computed tomography
CT	Calcitonin
CT	Clotting time
DAT	Direct antiglobulin test
DOPAC	3, 4-dihydroxyphenylacetic acid
DSA	Digital subtraction angiography
DVI	Digital vascular imaging
E_2	Estradiol
E_3	Estriol
EA	Early antigen
EBNA	Epstein-Barr nuclear antigen
ECG	Electrocardiogram
ECHO	Echocardiogram
ECT	Emissions computed tomography
ECT	Euglobulin clot test
EDS	Word discrimination score
EEG	Electroencephalography
EFM	Electronic fetal monitoring
EGD	Esophagogastroduodenoscopy
EIA	Enzyme immunoassay
EKG	Electrocardiogram
ELISA	Enzyme-linked immunosorbent assay
EMG	Electromyography
ENG	Electronystagmography
EP	Erythropoietin

EPS	Electrophysiology studies
ERCP	Endoscopic retrograde cholangiopancreatography
ER/PgR	Estrogen/progesterone assay
ERV	Expiratory reserve volume
ESR	Erythrocyte sedimentation rate
EUG	Excretory urogram
EUS	Endoscopic ultrasonography
FANA	Fluorescent antinuclear antibody
FBP	Fibrin breakdown products
FBS	Fasting blood sugar
FDP	Fibrin degradation products
FEF	Forced midexpiratory flow
FEV	Forced expiratory volume
FNA	Fine needle aspiration
FNB	Fine needle biopsy
FRC	Functional residual capacity
FSH	Follicle-stimulating hormone
FSP	Fibrin split products
FT_3	Free triiodothyronine
FT_4	Free thyroxine
FTA-ABS	Fluorescent treponemal antibody absorption test
FVC	Forced vital capacity
GB	Gallbladder
GE	Gastroesophageal
GEST	Graded exercise testing
GEX	Graded exercise testing
GGT	Gamma glutamyltransferase
GH	Growth hormone
GHB	Glycohemoglobin
GLU	Glucose
GPT	Glutamate pyruvate transaminase
G-6-PD	Glucose-6-phosphate dehydrogenase
GTP	Gamma glutamyl transpeptidase
HAA	Hepatitis associated antigen
HAV, Ab	Hepatitis A antibody
HAVAb	Hepatitis A antibody
Hb	Hemoglobin
$Hb\ A_1$	Glycohemoglobin
HBcAb	Hepatitis B core antibody
HBeAb	Hepatitis Be antibody
HBeAg	Hepatitis Be antigen
HbF	Fetal hemoglobin
HBsAb	Hepatitis B surface antibody
HBsAg	Hepatitis B surface antigen
HBsAgAb	Hepatitis B surface antigen antibody
HCG	Human chorionic gonadotropin

HCO_3^-	Bicarbonate
Hct	Hematocrit
HDL	High-density lipoprotein
Hbg	Hemoglobin
5-HIAA	5-Hydroxyindoleacetic acid
HLA	Human leukocyte antigen
HSV	Herpes simplex virus
HVA	Homovanillic acid
I-ALP	Alkaline phosphatase isoenzymes
IADSA	Intraarterial digital subtraction angiography
IAT	Indirect antiglobulin test
IC	Inspiratory capacity
IF	Intrinsic factor
IgG	Immunoglobulin gamma G
IgM	Immunoglobulin gamma M
IRV	Inspiratory reserve volume
ITT	Insulin tolerance test
IUG	Intravenous urography
IVC	Intravenous cholangiography
IVDSA	Intravenous digital subtraction angiography
IVFA	Intravenous fluorescent angiography
IVP	Intravenous pyelogram
IVU	Intravenous urography
IVUS	Intravascular ultrasonography
K^+	Potassium
17-KGS	17-Ketogenic steroids
17-KS	17-Ketosteroids
LAP	Leucine aminopeptidase
LATS	Long-acting thyroid stimulator
LDH	Lactic dehydrogenase
LDL	Low-density lipoprotein
LDM	Low-dose myelography
LH	Luteinizing hormone
LP	Lumbar puncture
L/S	Lecithin/sphingomyelin
L-W	Lee-White clotting time
MAO	Maximum acid output
Mb	Myoglobulin
MBC	Maximum breathing capacity
MCH	Mean corpuscular hemoglobin
MCHC	Mean corpuscular hemoglobin
MCV	Mean corpuscular volume
Mg	Magnesium
MHA-TP	Microhemoagglutination assay–*treponema pallidum*
MMEF	Forced midexpiratory flow rate
MRI	Magnetic resonance imaging

MUGA	Multiple gated acquisitions angiography
MV	Minute volume
MVV	Maximum voluntary ventilation
5'N	5'-Nucleotidase
Na	Sodium
NAP	Neutrophil alkaline phosphate
NCS	Nerve conduction studies
NH_3	Ammonia
NPO	Nothing by mouth
NST	Nonstress testing
5'NT	5'-Nucleotidase
O & P	Ova and parasites
O_2 sat	Oxygen saturation
OF	Osmotic fragility
OGTT	Oral glucose tolerance test
P_4	Progesterone
PAO	Peak acid output
PAP	Prostatic acid phosphatase
PAP	Papanicolaou smear
PCA	Partial cell antibody
PCA	Polymerase chain reaction
P_{CO_2}	Partial pressure of carbon dioxide
Pcr	Plasma creatinine
PCR	Polymerase chain reaction
PCR	Pulse cuff recording
PCV	Packed cell volume
PDi	Transdiaphragmatic pressure
P_{ETCO_2}	End-tidal carbon dioxide pressure
pH	Partial pressure of hydrogen
PHE	Phenylalanine
$P_{I}max$	Maximum intrathoracic pressure
PKU	Phenylalanine
P_{O_2}	Partial pressure of oxygen
$PO_4^=$	Phosphate
PPD	Purified protein derivative
PRA	Plasma renin activity
PRL	Prolactin
PSA	Prostate-specific antigen
PT	Prothrombin time
PTC	Percutaneous transhepatic cholangiography
PTH	Parathyroid hormone
PTHC	Percutaneous transhepatic cholangiography
PTT	Partial thromboplastin time
PUBS	Percutaneous umbilical cord sampling
P_{VO_2}	Partial pressure of oxygen in the venous system
RAIU	Radioactive iodine uptake

RBC	Red blood cell
RDW	Red cell distribution width
RF	Rheumatoid factor
RIA	Radioimmunoassay
RPR	Rapid plasma reagin
RT_3U	Resin triiodothyronine uptake
RV	Residual volume
SACE	Serum angiotensin-converting enzyme
SAECG	Signal-averaged electrocardiogram
Sao_2	Arterial oxygen saturation
SGOT	Serum glutamic oxaloacetic transaminase
SGOT	Glutamate oxaloacetate transaminase, serum
SGPT	Serum glutamic-pyruvic transaminase
SHBD	Serum alpha-hydroxybutyrate dehydrogenase
SPECT	Single photon emission computed tomography
SRT	Speech reception threshold
STH	Growth hormone; somatotropin
Svo_2	Oxygen saturation in the venous system
T-ALP	Total alkaline phosphatase
T_3	Triiodothyronine
T_4	Thyroxine
TBG	Thyroxine-binding globulin
T & C	Type and cross match
TEE	Transesophageal echocardiography
TIBC	Total iron-binding capacity
TLC	Total lung capacity
TP	Total protein
TRH	Thyroid-releasing hormone
TSH	Thyroid-stimulating hormone
TUS	Transluminal ultrasound
TV	Tidal volume
UA	Urinalysis
V/Q	Ventilation/perfusion
VA	Visual acuity
VC	Vital capacity
VCA	Viral capsid antigen
VCG	Vectorcardiogram
V_D	Dead space volume
VDRL	Venereal Disease Research Laboratory
VEST	Ventricular extrastimulus testing
VMA	Vanillylmandelic acid
WBC	White blood cell

Table of Symbols and Units of Measurements

α	alpha
cc	cubic centimeter
cm	centimeter
dl	deciliter
γ	gamma
g	gram
gm	gram
IU	international unit
kg	kilogram
L	liter
μg	microgram
mEq	milliequivalent
mg	milligram
mIU	milliinternational unit
ml	milliliter
mm	millimeter
mm Hg	millimeters of mercury
mmol	millimole
mOsm	milliosmole
mu	micro (μ)
ng	nanogram
%	percentage

pg	picogram
SI	Système International (international system)
U	unit
μ	micro

Normal Values: Whole Blood, Serum, and Plasma Tests

TABLE E-1
NORMAL VALUES: WHOLE BLOOD, SERUM, AND PLASMA TESTS

Name of Test	Conventional Values	SI Units	Chapter No.
Activated partial thromboplastin time			
Average value	25–35 seconds	Same	6
Newborn	<90 seconds	Same	6
Adrenocorticotropic hormone			
In A.M.	25–100 pg/ml	25–100 ng/L	19
In P.M.	0–50 pg/ml	0–50 ng/L	19
Adrenocorticotropic hormone stimulation test: a rise of plasma cortisol level within 30–60 minutes	≥18 µg/dl	≥497 nmol/L	19
Alanine aminotransferase			
Average adult range	10–35 IU/L at 37° C	Same	18
Newborn–1 year	13–45 IU/L at 37° C	Same	18
Albumin			
Adult >60 years	3.4–4.8 g/dl	34–48 g/L	18
Adult <60 years	3.5–5 g/dl	35–50 g/L	18
Child	3.2–5.4 g/dl	32–54 g/L	18
Newborn	2.8–4.4 g/dl	28–44 g/L	18
Albumin:globulin ratio	>1	Same	18
Aldosterone			
Adult—Average sodium diet			
Supine	3–10 ng/dl	0.08–0.27 nmol/L	19
Upright	5–30 ng/dl	0.14–0.83 nmol/L	19
After fluorocortisone suppression or intravenous infusion	<4 ng/dl	<0.11 nmol/L	19
Adrenal vein	200–800 ng/dl	5.54–22.16 nmol/L	19
Child			
11–15 years	<5–50 ng/dl	<0.14–1.39 nmol/L	19
3–5 years	<5–80 ng/dl	<0.14–2.22 nmol/L	19
1 week–1 year	1–160 ng/dl	0.03–4.43 nmol/L	19
Alkaline phosphatase			
Adult	4.5–13 King-Armstrong units/dl 1.4–4.4 Bodansky units 10–30 King-Armstrong units/dl	32–92 U/L	18
Infant	71–213 U/L		18

Table continued on following page

TABLE E-1
NORMAL VALUES: WHOLE BLOOD, SERUM, AND PLASMA TESTS *Continued*

Name of Test	Conventional Values	SI Units	Chapter No.
Alkaline phosphatase isoenzymes	*Percent Inactivation* 16 Minutes at 55° C	*Fractional Inactivation* 16 Minutes at 55° C	18
Liver	50–70	0.5–0.7	18
Bone	90–100	0.9–1	18
Intestine	50–60	0.5–0.6	18
Placenta	0	0	18
Regan	0	0	18
Alpha₁-fetoprotein			
Adult	2–16 ng/ml	2–16 μg/L	18
Normal pregnancy	550 ng/ml	550 μg/L	18
Ammonia			
Adult	15–45 μg/dl	11–22 μmol/L	18
Neonate	90–150 μg/dl	64–107 μmol/L	18
Amylase			
Adult	60–180 Somogyi units	25–125 U/L	18
Neonate	5–65 U/L	Same	18
Androstenedione			
Adult male	75–205 ng/dl	2.6–7.2 nmol/L	21
Adult female	85–275 ng/dl	3–9.6 nmol/L	21
Child 10–17 years	8–240 ng/dl	0.3–8.4 nmol/L	21
Newborn	20–290 ng/dl	0.7–10.1 nmol/L	21
Angiotensin-converting enzyme			
Male	12–36 IU/L	Same	13
Female	10–30 IU/L	Same	13
Anion gap	10–15 mEq/L	10–15 mmol/L	13
Anti-DNA antibody	Negative	Same	23
Radioimmunoassay method	<10% binding	<0.1 binding fraction	23
Enzyme immunoassay method	<250 U/L	Same	23
Indirect immunofluorescent method	<1:10	Same	23
Antiglobulin test, direct	Negative	Same	16
Antiglobulin test, indirect	Negative	Same	16
Antinuclear antibody	Negative at a 1:20 dilution	Same	23
Antithrombin III	21–30 mg/dl	210–300 mg/L	6
	86–113%	86–113 AU	6
Aspartate aminotransferase			
Adult	8–20 U/L	Same	14,18
Newborn	16–72 U/L	Same	14,18

Test			Reference
Bilirubin, direct			
Adult	0–0.4 mg/dl	<5 µmol/L	18
Bilirubin, indirect			
Adult	0.2–0.8 mg/dl	3.4–13.6 µmol/L	18
Bilirubin, total			
Adult	0.3–1 mg/dl	5–17 µmol/L	18
Child	0.2–0.8 mg/dl	3.4–13.6 µmol/L	18
Full-term neonate	6–10 mg/dl	103–171 µmol/L	18
Premature neonate*	<12 mg/dl	<205 µmol/L	18
Blood gases, arterial			
pH	7.35–7.45	7.35–7.45	13
P_{CO_2}	35–40 mm Hg	4.7–5.3 kPa	13
HCO_3^-	21–28 mEq/L	21–28 mmol/L	13
P_{O_2}			
Adult	80–100 mm Hg	10.6–13.3 kPa	13
Newborn	60–70 mm Hg	8–10.33 kPa	13
Oxygen saturation			
Adult	>95%	Fraction saturated: >0.95	13
Newborn	40–90%	Fraction saturated: 0.4–0.9	13
Base excess	±2 mEq/L	±2 mmol/L	13
Blood gases, mixed venous			
pH	7.33–7.43	7.35 ± 0.05	13
P_{CO_2}	40–45 mm Hg	5.3–6 kPa	13
HCO_3^-	24–28 mm Hg	24–28 mmol/L	13
Blood volume, total	60–80 ml/kg	Same	16
Calcitonin, serum			
Adult	150 pg/ml	150 ng/L	19
Infant (cord blood)	25–150 pg/ml	25–150 ng/L	19
Infant (7 days old)	70–350 pg/ml	70–350 ng/L	19
Calcitonin, plasma			
Male	≤19 pg/ml	≤19 ng/L	19
Female	≤14 pg/ml	≤14 pg/L	19
Calcium, total			
Adult	8.2–10.2 mg/dl	2.05–2.54 mmol/L	20
Child, 1 month–1 year	8.6–11.2 mg/dl	2.15–2.79 mmol/L	20
Newborn–1 month	7–11.5 mg/dl	1.75–2.87 mmol/L	20
Calcium, ionized	44–55% of total serum calcium	0.45–0.55 fraction of serum calcium	19
Adult, serum	4.65–5.28 mg/dl	1.16–1.32 mmol/L	19
Child, serum	4.8–5.52 mg/dl	1.2–1.38 mmol/L	19

*The values for premature neonates vary according to the degree of prematurity.

Table continued on following page

TABLE E-1
NORMAL VALUES: WHOLE BLOOD, SERUM, AND PLASMA TESTS *Continued*

Name of Test	Conventional Values	SI Units	Chapter No.
Cancer antigen 125	<35 U/ml	<35 kU/L	21
Carbohydrate antigen 19-9			17
Adult	<37 U/ml	<37 kU/L	
Carbon dioxide, total			
Adult, venous	22–26 mEq/L	22–26 mmol/L	5
Adult, arterial	19–24 mEq/L	19–24 mmol/L	5
Infant, capillary	20–28 mEq/L	20–28 mmol/L	5
Carcinoembryonic antigen			
Adult, nonsmoker	<2.5 ng/ml	2.5 µg/L	17
Adult, smoker	Up to 5 ng/ml	Up to 5 µg/L	17
Carotene			
Adult	40–200 µg/dl	0.7–3.7 µmol/L	18
Infants	<60 µg/dl	<1.52 µmol/L	18
Catecholamines (standing)*			
Epinephrine	<900 pg/ml	<4914 pmol/L	19
Norepinephrine	125–700 pg/ml	739–4137 nmol/L	19
Dopamine	<87 pg/ml	<475 pmol/L	19
Ceruloplasmin			
Adult	20–40 mg/dl	200–350 mg/L	18
Neonate–3 months	5–18 mg/dl	50–180 mg/L	18
Chloride			
Adult	98–107 mEq/L	98–107 mmol/L	5
Newborn	98–113 mEq/L	98–113 mmol/L	5
Premature infant	95–110 mEq/L	95–110 mmol/L	5
Cholesterol, total	120–200 mg/dl	3.11–5.18 mmol/L	14
Clot retraction time	1–24 hours	Same	6
Average time	4 hours	Same	6
Clotting time	8–15 minutes	Same	6
Coagulation factor assay (general values)	50–150%	50–150 AU	16
Complement, total	75–160 U/ml	75–160 kU/L	16

Test	Conventional Units	SI Units	Ref.
Complete blood count			
Hematocrit			
Male	40–54%	0.4–0.59 (volume fraction)	4
Female	38–47%	0.38–0.47 (volume fraction)	4
Hemoglobin			
Male	13.5–18 g/dl	135–180 g/L	4
Female	12–16 g/dl	120–160 d/L	4
Red cell count			
Male	$4.6-6.2 \times 10^6/\mu l$	$4.6-6.2 \times 10^{12}/L$	4
Female	$4.2-5.4 \times 10^6/\mu l$	$4.2-5.4 \times 10^{12}/L$	4
Red cell indices			
Mean corpuscular volume	$80-96 \ \mu m^3$	80–96 fL	4
Mean corpuscular hemoglobin	27–31 pg	27–31 pg	4
Mean corpuscular hemoglobin concentration	32–36%	0.32–0.36 (mean concentration fraction)	4
Red cell distribution width	13.1%	—	4
White cell count	$4.5-11 \times 10^3/\mu l$	$4.5-11 \times 10^9/L$	4
Platelets			
Adult	150,000–450,000 cells/L	$150-450 \times 10^9/L$	4
Newborn	84,000–478,000 cells/L	$84-478 \times 10^9/L$	4
Cortisol			
8 A.M.–10 A.M.	5–23 µg/dl	138–635 nmol/L	19
4 P.M.–6 P.M.	3–13 µg/dl	83–359 nmol/L	19
C-reactive protein	<1 mg/dl	<10 mg/L	23
Creatinine			
Adult male	0.7–1.3 mg/dl	62–115 µmol/L	5
Adult female	0.6–1.1 mg/dl	53–97 µmol/L	5
Newborn	0.3–1 mg/dl	27–88 µmol/L	5
Creatine phosphokinase			
Adult male	38–175 U/L	Same	14
Adult female	25–135 U/L	Same	14
Child, male	35–185 U/L	Same	14
Child, female	50–100 U/L	Same	14
Newborn	10–200 U/L	Same	14

*Values are lower when the patient is in a supine position.

Table continued on following page

TABLE E-1
NORMAL VALUES: WHOLE BLOOD, SERUM, AND PLASMA TESTS *Continued*

Name of Test	Conventional Values	SI Units	Chapter No.
Isoenzymes			
Creatine phosphokinase—MM	5–70 U/L	Same	14
	90–97% (of total CPK)	0.9–0.97 (fraction of total creatine phosphokinase)	14
Creatine phosphokinase—MB	0–7 U/L	Same	14
	0–6% of total creatine phosphokinase	0–0.06 (fraction of total creatine phosphokinase)	14
Creatine phosphokinase—BB	0–3 U/L	Same	14
	0–3%	0–0.03 (fraction of total creatine phosphokinase)	14
D-Dimer	<250 ng/ml	<250 μg/L	6
	No D-dimer fragments are present	Same	6
Dexamethasone overnight, single-dose suppression test			
Plasma cortisol	Suppression to <5 μg/dl	Suppression to <138 nmol/L	19
D-Xylose absorption test			
Child—1 hour	>30 mg/dl	>2 mmol/L	17
Adult (2 hours, 5-g dose)	>20 mg/dl	>1.33 mmol/L	17
Adult (2 hours, 25-g dose)	>25 mg/dl	>1.67 mmol/L	17
Epstein–Barr titer			
Viral capsid antigen—IgM	<1:10	Same	7
Viral capsid antigen—IgG	<1:10	Same	7
Epstein–Barr antinuclear antibody	<1:5	Same	7
Early antigen	<1:10	Same	7
Erythrocyte sedimentation rate			
Adult			
<50-year-old male	0–15 mm/hour	Same	23
<50-year-old female	0–20 mm/hour	Same	23
Adult			
>50-year-old male	0–20 mm/hour	Same	23
>50-year-old female	0–30 mm/hour	Same	23
Child	0–10 mm/hour	Same	23

Test	Conventional	SI	Reference
Erythropoietin	5–36 μU/ml	5–35 IU/L	20
Estradiol			
Premenopausal female	30–400 pg/ml	110–1468 pmol/L	21
Postmenopausal female	0–30 pg/ml	0–110 pmol/L	21
Male	10–50 pg/ml	37–184 pmol/L	21
Estriol, pregnancy			
28–30 weeks	38–140 ng/ml	132–486 nmol/L	21
32–34 weeks	35–260 ng/ml	121–902 nmol/L	21
36–38 weeks	48–570 ng/ml	167–1978 nmol/L	21
40 weeks	95–460 ng/ml	330–1596 nmol/L	21
Euglobin clot lysis	1.5–4 hours	Same	6
Factor II	0.5–1.5 U/ml	0.5–1.5 kU/L	6
	60–150%	60–150 AU	6
Factor V	0.5–2 U/ml	0.5–2 kU/L	6
	60–150%	60–150 AU	6
Factor VII	65–135%	65–135 AU	6
Factor VIII	60–145%	60–145 AU	6
Factor IX	60–140%	60–140 AU	6
Factor X	60–130%	60–130 AU	6
Factor XI	60–135%	60–135 AU	6
Factor XII	60–150%	60–150 AU	6
Factor XIII	Clot is stable in 5 mol of urea for 24 hours	Same	6
Ferritin			
Adult male	20–250 ng/ml	20–250 μg/L	16
Adult female	10–120 ng/ml	10–120 μg/L	16
Newborn	25–200 ng/ml	25–200 μg/L	16
Fibrinogen			
Adult	200–400 mg/dl	2–4 g/L	6
Newborn	125–300 mg/dl	1.25–3 g/L	6
Fibrin split products	<10 μg/ml	<10 mg/L	6
5'-Nucleotidase (adult)	2–17 IU/L	Same	18
Follicle-stimulating hormone			
Adult male	1–7 mU/ml	1–7 U/L	21
Adult female			
Follicular phase	1–9 mU/ml	1–9 U/L	21
Midcycle peak	6–26 mU/ml	6–26 U/L	21
Luteal phase	1–9 mU/ml	1–9 U/L	21

Table continued on following page

TABLE E–1
NORMAL VALUES: WHOLE BLOOD, SERUM, AND PLASMA TESTS *Continued*

Name of Test	Conventional Values	SI Units	Chapter No.
Gamma-glutamyl transferase			
Average adult range	5–40 IU/L	Same	18
Male adult	22.1 ± 11.7 IU/L	Same	18
Female adult	15.4 ± 6.58 IU/L	Same	18
Gastrin			
Adult male	<100 pg/ml	<100 ng/L	17
Adult female	<75 pg/ml	<75 ng/L	17
Newborn	120–183 pg/ml	120–183 ng/L	17
Globulin	2.8–4.4 g/dl	28–44 g/L	18
Glucagon, fasting	50–100 pg/ml	25 ng/L	19
Glucose, fasting			
Adult			
Whole blood	60–110 mg/dl	3.3–6.1 mmol/L	19
Serum, plasma	70–120 mg/dl	3.9–6.7 mmol/L	19
Elderly	80–150 mg/dl	4.4–8.3 mmol/L	19
Child, <2 years old	60–100 mg/dl	3.3–5.6 mmol/L	19
Infant	40–90 mg/dl	2.2–5 mmol/L	19
Newborn	30–60 mg/dl	1.7–3.3 mmol/L	19
Glucose monitoring (capillary blood)	60–110 mg/dl	3.3–6.1 mmol/L	19
Glucose-6-phosphate dehydrogenase screen	Enzyme activity is present	Same	16
Glucose tolerance test, oral (adult fasting)			
Baseline fasting blood glucose	70–105 mg/dl	3.9–5.8 mmol/L	19
30-minute fasting blood glucose	110–170 mg/dl	6.1–9.4 mmol/L	19
60-minute fasting blood glucose	120–170 mg/dl	6.7–9.4 mmol/L	19
90-minute fasting blood glucose	100–140 mg/dl	5.6–7.8 mmol/L	19
120-minute fasting blood glucose	70–120 mg/dl	3.9–6.7 mmol/L	19
Glucose, 2-hour postprandial	<140 mg/dl	<7.78 mmol/L	19
Glycosylated hemoglobin assay	5–8% of total hemoglobin	0.05–0.08 fraction of total hemoglobin	19
Growth hormone			
Adult			
Male	0–5 ng/ml	0–5 µg/L	19
Female	0–10 ng/ml	0–10 µg/L	19
Child	0–16 ng/ml	0–16 µg/L	19

Test	SI Reference Values	Conventional Reference Values	
Growth hormone stimulation test			
With arginine	>7 µg/L	>7 ng/ml	19
With insulin	>20 µg/L	>20 ng/mL	19
Growth hormone suppression test	<3 µg/L	<3 ng/ml	19
Hematocrit			
Male	0.4–0.59 (volume fraction)	40–54%	4
Female	0.38–0.47 (volume fraction)	38–47%	4
Hemoglobin			
Male	135–180 g/L	13.5–18 g/dl	4
Female	120–160 g/L	12–16 g/dl	4
Hemoglobin electrophoresis			
Hb A	0.95–0.98 Hb fraction	95–98%	16
Hb A_2	0.015–0.035 Hb fraction	1.5–3.5%	16
Hb F	0–0.02 Hb fraction	0–2%	16
Hb C	Same	Absent	16
Hb S	Same	Absent	16
Hemoglobin, fetal			
Adult	<0.02 mass fraction Hb F	<2% Hb F	16
Newborn	0.77 ± 0.073 mass fraction Hb F	77 ± 7.3% Hb F	16
Hepatitis A antibody	Same	Negative	18
Hepatitis B core antibody	Same	Negative	18
Hepatitis Be antibody	Same	Negative	18
Hepatitis Be antigen	Same	Negative	18
Hepatitis B surface antigen	Same	Negative	18
Hepatitis C antibody	Same	Negative	18
Hepatitis delta antibody	Same	Negative	18
High-density lipoprotein cholesterol			
Male	1.24–1.27 mmol/L	44–45 mg/dl	14
Female	1.425 mmol/L	55 mg/dl	14
Histoplasmosis serologic study			
Complement fixation titer	Same	<1:4	
Immunodiffusion test	Same	Negative	7
Human immunodeficiency virus serologic study	Same	Negative	7

Table continued on following page

TABLE E-1
NORMAL VALUES: WHOLE BLOOD, SERUM, AND PLASMA TESTS *Continued*

Name of Test	Conventional Values	SI Units	Chapter No.
Human chorionic gonadotrophin			
Male and nonpregnant female	<5 mU/ml	<5 U/L	21
Pregnant female			
1 week gestation	5–50 mU/ml	5050 U/L	21
4 weeks' gestation	1000–30,000 mU/ml	1000–30,000 U/L	21
6–8 weeks' gestation	12,000–270,000 mU/ml	12,000–270,000 U/L	21
12 weeks' gestation	15,000–270,000 mU/ml	15,000–270,000 U/L	21
Human leukocyte antigen	No destruction of lymphocytes	Same	16
Insulin (fasting)			
Adult	5–25 μU/ml	34–172 pmol/L	19
Newborn	3–20 μU/ml	21–138 pmol/L	19
1 hour after eating	50–130 μU/ml	347.3–902.8 pmol/L	19
2 hours after eating	<30 μU/ml	<208.4 pmol/L	19
Intrinsic factor antibodies	Negative	Same	16
Iron			
Adult male	65–175 μg/dl	11.6–31.3 μmol/L	16
Adult female	50–170 μg/dl	9–30.4 μmol/L	16
Newborn	100–250 μg/dl	17.9–44.8 μmol/L	16
Iron-binding capacity, total	218–385 μg/dl	39–69 μmol/L	16
Ketones	Negative	Same	19
Lactate dehydrogenase	70–200 IU/L	Same	14
Lactate dehydrogenase isoenzymes			
LDH$_1$	14–26%	0.14–0.26 (fraction of total LDH)	14
LDH$_2$	29–39%	0.29–0.39 (fraction of total LDH)	14
LDH$_3$	20–26%	0.2–0.26 (fraction of total LDH)	14
LDH$_4$	8–16%	0.08–0.16 (fraction of total LDH)	14
LDH$_5$	6–16%	0.06–0.16 (fraction of total LDH)	14
Lactic acid	1–2 mEq/L	1–2 mmol/L	13
Lactose tolerance test, blood glucose	>20–30 mg/dl	1.1–1.7 mmol/L	17

Test			
Low-density lipoprotein:high-density lipoprotein	<3	Same	14
LE cell test	Negative	Same	23
Leucine aminopeptidase			
Adult male	80–200 U/ml (Goldberg-Rutenberg units)	19.2–48.0 U/L	18
Adult female	75–185 U/ml (Goldberg-Rutenberg units)	18–44 U/L	18
Lipase (adult)	<200 U/L	Same	18
Lipids, total	400–800 mg/dl	4–8 g/L	14
Long-acting thyroid stimulation	None; no long-acting thyroid stimulator present	Same	19
Low-density lipoprotein cholesterol	<130 mg/dl	<3.37 mmol/L	14
Luteinizing hormone			
Adult male	1–8 mU/ml	1–8 U/L	21
Adult female			
Follicular phase	1–12 mU/ml	1–12 U/L	21
Midcycle peak	16–104 mU/ml	16–104 U/L	21
Luteal phase	1–12 mU/ml	1–12 U/L	21
Postmenopausal	16–66 mU/ml	16–66 U/L	21
Child, 6 months–10 years	1–5 mU/ml	1–5 U/L	21
Magnesium			
Adult	1.3–2.1 mEq/L	0.65–1.05 mmol/L	20
Child			
12–20 years	1.56 ± 0.21 mEq/L	0.78 ± 0.11 mmol/L	20
6–12 years	1.56 ± 0.18 mEq/L	0.78 ± 0.09 mmol/L	20
5 months–6 years	1.65 ± 0.23 mEq/L	0.83 ± 0.12 mmol/L	20
Newborn–4 days	1.2–1.8 mEq/L	0.6–0.9 mmol/L	20
Malaria smear	No organisms identified	Same	16
Metyrapone stimulation test (11-deoxycortisol)	>7 µg/dl	>200 nmolL	19
Microfilariae smear	No parasites visualized	Same	16
Mononucleosis tests			
Monotest	Negative; nonreactive	Same	7
Heterophil titer	<1:56	Same	7
Neutrophil alkaline phosphatase	Score: 40–130	Same	16

Table continued on following page

TABLE E–1
NORMAL VALUES: WHOLE BLOOD, SERUM, AND PLASMA TESTS *Continued*

Name of Test	Conventional Values	SI Units	Chapter No.
Osmolarity			
Adult	285–319 mOsm/kg H_2O	285–319 mmol/kg H_2O	19
Child	270–290 mOsm/kg H_2O	270–290 mmol/kg H_2O	19
Osmotic fragility			
Initial hemolysis of erythrocytes	0.45% NaCl	4.5 g/L NaCl	16
Complete hemolysis of erythrocytes	0.3% NaCl	3 g/L NaCl	16
Parathyroid hormone			
Intact parathyroid hormone	210–310 pg/ml	210–310 ng/L	19
N-terminal	230–630 pg/ml	230–630 ng/L	19
C-terminal	410–1760 pg/ml	410–1760 ng/L	19
Parietal cell antibody	Negative	Same	16
pH (fetal scalp)	7.25–7.35	Same	21
Phenylalanine			
Guthrie test	<2 mg/dl	121 µmol/L	20
Fluorometry method			
Adult	0.8–1.8 mg/dl	48–109 µmol/L	20
Normal newborn	1.2–3.4 mg/dl	73–206 µmol/L	20
Premature newborn	2–7.5 mg/dl	121–454 µmol/L	20
Phosphorus, serum			
Adult			
12–60 years	2.7–4.5 mg/dl	0.87–1.45 mmol/L	20
>60 years	2.3–3.7 mg/dl	0.74–1.2 mmol/L	20
Child			
2–12 years	4.5–5.5 mg/dl	1.45–1.78 mmol/L	20
10 days–2 years	4.5–6.7 mg/dl	1.45–2.16 mmol/L	20
Infant 0–10 days	4.5–9 mg/dl	1.45–2.91 mmol/L	20
Premature infant	5.4–10.9 mg/dl	1.74–3.52 mmol/L	20
Cord blood	3.7–8.1 mg/dl	0.85–1.5 mmol/L	20
Phosphate, plasma (adult)	8.2–14.5 mg/dl	0.85–1.5 mmol/L	20
Plasma cell volume	40–50 ml/kg	Same	16
Platelet aggregation	3–5 minutes	Same	6
Platelet count			
Adult	150,000–450,000 cells/µl	150–450 × 10^9/L	4
Newborn	84,000–478,000 cells/µl	84–478 × 10^9/L	4

Test	Conventional units	SI units	Ref.
Potassium			
Adult	3.5–5 mEq/L	3.5–5.1 mmol/L	5
Newborn	3.7–5.9 mEq/L	3.7–5.9 mmol/L	5
Progesterone			
Adult male	13–97 ng/dl	0.4–3.1 nmol/L	21
Menstruating female			
Follicular phase	15–70 ng/dl	0.5–2.2 nmol/L	21
Luteal phase	200–2500 ng/dl	6.4–79.5 nmol/L	21
Pregnant female			
7–13 weeks' gestation	1025–4400 ng/dl	32.6–139.9 nmol/L	21
30–42 weeks' gestation	6500–22,900 ng/dl	206.7–728.2 nmol/L	21
Prolactin			
Adult	0–20 ng/ml	0–20 µg/L	21
Pregnancy			
Third trimester	34–306 ng/ml	34–306 µg/L	21
Lactating mother	<40 ng/ml	<40 µg/L	21
Newborn	<300 ng/ml	<300 µg/L	21
Prostate-specific antigen (male >15 years)	0.81 ± 0.89 ng/mL	0.81 ± 0.89 g/L	20
Prostatic acid phosphatase 4-Nitrophenylphosphate method (male)	0.13–0.63 U/L	2.2–10.5 U/L	20
Protein C	71–142%	0.71–1.42 fraction of whole	6
Protein electrophoresis	2.82–5.65 µg/ml	2.82–5.65 mg/L	
Adult			
Albumin	3.5–5 g/dl	35–50 g/L	18
Alpha$_1$-globulin	0.1–0.3 g/dl	1–3 g/L	18
Alpha$_2$-globulin	0.6–1 g/dl	6–10 g/L	18
Beta globulin	0.7–1.1 g/dl	7–11 g/L	18
Gamma globulin	0.8–1.6 g/dl	8–16 g/L	18
Child			
Albumin	3.6–5.2 g/dl	36–52 g/L	18
Alpha$_1$-globulin	0.1–0.4 g/dl	1–4 g/L	18
Alpha$_2$-globulin	0.5–1.2 g/dl	5–12 g/L	18
Beta globulin	0.5–1.2 g/dl	5–11 g/L	18
Gamma globulin	0.5–1.7 g/dl	5–17 g/L	18
Protein S	61–130%	0.61–1.3 fraction of whole	6

Table continued on following page

TABLE E-1
NORMAL VALUES: WHOLE BLOOD, SERUM, AND PLASMA TESTS *Continued*

Name of Test	Conventional Values	SI Units	Chapter No.
Protein, total			
Adult, ambulatory	6.4–8.3 g/dl	64–83 g/L	18
Adult, recumbent	6–7.8 g/dl	60–78 g/L	18
Newborn	4–7 g/dl	40–70 g/L	18
Prothrombin time			
Average	10–13 seconds	Same	6
Newborn–6 months	13–18 seconds	Same	6
Red cell volume			
Male	25–35 ml/kg	Same	16
Female	20–30 ml/kg	Same	16
Renin, plasma			
Supine	12–79 mU/L	Same	19
Upright	13–114 mU/L	Same	19
Reticulocyte count			
Adult	0.5–1.5%	0.005–0.015 number fraction	4
	25,000–75,000/μl	$25–75 \times 10^9$/L	4
Newborn	1.1–4.5%	0.011–0.045 number fraction	4
Rheumatoid factor	Negative	Same	23
Serotonin	50–175 ng/ml	0.28–0.99 μmol/L	17
Sickle cell tests	Negative	Same	16
Sodium			
Adult	136–145 mEq/L	136–145 mmol/L	5
Newborn	133–146 mEq/L	133–146 mmol/L	5
Syphilis serologic studies			
Venereal Disease Research Laboratory	Negative; nonreactive	Same	7
Rapid plasma reagin	Negative; nonreactive	Same	7
Fluorescent treponemal antibody absorption test	Negative; nonreactive	Same	7
Microhemagglutination assay–*Treponema pallidum*	Negative; nonreactive	Same	7
Testosterone, free			
Adult male	52–280 pg/ml	180.4–971.6 pmol/L	21
Adult female	1.6–6.3 pg/ml	5.6–21.9 pmol/L	21
Child 1–10 years	0.15–0.66 pg/ml	0.5–2.1 pmol/L	21

Test	Conventional Units	SI Units	Reference
Testosterone, total			
Adult male	300–1000 ng/dl	10.4–34.7 nmol/L	21
Adult female	20–75 ng/dl	0.69–2.6 nmol/L	21
Child 1–10 years	<3–10 ng/dl	<0.1–0.35 nmol/L	21
Thyroid microsomal autoantibodies	Titer <1:1000; negative	Same	19
Thyroglobulin autoantibodies	Titer <1:1000; negative	Same	19
Thyrotropin			
Adult	0.4–8.9 µU/ml	0.4–8.9 mU/L	19
Newborn, whole blood	<20 µU/ml	<20 mU/L	19
Thyrotropin-releasing hormone test			
Thyroid-stimulating hormone value			
Male	14–24 µIU/ml	14–24 mIU/L	19
Female	16–26 µIU/ml	16–26 mIU/L	19
Thyroxine			
Adult	5–12 µg/dl	64.4–154.4 nmol/L	19
Child 1–10 years	6.4–15 µg/dl	82.4–193.1 nmol/L	19
Newborn	6.4–23.2 µg/ml	82.4–298.6 nmol/L	19
Thyroxine-binding globulin	16–34 µg/ml	16–34 mg/L	19
Thyroxine, free	0.9–1.7 ng/dl	11.5–21.8 pmol/L	19
Tolbutamide stimulation, serum insulin level	<195 µU/ml	1354 pmol/L	19
Toxoplasmosis serologic study	IgM antibody titer: <1:8	Same	7
Transferrin			
Adult <60 years	200–400 mg/dl	2–4 g/L	16
Newborn	130–275 mg/dl	1.3–2.75 g/L	16
Transferrin saturate	20–50%	Same	16
Triglycerides			
Male <40 years	46–316 mg/dl	0.52–3.57 mmol/L	14
Female <40 years	37–174 mg/dl	0.42–1.97 mmol/L	14
Male >50 years	75–313 mg/dl	0.85–3.54 mmol/L	14
Female >50 years	52–200 mg/dl	0.59–2.26 mmol/L	14
Triiodothyronine			
Adult	95–190 ng/dl	1.5–2 nmol/L	19
Child 1–10 years	94–269 ng/ml	1.4–4.1 nmol/L	19
Newborn	32–250 ng/ml	0.49–3.8 nmol/L	19
Triiodothyronine, free	0.2–0.52 ng/dl	3–8 pmol/L	19
Triiodothyronine resin uptake			
Adult	25–35% of total	0.25–0.35 fraction of total	19
Free thyroxine index	1.3–4.2	Same	19
Free triiodothyronine index	24–67	Same	19

Table continued on following page

TABLE E–1
NORMAL VALUES: WHOLE BLOOD, SERUM, AND PLASMA TESTS *Continued*

Name of Test	Conventional Values	SI Units	Chapter No.
Urea nitrogen			
Adult	5–20 mg/dl	1.8–7.1 mmol/L	5
Newborn–infant	4–16 mg/dl	1.4–5.7 mmol/L	5
Uric acid			
Adult <60 years	4.5–8 ng/dl	0.27–0.47 mmol/L	23
Adult male	2.5–6.2 ng/dl	0.15–0.37 mmol/L	23
Adult >60 years			
Male	4.2–8 ng/dl	0.25–0.47 mmol/L	23
Female	2.7–6.8 ng/dl	0.16–0.4 mmol/L	23
Child <12 years	2–5.5 ng/dl	0.12–0.32 mmol/L	23
Vasopressin			
With osmolarity of >290 mOsm/kg	2–12 pg/ml	1.85–11.1 pmol/L	19
With osmolarity of <290 mOsm/kg	<2 pg/ml	<1.85 pmol/L	19
Vitamin D, activated	25–45 pg/ml	60–180 nmol/L	19
White blood cell differential (adult),			
Segmented neutrophils	56%	0.56 (mean number fraction)	4
	1800–7800/μl	$1.8–7.8 \times 10^9$/L	4
Bands	3%	0.03 (mean number fraction)	4
	0–700/μl	$0–0.07 \times 10^9$/L	4
Eosinophils	2.7%	0.027 (mean number fraction)	4
	0–450/μl	$0–0.45 \times 10^9$/L	4
Basophils	0.3%	0.003 (mean number fraction)	4
	0–200/μl	$0–0.2 \times 10^9$/L	4
Lymphocytes	34%	0.34 (mean number fraction)	4
	1000–4800/μl	$1.0–4.8 \times 10^9$/L	4
Monocytes	4%	0.04 (mean number fraction)	4
	0–800/μl	$0–0.8 \times 10^9$/L	4

Normal Values: Urine Tests

TABLE F-1
NORMAL VALUES: URINE TESTS

Name of Test	Conventional Values	SI Units	Chapter No.
Aldosterone	2–26 μg/24 hours	6–72 nmol/24 hours	19
Calcium (adult)			
Normal calcium intake	100–300 mg/day	2.5–7.5 mmol/day	20
Infant and child	<6 mg/kg/day	<0.15 mmol/kg/day	20
Catecholamines			
Norepinephrine	15–56 μg/24 hours	88.6–331 nmol/24 hours	19
Epinephrine	<15 pg/ml	<82 nmol/24 hours	19
Dopamine	100–400 pg/ml	625–2750 nmol/24 hours	19
Vanillylmandelic acid	2–7 mg/24 hours	10–35 μmol/24 hours	19
Metanephrine	24–96 μg/24 hours	131–524 nmol/24 hours	19
Normetanephrine	75–375 μg/24 hours	409–2047 nmol/24 hours	19
Chloride			
Adult	110–250 mEq/24 hours	110–250 mmol/24 hours	20
Adult >60 years	95–195 mEq/24 hours	95–195 mmol/24 hours	20
Child 10–14 years			
Male	64–176 mEq/24 hours	64–176 mmol/24 hours	20
Female	36–173 mEq/24 hours	36–173 mmol/24 hours	20
Child 6–10 years			
Male	36–110 mEq/24 hours	36–110 mmol/24 hours	20
Female	18–74 mEq/24 hours	18–74 mmol/24 hours	20
Child <6 years	15–40 mEq/24 hours	15–40 mmol/24 hours	20
Infant	2–10 mEq/24 hours	2–10 mmol/24 hours	20
Cortisol, free (adult)	0–110 μg/24 hours	0–303.6 nmol/24 hours	19
Creatinine clearance			
Adult male	1–2 g/day	8.8–17.7 mmol/L	20
Adult female	0.8–1.8 g/day	7.1–15.9 mol/day	20
Child	70–140 ml/minute/1.73 m^2	1.17–2.33 ml/second/m^2	20
Dexamethasone suppression test, low dose (adult)			
17-hydroxycorticosteroid	<4 ng/24 hours	<138 nmol/L	19
Free cortisol	<4 ng/ml	<11.04 nmol/24 hours	19
D-Xylose absorption test			
Child	16–33% of ingested dose/5 hours	0.16–0.33 fraction of ingested dose/5 hours	17
Adult, 5-g dose	>1.2 g/5 hours	>8 mmol/L/5 hours	17
Adult, 25-g dose	>4 g/5 hours	>26.64 mmol/L/5 hours	17
Adult >65 years	3.5 g/5 hours	>23.31 mmol/L/5 hours	17

Test	Conventional	SI Units	Ref
Estriol, pregnancy			
28–30 weeks	5–18 mg/24 hours	17–62 µmol/L	21
32–34 weeks	2–26 mg/24 hours	24–90 µmol/L	21
36–38 weeks	10–36 mg/24 hours	35–125 µmol/L	21
40 weeks	13–42 mg/24 hours	45–146 µmol/L	21
Estrogens			
Postmenopausal female	<20 µg/24 hours	69 µmol/24 hours	21
Premenopausal female	15–80 µg/24 hours	52–277 µmol/24 hours	21
Male	15–40 µg/24 hours	52–139 µmol/24 hours	21
Child	<10 µg/24 hours	<35 µmol/24 hours	21
5-Hydroxyindoleacetic acid, quantitative, adult	1–7 mg/24 hours	5–37 µmol/24 hours	17
Glucose	Negative	Same	3,19
Fibrin split products	<0.25 µg/ml	<0.25 mg/L	6
Follicle-stimulating hormone			
Adult male	4–18 U/24 hours	Same	21
Female			
Follicular phase	3–12 U/24 hours	Same	21
Midcycle peak	8–60 U/24 hours	Same	21
Hemosiderin	Negative	Same	16
Human chorionic gonadotropin			
Male, nonpregnant female	Negative	Same	21
Pregnant female	Positive	Same	21
17-Hydroxycorticosteroids			
Adult male	4.5–12 mg/24 hours	12.4–33.1 µmol/24 hours	19
Adult female	2.5–10 mg/24 hours	6.9–27.6 µmol/24 hours	19
Child			
8–12 years	<4.5 mg/24 hours	<12.4 µmol/24 hours	19
<8 years	<1.5 mg/24 hours	<4.14 µmol/24 hours	19
17-Ketogenic steroids			
Male	4–14 mg/24 hours	13–49 µmol/24 hours	19
Female	2–12 mg/24 hours	7–42 µmol/24 hours	19
Child			
11–14 years	2–9 mg/24 hours	7–31 µmol/24 hours	19
<11 years	0.1–4 mg/24 hours	0.3–14 µmol/24 hours	19
Ketones	Negative	Same	3,19

Table continued on following page

TABLE F–1
NORMAL VALUES: URINE TESTS *Continued*

Name of Test	Conventional Values	SI Units	Chapter No.
17-Ketosteroids			
Male	10–25 mg/24 hours	37–87 μmol/24 hours	19
Female	6–14 mg/24 hours	21–49 μmol/24 hours	19
Child			
10–14 years	1–6 mg/24 hours	3–21 μmol/24 hours	19
<10 years	<3 mg/24 hours	<10 μmol/24 hours	19
Lactose tolerance test			
Urine lactose			
Adult	12–40 mg/dl/24 hours	0.7–2.2 mmol/L	17
Child	<1.5 mg/100 dl	—	17
Luteinizing hormone			
Adult male	9–23 U/24 hours	Same	21
Female	4–30 U/24 hours	Same	21
Male 1–10 years	<1–5.6 U/24 hours	Same	21
Female 1–10 years	1.4–4.9 U/24 hours	Same	21
Magnesium	7.3–12.2 mg/dl/day	3–5 mmol/day	20
Osmolarity			
Normal diet and fluid intake	500–800 mOsm/kg H_2O	500–800 mmol/kg H_2O	19
Range	50–1400 mOsm/kg H_2O	50–1400 mmol/kg H_2O	19
Ova and parasites	Negative	Same	7
Phenylalanine	Negative	Same	20
Potassium			
Adult	25–125 mEq/24 hours	25–125 mmol/24 hours	20
Child 10–14 years			
Male	22–57 mEq/24 hours	22–57 mmol/24 hours	20
Female	18–58 mEq/24 hours	18–58 mmol/24 hours	20
Child 6–10 years			
Male	17–54 mEq/24 hours	17–54 mmol/24 hours	20
Female	8–37 mEq/24 hours	8–37 mmol/24 hours	20
Infant	4.1–5.3 mEq/24 hours	4.1–5.3 mmol/24 hours	20
Pregnanetriol			
Adult	<2 mg/day	<5.9 μmol/day	21
Child			
0–6 years	<0.2 mg/day	<0.6 μmol/day	21
7–16 years	<0.3–1.1 mg/day	<0.9–3.3 μmol/day	21
Protein	40–150 mg/24 hours	Same	20
Protein electrophoresis	40–150 ng/24 hours	40–150 mg/24 hours	20

Test	Conventional units	SI units	Ref.
Schilling test			
Stage 1	10–40% cobalt-58, vitamin B$_{12}$ excretion/24 hours	0.1–0.4 fraction of dose excreted	16
Stage 2	0–42% cobalt-57, vitamin B$_{12}$, and intrinsic factor excretion/24 hours	0–0.42 fraction of dose excreted	16
Cobalt-57 : cobalt 58 ratio	0.7–1.3	Same	16
Sodium			
Adult	40–220 mEq/24 hours	40–220 mmol/24 hours	20
Child 10–14 years			
Male	63–117 mEq/24 hours	63–117 mmol/24 hours	20
Female	48–168 mEq/24 hours	48–168 mmol/24 hours	20
Child 6–10 years			
Male	41–115 mEq/24 hours	41–115 mmol/24 hours	20
Female	20–69 mEq/24 hours	20–69 mmol/24 hours	20
Uric acid (adult, average diet)	250–750 mg/24 hours	1.48–4.43 mmol/24 hours	20
Urinalysis			
Specific gravity	1.003–1.029	Same	3
pH	4.5–7.8	Same	3
Protein	Negative	Same	3
Bilirubin	Negative	Same	3
Urobilinogen	Normal	Same	3,18
Glucose	Negative	Same	3,19
Ketone	Negative	Same	3,19
Occult blood	Negative	Same	3
Red blood cells (male)	0–3/high-power field	Same	3
Red blood cells (female)	0–5/high-power field	Same	3
White blood cells	0–5/high-power field	Same	3
Bacteria	Negative	Same	3
Leukocyte esterase	Negative	Same	3
Casts	0–4 hyaline casts/low-power field	Same	3
Crystals	Few	Same	3
Urobilinogen			
Male	0.3–2.1 mg/2 hours	0.5–3.6 μmol/2 hours	3,18
Female	0.1–1.1 mg/2 hours	0.2–1.9 μmol/2 hours	3,18
Water deprivation			
Specific gravity	1.025–1.032	Same	19
Urine osmolarity	>800 mOsm/kg	>800 mmol/kg	19

Normal Values: Body Fluids

TABLE G–1
NORMAL VALUES: BODY FLUIDS

Body Fluid	Name of Test	Conventional Values	SI Units	Chapter No.
Amniotic fluid	Amniotic fluid analysis			
	Chromosome analysis	Normal karyotype	Same	21
	Alpha₁-fetoprotein	0.5–3 Multiples of median (MoM)	Same	21
	Acetylcholinesterase	Negative	Same	21
	Rh incompatibility	Negative/1+	Same	21
	Bilirubin	0.01–0.03 mg/dl	0.02–0.06 μmol/L	21
	Creatinine			
	36 weeks' gestation	1.6–1.8 mg/dl	141–159 μmol/L	21
	37–38 weeks' gestation	>2 mg/dl	>177 μmol/L	21
	Lecithin/sphingomyelin ratio	>2	Same	21
	Phosphatidylglycerol	Present	Same	21
	Pulmonary surfactant	Positive; foam stability index, >0.48	Same	21
	Meconium	Absent	Same	21
Cerebrospinal fluid	Cerebrospinal fluid analysis			
	Pressure	90–180 mm H_2O	Same	22
	Appearance	Clear, colorless	Same	22
	Leukocyte count			
	Adult	0–5 cells/μl	$0–5 \times 10^6$/L	22
	Child 5–18 years	0–10 cells/μl	$0–10 \times 10^6$/L	22
	Neonate–1 year	0–30 cells/μl	$0–30 \times 10^6$/L	22
	Lymphocytes (adult)	40–80%	0.4–0.8 fraction	22
	Monocytes	15–45%	0.15–0.45 fraction	22
	Neutrophils	0–6%	0–0.06 fraction	22
	Lymphocytes (neonate)	5–35%	0.05–0.35 fraction	22
	Monocytes	50–90%	0.5–0.9 fraction	22
	Neutrophils	0–8%	0–0.08 fraction	22
	Lactate	10–22 mg/dl	1.1–2.4 mmol/L	22
	Glucose	50–80 mg/dl	2.75–4.4 mmol/L	22
	Total protein	15–45 mg/dl	150–450 mg/L	22
	Albumin	10–30 mg/dl	100–300 mg/L	22
	IgG	1–4 mg/dl	10–40 mg/L	22
	Protein electrophoresis			
	Prealbumin	2–7%	0.02–0.07 fraction	22
	Albumin	56–76%	0.56–0.76 fraction	22

Table continued on following page

TABLE G–1
NORMAL VALUES: BODY FLUIDS *Continued*

Body Fluid	Name of Test	Conventional Values	SI Units	Chapter No.
	Alpha$_1$-globulin	2–7%	0.02–0.07 fraction	22
	Alpha$_2$-globulin	4–12%	0.04–0.12 fraction	22
	Beta globulin	8–18%	0.08–0.18 fraction	22
	Gamma globulin	3–12%	0.03–0.12 fraction	22
	Myelin–basic protein	0–5 µg/L	Same	22
Effusion fluid	Carcinoembryonic antigen			
	Adult, nonsmoker	<2.5 ng/ml	2.5 g/L	17
	Adult, smoker	Up to 5 ng/ml	Up to 5 g/L	17
Gastric secretion	Gastric analysis			
	pH	<2	<2	17
	Basal acid output			
	Male	4.2 mEq/hour	4.2 mmol/hour	17
	Female	1.8 mEq/hour	1.8 mmol/hour	17
	Maximal acid output			
	Male	22.6 mEq/hour	22.6 mmol/hour	17
	Female	15.2 mEq/hour	15.2 mmol/hour	17
	Peak acid output			
	Male	35 mEq/hour	35 mmol/hour	17
	Female	25 mEq/hour	25 mmol/hour	17
	Basal acid output:maximal acid output	<0.4 (40%)	<0.4 (40%)	17
Peritoneal fluid	Peritoneal fluid analysis			
	Appearance	Clear, odorless, pale yellow, scanty	Same	17
	Ammonia	<50 µg/dl	—	17
	Amylase	138–404 amylase units/L	Same	17
	Bacteria, fungi	None present	Same	17
	Cells	No malignant cells present	Same	17
	Glucose	70–90 mg/dl	3.89–4.99 mmol/L	17
	Protein	0.3–4.1 g/dl	3–41 g/L	17
	Red blood cells	None	None	17
	White blood cells	<300/µl	<300 × 10^6/L	17
Perspiration	Sweat test	5–40 mEq/L	5–40 mmol/L	18

Category	Test	Value	SI Value	Ref
Semen				
	Semen analysis			
	Appearance	Opalescent gray-white color	Same	21
	Volume	2–5 ml	0.002–0.005 L	21
	Liquefaction	10–60 minutes	Same	21
	pH	7.2–7.8	Same	21
	Acid phosphatase	>200 U/ejaculate	Same	21
	Citric acid	>52 μmol/ejaculate	Same	21
	Fructose	>13 μmol/ejaculate	Same	21
	Zinc	>2.4 μmol/ejaculate	Same	21
	Motility	>50%	>0.5 number fraction	21
	Concentration	$20–250 \times 10^6$/ml	$20–250 \times 10^9$/L	21
	Morphologic characteristics	>50% normal, mature spermatozoa	>0.5 number fraction	21
	Viability	>50% live spermatozoa	>0.5 number fraction	21
	Leukocytes	$<1 \times 10^6$/ml	$<1 \times 10^9$/L	21
Synovial fluid				
	Synovial fluid analysis			
	Appearance	Crystal clear, transparent, pale yellow	Same	23
	Viscosity	High	Same	23
	Volume	<3.5 ml	Same	23
	Red blood cells	Absent	Same	23
	White blood cells	$0–200$/mm^3	$0–200 \times 10^6$/L	23
	Nucleated cell count	<200 cells/μl	$<200 \times 10^6$ cells/L	23
	Granulocytes	<25% of nucleated cells	<0.25 of nucleated cells; number fraction of granulocytes	23
	Protein	3 g/dl	30 g/L	23
	Uric acid	<8 mg/dl	476 mol/L	23
	Glucose (fasting)	70–110 mg/dl	3.9–6.1 mmol/L	23
	Blood-synovial fluid glucose difference	<10 mg/dl	<0.56 mmol/L	23
	Fibrin clot	Negative or absent	Same	23
	Mucin clot	Positive or abundant	Same	23
	String test	Formation of a long string	Same	23
Vaginal secretions	Culture	No growth	Same	23
	Rheumatoid factor	Negative	Same	23
	Prostatic acid phosphatase	<2 U/L	Same	20

I N D E X

DIAGNOSTIC PROCEDURES